Frontiers in Interventional Cardiology

Frontiers in Interventional Cardiology

Edited by

Rafael Beyar MD DSc
Professor, Medicine and Biomedical Engineering
Director, Division of Invasive Cardiology,
Rambam Medical Center
Head, Heart System Research Center
Technion-Israel Institute of Technology
Haifa
Israel

Gad Keren MD FACC FESC
Professor of Medicine
Sackler Medical School
Tel Aviv University
Head, Intermediate Care Unit
and Non-Invasive Laboratory
Tel Aviv Medical Center
Tel Aviv
Israel

Martin Leon MD FACC
President and Chief Executive Officer
Cardiovascular Research Foundation
Washington Cardiology Center
Washington DC
USA

Patrick W Serruys MD PhD
FACC FESC
Professor of Interventional Cardiology
Catheterization Laboratory
Division of Cardiology
Thoraxcenter
Academic Hospital Dijkzigt
Rotterdam
The Netherlands

With the technical assistance of

Deborah E. Shapiro LPN
Heart System Research Center
Technion-Israel Institute of Technology
Haifa
Israel

Mosby

St. Louis Baltimore Boston Carlsbad Chicago Naples New York Philadelphia Portland
London Madrid Mexico City Singapore Sydney Tokyo Toronto Wiesbaden

MARTIN DUNITZ

© Martin Dunitz Ltd 1997

First published in the United Kingdom in 1997 by
Martin Dunitz Ltd
The Livery House
7-9 Pratt Street
London NW1 OAE

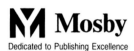
Mosby
Dedicated to Publishing Excellence

A Times Mirror Company

Distributed in the U.S.A. and Canada by

Mosby–Year Book
11830 Westline Industrial Drive
St. Louis, Missouri 63146

Times Mirror Professional Publishing Ltd.
130 Flaska Drive
Markham, Ontario L6G 1B8

A CIP catalogue record for this book is available from the British Library

ISBN 1-85317-487-4

Composition by Wearset, Boldon, Tyne and Wear
Printed and bound in Spain by Grafos, S.A. Arte sobre papel

We dedicate *Frontiers in Interventional Cardiology* to

our families for their infinite patience and love

our students and colleagues for their intellectual stimulation and hard work

our patients for their trust and courage as we pursue new investigational therapies

Contents

List of Contributors

Sharon Aboulafia BSc
Cardiovascular Molecular Biology Laboratory, Cardiology Division, Soroka Medical Center, Faculty of Health Sciences, Ben Gurion University of the Negev, Beer Sheva 84105, Israel.
20. Growth factors: a future role in interventional cardiology?

Tatsuro Akiyama MD
Cardiac Catheterization Laboratory, Centro Cuore Columbus, 20145 Milano, Italy.
32. Intracoronary Doppler: the technique and clinical applications

Max Amor MD
Director, Unité de Chirurgie et Cardiologie Interventionnelle (UCCI), Polyclinique d'Essey-les-Nancy, 54270 Essey-les-Nancy, France.
34. Tools in peripheral interventions

Takayuki Asahara MD
Department of Biomedical Research, St Elizabeth's Medical Center, Tufts University School of Medicine, Boston MA 02135, USA.
19. Arterial gene transfer for therapeutic angiogenesis: early clinical results

Alexander Battler MD FACC
Professor of Medicine/Cardiology, Andre Feher Chair of Cardiology, Chairman, Cardiac Research Center, Director, Cardiology Division, Soroka Medical Center, Faculty of Health Sciences, Ben Gurion University of the Negev, Beer Sheva 84105, Israel.
20. Growth factors: a future role in interventional cardiology?

Dietrich Baumgart MD
Research Fellow, Abteilung für Kardiologie, Zentrum für Innere Medizin, Universitätsklinikum Essen, 45122 Essen, Germany.
23. Analysis of pathogenesis of atherosclerosis by intravascular ultrasound

Christophe Bauters MD
Professor of Medicine (Cardiology), Service de Cardiologie B & Hémodynamique, Hopital Cardiologique, 59037, Lille, France.
24. Coronary angioscopy

Lee Benson MD
Professor of Paediatrics (Cardiology), and Director, The Variety Club Cardiac Catheterization Laboratory, The Hospital for Sick Children, University of Toronto School of Medicine, Toronto ON, Canada.
38. Interventional pediatric cardiology: an overview

Michel E Bertrand MD FRCP FACC FESC
Professor of Cardiology, Service de Cardiologie B & Hémodynamique, Hopital Cardiologique, 59037, Lille, France.
24. Coronary angioscopy

Rafael Beyar MD DSc FACC
Professor, Faculty of Medicine and Department of Biomedical Engineering; Head, Heart System Research Center, Technion Israel Institute of Technology; and Director, Division of Invasive Cardiology, Rambam Medical Center, Haifa 31096, Israel.
8. Functional design characteristics and clinical results with balloon expandable and self-expanding stents
31. Coronary flow dynamics: physiological principles for the interventional cardiologist

Richard Blair MD
Departments of Medicine, Biomedical Research, Radiology and Surgery, St Elizabeth's Medical Center, Tufts University School of Medicine, Boston MA 02135, USA.
19. Arterial gene transfer for therapeutic angiogenesis: early clinical results

Arnon Blum MD
Catheterization Laboratory, Department of Cardiology, Tel Aviv Medical Center, Tel Aviv 64239, Israel.
22. The role of inflammation in atherosclerosis

Brigitta C Brott MD
Department of Cardiology, Vanderbilt University Medical Center, Nashville TN 37232, USA.
17. The role of the adventitia and neointima after angioplasty

Anoop Chauhan MD MRCP
Papworth Hospital, Papworth Everard, Cambridge CB3 8RE, UK; and Vancouver General Hospital, Vancouver BC V5Z 4E4, Canada.
11. Belief and bias: insights from comparative trials of whether to stent or not

Antonio Colombo MD FESC FACC
Director, Cardiac Catheterization Laboratory, Centro Cuore
Columbus, 20145 Milano, Italy, and Director,
Investigational Angioplasty, Lenox Hill Hospital, New York
NY, USA.
7. The current practice of coronary stenting
*32. Intracoronary Doppler: the technique and clinical
applications*

Gianni Cuman MD
Cardiac Catheterization Laboratory, Centro Cuore
Columbus, 20145 Milano, Italy.
*32. Intracoronary Doppler: the technique and clinical
applications*

Ivan De Scheerder MD PhD
Professor, Invasive Cardiology, Department of Cardiology,
Katholieke Universiteit Leuven, Campus Gasthuisberg, BE-
3000 Leuven, Belgium.
18. Local drug delivery with stents

Lucia di Francesco MD
Cardiac Catheterization Laboratory, Centro Cuore
Columbus, 20145 Milano, Italy.
*32. Intracoronary Doppler: the technique and clinical
applications*

Carlo di Mario MD PhD FESC FACC
Director of Clinical Research, Cardiac Catheterization
Laboratory, Centro Cuore Columbus, 20145 Milano, Italy.
*32. Intracoronary Doppler: the technique and clinical
applications*

Gerald Dorros MD FACC FESC FSCAI
The William Dorros–Isadore Feuer Interventional
Cardiovascular Disease Foundation Ltd, Milwaukee WI
53215, USA.
*33. Peripheral angioplasty: a perspective for now and the
future*

Elazer R Edelman MD PhD FACC
Thomas D and Virginia W Cabot Associate Professor and
Director, Harvard-MIT Biomedical Engineering Center,
Harvard-MIT Division of Health Sciences and Technology,
Cambridge MA; and Cardiovascular Division, Department
of Medicine, Brigham and Women's Hospital, Boston MA
02115, USA.
10. Stent design and the biologic response

Raimund Erbel MD FESC FACC
University Professor of Medicine/Cardiology, Director,
Abteilung für Kardiologie, Zentrum für Innere Medizin,
Universitätsklinikum Essen, 45122 Essen, Germany.
*23. Analysis of pathogenesis of atherosclerosis by
intravascular ultrasound*

Gérard Ethevenot MD
Cardiology Department, Hopital Central, 54000 Nancy,
France.
34. Tools in peripheral interventions

Jean Fajadet MD
Unité de Cardiologie Interventionnelle, Clinique Pasteur,
31076 Toulouse, France.
*9. Seven years of coronary stenting: evolution of
therapeutics, techniques and results*

Andrew Farb MD
Department of Cardiovascular Pathology, Armed Forces
Institute of Pathology, Washington DC 20306, USA.
*17. The role of the adventitia and neointima after
angioplasty*

Moshe Y Flugelman MD
Laboratory of Molecular Cardiology, Department of
Cardiology, Lady Davis Carmel Medical Center and the
Bruce Rappaport School of Medicine, Technion IIT, Haifa
34362, Israel.
21. Genetic engineering of stents

David P Foley MB BCh PhD MRCPI
Clinical Director, Department of Coronary Diagnostics and
Intervention, Division of Cardiology, Thoraxcentre,
Academic Hospital Rotterdam–Dijkzigt, 3015 GD
Rotterdam, The Netherlands.
2. Stenting for multivessel disease

Joseph Garasic MD
Harvard-MIT Division of Health Sciences and Technology,
Cambridge MA; and Cardiovascular Division, Department
of Medicine, Brigham and Women's Hospital, Boston MA
02115, USA.
10. Stent design and the biologic response

Junbo Ge MD
Director, Intravascular Ultrasound Laboratory, Abteilung
für Kardiologie, Zentrum für Innere Medizin,
Universitätsklinikum Essen, 45122 Essen, Germany.
*23. Analysis of pathogenesis of atherosclerosis by
intravascular ultrasound*

Günther Görge MD
Privatdozent, Fellow, Abteilung für Kardiologie, Zentrum
für Innere Medizin, Universitätsklinikum Essen, 45122
Essen, Germany.
*23. Analysis of pathogenesis of atherosclerosis by
intravascular ultrasound*

Laura Haley BS
Department of Biomedical Research, St Elizabeth's Medical Center, Tufts University School of Medicine, Boston MA 02135, USA.
19. Arterial gene transfer for therapeutic angiogenesis: early clinical results

David A Halon MB ChB
Department of Cardiology, Lady Davis Carmel Medical Center, Haifa 34362, Israel.
21. Genetic engineering of stents

Jaap N Hamburger MD
Department of Coronary Diagnostics and Intervention, Division of Cardiology, Thoraxcentre, Academic Hospital Rotterdam–Dijkzigt, 3015 GD Rotterdam, The Netherlands.
6. Laser guidewire for recanalization of chronic total occlusions

Haim Hammerman MD
Senior Lecturer in Cardiology, Rappaport Faculty of Medicine, Technion Israel Institute of Technology, and Director, Intensive Coronary Care Unit, Rambam Medical Center, Haifa 31096, Israel.
5. Thrombolytic vs interventional treatment in acute myocardial infarction

David Hasdai MD
Clinical Fellow, Division of Cardiovascular Diseases and Internal Medicine, Mayo Clinic, Rochester MN 55905, USA.
30. Lessons from coronary flow reserve in clinical practice

Michael Haude MD
Head, Catheterization Laboratory, Abteilung für Kardiologie, Zentrum für Innere Medizin, Universitätsklinikum Essen, 45122 Essen, Germany.
23. Analysis of pathogenesis of atherosclerosis by intravascular ultrasound

Isabelle Henry MD
Cabinet de Cardiologie et d'Explorations Vasculaires, Cardiologie Interventionnelle, Policlinique d'Essey-les-Nancy, 54270 Essey-les-Nancy, France.
34. Tools in peripheral interventions

Michel Henry MD
Director, Unité de Chirurgie et Cardiologie Interventionnelle (UCCI), Polyclinique d'Essey-les-Nancy, 54270 Essey-les-Nancy, France.
34. Tools in peripheral interventions

Walter R M Hermans MD
Department of Coronary Diagnostics and Intervention, Division of Cardiology, Thoraxcentre, Academic Hospital Rotterdam–Dijkzigt, 3015 GD Rotterdam, The Netherlands.
2. Stenting for multivessel disease

Richard R Heuser MD
Director, Research and Education, Arizona Heart Institute & Foundation, and Medical Director, Cardiac Catheterization Laboratory, Columbia Medical Center Phoenix, Phoenix AZ 85006, USA.
35. Peripheral stenting for the cardiologist

Ziyad M Hijazi MD MPH FACC
Associate Professor of Pediatrics and Medicine, Division of Pediatric Cardiology, Tufts University School of Medicine, New England Medical Center, Boston MA 02111, USA.
40. Transcatheter closure of atrial septal defects and patent foramen ovale: Angel Wings device

David R Holmes Jr MD
Professor of Medicine, Mayo Medical School, Consultant in Cardiovascular Diseases and Internal Medicine, Mayo Clinic, Rochester MN 55905, USA.
3. Complex coronary interventions: chronic total occlusions and bifurction disease

Mun K Hong MD
Director, Experimental Physiology and Pharmacology, Department of Internal Medicine, Division of Cardiology, Washington Hospital Center, Washington DC 20010, USA.
4. Treatment for saphenous vein grafts

Jeffrey M Isner MD
Chief, Cardiovascular Research, Departments of Medicine and Biomedical Research, St Elizabeth's Medical Center, Tufts University School of Medicine, Boston MA 02135, USA.
19. Arterial gene transfer for therapeutic angiogenesis: early clinical results

Shigenori Ito MD
Department of Internal Medicine, Division of Cardiology, Washington Hospital Center, Washington DC 20010, USA.
27. A practical approach to quantitative coronary angiography

Michael R Jaff DO FACP FACC
The William Dorros–Isadore Feuer Interventional Cardiovascular Disease Foundation Ltd, Milwaukee WI 53215, USA.
33. Peripheral angioplasty: a perspective for now and the future

Allan Jeremias MD
Resident, Abteilung für Kardiologie, Zentrum für Innere Medizin, Universitätsklinikum Essen, 45122 Essen, Germany.
23. Analysis of pathogenesis of atherosclerosis by intravascular ultrasound

Kenneth M Kent MD PhD
Director, Cardiology Research Foundation, and Department of Internal Medicine, Division of Cardiology, Washington Hospital Center, Washington DC 20010, USA.
4. Treatment for saphenous vein grafts
16. Arterial remodeling as a mechanism of restenosis following interventional coronary procedures: evidence from serial intravascular ultrasound studies

Gad Keren MD FACC FESC
Professor of Cardiology, Tel Aviv Sourasky Medical Center, Sackler Medical School of Medicine, Tel Aviv University, Tel Aviv 64239, Israel.
25. Intravascular ultrasound imaging: an update

Iris Keren-Tal PhD
Laboratory of Molecular Cardiology, Department of Cardiology, Lady Davis Carmel Medical Center and the Bruce Rappaport School of Medicine, Technion IIT, Haifa 34362, Israel.
21. Genetic engineering of stents

Morton J Kern MD
Professor of Medicine, St Louis University, and Director, J G Mudd Cardiac Catheterization Laboratory, St Louis University Health Sciences Center, St Louis MO 63110, USA.
29. Current status of translesional coronary physiology: decisions regarding coronary interventions in the catheterization laboratory

Spencer B King III MD
Professor of Medicine (Cardiology) and Director, Interventional Cardiology, Emory University Hospital, Atlanta GA 30322, USA.
1. Angioplasty, stenting or surgery?
13. Radiation for restenosis: an overview

Yoshio Kobayashi MD
Cardiac Catheterization Laboratory, Centro Cuore Columbus, 20145 Milano, Italy.
32. Intracoronary Doppler: the technique and clinical applications

Konstantinos G Kostopoulos MD
Department of Cardiology, Katholieke Universiteit Leuven, Campus Gasthuisberg, BE-3000 Leuven, Belgium.
18. Local drug delivery with stents

Jean-Marc Lablanche MD FACC FESC
Professor of Cardiology, Service de Cardiologie B & Hémodynamique, Hopital Cardiologique, 59037, Lille, France.
24. Coronary angioscopy

John R Laird MD
Department of Internal Medicine, Division of Cardiology, Washington Hospital Center, Washington DC 20010, USA.
12. Anticoagulation strategies after stenting

Alexandra J Lansky MD
Department of Internal Medicine, Division of Cardiology, Washington Hospital Center, Washington DC 20010, USA.
12. Anticoagulation strategies after stenting
27. A practical approach to quantitative coronary angiography

Martin B Leon MD FACC
Clinical Professor of Medicine, Georgetown University Medical Center, and President and CEO, Cardiovascular Research and Education, Cardiology Research Foundation, Washington Hospital Center, Washington DC 20010, USA.
4. Treatment for saphenous vein grafts
8. Functional design characteristics and clinical results with balloon expandable and self-expanding stents
12. Anticoagulation strategies after stenting
16. Arterial remodeling as a mechanism of restenosis following interventional coronary procedures: evidence from serial intravascular ultrasound studies

Jonathan Leor MD FACC
Acting Director ICCU, and Associate Director, Cardiology Division, Soroka Medical Center, Faculty of Health Sciences, Ben Gurion University of the Negev, Beer Sheva 84105, Israel.
20. Growth factors: a future role in interventional cardiology?

Amir Lerman MD
Associate Professor, Division of Cardiovascular Diseases and Internal Medicine, Mayo Clinic, Rochester MN 55905, USA.
30. Lessons from coronary flow reserve in clinical practice

Basil S Lewis MD FRCP
Professor of Medicine, Bruce Rappaport School of Medicine, Technion IIT, and Director, Department of Cardiology, Lady Davis Carmel Medical Center, Haifa 34362, Israel.
21. Genetic engineering of stents

Fengqi Liu MD
Cardiologist, Abteilung für Kardiologie, Zentrum für Innere Medizin, Universitätsklinikum Essen, 45122 Essen, Germany.
23. Analysis of pathogenesis of atherosclerosis by intravascular ultrasound

Eugène P McFadden MB BCh MRCP FACC FESC
Practicien Hospitalier, Service de Cardiologie B & Hémodynamique, Hopital Cardiologique, 59037, Lille, France.
24. Coronary angioscopy

Jean Marco MD
Professor, Unité de Cardiologie Interventionnelle, Clinique Pasteur, 31076 Toulouse, France.
9. Seven years of coronary stenting: evolution of therapeutics, techniques and results

Gerald R Marx MD
Associate Professor of Pediatrics, Division of Pediatric Cardiology, Department of Pediatrics, Floating Hospital for Children at New England Medical Center, Tufts University School of Medicine, Boston MA 02111, USA.
40. Transcatheter closure of atrial septal defects and patent foramen ovale: Angel Wings device

Hylton I Miller MD
Director, Catheterization Laboratory, Department of Cardiology, Tel Aviv Medical Center, Tel Aviv 64239, Israel.
22. The role of inflammation in atherosclerosis

Gary S Mintz MD
Director, Coronary Ultrasound Programme, Intravascular Ultrasound Imaging and Cardiac Catheterization Laboratories, Washington Hospital Center, Washington DC 20010, USA.
16. Arterial remodeling as a mechanism of restenosis following interventional coronary procedures: evidence from serial intravascular ultrasound studies

Harald Mudra MD
Medizinische Klinik, Klinikum Innenstadt der Universität München, Kardiologische Abteilung, 80336 München, Germany.
28. The role of intravascular ultrasound in coronary stenting

Masakiyo Nobuyoshi MD
Vice Medical Director and Director, Department of Cardiology, Kokura Memoral Hospital, Kitakyushu 802, Japan.
15. Time course of geometrical remodeling after angioplasty

David Nykanen MD
Assistant Professor of Paediatrics (Cardiology), The Hospital for Sick Children, University of Toronto School of Medicine, Toronto ON, Canada.
38. Interventional pediatric cardiology: an overview

Juan C Parodi MD
Chief, Department of Vascular Surgery, Instituto Cardiovascular de Buenos Aires, and Vice Director, Post-Graduate Training Program in Cardiovascular Surgery, Universidad de Buenos Aires, Buenos Aires, Argentina.
36. The use of stent grafts in arterial pathologies: an overview after review of 147 clinical cases

Ian M Penn MB BS FRACP FRCP FACC
Clinical Associate Professor, Department of Medicine, University of British Columbia, and Director, Interventional Cardiology, Larel Cardiology, Vancouver Hospital and Health Sciences Centre, Vancouver BC V5Z 1L7, Canada.
11. Belief and bias: insights from comparative trials of whether to stent or not

Augusto D Pichard MD
Intravascular Ultrasound Imaging and Cardiac Catheterization Laboratories, Washington Hospital Center, Washington DC 20010, USA.
16. Arterial remodeling as a mechanism of restenosis following interventional coronary procedures: evidence from serial intravascular ultrasound studies

Ann Pieczek RN
Departments of Medicine and Biomedical Research, St Elizabeth's Medical Center, Tufts University School of Medicine, Boston MA 02135, USA.
19. Arterial gene transfer for therapeutic angiogenesis: early clinical results

Jeffrey J Popma MD
Executive Director and Director, Angiographic Core Laboratory and Data Coordinating Center, Cardiology Research Foundation, and Department of Internal Medicine, Division of Cardiology, Washington Hospital Center, Washington DC 20010, USA.
12. Anticoagulation strategies after stenting
16. Arterial remodeling as a mechanism of restenosis following interventional coronary procedures: evidence from serial intravascular ultrasound studies
27. A practical approach to quantitative coronary angiography

Bernhard Reimers MD
Cardiac Catheterization Laboratory, Centro Cuore Columbus, 20145 Milano, Italy.
32. Intracoronary Doppler: the technique and clinical applications

xvi List of Contributors

Campbell Rogers MD FACC
Harvard-MIT Division of Health Sciences and Technology,
Cambridge MA; and Assistant Professor of Medicine,
Cardiac Catheterization Laboratory and Coronary Care
Unit, Cardiovascular Division, Department of Medicine,
Brigham and Women's Hospital, Boston MA 02115, USA.
10. Stent design and the biologic response

Tiberio Rosenfeld MD
Head, Heart Institute, Haemek Medical Center, 18101
Afula, Israel.
*37. Balloon mitral valvuloplasty: a single Israeli center
experience*

Stephen Sack MD
Fellow, Abteilung für Kardiologie, Zentrum für Innere
Medizin, Universitätsklinikum Essen, 45122 Essen,
Germany.
*23. Analysis of pathogenesis of atherosclerosis by
intravascular ultrasound*

Giuseppe Sangiorgi MD
Research Associate, Department of Cardiology, Mayo
Clinic, Rochester MN 55905, USA.
*17. The role of the adventitia and neointima after
angioplasty*

Lowell F Satler MD
Director, Cardiology Research Foundation, and
Intravascular Ultrasound Imaging and Cardiac
Catheterization Laboratories, Washington Hospital Center,
Washington DC 20010, USA.
*16. Arterial remodeling as a mechanism of restenosis
following interventional coronary procedures: evidence
from serial intravascular ultrasound studies*

Jorge F Saucedo MD
Department of Internal Medicine, Division of Cardiology,
Washington Hospital Center, Washington DC 20010, USA.
*27. A practical approach to quantitative coronary
angiography*

Robert Schainfeld DO
Department of Medicine, St Elizabeth's Medical Center,
Tufts University School of Medicine, Boston MA 02135,
USA.
*19. Arterial gene transfer for therapeutic angiogenesis:
early clinical results*

Robert S Schwartz MD
Professor of Medicine, Department of Cardiology, Mayo
Clinic, Rochester MN 55905, USA.
*17. The role of the adventitia and neointima after
angioplasty*

Douglas Scott MD
Department of Cardiology, Georgetown University,
Washington DC 20007, USA.
*17. The role of the adventitia and neointima after
angioplasty*

Patrick W Serruys MD PhD FACC FESC
Professor of Interventional Cardiology, Interuniversity
Cardiological Institute of The Netherlands and Erasmus
University, Thoraxcentre, Academic Hospital
Rotterdam–Dijkzigt, 3015 GD Rotterdam, The
Netherlands.
2. Stenting for multivessel disease
*6. Laser guidewire for recanalization of chronic total
occlusions*
*26. Three-dimensional intravascular ultrasound in
interventional cardiology*

Yoav Turgeman MD
Deputy Head, Heart Institute, Haemek Medical Center,
18101 Afula, Israel.
*37. Balloon mitral valvuloplasty: a single Israeli center
experience*

Kiril Tzvetanov MD
Clinique Cardiologique, Cabinet de Cardiologie et
d'Explorations Vasculaires, Cardiologie Interventionnelle,
Policlinique d'Essey-les-Nancy, 54270 Essey-les-Nancy,
France.
34. Tools in peripheral interventions

Eric van Belle MD
Assistant Professor of Medicine, Service de Cardiologie B &
Hémodynamique, Hopital Cardiologique, 59037, Lille,
France.
24. Coronary angioscopy

Renu Virmani MD
Chairman, Department of Cardiovascular Pathology,
Armed Forces Institute of Pathology, Washington DC
20306, USA.
*17. The role of the adventitia and neointima after
angioplasty*

Clemens von Birgelen MD
Clinical Research Fellow, Cardiac Catheterization and
Intracoronary Imaging Laboratory, Thoraxcentre, Academic
Hospital Rotterdam–Dijkzigt, Erasmus Universiteit
Rotterdam, 3015 GD Rotterdam, The Netherlands.
*26. Three-dimensional intravascular ultrasound in
interventional cardiology*

Ron Waksman MD FACC
Director, Experimental Angioplasty and Vascular
Brachytherapy, Cardiology Research Foundation,
Washington Hospital Center, Washington DC 20010, USA.
14. Intracoronary radiation: does it really work?

Kai Wang MD
Katholieke Universiteit Leuven, Campus Gasthuisberg, BE-
3000 Leuven, Belgium.
18. Local drug delivery with stents

Anat Weisz PhD
Laboratory of Molecular Cardiology, Department of
Cardiology, Lady Davis Carmel Medical Center and the
Bruce Rappaport School of Medicine, Technion IIT, Haifa
34362, Israel.
21. Genetic engineering of stents

Benjamin Zeevi MD
Cardiac Catheterization Unit, Cardiology Institute,
Schneider Children's Medical Center of Israel, Beilinson
Campus, Petah Tiqva, and Sackler Faculty of Medicine, Tel
Aviv University, Tel Aviv 49202, Israel.
*39. Transcatheter closure of patent ductus arteriosus as a
pathfinder for interventional pediatric cardiology*

Preface

With the first coronary balloon angioplasty performed in 1977 by the late Andreas Grüntzig, interventional cardiology was born. Since that time, the field of interventional cardiology has progressed hand-in-hand with technology, combining innovative catheter-based technologies and vascular pathobiology with new frontiers in pharmaceutical and molecular biology research. The field is constantly growing and combines various interrelated disciplines such as:

- classical interventional adult cardiology,
- interventional pediatric cardiology,
- interventional angiology, involving treatment of vessels other than those of the heart.

While each discipline bears its own uniqueness and expertise, they share many common features; thus, bringing them all together is of practical and scientific importance.

Two years ago the *First International Meeting on Interventional Cardiology* was held in Jerusalem, and was dedicated to clinical and basic science along the lines sketched above. *Frontiers in Interventional Cardiology* evolved from that meeting and is derived from the scientific program of the *Second International Meeting in Interventional Cardiology* (Jerusalem, 1997). These international symposiums, as well as this volume, have emerged from the need to accelerate basic and clinical research initiatives and to optimize patient care strategies. With the rapidly growing knowledge in the field of interventional cardiology, it is of utmost importance to enhance the flow of information and ideas among the deeply committed researchers and clinicians who are involved in this field. This volume addresses pertinent issues in basic and clinical research in this rapidly progressive and exciting field. *Frontiers in Interventional Cardiology* covers the frontiers of conventional and new device angioplasty modalities, including "plain old" balloon angioplasty and various atherectomy techniques, and features innovative topics in clinical investigation and basic research on stents. Old and new imaging technologies, drug therapies, experimental physiology and coronary flow, endothelial function, and molecular biology related to various aspects of the coronary vasculature are also covered.

Up-to-date comprehensive scientific, clinical and technological reviews, written by the leading world experts on the related topics, are provided. This book comprises 40 chapters covering eight major topics.

Section I covers the changing clinical trends in interventional cardiology, providing the reader with comprehensive reviews of the current clinical trends utilizing the old and new devices, and taking into account the constantly changing indications for different treatment modalities.

Section II covers the rapidly changing field of stenting, addresses various stent designs, the current practice of stenting, and new research, oriented to fight the proliferative response – the enemy of stenting.

Restenosis, the Achilles' heel of angioplasty and arterial remodeling, and an important mechanism following balloon injury, is discussed in Section III. Various drug treatments, new devices, as well as brachytherapy, all aimed at reducing stenoses, are also discussed.

Understanding and modification of the vascular biological response to 'mechanical' interventions can be another solution to restenosis, as discussed in Section IV. Arterial gene therapy and molecular biology techniques will shape the future of interventional cardiology.

New imaging modalities, Section V, continue to evolve, providing the operator with better 'eyes' to understand the impact of mechanical devices and to study the mechanisms of the pathological processes during and following interventions.

Coronary physiology, discussed in Section VI, is now an integral part of the catheterization laboratory, with miniaturization technology allowing for Doppler blood flow as well as pressure measurements using an angioplasty wire. Coronary flow reserve is the physiologic link between the geometry of the lesion and the microvascular response. Its role in guiding interventions is discussed in detail.

Peripheral and general vascular interventions are described in Section VII.

Finally, pediatric interventions, Section VIII, are extensively covered, describing the innovative and percutaneous techniques to treat the specific pediatric cardiological diseases.

This book could not have been written without the contribution and enthusiasm of the distinguished scientists in the field. The time and effort put into this volume are directed towards the progress of science and technology in the aid of medicine. Such progress helps lead the way to enormous changes and advances in treatment strategies in this therapeutic field, and joins the fight against this most prevalent disease in the modern western world.

Indeed, the field of interventional cardiology has come a long way since the pioneering work of Andreas Grüntzig, with prolific research leading to ever widening new dimensions. However, we are still on the verge of what continues to be a rapid expansion of knowledge regarding the pathobiology of interventional cardiology. The constant progress of technology, the new horizons opened by molecular biology, and the innovative mind and spirit of investigators in the field will continue to lead the way. This first volume, *Frontiers in Interventional Cardiology*, is intended to provide an overview of the field and its innovations, as well as to effect it and help set standards for the years to come, for the benefit of the patients in our care.

Rafael Beyar
Gad Keren
Martin B Leon
Patrick W Serruys
June 1997

I

Clinical Trends in Interventional Cardiology

1

Angioplasty, stenting or surgery?

Spencer B King III

Introduction

The title of this chapter suggests that we are comparing three different strategies for revascularization. In truth, there are only two strategies; in current clinical practice the comma between angioplasty and surgery must be removed. Whereas balloon angioplasty and stenting have been compared in a competitive way in randomized trials,[1,2] in clinical practice the techniques are no longer viewed as competitive but complementary. Certainly, opinion varies on the appropriate use of stents. Some operators take the position that stents should be used in all lesions possible, while others hold to the practice of provisional stenting, i.e., placing stents when the angioplasty result is not excellent or the desired minimal lumen diameter is not achieved. In this regard, we must also expand the word angioplasty to include all devices used in modifying the inner lumen of the obstructed vessel. Therefore, included in this discussion, under the term angioplasty, is the use of balloons, directional atherectomy devices, rotary ablation, transluminal extraction catheter (TEC) atherectomy and laser procedures, as well as stenting. These interventional procedures, like surgery, require several tools and therefore the term angioplasty will refer to all interventional techniques, and surgery will refer to all surgical techniques.

Angioplasty or surgery?

How do we choose between angioplasty or surgery today? An obvious concern is the completeness of revascularization. In patients with single-vessel disease, complete revascularization is almost always planned using either technique. Gruentzig's original approach was to select patients with severely symptomatic single-vessel disease who were destined for surgery, and to offer a less invasive approach. Over the years, this strategy has proven so effective that there is little debate over the intervention of choice in single-vessel disease when an intervention is warranted.

It is in more complex forms of multivessel disease that the debate arises. Complete revascularization in multivessel disease has become a tenet of surgical opinion. Incomplete revascularization has been associated with a less optimal outcome in patients who undergo bypass surgery. Often this is unavoidable because of the nature of the disease, but incomplete revascularization has been shown to be a predictor of diminished long-term survival. Jones et al.[3] reported a series of multivessel disease patients who underwent surgery at Emory. This study of 3481 patients divided the subjects into those with complete and incomplete revascularization. Those with incomplete revascularization showed a somewhat lower ejection fraction and more extensive coronary obstructions. However, fewer grafts were placed in patients with incomplete revascularization (2.6 per patient) as compared to complete revascularization patients (3.2 per patient). The major predictors of incompleteness of revascularization were the number of vessels involved and the ejection fraction.

Long-term follow-up of these patients showed that

freedom from angina and survival were superior in those who could have complete revascularization. Ten-year survival was 81% in those with complete revascularization and 72% in those with incomplete revascularization. This difference remained after correcting for baseline features.

Completeness of revascularization

We have been less successful in correlating completeness of revascularization with outcome in patients who have interventional procedures. An observational study was performed on patients undergoing angioplasty or surgery with two-vessel disease and followed for 5 years.[4] Four hundred and seventeen angioplasty patients and 503 bypass surgery patients were examined. They had obvious different baseline features with angioplasty patients being younger, having less diabetes and less prior myocardial infarction or severe angina. The left anterior descending artery (LAD) involvement was less and the ejection fraction was higher in the angioplasty group. Although completeness of revascularization was not directly assessed, there were 3.4 grafts placed per patient in the surgery group, and only 1.5 lesions dilated in the angioplasty group, indicating several more complete attempts in the surgery patients. The raw survival figures at 5 years show that angioplasty was superior; however, when correcting for baseline differences, there was no survival difference. No study has ever been carried out comparing intentional incomplete revascularization and therefore all such observations are fraught with a great deal of bias. There is also a clear difference in the goals for revascularization in patients undergoing surgery compared to angioplasty. Surgery patients commonly have every lesion bypassed since the hope is that there will not be another operation for a significant period of time. Angioplasty, on the other hand, has the opportunity of being repeated at any time and therefore operators do not feel compelled to open less severe stenoses.

The Emory Angioplasty vs. Surgery Trial (EAST), which will be examined later, did give insight into the difference in completeness of revascularization achieved with angioplasty and surgery in a randomized context.[5] Revascularization was at the discretion of the surgeon or the angioplasty operator with the goal being to revascularize all significantly ischemic regions by angioplasty, when possible. Following the initial baseline procedure, 71% of the obstructed index segments were revascularized by angioplasty and virtually 100% were bypassed with surgical grafts. Coronary angiograms were performed at 1 year and 3 years and showed that sustained revascularization had been accomplished in 88% of the index segments of the surgery group patients compared to 59% of the angioplasty group

patients. By 3 years this difference had narrowed because of repeat interventional procedures so that 87% of surgical index segments per patient were revascularized compared to 70% of index segments for the angioplasty patients. Further analysis of this data showed that when considering only severe remaining stenoses, the difference between the surgery and angioplasty group had disappeared entirely by 3 years, indicating that there was little difference in the potential for severe ischemia between the two populations. This randomized trial, however, required that patients be suitable candidates for angioplasty and excluded most patients with total occlusions, a subset in which angioplasty has much less potential to provide complete revascularization.

Comparison of clinical outcomes of angioplasty vs. surgery

Multiple observational studies have compared angioplasty and surgical patients.[6-10] Most of the angioplasty series were weighted towards the patients with two-vessel disease and better left ventricular function. These studies, not surprisingly, showed similar survival figures, a much shorter hospital stay for percutaneous transluminal coronary angioplasty (PTCA) patients and a need for more repeat procedures among PTCA patients.

Nine randomized trials have now been carried out to assess angioplasty directly compared to bypass surgery. Most of these involve patients with multivessel disease and a few of them also include single-vessel patients. A meta-analysis of eight of the trials[11] showed no difference in in-hospital or one-year mortality for the patients randomized to angioplasty or surgery. The same was true for the incidence of myocardial infarction. The three trials that included single-vessel patients showed a one-year mortality for surgical patients of 0.3% and PTCA of 1.9%. For those six trials of multivessel patients, the 1-year mortality for the coronary artery bypass graft surgery (CABG) group was 2.8% and PTCA 3.1%. None of these were statistically different. Repeat angioplasty, however, was much more common in the angioplasty group. Repeat intervention, either angioplasty or surgery, was required in 33% of the angioplasty randomized patients and only 3% of the patients randomized to surgery. I would therefore like to explore some of the lessons learnt from several of these randomized trials.

The Emory Angioplasty vs. Surgery Trial, which was the first multivessel trial to be initiated in the USA, was sponsored by the National Heart, Lung and Blood Institute;[5] 392 patients with multivessel disease were randomized. Forty percent had three-vessel disease and 60% two-vessel disease. Follow-up included 1-year and 3-year thallium scans and angiograms. The endpoint of this trial was a composite of death, Q-wave myocardial infarction or a large ischemic defect found on thallium scanning. There were no differences in this primary endpoint at 1 year or 3 years and no differences have emerged in mortality, now followed to 5 years. The main differences in the trial related to the need for repeat revascularization. At 3 years, 1% of the surgery patients required repeat surgery and 13% required PTCA. During the same time frame, 22% of the PTCA patients required surgery and 41% required repeat PTCA. Despite this additional intervention in the angioplasty group, angina was more frequent in those patients (20% vs. 12% in the surgical cohort).

The Bypass Angioplasty Revascularization Investigation (BARI) was a multicenter study started approximately one year after EAST and involved 18 centers;[12] 914 patients were assigned to surgery and 915 to angioplasty. Those patients have now been followed over 5 years. The in-hospital mortality rates were 1.3% for surgery and 1.1% for angioplasty; 5-year survival was 89.3% for surgery and 86.3% for angioplasty ($p = 0.19$). By the 5-year endpoint, 8% of the surgery patients had undergone an additional revascularization procedure as compared with 54% of the angioplasty assigned patients. The baseline features in the BARI trial were very similar to EAST with 41% triple-vessel disease, with the same entry age, approximately 62 years. An important substudy of the BARI trial was performed in those patients who had diabetes and were on either oral therapy or insulin. In that group of 353 patients, 5-year survival was 80.6% in the surgery patients compared with only 65.5% in the angioplasty patients ($p = 0.003$). A similar difference was not seen in a small number of patients (59 diabetic patients) in the EAST trial,[13] nor have differences been seen in the registry of the BARI nonrandomized patients who had diabetes.

The Coronary Angioplasty vs. Bypass Revascularization Investigation (CABRI) was conducted in Europe and randomized 1054 patients.[14] At 1 year there were no differences in death or myocardial infarction (1-year mortality, surgery 2.7%, angioplasty 3.9%). Long-term follow-up of diabetic patients in this trial supports the conclusion from BARI that multivessel patients with diabetes seem to be having a better survival with surgical intervention.

The Randomized Intervention Treatment of Angina trial (RITA) enrolled 1011 patients with a combined endpoint of death or myocardial infarction at 5 years.[15] This study cannot be directly compared to EAST, BARI and CABRI because approximately half the patients had single-vessel disease. The $2\frac{1}{2}$ year follow-up showed no difference in mortality (3.6% for surgery vs. 3.1% for angioplasty). Angina remained more common in the angioplasty group at 2 years (31% in the angioplasty patients and 21% in the surgery patients); however, class III and IV angina were not different (6% in each group).

The other randomized trials were the Argentine randomized trial of angioplasty vs. surgery (ERACI)[16] which evaluated patients with multivessel disease, the German Angioplasty Bypass Investigation (GABI)[17] which was a multicenter trial comparing patients in whom complete revascularization was possible and included 18% triple-vessel disease, the Toulouse trial of two- and three-vessel disease,[18] and two single-vessel trials, the Medicine Angioplasty or Surgery Study (MASS) from Brazil limited to isolated LAD stenoses and normal ejection fraction,[19] and the Lausanne trial limited to ostial or proximal LAD stenoses.[20]

Whereas randomized trials give significant insight into the value of a therapy without selection bias, they are limited in two important ways. One is that, by definition, they must deal with a defined group of patients and in many cases such as these multivessel coronary disease trials, a great number of patients are excluded. For that reason, continued observational studies will be important to judge the value of interventional therapies in other subsets. Secondly, randomized trials remove bias in the selection process. Such bias may be based on features that are unmeasured and yet predict in some way the early and long-term outcome of patients undergoing these procedures. Such information arose in the registry of the EAST trial. In that trial, in addition to the 392 patients randomized, there were 450 patients who were eligible for the trial but were not randomized because of patient or referring physician refusal. Whereas all those patients met the entry criteria and the baseline features were similar to the randomized patients (40% triple-vessel disease, age 62, ejection fraction 60, prior myocardial infarction (MI) 40%, diabetes 22%, hypertension 52%, congestive heart failure 3%), there were some small differences with more randomized patients having class IV angina (62% vs. 53%), more being on intravenous heparin (32% vs. 22%) and fewer having a college education (32% vs. 49%). The major difference, however, between the two groups was that one was randomized and the other had their treatment selected by the attending physicians. There may have been subtle differences that drove that selection process including unmeasured lesion characteristics, difficulty of angioplasty approach, etc. The results reflected a superior survival for the entire cohort of patients in the registry (96.4% as compared with those in the randomized cohort 93.4%, $p = 0.044$). It can be argued that physician judgment in making this selection was important or that there were unmeasured baseline differences between the two groups which accounted for these differences. In reality, it does not matter which conclusion is drawn, but it does point to the importance of following the outcome of patients who are eligible but who do not participate in randomized trials in order to understand more fully the outcomes of therapy.

New devices

All the trials that have been discussed herein compare balloon angioplasty to bypass surgery. No trials have been conducted to date against surgery which utilize the new devices developed in the early 1990s to offset the limitations of balloon angioplasty. Directional coronary atherectomy was the first new device to come into wide use. Direct comparative studies against balloon angioplasty (CAVEAT and C-CAT)[21,22] failed to show any major advantage for directional atherectomy over balloon angioplasty. Subsequently the Balloon vs. Optimal Atherectomy Trial (BOAT) has shown, with more complete removal of tissue, an improved restenosis rate for directional atherectomy compared to the balloon for the type of lesions that were tested (oral presentation, American Heart Association meeting, New Orleans, LA, USA, 1996). It should be remembered that many of the primary uses of directional atherectomy, such as in ostial lesions and in bifurcations, were not tested in the BOAT trial since this was not an inclusion.

Heavily calcified and fibrotic lesions were helped considerably by the use of the rotary ablation technique. Although Rotablator has not been shown to reduce restenosis in any trial, it has enabled the extension of angioplasty to some lesions that could not otherwise be treated.[23] Laser angioplasty has not found wide acceptance but is still used in some centers for debulking long lesions, treating vein grafts and the opening of total occlusions via use of an experimental laser guidewire.

However, the most successful technology for augmenting angioplasty has been the use of intracoronary stents. The wide acceptance of stenting in angioplasty is indicated by the use pattern of stents throughout the world. Stent utilization varies from 20 to 70% in centers within the USA and sometimes even higher outside the USA, where more stents are available. Although stenting has been widely accepted and used, the data showing the superiority of stents to other interventions remain somewhat limited. Stenting, in most cases, leaves a more impressive initial result than balloon angioplasty, but the primary goal of stenting is to reduce the long-term restenosis rate so that a more lasting benefit can be obtained. The effect on restenosis was studied in two landmark trials: the Stent Restenosis Study (STRESS)[1] and the Belgium–Netherlands Stent Trial (BENESTENT).[2] These trials evaluated the Palmaz–Schatz stent compared to balloon angioplasty in lesions which could be covered by one stent located in vessels larger than 3 mm in diameter. In these two studies, stent restenosis was reduced (BENESTENT 32% for balloon to 22% for stents and in STRESS from 42% for balloon to 32% for stent). The anticoagulation regimen used in both these trials was vigorous heparinization followed by coumadin therapy and aspirin. Both trials were associated with higher bleeding complication rates in the stent group,

longer hospitalization and likely higher costs. Subsequently, most centers throughout the world have abandoned coumadin anticoagulation and gone to a program of pure antiplatelet therapy following the initial heparin anticoagulation. Patients are being treated with aspirin and ticlopidine and stent deployment is being assured with the use of high-pressure post-stent balloon inflation. Using these new strategies, the BENESTENT II trial was carried out and resulted in a significant reduction in bleeding complications, as well as improvement in acute vessel closure. A move to change the post-stent therapy to aspirin alone was muted by the results of the STARS trial which showed that acute closure events were remarkably low (0.6% in the aspirin/ticlopidine cohort, but 3% in the aspirin alone cohort) (oral presentation, American Heart Association meeting, New Orleans, LA, USA, 1996).

Whereas these trials have tested stents only in relatively ideal lesions, stenting is used much more extensively in situations where the benefit on restenosis prevention has not been proven. These include small vessels, long lesions, ostial and bifurcation lesions, restenotic lesions and vein grafts.

One trial of patients with high-risk features such as prior bypass surgery and significant left ventricular dysfunction is being conducted in the US veterans' hospitals. Trials utilizing the new technologies have also begun. Two trials test interventional techniques using stents. The ARTS trial, sponsored by Cordis, a Johnson & Johnson Co, is designed to study patients who are suitable to have at least two stents placed. These patients are then randomized to bypass surgery or an intervention with stent placement. The other trial, stent or surgery (SOS), is a strategy trial of patients with stenting of some lesions possible. Multiple stent manufacturers are supporting this trial. Both these trials allow other interventional techniques as required. The outcome of these trials awaits their completion. An important endpoint will be the economic impact of the two approaches. Can the improved results of interventions with the addition of stenting offset the higher costs of the initial procedure? Will improved surgical techniques, especially early extubation and early hospital discharge, narrow the economic gap between surgery and angioplasty?

Conclusions

Apart from clinical trials, selection of a revascularization procedure will continue to be based on which approach is likely to achieve a satisfactory acute and long-term success, in addition to safety concerns. In the majority of cases, this is relatively clear. If effective methods of treating small vessels, long lesions, ostial and bifurcation disease, restenotic lesions and vein grafts will be established, then the number of patients referred for interventional therapy will increase. If surgical techniques become even less invasive and minimally invasive techniques prove reliable for multivessel disease patients, then surgical approaches will flourish. One must remember, however, that the singular advantage that bypass grafting has over interventional techniques is the more lasting result. A solution to restenosis will firmly establish angioplasty techniques as the treatment of choice.

References

1 Fischman DL, Leon MB, Baim DS. A randomized comparison of coronary stent placement and balloon angioplasty in the treatment of coronary artery disease. *N Engl J Med* 1994; **331**: 496–501.

2 Serruys PW, de Jaegere P, Kiemeneij F, *et al.* A comparison of balloon-expandable stent implantation with balloon angioplasty in patients with coronary artery disease. *N Engl J Med* 1994; **331**: 489–95.

3 Jones EL, Craver JM, Guyton RA, *et al.* Importance of complete revascularization in performance of the coronary bypass operation. *Am J Cardiol* 1983; **51**: 7–12.

4 Weintraub WS, King SB III, Jones EL, *et al.* Coronary surgery and coronary angioplasty in patients with two vessel coronary artery disease. *Am J Cardiol* 1993; **71**: 511–17.

5 King SB III, Lembo NJ, Weintraub WS, *et al.* A randomized trial comparing coronary angioplasty with coronary bypass surgery. *N Engl J Med* 1994; **331**: 1044–50.

6 Holmes DR, Berger PB. Complex and multivessel dilatation. In: Topol EJ (ed.), *Textbook of Interventional Cardiology* (Philadelphia, PA: WB Saunders, 1994): 231–50.

7 Mark DB, Nelson CL, Califf RM, *et al.* Continuing evolution of therapy for coronary artery disease. Initial results from the era of coronary angioplasty. *Circulation* 1994; **89**: 2015–25.

8 Hartz AJ, Kuhn EM, Pryer DB, *et al.* Mortality after coronary angioplasty and coronary artery bypass surgery (the National Medicare Experience). *Am J Cardiol* 1992; **70**: 179–85.

9 Weintraub WS, Jones EL, King SB III, *et al.* Changing use of coronary angioplasty and coronary bypass surgery in the treatment of chronic coronary artery disease. *Am J Cardiol* 1990; **65**: 183–8.

10 O'Keefe JH, Allan JJ, McCallister BD, *et al.* Angioplasty versus bypass surgery for multivessel coronary artery disease with left ventricular ejection fraction ≤40 percent. *Am J Cardiol* 1993; **71**: 897–901.

11 Pocock SJ, Henderson RA, Rickards AF, *et al.* Meta-analysis of randomised trials comparing coronary angioplasty with bypass surgery. *Lancet* 1995; **345**: 1184–9.

12 The Bypass Angioplasty Revascularization Investigation (BARI) Investigators. Comparison of coronary bypass surgery with angioplasty in patients with multivessel disease. *N Engl J Med* 1996; **335**: 217–25.

13 Kosinski AS, Barnhart HX, Weintraub WS, *et al.* Five year outcome after coronary surgery or coronary angioplasty: results from the Emory Angioplasty vs. Surgery Trial (EAST). *Circulation* 1995; **19(Suppl I)**: I-543 (abstract).

14 CABRI trial Participants. Coronary Angioplasty vs. Bypass Revascularisation Investigation (CABRI) results during the first year. *Lancet* 1995; **346**: 1179–83.

15 RITA Trial Participants. Coronary angioplasty versus coronary artery bypass surgery: the Randomised Intervention Treatment of Angina (RITA) trial. *Lancet* 1993; **341**: 573–80.

16 Rodriguez A, Boullon F, Perez-Balino N, *et al.* Argentine randomized trial of percutaneous transluminal coronary angioplasty versus coronary artery bypass surgery in multivessel disease (ERACI): in-hospital results and 1-year follow-up. *J Am Coll Cardiol* 1993; **33**: 1060–7.

17 Hamm CW, Reimers J, Ischinger T, *et al.* A randomized study of coronary angioplasty compared with bypass surgery in patients with symptomatic multivessel coronary artery disease. *N Engl J Med* 1994; **331**: 1037–43.

18 Puel J, Karouny E, Marco F, *et al.* Angioplasty versus surgery in multivessel disease: immediate results and in-hospital outcome in a randomized prospective study. *Circulation* 1992; **86 (Suppl I)**: 372.

19 Hueb W, Arie S, Oliveira SA, *et al.* Surgery, angioplasty or medical therapy in severe isolated proximal left anterior descending artery stenosis: initial results of a randomized trial. *Circulation* 1992; **86 (Suppl I)**: 717.

20 Goy JJ, Eeckhout E, Burnand B, *et al.* Coronary angioplasty versus left internal mammary artery grafting for isolated proximal left anterior descending artery stenosis. *Lancet* 1994; **343**: 1449–53.

21 Topol EJ, Leya F, Pinkerton CA, *et al.* A comparison of directional coronary atherectomy with coronary angioplasty in patients with coronary artery disease. *N Engl J Med* 1993; **329**: 221–7.

22 Adelman AG, Cohen EA, Kimball BP, *et al.* A comparison of directional atherectomy with balloon angioplasty for lesions of the left anterior descending coronary artery. *N Engl J Med* 1993; **329**: 228–33.

23 Teirstein PS, Warth DC, Haq N, *et al.* High speed rotational coronary atherectomy for patients with diffuse coronary artery disease. *J Am Coll Cardiol* 1991; **18**: 1694–701.

2

Stenting for multivessel disease

David P Foley, Walter RM Hermans and Patrick W Serruys

Introduction

Elective coronary stent implantation is now an accepted therapeutic strategy for patients with single vessel coronary artery disease. The improved clinical and angiographic results over balloon angioplasty, in the acute phase, have been shown to be maintained after 6 months follow-up;[1,2] after 1 year, clinical status is significantly more favourable among stented patients.[3] Furthermore, there is now three-year follow-up angiographic evidence that the luminal geometry of stented coronary segments does not tend to deteriorate further after 6 months and, if anything, may actually improve with time.[4] These findings appear to consolidate the place of stent implantation in the treatment of obstructive coronary artery disease. A wide variety of new stents available for clinical use outside the USA are now being somewhat empirically applied to all types of coronary lesions in all clinical settings. Perhaps this development is a testament to the effectiveness of stent implantation in the acute setting, in achieving a visually pleasing geometric coronary lumen. Nevertheless, since there are as yet no clinical trials examining the effects of stent implantation in longer coronary lesions, bifurcation lesions, coronary bypass graft lesions, unstable angina, acute myocardial infarction and no trials providing information on the long-term effects of stent implantation, the dangers of 'stentomania' may yet become apparent. We should, perhaps, be more cautious with the use of these permanent indwelling prostheses.

Accordingly, it seems logical to evaluate the stent comparatively as a panacea, with the gold standard revascularization therapy—coronary artery bypass graft surgery. One apparently logical extension of the indication for stenting is

for treatment of multivessel disease suitable for percutaneous revascularization. Over the past decade, balloon angioplasty has been subjected to exhaustive clinical comparisons with coronary artery bypass graft surgery (CABG) for treatment of multivessel disease. The outcomes of the large randomized trials are similar, showing no difference in the major end-points of mortality and transmural myocardial infarction, but a significantly higher 're-intervention rate' in the balloon angioplasty treated patients within the first year. Longer term follow-up reveals a similar clinical outcome regarding event-free survival and freedom from angina after the first year.[6-10] The outcomes of these randomized trials are similar: they show no significant difference in the major end-points of mortality and Q-waver (transmural) myocardial infarction within the first 5 years (BARI) but already within the first year a significantly higher 'reintervention rate' in the balloon angioplasty-treated patients. The conclusion of the BARI study—the most recently completed and the largest of the PTCA versus CABG trials—that angioplasty offers a reasonable alternative with an expectation of similar overall survival rates, free of Q-wave myocardial infarction, is indeed gratifying for the interventional cardiologist, since most interventional cardiologists believe that their techniques are now much better than during the period when these trials were ongoing. Since stent implantation is shown to reduce the need for re-intervention in the first year compared with balloon angioplasty, and given the ongoing developments in stent design, stent coatings, the techniques of implantation and in adjunctive pharmacological therapy to increase safety of angioplasty in general (GPIIb/IIIa antagonists, ticlopidine, clopidogrel etc.), it now seems logical to instigate a randomized trial comparing stent implantation with bypass graft surgery in multivessel coronary artery disease.

As a prelude to such a trial, we initiated a prospective single centre study at the Thoraxcentre to evaluate the safety and efficacy of multivessel stenting, with long-term follow-up of the patients, as well as to investigate cost aspects. We present here a description of this single centre study, including the acute and in-hospital results and the available 6-month clinical outcome, as a basis for the planned randomized Arterial Revascularization Therapy Study (ARTS), due to commence in mid-1997.

Methodology

This single centre study consists of a safety and efficacy type investigation to evaluate whether multivessel coronary stenting is practicable, in terms of safety and feasibility of complete revascularization in a single or staged session (with such factors as procedural duration, patient tolerance, volume of contrast material, planning logistics, need for use of other devices, etc.), completeness and effectiveness of revascularization (acute, medium and long-term clinical and angiographic follow-up), and financial implications.

To ensure practical clinical relevance, all patients being referred to our department with multivessel disease are considered for inclusion. Our group, consisting of interventional cardiologists, clinical cardiologists and cardiac surgeons, routinely discusses all patients referred for elective or urgent angioplasty. Thus, patients with multivessel disease referred to the cardiology group (as opposed to those referred directly for surgery, from the cardiologists of the region), where all significant lesions are considered amenable to stent implantation and all diseased vessels are considered equally suitable for bypass grafting, in the presence of no contraindications to bypass surgery, are proposed for inclusion in this study. Patients with unstable angina, long lesions, bifurcation lesions, total occlusion, coronary calcification or thrombus are not excluded, if the target lesions are considered by us, in the evolving practice of coronary intervention, amenable to percutaneous revascularization and eventual stent implantation. The final decision to proceed with our proposal is left to the referring cardiologist after discussion with our group and the patient. According to the preference of the interventional cardiologist, patients who give written informed consent are treated by stent implantation following general comprehensive discussion within the group, with regard to the strategy and especially regarding the need for employing a staged procedure (during the same hospital admission), the use of adjunctive devices, pre-treatment with ReoPro (Eli Lilly), the type and length of stents to be used, and the order in which lesions should be treated. During the treatment period, a total of 20 different stent types are available for

use at the Thoraxcentre, providing a wide variety of choice of materials, designs and lengths. In addition, a laser guidewire for recanalization of chronic occlusions, and a Possis Angiojet thrombectomy catheter for removal of established or fresh bulky thrombus, standard excimer laser angioplasty, directional atherectomy, pullback atherectomy and Rotablator, are available for use.

Patients with stable angina are routinely admitted from home the day prior to intervention, continuing on their routine medications. Patients with unstable angina, referred from other hospitals in the region for intervention, are usually transferred to the 'step-down' care unit of our department 2–4 hours prior to the planned intervention. Patients with unstable angina in our department are transferred directly to the intervention suite for the procedure. Virtually all patients with unstable angina awaiting intervention were receiving intravenous nitroglycerine and heparin, as well as aspirin and double or triple oral antianginal therapy. All procedures are performed via the femoral artery, using 8F guiding catheters. Pre-medication consists of heparin 10,000 units and further 5000 units bolus per hour thereafter, based on hourly activated clotting time measurements and aspirin 250 mg intravenously. Intravenous ReoPro is used for patients with known intracoronary thrombus, or felt to be at particular risk (a total of 25% received ReoPro, which was usually commenced at the beginning of the procedure, but in about one third of cases, during the procedure). Ticlopidine therapy is started before the procedure where possible, or at least before, or shortly after stent implantation (loading dose of 1 g, followed by 500 mg daily for 1 month).

After adequate pre-dilatation and stent placement, routine post-dilatation is performed to 14–24 atmospheres using semi- or non-compliant balloons with a target balloon:artery ratio of 1.1–1.2. Intra-coronary ultrasound guidance is used, where it is felt to be of clinical value, and according to the preference of the operator.

Results

Between September 1995 and November 1996, a total of 85 patients were included (58 (68%) male, 27 (32%) female; mean age 58.7 years, range 35–85). It is noteworthy that 70% of the patients were referred for treatment of post-infarct or unstable angina, requiring urgent revascularization during hospital admission; the rest were treated for elective indications. Patient demographics are shown in Table 2.1. Triple vessel stenting was required in seven patients, double vessel in 66 and single or double native vessel plus single or double vein graft or internal mammary artery graft stenting in 12 patients. Mean vessel diameter was 2.68 ± 0.50-mm, mean lesion length was 16.0 ± 14.8-mm, minimal pre-PTCA diameter 0.80 ± 0.38

Table 2.1 Patient demographics in the single centre trial.

	n (%)
Male/female	58 (68%)/27 (32%)
Mean age	58.7 years
Diabetes	13%
Hypercholesterolemia	53%
Peripheral vascular disease	14%
Family history	40%
Current smoking	37%
Prior myocardial infarction	59%
anterior	40%
inferior	34%
unknown	26%
Prior CABG	20%
Prior PTCA	18%
Stable angina	28%
Unstable angina	72%
Canadian Cardiovascular Class	
II	11%
III	33%
IV	66%
Three-vessel disease	26%
Two-vessel disease	74%
Primary/restenosis lesion	92%/8%
Left ventricular function:	
normal	69%
impaired	19%
severely impaired	6%
not documented	6%
Surgical 'standby' agreed	88%

CABG, coronary artery bypass graft surgery; PTCA, percutaneous transluminal coronary angioplasty

Table 2.2 Angiographic baseline and procedural characteristics in the single centre trial.

Vessel combination treated:	n (%)
3 vessels	7 (9%)
LAD + RCA	20 (22%)
LAD + LCX	28 (33%)
RCA + LCX	17 (20%)
LMain + RCA	1 (1%)
Bypass(es) + native(s)	12 (15%)
Mean number of lesions/patient stented	2.8
Mean number of stents/patient	3.5
Mean number of balloons/patient	4.2
Lesion type (ACC/AHA): A	18%
B1	45%
B2	23%
C	14%
Total occlusion pre-procedure	12%
Intracoronary thrombus pre-procedure	7%
Reference vessel diameter	2.68 ± 0.50 mm
Minimal luminal diameter pre-procedure	0.80 ± 0.38 mm
Minimal luminal diameter post-procedure	2.73 ± 0.42 mm
% Diameter stenosis pre-procedure	72 ± 11%
% Diameter stenosis post-procedure	12 ± 7%

LAD, left anterior descending artery; RCA, right coronary artery; LCX, left circumflex artery; LMain, left main stem

mm increasing to 2.73 ± 0.42-mm post-procedure. Thus a negative diameter stenosis compared with the pre-procedural reference vessel diameter is obtained, but since the conventionally used reference diameter is the post-procedural reference diameter, and since this is increased by the influence of stent implantation on the entire segment (3.02-mm in the present series, compared with 2.68-mm pre-procedure) the mean post-procedural diameter stenosis was 12 ± 7%, a satisfactory result (Table 2.2). In 12 patients the procedure was staged over two sessions, 1–7 days apart. Mean procedure time was 171 min (45–255 min) and mean contrast volume was 805 ml. Reo-Pro was used in 25% of the patients. The only in-hospital major adverse cardiac events were 1% emergency CABG (tamponade after perforation under ReoPro use) and 8% non-Q-wave myocardial infarction (creatine phosphokinase, (CPK) 3 times above normal) in 8% of patients. Of the

patients having double vessel native coronary stenting, the combination of stented left anterior descending (LAD) and circumflex arteries was—42%, in the LAD and right coronary arteries (RCA)—34%, and in the RCA and circumflex—23%, with one patient undergoing stenting of the left main stem and RCA. A mean of 3.5 stents per patient was used, ranging in individual length from 6-mm (AVE Micro II) to 60-mm (Schneider Wallstent) and a nominal diameter from 1.5-mm (Boston Scientific NIR '5 cell') to 6-mm (Schneider Wallstent). The following stent types were employed:

- Boston Scientific NIR,
- Cordis, a Johnson & Johnson Palmaz–Schatz and Crown,
- AVE Micro II and GFX,
- Schneider Wallstent, Wellstent and Magic stent,
- Medtronic beStent and Wiktor stent,
- Cook Gianurco–Roubin Flex II,
- Advanced Cardiovascular Systems Multilink stent,
- Global Therapeutics Freedom,
- ACT I stent,
- Devon Puva and Pura-Vario,
- Angiodynamics Angiostent,
- Instent Cardiocoil stent.

In addition, a mean of 4.2 balloons per patient were used. In 15% of patients, the procedure was staged over two sessions, ranging from 1 day to 1 week apart, for reasons including patient preference, compromised renal function, borderline left ventricular function and particularly complex interventions with a predicted duration longer than 4 hours. The average procedural duration was 171 min, with a range of 65–465 min. The longest duration was a staged procedure of considerable complexity, involving laser wire recanalization of a chronic total occlusion, in separate sessions 24 hours apart, of both the LAD and circumflex artery, and additional stenting of a trifurcation lesion in the circumflex artery. A mean of 845 ml of contrast was used per patient with a range of 400–1800 ml.

A successful procedural outcome was achieved in 84 patients (Fig. 2.1), defined as successful placement of a stent in all target lesions, with a 20% or more reduction of stenosis determined by on-line quantitative angiography (QCA) (with or without additional intracoronary ultrasound evaluation as deemed necessary by the responsible physician, in which case criteria of complete stent apposition, symmetry score ≥0.9 and minimal luminal cross sectional area ≥90% of the distal reference area are met). One patient (64-year-old male with Braunwald Class III unstable angina) was sent for emergency surgery because of perforation of the LAD after high pressure post-dilatation, which could not be closed by prolonged inflation of a perfusion balloon, presumably due to the concomitant use of ReoPro. In fact this patient had been proposed for surgery because of the diffuse nature of the obstructive disease in his LAD and right coronary arteries, but he refused surgery and requested angioplasty with stent implantation, despite the attendant increased risk of complications. To illustrate the fragility of outcome in this type of patient, the right coronary artery had been successfully stented and the long irregular and calcified lesion in the LAD had also been carefully dilated, stented and reasonably satisfactorily post-dilated. However, with QCA measurement of the segment, the distal part of the stent in the LAD had a mean luminal diameter (MLD) of 1.9-mm. Additional dilatation with a short semi-compliant balloon was felt to be indicated and it was this extra dilatation that perforated the artery requiring surgery. In another patient with Braunwald Class III B unstable angina, the distal LAD was partially occluded by embolization of material. Despite successful stenting of the target lesions, and despite optimal anticoagulation and aggressive anti-platelet therapy with intravenous ReoPro and oral ticlopidine, a small non-Q-wave myocardial infarction developed with a peak CPK of 800iu (MB of 10%). In another five patients a creatine kinase increase to more than three times the upper limit was observed and diagnosis of non-Q-wave myocardial infarction was made (total of 7% incidence of non-Q-wave MI during the in-hospital phase). A 54-year-old female treated for Braunwald Class III B unstable angina experienced recurrence of chest pain

at rest 12 hours after successful stenting of the LAD and right coronary artery, which led to recatheterization within 24 hours of the procedure, with no significant stenosis. All other patients experienced no adverse cardiac events during the in-hospital stay.

In four patients, the Spectranetics Primo laser guidewire was used to recanalize a chronically occluded target lesion prior to multivessel stenting; in two patients the Possis Medical Angiojet thrombectomy catheter was used to remove bulky intracoronary thrombus prior to stenting; in one patient directional atherectomy was performed prior to stenting and in another patient the Arrow Pullback Atherectomy Catheter was used to debulk one of the target lesions before stent implantation. In general, sheaths were removed 4–6 hours after the procedure, except for cases where heparin infusion was kept overnight, according to individual physician preferences. Two patients experienced bleeding, requiring transfusion (one with gastrointestinal bleeding; the other with access site bleeding). Neither patient experienced adverse sequela and surgical intervention was not required. In-hospital stay averaged 2.2 days after treatment.

Follow-up

Of 60 patients eligible for 6-month clinical follow-up, 70% were event free. A 68-year-old female patient died from pneumonia, as a result of prolonged mechanical respiration following emergency surgery for intracerebral haemorrhage, which suddenly occurred 12 hours after re-PTCA with additional stent implantation and initiation of ReoPro infusion, for extensive diffuse restenosis with previously placed stents in a dominant right coronary artery. Incidentally, this was the first patient with fatal bleeding associated with use of ReoPro at the Thoraxcentre, after some 150–200 patients had already been so treated using the original concomitant heparin regime. To date, no patient has experienced a Q-wave myocardial infarction or undergone bypass surgery (apart from the patient who had surgery because of intra-procedural coronary perforation with persistent bleeding, related to ReoPro). Thirty percent of patients have undergone re-intervention, of whom 30% had restenosis of more than one lesion (Fig. 2.2); 70% were restricted to one lesion. Of the 70% of patients who remained event free, 10% are symptomatic Canadian Cardiovascular Society (CCS) class 2 and the remainder are symptom free.

Cost

The average procedural cost of disposables per patient (according to the market price of the materials) was 14,500 Dutch guilders (Dfl).

Discussion of the study strategy and results and introduction of the ARTS trial

In evaluating the potential impact of a strategy of elective multivessel stenting in multivessel disease, we wanted to be minimally restrictive in our patient inclusion, in order to make the study clinically relevant and representative of daily practice. However, this strategy has an inherent risk of greater acute complications and potentially unimpressive long-term results, which might thus be damaging to the inauguration of a randomized trial comparing this strategy with bypass graft surgery. In spite of the extremely high prevalence of unstable angina and the acceptance of a large percentage of target lesions, which would have been excluded from virtually all clinical trials on stenting up to now (vessel size less than 3-mm, lesions longer than 15-mm, presence of thrombus, chronic total occlusion, recent myocardial infarction etc), multivessel stenting was acutely successful in all but one patient who had to be sent for surgery due to coronary perforation exacerbated with ReoPro use. Therefore, despite good percutaneous revascularization, surgery was needed to treat the perforation. These data demonstrate the feasibility and efficacy of the strategy of stenting for multivessel disease, despite adverse clinical and lesion characteristics. Improvement in the acute and 6-month clinical outcome of angioplasty in unstable angina, associated with the use of platelet GPIIB/IIA antagonism, is highly likely to improve the safety of stenting in unstable angina and may further improve results in stable angina, especially in patients with less favourable morphologies. Obviously, we must await the randomized trial before pronouncing the likely benefits, given the sometimes catastrophic side-effects, that occurred in two patients (one with a fatal outcome after cerebral haemorrhage and the other needing emergency surgery for tamponade after coronary perforation).

Our group has also used a strategy of what could be called tailored stenting. That is possible with the large variety of available stent designs, lengths and diameters. Thus, we were able, in most cases, to select one stent per lesion, based on the on-line QCA measurements of the target lesion. Therefore, we frequently used combinations of different stent types in the same patient and also occasionally, different stent types in the same vessel for different lesions. Thus a segment requiring a stent 35-mm or longer could be treated by a 35-mm ACS Multilink, a 39-mm AVE, a 40-mm Gianturco–Roubin II, a 40-mm Freedom, a 35-mm beStent or a long Magic Wallstent. Depending on the need to preserve the ostium of an important sidebranch, the tortuosity of the segment or of the need for stronger support, the appropriate stent could be chosen. The NIR 32-mm, Cordis, a Johnson & Johnson Crown 30-mm, Jostent 32-mm, Biocompatibles 32-mm, AVE 30-mm, Freedom 30-mm or Magic Wallstent, could be used for lesions in the region of 30-mm. Accordingly, routine application of QCA to the least foreshortened view of the target lesion can be used for selection of the appropriate length and diameter of stent from the wide variety available (outside North America). Therefore, the need for multiple stents per lesion should no longer be mandatory when adopting a policy of multivessel stenting for all patients with at least one long lesion.

The long-term outcome, the cost-effectiveness, and the applicability to the average patient group referred for revascularization of multivessel disease remains to be determined. Clearly, a selection process must take place in the future to exclude patients not suitable for stenting, but, at the rate of current growth in applications and increasing usability of stents, which allows access to side branches, more flexible and longer stents, less thrombogenic and coated stents and stents with less metal surface, for smaller vessels, the selectivity is becoming less exclusive. As outlined above, we have already made our inclusion criteria as broad as possible to make our evaluation clinically relevant. Nonetheless, because all patients referred for revascularization from our region do not go through a central triage process, our group is not in a position to estimate what percentage of the total group of patients undergoing revascularization for multivessel disease is represented by the patients described here. The only way to provide such data, will be to use a 'screening log' wherein all patients referred from the region to our centre are logged in, with their diagnosis, recommended treatment strategy and ultimate strategy, and the reasons for not undergoing multivessel stenting. In multicentre restenosis prevention trials co-ordinated by Cardialysis, Rotterdam, this policy has been applied and the results certainly make interesting reading, mostly showing that, at least in angioplasty/restenosis or stent/balloon angioplasty studies, it is unusual to have more than 15% of the patient workload of a given interventional department being considered eligible for the trial. Of course, this finding is often cited as rendering the findings of certain trials such as BENESTENT and STRESS inapplicable to the general patient population, since they are not representative of the majority of treated patients. It is also interesting to note, however, that the boom in stent implantation in the past 2 years, with empirical application to wide varieties of coronary pathology, is largely justified by most clinicians on the basis of the BENESTENT and STRESS trials.

In our patient population, 60 of the 84 patients having successful multivessel stenting have completed 6-month clinical follow-up; 30% required re-intervention of one or more lesions. This figure is superficially unsatisfactory, being somewhat higher than BENESTENT and STRESS and considerably higher than BENESTENT II, which allowed multivessel intervention. Yet, this is the price we paid for a broad inclusion in this study, since we were concerned with

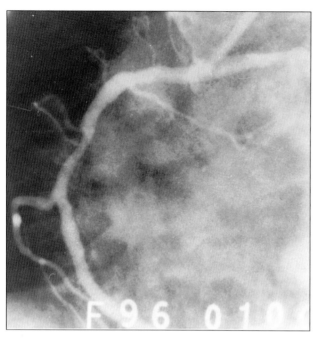

a

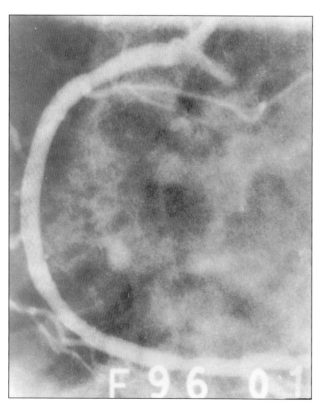

b

Figure 2.1

Angiograms before (a and d), after (b and e) and at 6-month follow-up (c and f) after stent implantation of the right coronary artery in the left anterior oblique projection (a, b and c) and the circumflex (d, e and f), and recanalization and stent implantation in the left anterior descending coronary artery (d, e and f), in the right anterior oblique projection, in a 39-year-old extremely obese (125 kg, 18 cm in height) non-insulin dependent diabetic, referred to The Thoraxcentre for revascularization because of unstable angina, Braunwald class IIIB. Because of his age and obesity, he was proposed for recanalization of the LAD and if successful, stenting of the right and circumflex. Since the LAD was collaterally filled from the diseased right coronary artery, this was first pre-dilated and stented with a self-expanding Wallstent post-dilated with a 3.5 mm balloon to 18 atmospheres (b). Thereafter, the occluded LAD (double arrow in d), was visualized by employing simultaneous bilateral coronary injections (using bilateral femoral arterial access and biplane angiography, as described in Chapter 6) and was successfully recanalized using the Primo laser wire (Spectranetics). This was followed by balloon dilatation and placement of a hand crimped Palmaz–Schatz PS-204 stent on a 3.0 mm semi-compliant balloon, dilated to 18 atmospheres (e, double arrow). The short circumflex lesion, shown by the single arrow in (d), was stented using an AVE Micro-II stent. After post-dilatation, there was a localized perforation with tamponade, which was successfully managed by immediate pericardiocentesis and prolonged balloon inflation. Because of the tamponade, the patient was observed for 24 hours in the Coronary Care Unit; the drain was removed 12 hours post-procedure, since no leakage had been observed and Echo control revealed no pericardial fluid. Despite the tamponade, the patient was further treated with aspirin and ticlopidine for 30 days. Because of his age and risk factors, despite being asymptomatic and with a negative maximal exercise test he was recatheterized after six months, with excellent angiographic results, as displayed in (c) and (f).

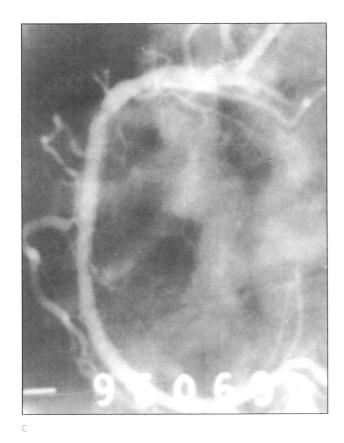

c

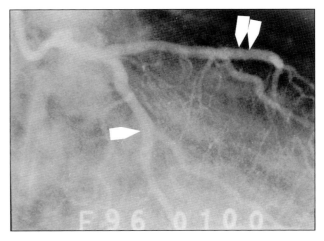

e

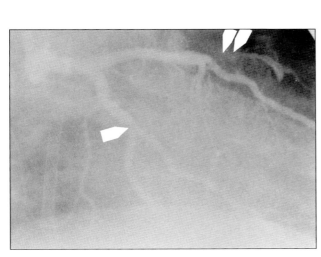

d

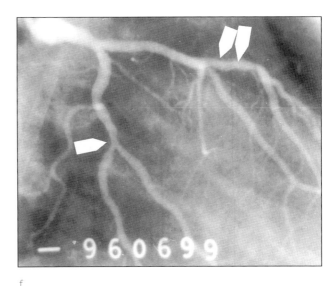

f

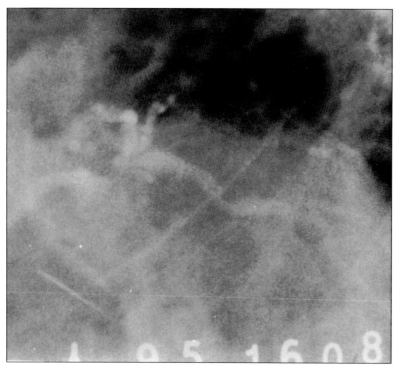

a

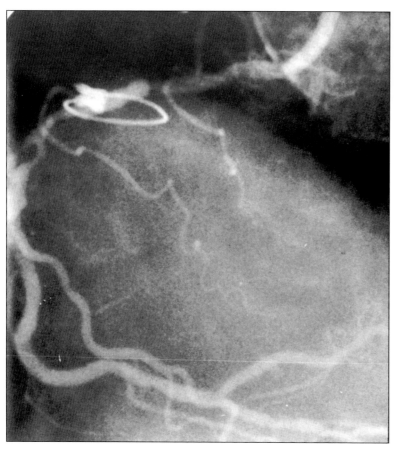

b

Figure 2.2

Pre- (a and b) and post- (c and d) procedural angiograms of a 73-year-old female with severe intractable unstable angina pectoris, despite adequate betablockade (resting heart rate 48/min) and aggressive calcium antagonism and intravenous nitrate use (resting systemic blood pressure 105/65-mmHg), aspirin and intravenous heparin therapy. Despite the sub-total left main coronary stenosis (shown in Figure 2.2a in the left inferior oblique projection) with TIMI 2 flow in the left coronary artery, with good left ventricular function, surgery was considered to be extremely high risk because of her age, prior aortic valve replacement, impaired pulmonary function (forced vital capacity and forced expiratory volume in 1 second 60% of expected for age and body mass) and prior history of transient ischemic attacks, with documented bilateral severe carotid stenosis. Accordingly, it was decided to perform elective stent implantation of the left main and of the long severe irregular lesion of the right coronary artery (b). On-line QCA revealed a reference diameter of 3.44-mm and lesion length of 12-mm in the left main. Guidewires were placed in both the LAD and circumflex and after pre-dilatation with a 3.5/16-mm compliant balloon, a hand-crimped 15-mm beStent was placed in the left-main, making use of the end radio-opaque markers of the beStent for precise placement to avoid overlapping the ostium of the circumflex artery. Post-dilatation was performed using a 15-mm/3.5-mm Speedino balloon (Schneider). The right coronary lesion measured 36 mm in length, with a reference diameter of 2.8-mm. Pre-dilation was performed with a 3-mm/40-mm Cordis Passage and a 39-mm long/3-mm diameter AVE stent was placed and post-dilated with a 3.0-mm/20-mm Schneider Speedy to 18 atmospheres. The procedure was completed in 80 minutes. The patient was discontinued from heparin and nitrate and ticlopidine was initiated for 30 days. After 4 months, the patient complained of progressive recurrence of symptoms on minimal exertion and re-catheterization revealed severe focal restenosis of both lesions which were successfully treated by re-balloon angioplasty to greater than 18 atmospheres using similarly sized balloons as initially. Eight months later she remains clinically asymptomatic.

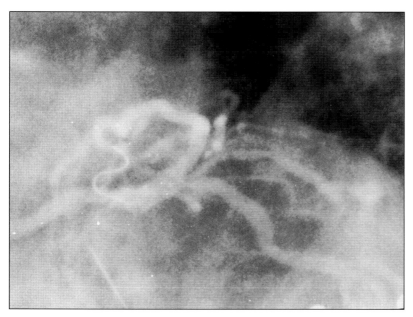

c

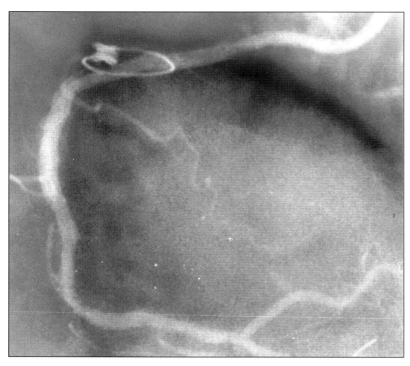

d

broad applicability of the treatment strategy. To our knowledge, no other coronary intervention study has previously included such a high proportion of 'high risk' patients, so there are no comparative standards. The control groups in the CAPTURE and EPIC trials may be somewhat comparable regarding clinical syndromes, although these trials did not allow inclusion of patients requiring multivessel intervention, or patients with bypass graft lesions. In these trials, nevertheless, the re-intervention rates at 6 months was approximately 30%, in both control and treatment groups. Therefore, the results of this study must be considered acceptable, since ReoPro was used in only 25% of patients despite unstable angina being the indication in 70% and since 16% of the patients had stenting of a bypass graft as part of their multivessel stent therapy. In addition, the mean pre-treatment vessel diameter was very small (2.63-mm), which is conventionally considered not suitable for stenting. We have previously demonstrated the adverse influence of small vessel size on late restenosis. This factor may play an important role in the 30% re-intervention rate in ARTS. Obviously, serial angiographic follow-up will be required to evaluate the factors influencing late restenosis, but for logistic reasons and with respect to patients' preferences, we have not required systematic angiographic follow-up, although a considerable proportion of patients will be undergoing angiographic follow up at 6 months and those results will be of major interest. Nevertheless, with complete clinical follow-up it will be possible to evaluate all the available baseline, angiographic and procedural factors related to a better or worse outcome. At this time, accounting for the complexity of the treated patient group, the acute results of multivessel stenting applied to all patients with symptomatic multivessel disease show the procedure to be safe and effective in achieving complete revascularization. With the presence of a high proportion of risk factors for restenosis in such a population, a re-intervention rate of 30% can be expected and it is left to the clinician and patient to decide if this type of statistic is acceptable when undertaking the treatment.

With the additional application of therapies that are currently under investigation (e.g. heparin or other stent coatings, peri- and post-procedural ReoPro, local drug delivery of various active agents, local brachytherapy, and endothelial cell sodding to name a few), it is possible that adjunctive therapy at the time of stenting, or the use of coated or radioactive stents, may reduce the proliferative response after stenting,[13] thus reducing the re-intervention rate. Accordingly, our data must be considered encouraging, particularly the acute procedural success, low incidence of in-hospital problems and short hospital stay, despite the unstable antecedent presentation in so many patients. The time is therefore ripe for a major evaluation of the efficacy of multivessel stenting and its cost-effectiveness compared with the gold standard of bypass graft surgery, and presents the rationale for the ARTS trial.

The limitations of the single centre study

This evaluation is a prospective single centre study intended to examine real-world applicability of multivessel stenting to multivessel disease; as such it is limited by the selection bias of the individual interventionalists. The clinical spectrum of the trial's patients illustrates that the study included the high rather than low risk patients. There was no protocol defining inclusion and exclusion criteria, therapeutic principles, and follow-up evaluations. However, as a single group with a common *modus operandi* strengthened by weekly case discussions, detailed therapeutic recommendation on each patient's 'surgical/intervention card', and routine responsibility of senior interventionalists for complex cases, the limitation of the lack of such a protocol in streamlining the treatment strategy is minimal. The only advantage provided by such 'trial documents' would be to have an additional case record form to facilitate data collection and storage. Inclusion of patients having a bypass graft and native vessel stented as multivessel stenting introduces additional heterogeneity, but, again leaning towards the high risk patient, since the risks associated with bypass graft angioplasty are higher than native vessel in both the short and long-term. It is also of importance to point out that these patients were all considered candidates for re-operation, which is an important aspect of this study, i.e. evaluating the efficacy of multivessel stenting in operable patients. Patients with no significant lesion in the LAD having stenting of right coronary and circumflex lesions, could be considered not representative of the type of patient who would be considered for bypass surgery. However, this is widely variable between centres and referring cardiologists, and this possibly 'low risk' sub-group (20% in this series) is more than compensated by the high risk features already mentioned. Twelve percent of the patients were not considered candidates for elective bypass surgery and were thus treated by stenting with standby surgery only in the event of a life threatening complication.

Introduction to the randomized ARTS trial

The ARTS—Arterial Revascularization Therapy Study—commenced patient recruitment at 80 centres throughout Europe on 1 April 1997. Institution of this trial was prompted by the progressive empirical application of stenting to multivessel disease, now anecdotally reported by most high volume interventional centres, although minimal if any published reports describing results or justifying this practice exist at this time. The results of the single centre study presented in this report are not used to justify the performance of a trial. Rather, the fact that we are carrying out this prospective study, coupled with the known trends in other countries and the results of many balloon angioplasty versus surgery trials, are more than adequate impetus to stimulate interventionalists, surgeons and the stent industry to design a suitable trial. This trial required one year of preparatory discussions between European interventional cardiologists and cardiac surgeons before the protocol design could be finalized. Interestingly, the cardiologists were in general agreement to a sponsorship proposal by Cordis, a Johnson & Johnson Co, thus restricting themselves to the use of the Crown stents. Though in their daily practice, they may now be accustomed to a wider choice of stent, as shown by our practice in this study. The surgeons, however, were in broad disagreement regarding the surgical techniques, with some requiring a general policy of total arterial revascularization and others considering it unrealistic to apply to 80 investigating centres where routine surgical practice is not uniform. Eventually, it was agreed that the LAD should receive an arterial conduit in all patients, and that complete arterial revascularization would be left to the discretion of the surgeon. An extensive protocol description of the multiple choices available depending on the existing pathology of the included patient is intended to guide investigators.

Investigative centres for the ARTS trial were chosen on the basis of a minimum requirement of an annual performance of at least 750 bypass operations and 750 percutaneous coronary interventions, of which 40% were stent procedures, with 15–20% being multivessel stenting. Therefore, about 45–60 patients per year had to be treated by multivessel stenting, providing an adequate caseload to guarantee the minimal inclusion of one patient per week when coupled with the weekly CABG workload of the surgical group. The inclusion requirement is one randomized patient per week, so that the inclusion period should be complete within 6 months.

Case record forms are used to record all relevant information concerning the therapeutic procedure, the in-hospital stay and clinical follow-up at 6 months, 1 year and then annually to 5 years and again at 10 years. The major clinical endpoints are:

- death,
- myocardial infarction,
- re-intervention (percutaneous or surgical),

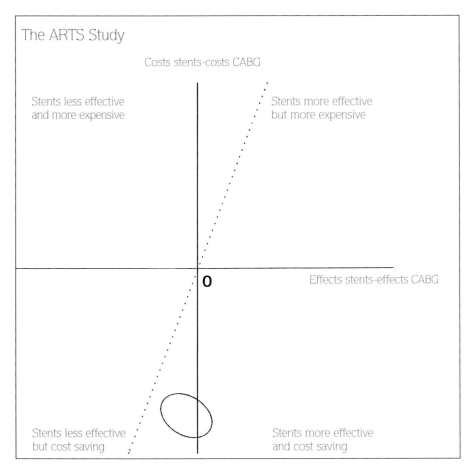

Figure 2.3
Illustration of the potential cost-effective outcome of the ARTS trial (or any trial comparing two treatment strategies). We hypothesize that stents will be less effective but also less costly than bypass surgery. For this to be confirmed in the trial, the relationship between cost and effect must emerge as shown. This simple graphic method of display may be used to summarize the outcome of cost-effectiveness comparisons.

- cerebrovascular events occurring during the follow-up period.

Quality of life and recurrence of symptoms will also be documented. All costs incurred in treatment and follow-up evaluations of each patient will be documented, so that ultimately, age adjusted quality of life years saved by the revascularization will be calculated using standard methodology. The final hypothesis is that multivessel stenting will be more cost-effective than bypass surgery, although it is not expected that multivessel stenting will be more effective than surgery in reducing the rate of major clinical events during follow-up. Thus, this is an unusual clinical trial, where the clinical outcome is already expected before commencing and the real evaluation concerns cost-effectiveness of therapy, which to a greater or lesser degree, hinges on how the purchase price of stents changes in the coming period (Fig. 2.3).

Conclusion

The CABRI, RITA, EAST, BARI, ERACI and other similar studies have laid the ground for the use of percutaneous technology in variable coronary disease cohorts, yet those seminal studies were limited to balloon angioplasty. Therefore, their conclusions regarding the incompleteness of revascularization and the higher reintervention rates within the first year in the percutaneously treated patients needs to be re-evaluated with the current use of stents. The ARTS trial should ultimately provide the platform for objective evaluation of the true place of percutaneous revascularization, facing the 21st century. Our enthusiasm for this type of patient management is growing apparently at a much greater rate than our budgetary allowance. Let us therefore hope that healthy competition between the manufacturers of the various interventional devices will lead to appropriate reduction in currently unjustifiably excessive costs, so that we can continue to develop new therapeutic strategies aimed at improving patient care, free of the currently inevitable millstone of financial constraints.

Acknowledgements

The authors have written this chapter on behalf of the Department of Coronary Diagnostics and Intervention, Thoraxcentre, Academic Hospital Dijkzigt, Rotterdam, The Netherlands.

References

1 Serruya PW, de Jaegere P, Kiemeneij F, et al. for the BENESTENT study group. A comparison of balloon-expandable stent implantation with balloon angioplasty in patients with coronary artery disease. N Eng J Med 1994; **331**: 489–95.

2 Fischman DL, Leon MB, Baim DS, et al. for the STRESS investigators. A randomized comparison of coronary artery stent placement and balloon angioplasty in the treatment of coronary artery disease. N Eng J Med 1994; **331**: 496–501.

3 Macaya C, Serruys PW, Ruygrok P, et al. Continued benefit of coronary stenting versus balloon angioplasty: one year clinical follow up of the BENESTENT trial. J Am Coll Cardiol 1996; **27**: 255–61.

4 Kimura T, Yokoi H, Nakagawa Y, et al. Three year follow up after implantation of metallic coronary artery stents. N Eng J Med 1996; **334**: 561–6.

5 Colombo A, Hall P, Nakamura S, et al. Intracoronary stenting without anticoagulation accomplished with ultrasound guidance. Circulation 1995; **91**: 1676–88.

6 RITA trial participants. Coronary angioplasty versus coronary artery bypass surgery: The Randomized Intervention Treatment of Angina (RITA) trial. Lancet 1993; **341**: 573–80.

7 Ham CW, Reimers J, Ischinger T, et al. A randomized study of coronary angioplasty compared with bypass surgery in patients with symptomatic multivessel disease. New Eng J Med 1994; **331**: 1037–43.

8 King SB III, Lembo NJ, Weintraub WS, et al. A randomized trial comparing coronary angioplasty with coronary bypass surgery. New Eng J Med 1994; **331**: 1044–50.

9 CABRI Trial Participants. First year results of CABRI (Coronary Angioplasty versus Bypass Revascularization Investigation). Lancet 1995; **346**: 1179–84.

10 The Bypass Angioplasty Revascularization Investigation (BARI) Investigators. Comparison of coronary bypass surgery with angioplasty in patients with multivessel disease. New Eng J Med 1996; **335**: 217–35.

3

Complex coronary interventions: chronic total occlusions and bifurcation disease

David R Holmes Jr

Introduction

The number of options for patients undergoing a percutaneous approach for the treatment of coronary artery disease continues to increase. These expanded options allow more patients to be treated and improves the initial outcome. Whether the long-term outcome can be improved requires further study. Among several different lesion subsets which cause particular concern for the interventional cardiologist, two are among the most problematic: 1) chronic total occlusions; and 2) bifurcation lesions. At the present time, approaches to these specific lesion subtypes have not been satisfactorily resolved.

Chronic total occlusions

The presence of a chronic total occlusion supplying viable myocardium is one of the most common lesions for surgical revascularization. A solution to this problem would markedly increase the number of patients who could benefit from a percutaneous approach.

There is an increasing amount of information available on the pathology of chronic total occlusion. Srivatsa et al.[1] studied the age-related changes and histologic composition and the neovascular channel patterns in an autopsy series of 96 angiographic chronic total occlusions from 61 patients who had undergone coronary angiography within 3 months of death. Acute occlusions were excluded. Of interest, although all the patients had occlusion documented by angiography, not all were occluded at the time of autopsy—in fact, the majority (78%) were less than 99% occluded by histologic assessment; 25% were 90–95% occluded; 24% were 96–98% occluded; 29% were 99% occluded; and only 22% were completely occluded. Angiographic occlusions may therefore be subtotal, which increases the potential for successful intervention. There was a relationship between the age of the occlusion and the histopathology. Cholesterol and foam cell-laden intimal plaques were seen more frequently in younger lesions while fibrocalcific intimal plaques increased with the age of the chronic total occlusion ($p = 0.008$). Cellular inflammation and neovascularization within the arterial wall were common in all chronic total occlusions. Neovascularization was particularly abundant; intimal plaque revascularization channels arose from the adventitial vasa vasorum and were related to the cellular inflammation.

These histopathologic findings have direct relevance to interventional cardiology and may explain the relationship between the success rate and age of occlusion; as has been reported,[2-4] older occlusions are harder to cross and treat successfully. The presence of prominent neovascularization within the intimal plaque may also explain why really fine wires (0.010-inch) may sometimes be successful in crossing a chronic total occlusion when other larger, stiffer wires have failed.

The major problem with chronic total occlusion is the inability to obtain access to the distal vascular bed; this is the rate-limiting step. Once the guidewire has successfully traversed the occlusion, the procedure can usually be completed successfully. Multiple large-series documented a success rate of approximately 60–65%.[2-5] Specific angiographic features associated with improved outcome have been identified and include short duration of occlusion, short length, absence of side-branches at the site of occlusion and a tapered entry point. There is also a definite learning curve involving optimal case selection as well as the specific technical approach.

The other problem with chronic total occlusion is the potential for reocclusion and/or restenosis. In the multicenter MARCATOR study[6] of 1436 patients, a chronic total occlusion was successfully treated in 139. There were significant differences between those patients treated for subtotal stenosis and those treated for chronic total occlusions. Patients in whom a chronic total occlusion had been present had a smaller reference vessel diameter (2.5 mm vs. 2.7 mm; $p < 0.0001$), smaller minimal lumen diameter (1.5 mm vs. 1.7 mm; $p = 0.0001$) and a greater residual diameter stenosis (37% vs. 34%; $p = 0.0004$). The striking finding on angiographic follow-up was that recurrent occlusion was more likely in patients with initial chronic total occlusion than in patients with an initial subtotal stenosis (19% vs. 7%; $p = 0.001$). Overall, the restenosis rate was 46% in patients with a chronic total occlusion. This increase in reocclusion rates, as well as a higher restenosis rate in general, has been previously documented.[6]

Despite the increased success rate and increased potential for reocclusion, there has been considerable enthusiasm for percutaneous treatment in these patients as the risks of the procedure are less than in patients with subtotal stenosis; in addition, with successful procedures, surgery can be avoided.[2,7]

To optimize the potential for success, a number of technical approaches should be used (Table 3.1). It is essential to visualize, if possible, the course of the distal bed either through injection of the collateral supplying vessels or through review of old films when the artery was still patent. If possible, simultaneous bilateral coronary arterial injection should be used to guide the procedure. These can help to guide the wire and insure that it is intraluminal. This adds to the complexity of the procedure but also adds to the potential for success. Biplane angiography is also very helpful. A stable guiding catheter position should be acquired and then a small catheter as a platform to deliver a variety of guidewires. This latter catheter could be a small balloon catheter, a probing sheath or a transfer catheter. Selection of the specific wire depends upon the operator's preference as well as specific anatomy. In a functional total occlusion, a 0.010-inch wire may pass with relative ease. If that is not successful, then a heavier wire, usually an intermediate 0.014-inch wire, is selected. This could be followed by increasingly stiff and heavy wires as the case may be. While there has been great interest in the olive-tipped Magnum wire (Schneider Europe) AG, Bülach, Switzerland, its utility varies. A variety of hydrophilic wires is also available and may be of help, although they decrease the tactile sense of the operator and may pass subintimally more frequently.

Table 3.1 Optimizing approach to chronic total occlusion.
• Initial patient/lesion selection—attempt only lesions that really merit being done
• Distinguish functional total from total occlusion
• Visualize course of distal vessel:
– review of old angiograms
– bilateral coronary injection to fill collaterals
• Biplane angiography
• Stable guiding catheter and wire delivery platform
• Guidewire selection:
– progression from thinner wires .010 in to start for functional total to thicker heavier wires
– progression from very steerable but flexible wires to standard wires
– consider laser guidewire
• Careful movement to avoid subintimal guidewire passage
• Persistence
• Following successful completion: if vessel adequate size—stent placement

There are two most important issues for approaching chronic total occlusions:

1 The time, expense and resource utilization of approaching these lesions are increased.[8] If a chronic total occlusion is to be approached, the operator should be prepared to spend the time and resources or the chronic total occlusion should not even be attempted.

2 The first approach to the chronic total occlusion can determine the eventual outcome. If a long subintimal guidewire passage is produced, it may dramatically decrease the subsequent success rate. These procedures are complex and should be treated by a very experienced coronary interventionist. These are not to be considered training cases.

Once the guidewire has been passed into the distal lumen, usually the procedure can be successfully finished, although in approximately 15% of cases, it may not be possible to pass a balloon. In these latter cases, the guidewire position in the distal lumen should be substantiated if possible; sometimes a distal injection can be helpful to document intraluminal position. The smallest possible balloon catheter should be used if there are problems crossing the occlusion after the guidewire has passed through it initially. The importance of a good stable guiding catheter cannot be overstressed in this situation. Another approach is the use of excimer laser. While this technology is seldom used, it has been shown to be very effective for long chronic total occlusions.

The most promising new approach to chronic total occlusion is the use of the laser guidewire: a 0.018-inch wire which can be used to create an initial pilot channel. Initial data from European and North American centers have been quite favorable.[9,10] In initial series of patients in whom a conventional approach to chronic total occlusion had been tried and failed, the Total guidewire was successful in 55–61%. For this procedure, visualization of the course of the distal arterial bed by collateral injection is essential. It is also essential to move slowly and carefully, reorienting the catheter as needed. Again, as with all chronic total occlusions, these procedures are often lengthy and associated with large contrast volume and resource consumption. Following successful placement of the laser guidewire in the distal vessel, the laser wire can be used to deliver a balloon or to deliver a larger laser catheter.

Following successful dilatation, consideration should be given to stent implantation. Preliminary data from registry experiences and small randomized trials indicate that stent implantation in this setting may be associated with improved outcome with decreased recurrent occlusion. Stents should only be implanted, however, if the vessel has good TIMI III outflow and if the vessel is greater than or equal to 2.75–3.00 mm. Small vessel occlusions with poor distal runoff should not be stented.

Bifurcation lesions

Bifurcation lesions remain among the most difficult lesions to treat in interventional cardiology. There are several different anatomical subsets of lesions which can be considered as bifurcation lesions. Treatment of these groups of lesions involves consideration of the size of the target vessel and branch, presence of ostial stenosis in the branch, angulation, plaque volume and potential for plaque shift, and presence of calcification within the target lesions and vessels (Table 3.2).

From the earliest days of interventional cardiology, the problems of bifurcation lesions have been documented. Specifically, the problem of branch vessel occlusion after balloon dilatation of the main vessel, which was increased to an incidence of approximately 30% if there was a stenosis at the origin of the branch.[11] Such a branch vessel occlusion, depending on the size of the vessel, could result in angina or non-Q-wave myocardial infarction. In addition,

Table 3.2 Assessment of bifurcation lesions.

- Size of target vessel and branch
- Presence of ostial branch stenosis
- Location of branch vessel relative to target stenosis
- Calcification within stenoses
- Proximal tortuosity
- Angulation of side-branch
- Potential for plaque shifting

there is the problem of inadequate dilatation due to elastic recoil of either the branch or the main vessel.

A number of conventional balloon-based techniques have been developed including safety guidewires (Table 3.3).[12–14] These techniques were matched to the specific lesion. If the branch vessel was small, nothing was done. If the branch vessel was larger, safety guidewires were sometimes used to allow access to the side-branch. Sequential balloon dilatation was occasionally performed in this matter as well as simultaneous balloon dilatation. Even with these approaches, the outcome was often suboptimal. This has led to the development of new approaches which involve new devices both for debulking the lesion and mechanically scaffolding them. Use of these new approaches makes consideration of the issues in Table 3.2 even more important.

There are three devices useful for debulking branch lesions: directional coronary atherectomy, rotational

Table 3.3 Bifurcation lesion (conventional dilatation).

- Small branch—benign neglect
- Large branch without stenosis:

  – benign neglect
  – safety guidewire

- Large branch with significant stenosis:

  – sequential balloon dilatation
  – simultaneous balloon dilatation

Table 3.4 Bifurcation lesions (directional coronary atherectomy).

- Direct cutter away from branch:
  - low or no pressure
- Safety wire usually not needed (if used—Nitinol to prevent wire damage)
- After atherectomy, document effect on branch vessel stenosis:
  - if branch vessel requires treatment, it can be performed with DCA if vessel is ≥3.0 mm, noncalcified and has a favorable take-off
- Document optimal angiographic result of both vessel and branch

Table 3.5 Bifurcation lesions (rotational atherectomy).

- Sequential burr sizing
- Identify most difficult access vessel and treat first
- Stand-alone rotablation or low-pressure balloon inflation
- Control angiography to assess other vessel
- Repeat rotational atherectomy on other vessel
- Document optimal angiography result of both target vessel and branch

atherectomy and excimer laser particularly with an eccentric laser catheter. Selection of the specific device and matching it to the specific lesion is complex. There is limited well controlled scientific data on outcome.

Directional atherectomy has the advantage that the device can be oriented to avoid the ostium of the side-branch to improve the flow initially (Table 3.4).[15–17] After some guided debulking, the lesion can be reassessed. Typically, a safety wire is not used in the branch vessel because of concerns of cutting the wire, and also, it is not usually needed. If a safety guidewire is used, it should be Nitinol to prevent wire damage by the cutter. If a safety wire is not used, even if there is branch vessel occlusion, it can usually be recrossed with relative ease. Both branches of the bifurcation can be treated provided that the angle into the branch (for example, a large diagonal) is not acute.

Directional atherectomy has limitations, however, because of its size and inflexibility. In addition, if the lesion is calcified, directional coronary atherectomy is usually not as successful. It does remain a useful technique for large, proximal, nontortuous bifurcation lesions such as those involving the left anterior descending and the diagonal arteries.

Eccentric directional laser is also an excellent approach in selected patients. There is very limited data available with this approach because lasers are currently infrequently used.[18] With this technique, a safety wire is rarely used. By virtue of its design, the device can be turned using fluoroscopic control and oriented towards eccentric plaque allowing for selective ablation of the bifurcation lesions.

This device is more flexible and smaller than directional atherectomy so it can be more readily and easily positioned. It has the disadvantage that it does not ablate calcium. In addition, it has the problem of relatively unpredictable arterial dissections.

The current ideal and most widely applicable technique for debulking bifurcation lesions is rotational atherectomy which can be used even with calcified lesions. A safety wire is not possible with this technique, so preplanning is extremely important. There are several approaches depending upon operator experience and the specific anatomic features present, including the size of the vessel and take-off as well as the location of the plaque (Table 3.5).

For ostial bifurcation lesions the author usually selects a small burr size (i.e. 1.25 mm). After the initial passage, repeat angiography is performed. If the other branch remains patent, then a larger burr size can be used to treat the initial lesion. One potential strategy is to achieve maximal ablation so that postrotablator dilatation is either minimized or can be avoided altogether. If postrotablator dilatation is performed, low pressure should be used. Even if low-pressure dilatation is used, occlusion of the other branch may occur.

After the initial lesion is treated, the other branch is approached using a similar strategy of sequential rotablator burrs, and then dilatation with low pressure. After treatment of each branch, control angiography should be performed to evaluate the effects of treatment on the other lesion. On occasion, the initial lesion may be compromised during treatment of the other vessel; this can be minimized by optimal debulking and then administration of drugs to minimize coronary spasm.

Deciding which lesion to treat first is an important consideration. An approach that has proven to be successful in the author's experience is to position the guidewire in that bifurcation branch which appears to be most difficult to access: for example, if there is an acute angle of the large diagonal with an ostial stenosis, and the continuing left anterior descending is straight, the diagonal branch is treated first. If occlusion of the left anterior descending occurs during rotablator of the diagonal, it is easier in this setting to pass the guidewire through the left anterior descending because it is not as angulated. After the diagonal is well treated, then the guidewire can be moved to the left anterior descending and that vessel can then be treated. Following rotablator therapy, adjunctive low-pressure dilatation can be performed.

In a consecutive series of 16 patients treated by Rotablator for bifurcation lesions at the author's institution, the most common vascular territory involved was the left anterior descending/diagonal coronary artery.[19] In all patients, a successful angiographic result was achieved with a residual stenosis of 30% or less in all bifurcation limbs. No patient required surgery or suffered a Q-wave myocardial infarction. One patient had a non-Q-wave myocardial infarction. While this is not a randomized series, the results are encouraging.

Stenting

There is increased interest in stenting for bifurcation lesions (Table 3.6).[20–26] This is complex, in part because there are no ideal stents for this application. Considerations for bifurcation stenting include vessel size, precise stent placement, the ability to access a side-branch through a stent and stent deformation. As is true with the ablative techniques, if the side-branch is small, a stent can be placed across the branch. It usually does not result in any clinical problem even if occlusion occurs. In several longitudinal studies, even if there is side-branch occlusion, it may be transient and patency may return. If the side-branch is larger, it is more problematic.

There are several potential approaches which have been described graphically as 'fork stenting', 'T stenting' or 'Y stenting'.

Table 3.6 Bifurcation lesions (stenting).

- Small vessel—benign neglect
- Large branch without stenosis:
  - coil stent
  - noncoil stent with side-branch access—? at articulation site
  - safety wire along side stent occasionally useful
  - withdraw safety wire prior to high-pressure dilatation
- Large branch with significant stenosis:
  - 'T stent'
  - 'Y stent'
  - 'Fork stent'
  - dilate branch, stent target vessel

Stenting a target lesion in proximity to the ostium of a significant branch

In this setting, a stent which allows access to the side-branch is optimal. Flexible coil stents are easiest for this application. Access through them after they have been fully deployed is usually not very difficult. Care must be taken to avoid damage to the stent when passing a balloon into the side-branch to be dilated. In general, the balloon should not be completely passed through the stent; in addition, a balloon which rewraps well upon deflation is helpful, so that during withdrawal, the stent is not damaged or dislodged. There is more concern with current noncoil stents, particularly the Johnson and Johnson Interventional Systems stent. While this can be crossed after deployment to access side-branches, this maneuver is difficult. If possible, the articulation should be placed at the origin of the branch to optimize access. It remains very important to use low-profile balloons which rewrap well upon deflation and avoid passing the balloon into the bifurcation beyond the lateral border of the stent. If, after dilatation of the side-branch, there is difficulty in withdrawing the balloon, more time and vigorous balloon aspiration should be attempted; continued gentle traction usually solves the problem. On occasion, however, the stent may still be damaged. This can usually be solved by redilating the stent. Newer stent designs make side-branch access easier.

Stenting the side-branch and the main vessel

This procedure is complex. It should only be used by experienced interventional cardiologists in large vessels of 3.0 mm or more. Branch vessels 2.5 mm or smaller, at the present time with current technology, do not merit stenting because of general suboptimal results.

A variety of approaches is possible. For these approaches, very precise localization of the stent is essential as well as careful consideration of the angle of the lesion. Perhaps the easiest is placement of a short stent in the bifurcation branch making sure that the proximal stent comes up to but does not encroach on the lumen of the main vessel. During this time, a safety wire can be placed down the main vessel although it may not be required. Following side-branch stenting, the other stenosis is treated. Conventional dilatation is then performed at the side-branch ostium to smooth off the stent end. The main branch is then stented with postdeployment high-pressure dilatation.

There are a number of creative ideas to simultaneous delivery of the stents to obviate the potential of misplacement at the ostial location. These are, however, awkward. Bifurcated stents are currently being developed. Their eventual role will depend upon their adaptability to the wide variation in anatomic configurations of this difficult group of patients.

Conclusions

Many of the problems of interventional cardiology have been successfully addressed with technologic device improvements, improved operator experience and the development of effective adjunctive medications. Some specific problems remain, including chronic total occlusion and bifurcation lesions. While there have been improvements in increasing the early success rates in these lesions, further work remains.

References

1 Srivatsa SS, Edwards WD, Boos CM, et al. Histologic correlates of angiographic chronic total coronary artery occlusions: influence of occlusion duration on neovascular channel patterns and intimal plaque composition. J Am Coll Cardiol, in press.

2 Bell MR, Berger PB, Bresnahan JF. Initial and long-term outcome of 354 patients after coronary balloon angioplasty of total coronary artery occlusions. Circulation 1992; **85**: 1003–11.

3 Stone GW, Rutherford BD, McConahay DR, et al. Procedural outcome of angioplasty for total coronary artery occlusion: an analysis of 971 lesions in 905 patients. J Am Coll Cardiol 1990; **61**: 23G–28G.

4 Ivanhoe RJ, Weintraub WS, Douglas JS jr, et al. Percutaneous transluminal coronary angioplasty of chronic total occlusions: primary success, restenosis, and long-term clinical follow-up. Circulation 1992; **85**: 106–15.

5 Serruys PW, Umans, V, Heyndrickx GR, et al. Elective PTCA of totally occluded coronary arteries not associated with acute myocardial infarction: short-term and long-term results. Eur Heart J 1985; **6**: 2–12.

6 Berger PB, Holmes DR jr, Ohman EM, et al. For the MARCATOR Investigators. Restenosis, reocclusion and adverse cardiovascular events after successful balloon angioplasty of occluded versus nonoccluded coronary arteries: results from the Multicenter American Research Trial with Cilazapril after angioplasty to prevent transluminal coronary obstruction and restenosis (MARCATOR). J Am Coll Cardiol 1996; **27**: 1:1–7.

7 Warren RJ, Black AJ, Valentine PA, et al. Coronary angioplasty for chronic total occlusion reduces the need for subsequent coronary bypass surgery. Am Heart J 1990; **120**: 270–4.

8 Bell MR, Menke KK, Berger PB, et al. Balloon angioplasty of chronic total coronary occlusions: what does it cost in radiation exposure, time and materials? Cathet Cardiovasc Diag 1992; **25**: 10–15.

9 Hamburger JN, de Feyter PJ. Recanalization of chronic total occlusions using a laser guidewire: the first 100 patients in a single center experience. Circulation 1996; **94**: L-618A.

10 Laird JR, Oesterle S, Eigler N, et al. Predictors of successful recanalization of refractory total occlusions with the laser wire. Circulation 1996; **94**: L-618A.

11 Meier B, Gruentzig AR, King SB, et al. Risk of side branch occlusion during coronary angioplasty. Am J Cardiol 1984; **53**: 10–14.

12 Pinkerton CA, Slack JD. Complex coronary angioplasty: a technique for dilatation of bifurcation stenoses. Angiography 1985; **36**: 543–8.

13 Zack PM, Ischinger T. Experience with a technique for coronary angioplasty of bifurcational lesions. Cathet Cardiovasc Diagn 1984; **10**: 433–43.

14 Renkin J, Wijus W, Hanet C, et al. Angioplasty of coronary bifurcation stenosis: immediate and long term results of the protecting branch technique. Cathet Cardiovasc Diagn 1991; **22**: 167–73.

15 Lewis BE, Leya FA, Johnson SA, *et al.* Assessment of outcome of bifurcation lesions treated in the CAVEAT Trial. *J Invas Cardiol* 1995; **7**: 251–8.

16 Mansour M, Fishman RF, Kuntz RE, *et al.* Feasibility of direction atherectomy for the treatment of bifurcation lesions. *Current Science* 1992; **3–8**: 761–5.

17 Lewis BE, Leya FS, Johnson SA, *et al.* Acute procedural results in the treatment of thirty coronary artery bifurcation lesions with a double wire atherectomy technique for side branch protection. *Am Heart J* 1994; **127**: 1600–7.

18 Ghazzal ZB, Shefer A, Litvack F, *et al.* The new directional laser catheter (DLC): early results from a multicenter experience. *Circulation* 1992; **86**: L-654.

19 Rihal CS, Garratt KN, Holmes DR jr. Rotational atherectomy for bifurcation lesions of the coronary circulation: technique and initial experience (pers. comm.).

20 Fort S, Lazzam C, Schwartz L. Coronary 'Y' stenting: a technique for angioplasty of bifurcation stenoses. *Can J Cardiol* 1996, **12**: 678–84.

21 Colombo A, Gaglione A, Nakmaura S, *et al.* 'Kissing' stents for bifurcational coronary lesion. *Cathet Cardiovasc Diagn* 1993; **30**: 327–30.

22 Nakamura S, Hall P, Maiello L, *et al.* Techniques for Palmaz–Schatz stent deployment in lesions with a large side branch. *Cathet Cardiovasc Diagn* 1995; **30**: 353–61.

23 Carrie D, Karouny E, Chouairi S, *et al.* 'T' shaped stent placement: a technique for the treatment of dissected bifurcation lesions. *Cathet Cardiovasc Diagn* 1996; **37**: 311–13.

24 Baim DS. Is bifurcation stenting the answer? *Cathet Cardiovasc Diagn* 1996; **37**: 314–16.

25 Fishman DL, Savage MP, Leon MB, *et al.* Fate of lesion related side branches after coronary artery stenting. *J Am Coll Cardiol* 1993; **22**: 1641–6.

26 Oda H, Ito E, Mida T, *et al.* 'Fork' stenting for bifurcation lesion. *J Interven Cardiol* 1996; **9**: 445–54.

4

Treatment for saphenous vein grafts

Mun K Hong, Martin B Leon and Kenneth M Kent

Introduction

Although coronary artery bypass surgery (CABG) is an effective revascularization procedure, its long-term benefit is limited by saphenous vein graft (SVG) failure. It has been established that approximately 50% of the SVGs will be occluded between 5 and 10 years after CABG.[1-8] Furthermore, repeat CABG is not an ideal option owing to higher morbidity and mortality, as well as less symptom improvement, compared with the original surgery.[9-11]

Thus, percutaneous transluminal balloon angioplasty (PTCA) has been used since the beginning of the technique as an alternative to repeat CABG in selected patients with recurrent ischemia resulting from SVG disease.[12] A recent review of 16 contemporary PTCA series in SVGs comprising 1571 patients by de Feyter et al.[13] reported an overall 88% procedural success rate. In aggregate, ischemic complications were infrequent and included death (<1%), myocardial infarction (4%), CABG (2%) and distal embolization (<3%). Overall procedure success was slightly lower in lesions involving the proximal (86%) versus mid (93%) and distal (90%) segments; proximal lesions also tended to have higher rates of angiographic restenosis (58% vs. 52% and 28% for mid and distal segments, respectively). Several variables have been associated with an increased risk of complications after PTCA of SVG lesions; these factors include older SVGs (≥36 months in age),[14-16] diffusely diseased SVGs,[17] totally occluded grafts,[18-20] and those grafts containing intraluminal thrombus, principally due to increased lesion friability and propensity to distal embolization.[21,22] Therefore, PTCA has a limited role for these complex SVG lesions, although it

remains the treatment of choice for distal anastomotic lesions.

As a result of these limitations, new angioplasty devices have been used in patients with symptomatic SVG disease[23-50] for three general indications: 1) to improve the initial angiographic result compared with PTCA alone (e.g. directional atherectomy and stenting for aorto-ostial lesions); 2) to reduce procedural complications associated with PTCA of friable and diffusely diseased SVG lesions (e.g. transluminal extraction atherectomy for degenerated grafts); and 3) to reduce restenosis after a successful procedure (e.g. intragraft stents for ostial and body lesions). Over the past 6 years, the authors have adopted a lesion-specific approach to device selection in SVG lesions at the Washington Hospital Center[51] which has been evolving due to the availability of new devices as well as emergence of new data from both our single-center experience and those of randomized studies. Our general guidelines for device selection have included the following algorithm (Fig. 4.1): directional atherectomy (DCA) was selected for aorto-ostial lesions and for focal, eccentric lesions located in non-degenerated SVGs 3.0 mm or more in reference diameter. Since 1992, we have rarely used DCA in SVG due to the risk of distal embolization and CAVEAT II results.[41] Transluminal extraction catheter (TEC) was chosen for ostial lesions in degenerated SVGs, and for focal and diffuse lesions located in diffusely diseased or thrombus-containing SVGs 2.5 mm or more in reference diameter.[28] Its use was also limited to the early experience due to the risk of distal embolization (mostly with adjunct PTCA) and associated major ischemic complications.[39] Excimer laser (ELCA) was reserved for ostial or diffuse lesions in straight segments of

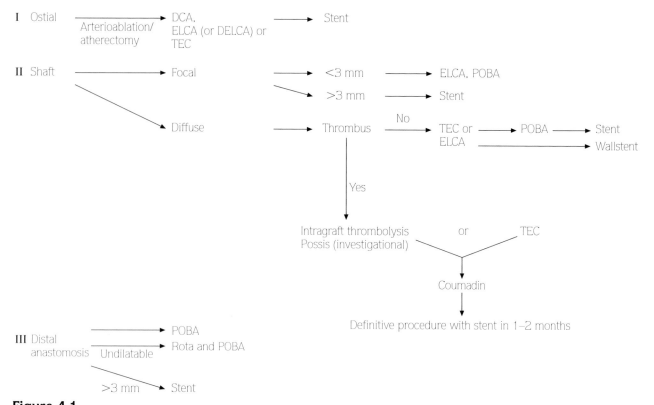

Figure 4.1
Lesion-specific, device selection approach to saphenous vein graft angioplasty. (DCA = directional coronary atherectomy; ELCA = excimer laser angioplasty; DELCA = directional ELCA; TEC = transluminal extraction catheter; Rota = rotational atherectomy.)

smaller SVGs (<3.0 mm) and, more recently, in degenerated SVGs, as a debulking device.[52] Lately, intragraft stenting has replaced all other modalities in SVGs 3.0 mm or more in reference diameter using 3.0–4.0-mm native coronary and 4.0–6.0-mm biliary (P104, P154 and PS204) tubular slotted stents for larger SVGs without significant inflow or outflow obstruction or intragraft thrombus.[40] Furthermore, with the refinement of optimal stent implantation techniques, both the length of hospital stay and procedural complications have been dramatically reduced without affecting the procedural success.[53] PTCA has been selected for lesions located at the distal anastomotic site, as an adjunct to thrombolytic therapy for thrombus-containing lesions, or for lesions with moderate or severe proximal SVG tortuosity or angulation precluding the use of larger new devices.

This chapter summarizes our single-center experience using this lesion-specific approach for treatment of SVG lesions and will address a few difficult lesion subsets (degenerated and aorto-ostial lesions).

Washington Hospital Center experience

The authors followed 1369 consecutive patients with 1898 SVG lesions treated at the Washington Hospital Center over a 5-year period ending in March 1996 (to allow for at least 6-month clinical follow-up). Patients presenting with acute myocardial infarction or cardiogenic shock, or undergoing bail-out or emergency angioplasty were excluded. During the study period, an additional 73 patients with 87 lesions were treated with rotational atherectomy (for undilatable distal anastomotic lesions), Possis device (for treatment of intragraft filling defects), Gianturco–Roubin stents (for the treatment of dissections in smaller SVGs), Dispatch catheter (for intragraft thrombus), CardioCoil stent (at a bend point), and peripheral Wallstent (for diffuse lesion), and they were not included in the analysis due to their limited sample size.

Based upon lesion-specific morphologic criteria,[51] the intended method of revascularization (PTCA, new device angioplasty or a combination of new device and adjunct

PTCA) was selected by the operator prior to the procedure and performed using methods described in detail elsewhere.[23–50]

Angiographic success was defined as a final diameter stenosis less than 50%. Procedural success was defined as angiographic success in the absence of major in-hospital complications (procedure-related death, emergency (ongoing ischemia) CABG, or Q-wave myocardial infarction). Major late cardiac events were reported using hierarchical events, including cardiac death, nonfatal Q-wave myocardial infarction, repeat CABG or repeat coronary angioplasty of the initial SVG lesion. Event-free survival (by patient) was defined as the freedom from death, Q-wave myocardial infarction or repeat revascularization during the follow-up period. Clinically driven (recurrent symptoms or exercise stress-testing demonstrating reversible ischemia), target-lesion revascularization was recorded for all study lesions that were treated with revascularization using CABG or repeat coronary angioplasty during the 12-month follow-up period.

Table 4.1 Baseline demographics and lesion characteristics of Washington Cardiology Center patients.

	1369 patients with 1898 lesions
Age (years)	66 ± 9
Male gender (%)	78
Unstable angina (%)	78
Graft age (months)	93 ± 50
Diabetes mellitus (%)	46
Hypertension (%)	62
LVEF	0.41 ± 0.13
Ostial location (%)	23
Lesion length (mm)	9.3 ± 7.2
Thrombus (%)	16
Degeneration (%)	31

Note:
LVEF = left ventricular ejection fraction.

Results

Baseline characteristics (Table 4.1)

The patients frequently presented with unstable angina (78%) and often had multiple cardiac risk factors (diabetes mellitus (46%), systemic hypertension (62%), one or more prior myocardial infarctions (65%)), and a reduced left ventricular function (ejection fraction = 0.41 ± 0.13). The average graft age was 93 ± 50 months.

Qualitative and quantitative angiographic analysis

The vast majority (88%) of lesions in this series had one or more adverse lesion characteristics using the modified American College of Cardiology/American Heart Association criteria;[54,55] approximately one third were 'C' lesions, most commonly due to the presence of SVG degeneration. Marked differences in preprocedural morphology were noted among the various devices used, attributable to the prespecified lesion-specific criteria for device selection. In general, PTCA was performed in the body and anastomotic sites of smaller SVGs (reference vessel diameter = 2.71 ± 0.90 mm). DCA was used in larger grafts (reference vessel diameter = 3.29 ± 0.63 mm), particularly those with lesions located in the graft ostium (59%).

Nearly two thirds of TEC procedures were performed in degenerated grafts; intragraft thrombus was frequently (45%) present. Intragraft stents were used in larger grafts (reference vessel diameter = 3.30 ± 0.64 mm), frequently for restenotic lesions (46%) in the ostium and body of both degenerated (26%) and nondegenerated (74%) grafts. Excimer laser angioplasty (ELCA) was used in relatively smaller grafts (reference vessel diameter = 2.81 ± 0.62 mm) and ostial (46%) or long (>10 mm) lesions (56%).

Procedural outcome (Table 4.2)

Overall angiographic success was achieved in 99% and procedural success in 97% of the patients. Cardiac death occurred in 0.9% of the patients, Q-wave myocardial infarction in 1.2% and emergency CABG in 0.6%. On the other hand, non-Q-wave myocardial infarction was frequent (15.9% of the patients).

Among the patient or lesion-related characteristics, the following were found to be univariate predictors of procedural failure (Table 4.3): initial TIMI 1 flow and intragraft thrombus. The only predictor on multivariate analysis was presence of intragraft thrombus.

Table 4.2 Procedural outcome.

	1369 patients with 1898 lesions
Angiographic success (%)	99
Procedural success (%)	97
Major ischemic complications (%)	2.2
Cardiac death (%)	0.9
Q-wave myocardial infarction (%)	1.2
Emergency CABG (%)	0.6
Non-Q-wave myocardial infarction (%)	15.9

Note:
CABG = coronary artery bypass surgery.

Table 4.3 Predictors of procedural failure.

	p value	Odds ratio
Univariate predictors		
Thrombus	0.01	3.0
TIMI 1 flow	0.03	3.5
Multivariate predictors		
Thrombus	0.04	2.6

Note:
TIMI = thrombolysis in myocardial infarction.

Table 4.4 Late clinical outcome.

	6 months (n = 1261)	12 months (n = 1040)
No event (%)	64.6	57.0
Any event (%)	35.4	43.0
Death (%)	8.4	10.2
Nonfatal Q-wave MI (%)	2.0	2.4
CABG (%)	5.3	6.4
PTCA (%)	19.7	23.9
Any TLR (%)	7.9	8.9
Repeat PTCA (%)	5.2	5.8
Repeat CABG (%)	3.0	3.5

Notes:
MI = myocardial infarction: CABG = coronary artery bypass surgery:
PTCA = percutaneous transluminal coronary angioplasty: TLR = target
lesion revascularization.

Late clinical outcome (Table 4.4)

All patients with successful procedure were followed for clinical status. At 6 months (follow-up in 95% of eligible patients), 35% of the patients had events. However, only 8% of these events were target lesion revascularization and the rest were unrelated to the treated graft. At 12 months (follow-up in 78% of eligible patients), the event rate increased to 43%, with 9% being target lesion revascularization. Therefore, many of the late events were unrelated to the angioplasty site.

Predictors of any late event or target lesion revascularization are summarized in Table 4.5. For any late event, the univariate predictors included diabetes mellitus and unstable angina, and multivariate predictors also included diabetes mellitus and unstable angina. For target lesion revascularization, the univariate predictors included restenotic lesion and unstable angina, and the multivariate predictors included ostial lesion location, unstable angina, prior myocardial infarction and left ventricular function.

In summary, in this single-center experience of 1369 patients (1898 lesions), the majority of whom were undergoing complex SVG angioplasty (mean graft age = 93 months; 88% type-B or C lesions; 78% unstable angina), a lesion-specific approach to balloon and new device selection resulted in an overall angiographic success and 97%

Table 4.5 Predictors of late events.

	p value	Odds ratio
Any late event		
Univariate predictors		
Unstable angina	0.0001	1.7
Diabetes mellitus	0.007	1.4
Multivariate predictors		
Diabetes mellitus	0.0001	1.9
Unstable angina	0.001	1.5
Any TLR		
Univariate predictors		
Prior PTCA	0.01	1.2
Unstable angina	0.02	1.6
Multivariate predictors		
Ostial location	0.0001	3.1
Prior MI	0.0001	1.0
LV EF	0.0002	28.3
Unstable angina	0.005	2.0

TLR = target lesion revascularization:
PTCA = percutaneous transluminal coronary angioplasty:
MI = myocardial infarction
LVEF = left ventricular ejection fraction

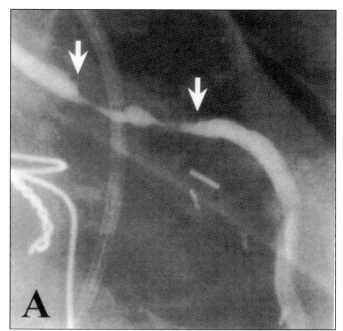
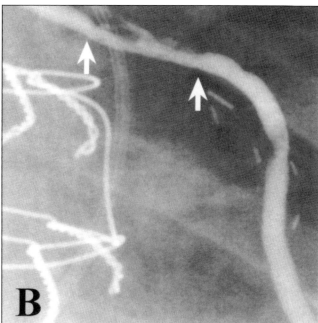
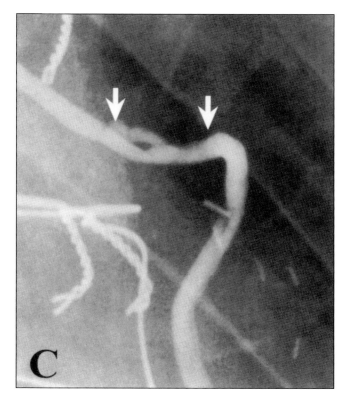
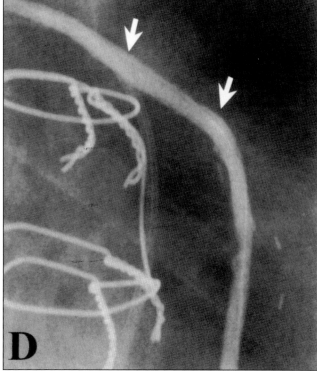

Figure 4.2

(a) Sequential lesions (lesion length = 23.5 mm) with luminal irregularity in a diffusely diseased saphenous vein graft (arrows indicate lesion sites in all panels). (b) Angiographic result following stand-alone TEC (final diameter stenosis = 45% by QCA), with improved lumen but more intimal disruption. (c) Healed intimal disruption on coumadin treatment for 1 month. There is residual stenosis with an ulceration (diameter stenosis = 60% of QCA). (d) Excellent angiographic result with staged stent (PS204 × 2 stents) implantation (final diameter stenosis = 10% by QCA).

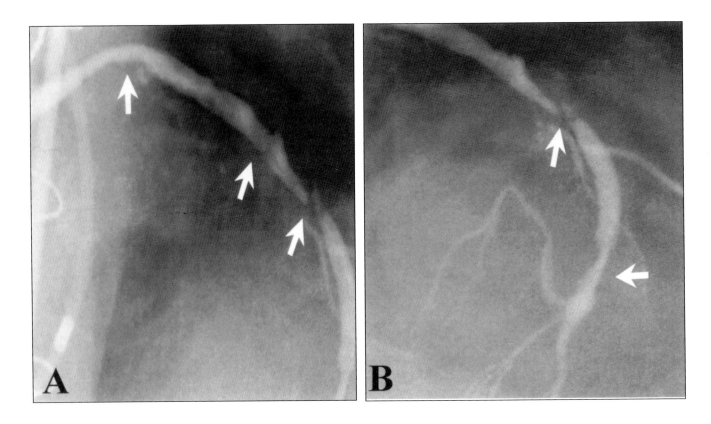

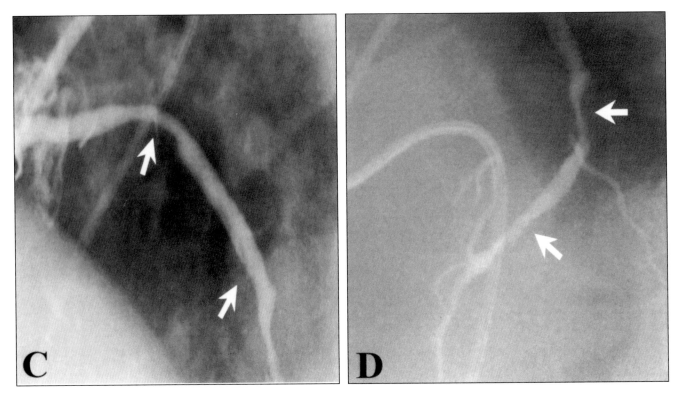

Figure 4.3

(a) and (b) Diffusely diseased saphenous vein graft, including ulcerated and possibly thrombus-containing lesions (arrows indicate lesion sites in all panels). (c) and (d) Improved lumen without distal embolization following initial debulking with 2.0-mm laser catheter. (e) and (f) Excellent final result after immediate, multiple stent implantation

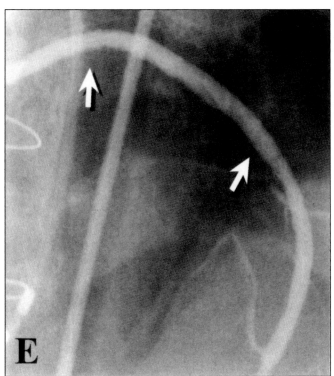

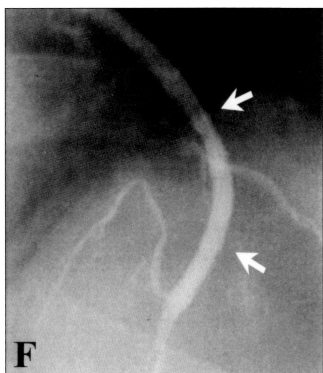

procedural success. Late target revascularization was required in 8% of patients within the first 6 months of follow-up after SVG angioplasty, related to the aorto-ostial location, unstable angina and prior MI with depressed left ventricular function.

Given the degree of complexity of SVG lesions included in this study, many of which were deemed unsuitable for conventional PTCA and in many cases, further interventional catheter-based therapy had been refused by experienced interventionalists, these results support the concept of a lesion-specific approach to balloon and new device selection for high-risk SVG angioplasty.

Treatment of degenerated SVG lesions

One of the most difficult SVG lesion subsets is the degenerated SVGs, with diffuse involvement of the SVG by the atherosclerotic process, frequently associated with intragraft filling defects. Our initial approach included thrombolytic therapy with both intragraft urokinase infusion and prolonged systemic urokinase infusion.[56] Although there

were improvements in the follow-up angiography, there was unacceptable incidence of intracranial and access-site bleeding complications. Thus, we then used TEC device with the hope of eliminating thrombolytic use and reducing distal embolization. Although it was mainly the adjunct PTCA responsible for distal embolization episodes, the ischemic complications were prohibitive,[39] with approximately 50% of the patients with distal embolization experiencing major ischemic complications, ranging from death in 27% to Q-wave myocardial infarction in another 27%. Thereafter, we adopted a staged strategy (Fig. 4.2), with initial recanalization performed with TEC only (with or without intragraft urokinase administration), followed by outpatient coumadinization for 1–2 months to organize intragraft thrombus, and definitive therapy with stenting 1–2 months after the TEC procedure.[57] This strategy completely eliminated the major ischemic complications during the initial procedure. However, one third of the patients refused to return for the second procedure (due to asymptomatic status) and there were rare occlusions between the procedures. Most recently, the authors have performed initial debulking with either TEC or ELCA, followed immediately by stenting (Fig. 4.3). The results have been encouraging, with 100% procedural success and rare distal embolization.[52]

Treatment of aorto-ostial lesions

Another difficult lesion subset, mainly due to the high restenosis rate, is the aorto-ostial stenoses (usually defined as within 3 mm of the proximal anastomosis). Except for a few studies with a small number of patients treated for aorto-ostial SVG lesions,[58,59] most new device studies suggest unacceptably high restenosis rates.[50] Review of our experience also demonstrates high restenosis rates,[60] even with stent use or device synergy (initial debulking followed by stent implantation).

Future directions

There are several new developments, which in the future may improve the treatment of SVG disease. Obviously, the best treatment of SVG disease is prevention, such as reduction in low-density lipoprotein[61] or using arterial conduits. Another approach would be pharmacologic therapy with antiproliferative agents, such as angiopeptin,[62] to reduce neointimal hyperplasia, the predominant mechanism of SVG attrition. Recent minimally invasive surgery with left internal mammary artery to left anterior descending coronary artery is an exciting development,[63] and if such a technique could be improved to allow other arterial conduits for bypass, this may eliminate the future problems with SVG degeneration. The possibility of improving myocardial perfusion with either surgical[64] or percutaneous transmyocardial revascularization[65] with laser therapy may provide an alternative to repeat CABG or high-risk PTCA. The use of long stents (e.g., Wallstent) may improve the acute and long-term results, possibly at a reasonable initial cost.[66] Covered stents, either with synthetic material[67] or autologous vein,[68] may also reduce the restenosis rates. Furthermore, the combination of adjunct pharmacology, including potent antiplatelet agents[69] or brachytherapy,[70] and stents may improve the long-term benefit of percutaneous treatment of SVG disease.

References

1   Lawrie GM, Lie JT, Morris GC, Beazley HL. Vein graft patency and intimal proliferation after aortocoronary bypass: early and long-term angiopathologic correlations. *Am J Cardiol* 1976; **38**: 856–62.

2   Fitzgibbon GM, Burton JR, Leach AJ. Coronary bypass graft fate: angiographic grading of 1400 consecutive grafts early after operation and of 1132 after one year. *Circulation* 1978; **57**: 1070–4.

3   Hamby RI, Aintablian A, Handler M, et al. Aortocoronary saphenous vein bypass grafts: long-term patency, mor-

phology and blood flow in patients with patent grafts early after surgery. *Circulation* 1979; **60**: 901–9.

4   Bourassa MG, Enjalbert M, Campeau L, Lesperance J. Progression of atherosclerosis in coronary arteries and bypass grafts: ten years later. *Am J Cardiol* 1984; **53**: 102C–107C.

5   Bourassa MG, Fisher LD, Campeau L, Gillespie MJ, McConney M, Lesperance J. Long-term fate of bypass grafts: the Coronary Artery Surgery Study (CASS) and Montreal Heart Institute experiences. *Circulation* 1985; **72 (Suppl V)**: V-71–V-78.

6   Seides SF, Borer JS, Kent KM, Rosing DR, McIntosh CL, Epstein SE. Long-term anatomic fate of coronary artery bypass grafts and functional status of patients five years after operation. *N Engl J Med* 1978; **298**: 1213–17.

7   Virmani R, Atkinson JB, Forman MB. Aortocoronary saphenous vein bypass grafts. *Cardiovasc Clin* 1988; **18**: 41–59.

8   Campeau L, Enjalbert M, Lesperance J, et al. The relation of risk factors to the development of atherosclerosis in saphenous-vein bypass grafts and the progression of disease in the native circulation. *N Engl J Med* 1984; **311**: 1329–32.

9   Loop FD, Cosgrove DM, Kramer JR, et al. Late clinical and arteriographic results in 500 coronary artery reoperations. *J Thorac Cardiovasc Surg* 1981; **81**: 675–85.

10 Shaff HV, Orzulak TA, Gersh BJ, et al. The morbidity and mortality of reoperation for coronary artery disease and analysis of late results with use of actuarial estimate of event-free interval. *J Thorac Cardiovasc Surg* 1983; **85**: 508–15.

11 Lytle BW, Loop FD, Cosgrove DM, et al. Fifteen hundred coronary reoperations: results and determinants of early and late survival. *J Thorac Cardiovasc Surg* 1987; **93**: 847–59.

12 Douglas JJ, Gruentzig A, King SB, et al. Percutaneous transluminal coronary angioplasty in patients with prior coronary bypass surgery. *J Am Coll Cardiol* 1983; **2**: 745–54.

13 de Feyter P, VanSuylen R, de Jaegere P, Topol E, Serruys P. Balloon angioplasty for the treatment of lesions in saphenous vein bypass grafts. *J Am Coll Cardiol* 1993; **21**: 1539–49.

14 Ernst S, van der Feltz T, Ascoop C, et al. Percutaneous transluminal coronary angioplasty in patients with prior coronary artery bypass grafting. *J Thorac Cardiovasc Surg* 1987; **93**: 268–75.

15 Reed D, Beller G, Nygaard T, Tedesco C, Watson D, Burwell L. The clinical efficacy and scintigraphic evaluation of post-coronary bypass patients undergoing transluminal

coronary angioplasty for recurrent angina pectoris. *Am Heart J* 1989; **117**: 60–71.

16 Plokker H, Meester B, Serruys P. The Dutch experience in percutaneous transluminal angioplasty of narrowed saphenous vein grafts used for aortocoronary bypass. *Am J Cardiol* 1991; **67**: 361–6.

17 El Gamal M, Bonnier H, Michels R, Heijman J, Stassen E. Percutaneous transluminal angioplasty of stenosed aortocoronary bypass grafts. *Br Heart J* 1984; **52**: 617–20.

18 de Feyter P, Serruys P, van den Brand M, Meester H, Beatt K, Suryapranata H. Percutaneous transluminal angioplasty of a totally occluded venous bypass graft: a challenge that should be resisted. *Am J Cardiol* 1989; **64**: 88–90.

19 McKeever L, Hartmann J, Bufalino V, et al. Acute myocardial infarction complicating recanalization of aortocoronary bypass grafts with urokinase therapy. *Am J Cardiol* 1989; **64**: 683–5.

20 Margolis J, Mogensen L, Mehta S, Chen CY, Krauthhamer D. Diffuse embolization following percutaneous transluminal coronary angioplasty of occluded vein grafts: the blush phenomenon. *Clin Cardiol* 1991; **14**: 489–93.

21 Platko W, Hollman J, Whitlow P, Franco I. Percutaneous transluminal angioplasty of saphenous vein graft stenosis: long-term follow-up. *J Am Coll Cardiol* 1989; **14**: 1645–50.

22 Meester B, Samson M, Suryapranata H, et al. Long-term follow-up after attempted angioplasty of saphenous vein grafts: the Thoraxcentre experience 1981–1988. *Eur Heart J* 1991; **12**: 648–53.

23 Urban P, Sigwart U, Golf S, Kaufmann U, Sadeghi H, Kappenberger L. Intravascular stenting for stenosis of aortocoronary venous bypass grafts. *J Am Coll Cardiol* 1989; **13**: 1085–91.

24 Kaufmann U, Garratt K, Vlietstra R, Holmes D. Transluminal atherectomy of saphenous vein aortocoronary bypass grafts. *Am J Cardiol* 1990; **65**: 1430–3.

25 Strumpf R, Mehta S, Ponder R, Heuser R. Palmaz–Schatz stent implantation in stenosed saphenous vein grafts: clinical and angiographic follow-up. *Am Heart J* 1992; **123**: 1329–36.

26 Keren G, Douek P, Oblon C, Bonner RF, Pichard AD, Leon MB. Atherosclerotic saphenous vein grafts treated with different interventional procedures assessed by intravascular ultrasound. *Am Heart J* 1992; **124**: 198–206.

27 Pomerantz R, Kuntz R, Carozza J, et al. Acute and long-term outcome of narrowed saphenous venous grafts treated by endoluminal stenting and directional atherectomy. *Am J Cardiol* 1992; **70**: 161–7.

28 Popma J, Leon M, Mintz G, et al. Results of coronary angioplasty using the transluminal extraction catheter. *Am J Cardiol* 1992; **70**: 1526–32

29 de Scheerder I, Strauss B, de Feyter P, et al. Stenting of venous bypass grafts: a new treatment modality for patients who are poor candidates for reintervention. *Am Heart J* 1992; **123**: 1046–54.

30 Cowley MJ, Whitlow PL, Baim DS, Hinohara T, Hall K, Simpson JB. Directional coronary atherectomy of saphenous vein graft narrowings: multicenter investigational experience. *Am J Cardiol* 1993; **72**: 30E–34E.

31 Safian RD, Grines CL, May MA, et al. Clinical and angiographic results of transluminal extraction coronary atherectomy in saphenous vein bypass grafts. *Circulation* 1994; **89**: 302–12.

32 Twidale N, Barth CW III, Kipperman RM, Bowles MH, Galichia JP. Acute results and long-term outcome of transluminal extraction catheter for saphenous vein graft stenoses. *Cathet Cardiovasc Diagn* 1994; **31**: 187–91.

33 Piana R, Moscucci M, Cohen D, et al. Palmaz–Schatz stenting for treatment of focal vein graft stenosis: immediate results and long-term outcome. *J Am Coll Cardiol* 1994; **23**: 1296–304.

34 Maiello L, Colombo A, Gianrossi R, Goldenberg S, Martini G, Finci L. Favourable results of treatment of narrowed saphenous vein grafts with Palmaz–Schatz stent implantation. *Eur Heart J* 1994; **15**: 1212–16.

35 Dorros G, Bates MC, Iyer S, et al. The use of Gianturco–Roubin flexible metallic coronary stents in old saphenous vein grafts: in-hospital outcome and 7 day angiographic patency. *Eur Heart J* 1994; **15**: 1456–62.

36 Bittl JA, Sanborn TA, Yardley DE, et al. Predictors of outcome of percutaneous excimer laser coronary angioplasty of saphenous vein bypass graft lesions. The Percutaneous Excimer Laser Coronary Angioplasty Registry. *Am J Cardiol* 1994; **74**: 144–8.

37 Fenton SH, Fischman DL, Savage MP, et al. Long-term angiographic and clinical outcome after implantation of balloon-expandable stents in aortocoronary saphenous vein grafts. *Am J Cardiol* 1994; **74**: 1187–91.

38 Litvack F, Eigler N, Margolis J, et al. Percutaneous excimer laser coronary angioplasty: Results in the first consecutive 3,000 patients. *J Am Coll Cardiol* 1994; **23**: 323–329.

39 Hong MK, Popma JJ, Pichard AD, et al. Clinical significance of distal embolization after transluminal extraction atherectomy in diffusely diseased saphenous vein grafts. *Am Heart J* 1994; **127**: 1496–503.

40 Wong SC, Popma JJ, Pichard AD, et al. A comparison of

clinical and angiographic outcomes after saphenous vein graft angioplasty using coronary versus 'biliary' tubular slotted stents. *Circulation* 1995; **91**: 339–50.

41   Holmes DR jr, Topol EJ, Califf RM, *et al.* A multicenter, randomized trial of coronary angioplasty versus directional atherectomy for patients with saphenous vein bypass graft lesions. *Circulation 1995;* **91**: 1966–74.

42   Meany TB, Leon MB, Kramer BL, *et al.* Transluminal extraction catheter for the treatment of diseased saphenous vein grafts: a multicenter experience. *Cathet Cardiovasc Diagn* 1995; **34**: 112–20.

43   Cardenas JR, Strumpf RK, Heuser RR. Rotational atherectomy in restenotic lesions at the distal saphenous vein graft anastomosis. *Cathet Cardiovasc Diagn* 1995; **36**: 53–7.

44   Strauss BH, Natarajan MK, Batchelor WB, *et al.* Early and late quantitative angiographic results of vein graft lesions treated by excimer laser with adjunctive balloon angioplasty. *Circulation* 1995; **92**: 348–56.

45   Wong SC, Baim DS, Schatz RA, *et al.* Immediate results and late outcomes after stent implantation in saphenous vein graft lesions: the multicenter US Palmaz–Schatz stent experience. The Palmaz–Schatz stent study group. *J Am Coll Cardiol* 1995; **26**: 704–12.

46   Rechavia E, Litvack F, Macko G, Eigler NL. Stent implantation of saphenous vein graft aorto-ostial lesions in patients with unstable ischemic syndromes: immediate angiographic results and long-term clinical outcome. *J Am Coll Cardiol* 1995; **25**: 866–70.

47   Abdel-Meguid AE, Whitlow PL, Simpfendorfer C, *et al.* Percutaneous revascularization of ostial saphenous vein graft stenoses. *J Am Coll Cardiol* 1995; **26**: 955–60.

48   Dooris M, Hoffmann M, Glazier S, *et al.* Comparative results of transluminal extraction coronary atherectomy in saphenous vein graft lesions with and without thrombus. *J Am Coll Cardiol* 1995; **25**: 1700–5.

49   Waksman R, Douglas JS, Scott NA, Ghazzal ZM, Yee-Peterson J, King SB III. Distal embolization is common after directional atherectomy in coronary arteries and saphenous vein grafts. *Am Heart J* 1995; **129**: 430–5.

50   Stephan WJ, Bates ER, Garratt KN, Hinohara T, Muller DW. Directional atherectomy of coronary and saphenous vein graft ostial stenoses. *Am J Cardiol* 1995; **75**: 1015–18.

51   Popma J, Leon M. A lesion specific approach to new device angioplasty. In: Topol E (ed.). *Textbook of Interventional Cardiology* (2nd edn). (Philadelphia PA: WB Saunders, 1994): 973–85.

52   Hong MK, Wong SC, Popma JJ, *et al.* Favorable results of debulking followed by immediate adjunct stent therapy for high risk saphenous vein graft lesions. *J Am Coll Cardiol* 1996; **27(Suppl A)**: 179A (abst).

53   Wong SC, Hong MK, Chuang YC, *et al.* The anti-platelet treatment after intravascular ultrasound guided optimal stent expansion (APLAUSE) trial. *Circulation* 1995; **92(Suppl I)**: I-795 (abst).

54   Ryan TJ and Subcommittee on Percutaneous Transluminal Coronary Angioplasty. Guidelines for percutaneous transluminal coronary angioplasty. *J Am Coll Cardiol* 1988; 12: 529–45.

55   Ellis S, Vandormael M, Cowley M, *et al.* Coronary morphologic and clinical determinants of procedural outcome with angioplasty for multivessel coronary disease. *Circulation* 1990; **82**: 1193–202.

56   Cospito PD, Popma JJ, Satler LF, Leon MB, Kent KM, Pichard AD. Prolonged intravenous urokinase infusion: an alternative pharmacologic approach in the treatment of thrombus-containing saphenous vein graft stenoses. *Cathet Cardiovasc Diagn* 1992; **26**: 291–4.

57   Hong MK, Pichard AD, Kent KM, *et al.* Assessing a strategy of stand-alone extraction atherectomy followed by staged stent placement in degenerated saphenous vein graft lesions. *J Am Coll Cardiol* 1995; **25(Suppl A)**: 394A (abst).

58   Zampieri P, Colombo A, Almagor Y, Maiello L, Finci L. Results of coronary stenting of ostial lesions. *Am J Cardiol* 1994; **73**: 901–3.

59   Kerwin PM, McKeever LS, Marek JC, Hartmann JR, Enger EL. Directional atherectomy of aorto-ostial stenoses. *Cathet Cardiovasc Diagn* 1993; **28(Suppl I)**: 17–25.

60   Wong SC, Popma JJ, Hong MK, *et al.* Procedural results and long term clinical outcomes in aorto-ostial saphenous vein graft lesions after new device angioplasty. *J Am Coll Cardiol* 1995; **25(Suppl A)**: 394A (abst).

61   The Post Coronary Artery Bypass Graft Trial Investigators. The effect of aggressive lowering of low-density lipoprotein cholesterol levels and low-dose anticoagulation on obstructive changes in saphenous-vein graft coronary-artery bypass grafts. *N Engl J Med* 1997; **336**: 153–62.

62   Calcagno D, Conte JV, Howell MH, Foegh ML. Peptide inhibition of neointimal hyperplasia in vein grafts. *J Vasc Surg* 1991; **13**: 475–9.

63   Benetti FJ, Ballester C, Sani G, Doonstra P, Grandjean J. Video assisted coronary bypass surgery. *J Card Surg* 1995; **10**: 620–5.

64   Frazier OH, Cooley DA, Kadipasaoglu KA, *et al.* Myocardial revascularization with laser. Preliminary findings. *Circulation* 1995; **92(Suppl II)**: II-58–II-65.

65   Oesterle SN, Walton AJ, Kernoff R, *et al*. Percutaneous trans-endocardial laser revascularization. *Circulation* 1995; **92(Suppl I)**: I-616 (abst).

66   Kelly PA, Kurbaan AS, Sigwart U. Total endovascular reconstruction of occluded saphenous vein grafts using coronary or peripheral Wallstents. *Circulation* 1996; **94(Suppl I)**: I-258 (abst).

67   Heuser RR, Reynolds GT, Papazoglou C, Diethrich EB, Mukherjee R. Compassionate endoluminal grafting for percutaneous treatment of aortocoronary SVG disease. *J Am Coll Cardiol* 1996; **27(Suppl A)**: 179A (abst).

68   Stefanadis C, Tsiamis E, Toutouzas K, *et al*. Autologous vein graft-coated stent for the treatment of coronary artery disease: immediate results after percutaneous implantation in humans. *J Am Coll Cardiol* 1996; **27(Suppl A)**: 179A (abst).

69   The EPIC Investigators. Use of monoclonal antibody directed against the platelet glycoprotein IIb/IIIa receptor in high-risk coronary angioplasty. *N Engl J Med* 1994; **330**: 956–61.

70   Teirstein PS, Massullo V, Jani S, *et al*. Radiation therapy following coronary stenting—6-month follow-up of a randomized clinical trial. *Circulation* 1996; **94(Suppl I)**: I-210 (abst).

5

Thrombolytic vs. interventional treatment in acute myocardial infarction

Haim Hammerman

Introduction

Coronary reperfusion is a well established and standard therapy for patients with acute myocardial infarction. Multiple techniques are available to reperfuse effectively the infarct-related artery. There is ample experimental data which demonstrate that early recanalization of the infarct-related artery will result in salvage of the ischemic myocardium at risk. The earlier this is performed, the greater will be the benefit. Large-scale randomized clinical studies have shown that early reperfusion is associated with less morbidity and lower mortality among patients suffering from ST-elevation myocardial infarction compared to late reperfusion or no reperfusion.[1,2]

There are two main modes to establish reperfusion in acute myocardial infarction: thrombolytic therapy and primary coronary angioplasty. Both techniques, primary (immediate) angioplasty and thrombolysis, are effective in recanalizing and restoring blood flow in the occluded coronary arteries; however, there is still a debate about which approach is better in acute evolving myocardial infarction. This chapter reviews the advantages and disadvantages of each approach and compares the two, based on currently available data.

Thrombolytic therapy

Large-scale placebo-controlled, randomized studies in almost 60,000 patients suffering from acute myocardial infarction have clearly demonstrated reduction of mortality and morbidity among patients treated with thrombolysis. If patients with myocardial infarction were treated within the first 6 hours of onset of pain, 26 lives per 1000 treated were saved. Better results were shown in patients treated within 3 hours of symptom onset compared to those treated later.[1,2]

GISSI-2 and ISIS-3 trials did not show any advantage on mortality of standard dose of t-PA as compared to streptokinase.[3,4] However the GUSTO Study demonstrated an advantage of t-PA over streptokinase when t-PA was used in the accelerated regimen. In this important trial, 30-day mortality among infarct patients was reduced to 6.3% with accelerated t-PA compared to 7.3% with streptokinase.[5]

These mega trials using intravenous thrombolytic agents teach us that thrombolytic therapy is very effective in improving mortality, easy to use, widely available, can be administered to large populations, and is relatively safe if given according to strict criteria. The GUSTO Study has shown in the accelerated t-PA regimen that TIMI 2 and 3 patency of coronary arteries could be achieved in 81% within 90 min. The mechanism of improved survival with accelerated t-PA is due to a more rapid reperfusion of the infarct-related coronary artery.[6]

As already stated, the most important determinant of clinical outcome in patients with myocardial infarction regarding reperfusion is early as possible thrombolytic therapy. The FTT Collaborative Group[1] showed that patients treated with thrombolysis very early derive the most benefit. In patients treated within 1 hour, 35 lives were saved per 1000 treated; between 2 and 3 hours, 25 lives per 1000; and between 4 and 6 hours from onset of symptoms only 19 lives per 1000 treated were saved. Today, a major goal of myocardial infarction management is to achieve very early thrombolysis by education to awareness of time and decreasing delay to therapy. The ease of implementing thrombolysis led to the Task Force recommendation that thrombolysis should be started within 30 min of arrival at hospital ('door-to-needle time').[7]

Primary coronary angioplasty

The evolution of mechanical reperfusion therapy by mode of coronary angioplasty set an alternative to thrombolytic therapy. There are no randomized controlled trials of primary coronary angioplasty vs. no reperfusion in acute myocardial infarction. The potential advantages of primary angioplasty over thrombolysis are high patency rates of coronary arteries (>90%), effective treatment of residual stenosis, avoidance of fibrinolytic complications, availability for patients with contraindications to thrombolysis and lower rates of recurrent ischemia and reinfarctions.

For the purpose of comparing primary angioplasty to thrombolysis, this review refers mostly to randomized studies, although it is worth while to mention a nonrandomized

summary of 2073 patients undergoing primary angioplasty in 10 centers. In this particular analysis, the mortality rate was 8.3%, with recurrent ischemia of only 4%.[8] This report is of limited value in view of the large differences in outcome between various centers and because patients in this study were selected on the basis of contraindications to thrombolysis and not in a randomized fashion.

Only five randomized studies have compared primary angioplasty with thrombolytic therapy in patients with acute myocardial infarction (Table 5.1).[9–13] The total number of patients in these studies was less than 1000. One of these studies compared angioplasty to intracoronary streptokinase, a study which is not relevant to the current comparison.[9]

In these studies primary angioplasty was reported to restore antegrade coronary flow in 88–95% of attempts. Zijlstra et al.[10] showed in a follow-up angiography weeks after infarction, coronary patency of 91% for patients with angioplasty and only 68% for those treated by streptokinase ($p = 0.001$). There was also less residual stenosis, fewer in-hospital adverse events (nonfatal infarction or death) and less recurrent ischemia. Similar results were observed by Gibbons et al.[11] who demonstrated less recurrent ischemia and revascularization among

Table 5.1 Outcome in randomized trials of primary angioplasty vs. thrombolysis in acute myocardial infarction.

Author	Therapy	Death	MI	LVEF
Grines et al.[12] (n = 395)	PTCA	5 (2.6%)	5 (2.6%)	53 ± 13
	t-PA	13 (6.5%) ($p < 0.10$)	13 (6.5%) ($p < 0.10$)	53 ± 13
Zijlstra et al.[10] (n = 142)	PTCA	0	0	51 ± 11
	STK	4 (6%)	9 (13%) ($p < 0.005$)	45 ± 12 ($p < 0.005$)
Gibbons et al.[11] (n = 103)	PTCA	4 (4.3%)	7 (15%)	53 ± 12
	t-PA	2 (3.6%)	20 (36%)	50 ± 11
Ribeiro et al.[13] (n = 100)	PTCA	3 (6%)	4 (8%)	59 ± 13
	STK	1 (2%)	5 (10%)	57 ± 13
Meta-analysis—Michels et al.[14]	PTCA	21/571 (3.7%)		
At 6 weeks	Thrombolysis	37/574 (6.4%)		
GUSTO 2 substudy— Ellis et al.[15,16] (preliminary) At 30 days	PTCA (n = 656)	6%	4%	
	t-PA (n = 573)	7% ($p = 0.37$)	6% ($p = 0.24$)	

angioplasty-treated patients. No difference was found in his study regarding left ventricular function, incidence of recurrent infarction and survival between groups. The PAMI trial[12] found a difference in favor of angioplasty in the primary endpoint (death and nonfatal reinfarction) between patients treated by primary angioplasty or alteplase—5.1% vs. 12.0% ($p = 0.02$).

Analysis of high-risk patients (older than 70 years with anterior infarction or tachycardia) revealed lower mortality in patients with angioplasty—2% compared to patients treated by thrombolysis—10% ($p = 0.01$). The benefit in survival was partly attributed to more cerebrovascular bleeding in the thrombolysis group. One of the small randomized studies by Ribeiro et al.[13] did not show any advantage of primary angioplasty in acute myocardial infarction. The authors even concluded that streptokinase may be preferred over primary angioplasty.

In a meta-analysis of studies comparing primary angioplasty and thrombolysis there was evidence of reduction of 6-week mortality and in combined outcome of short-term mortality and nonfatal reinfarction. Long-term data were not available from a sufficient number of patients (Table 5.1).[14] Only pooled data as summarized and presented by Grines,[15] including the meta-analysis[14] and the GUSTO IIb substudy,[16] demonstrated that primary angioplasty compared to thrombolysis was associated with a significant reduction in the rates of stroke (0.3% vs. 2.5%; $p = 0.007$), death and reinfarction (7.8% vs. 11.6%; $p = 0.002$).

The benefit in favor of primary angioplasty as presented in the meta-analysis data comes at the cost of performing angioplasty to a large population, i.e. all patients with acute myocardial infarction. Reeder et al.[17] compared the costs of immediate angioplasty vs. thrombolysis during a 12-month period. Although a trend was noted towards a briefer hospital stay and fewer late in-hospital procedures for patients treated initially with angioplasty compared to thrombolysis, the two strategies seem to have similar cost effectiveness. Goldman,[18] reviewing the cost and quality of life of the two strategies, summarizes that large-scale randomized trials are needed to determine which mode of therapy is more effective regarding cost and mortality.

Every et al.[19] reported in a community setting a comparison between the two strategies in treatment of acute myocardial infarction. There were 1050 patients in the angioplasty group and 2095 in the thrombolysis group. Patients in this study were not randomly assigned to each strategy and because of the potential for selection bias, several subgroup analyses were performed. These analyses included patients eligible for thrombolysis, high-risk patients and patients in the angioplasty group who were treated at hospitals with high volumes of angioplasty. In this relatively large-scale study, there was no significant difference in mortality during hospitalization or long-term follow-up between patients in the thrombolytic therapy group and those in the primary angioplasty group (hospital mortality 5.6% and

5.5%, respectively; $p = 0.93$). There was no significant difference in mortality between high-risk subgroups in the treatment strategies. The rates of procedures and costs were lower among patients in the thrombolysis group at the time of hospital discharge and after 3 years of follow-up.[19]

In the GUSTO-IIb study,[16] 1138 patients were randomly assigned to be treated by either primary angioplasty or thrombolysis with accelerated alteplase. Only a trend was observed in favor of angioplasty. Mortality was 5.7% vs. 7.0%, respectively, and a composite of death, reinfarction and disabling stroke was 9.6% vs. 13.1%, respectively. As mentioned before, only after pooling these data together with the meta-analysis data was a statistically significant difference shown between groups in favor of primary angioplasty.[16]

Controversy: how to reperfuse? To inflate or to infuse?

In view of the data presented, we are still faced with the controversial question of how to manage our patients with evolving myocardial infarction. I shall address this clinical question by summarizing the protagonist view in favor of thrombolysis, followed by the view in favor of primary angioplasty.

Thrombolysis vs. angioplasty

Thrombolysis in acute myocardial infarction proved itself as an effective therapy in many patients with an acceptable low rate of complications. Thrombolysis has been shown to limit infarct size, reduce morbidity, improve left ventricular function and reduce mortality. Data on primary angioplasty are limited and most of them lack statistical power to show advantage over thrombolysis regarding mortality. Every's report on more than 3000 patients failed to demonstrate any difference when comparing the two strategies.[19]

While thrombolysis is easy to perform and widely available, this is not the case for primary angioplasty. Less than 20% of hospitals in the USA and even less than 10% in other parts of the world are capable to perform angioplasty, and even fewer have the expertise and the logistics to perform emergency angioplasty. Although the transfer of patients to a hospital which performs angioplasty is possible, the time delay to reperfusion may outweigh the benefit.[20–22]

The real debate between the two modes of therapy arises only in a minority of the hospitals in which there are facilities to treat patients both ways. In the majority of the hospitals, no doubt, patients are treated by the only method available, thrombolysis, which is good and effective.

Even if the recommendations of the PAMI trial[12] are adapted, which are in favor of primary angioplasty, it is worth while to mention that patients treated by thrombolysis in this study had a worse outcome compared to outcome data for thrombolysis patients in other large-scale thrombolytic trials.

Since thrombolytic agents are improving and time to therapy will shorten, one can anticipate a better outcome for patients treated by thrombolysis. It is unlikely that the time to angioplasty will shorten or its availability will increase in the near future. Evidence to support this comes from multiple reports showing a greater time delay to angioplasty compared to thrombolysis.[10–13,19]

Angioplasty vs. thrombolysis

Primary coronary angioplasty in acute myocardial infarction can overcome the limitations of thrombolysis. It has been clearly demonstrated that angioplasty is associated with higher and better patency rates and less residual stenosis compared to thrombolysis. Patients treated with angioplasty are more likely to achieve TIMI 3 flow than patients treated by thrombolysis.[12,15] Additional advantages in favor of angioplasty are a high long-term patency rate of around 90%, reduction of the recurrent ischemia and reinfarction rate and a low rate of stroke—0.3%.

Angioplasty is of importance in patients with contraindications to thrombolysis, especially in those with a risk of bleeding. However, it should be stressed that this group benefits less from angioplasty as well, since these patients are sometimes unable to receive full antithrombotic therapy or antiplatelet therapy.

Recommendations of the ACC/AHA Task Force on practice guidelines

The ACC/AHA Task Force[7] expresses a serious concern that a routine policy of primary angioplasty will result in unacceptable delays in achieving reperfusion in a substantial number of patients and less than optimal outcomes if performed by less experienced operators. The task force clearly states the criteria and experience necessary for operators and centers to be eligible to perform primary angioplasty in acute myocardial infarction:

1 Balloon dilatation within 60–90 min of diagnosis.

2 Achieving TIMI 2 or 3 flow in more than 90% of patients.

3 Less than 5% emergency coronary artery bypass graft surgery (CABG).

4 Performance of angioplasty in 85% of patients brought to the laboratory.

5 Less than 12% mortality.

Therefore, primary angioplasty in acute myocardial infarction as an alternative to thrombolysis will be performed by skilled cardiologists who perform more than 75 procedures per year in centers with more than 200 angioplasties per year.

There is weight of evidence in favor of primary angioplasty as a mode of reperfusion in patients who have a risk of a bleeding contraindication to thrombolytic therapy and for patients in cardiogenic shock. Usefulness and efficacy is less established by evidence in patients who fail to qualify for thrombolysis for reasons other than a risk of bleeding contraindication.

Since up to 5% of patients referred to primary angioplasty may require emergency surgical intervention, angioplasty should be performed in hospitals capable of emergency cardiac surgery or they should rapidly transfer such patients to a nearby facility with a cardiac surgery.

Conclusion

From data currently available, it can be concluded that in highly skilled centers primary angioplasty in acute myocardial infarction is a safe and at least a good alternative to thrombolysis, with superiority only in 'soft' endpoints, such as recanalization rate and recurrent ischemia.

Both strategies are improving rapidly, and apparently in the near future, one would have to compare primary angioplasty and stenting vs. newer thrombolytic agents and new adjunctive agents. Still, it must be remembered that thrombolysis is a widespread, easy-to-use and simple mode of therapy compared to angioplasty, which requires high skill and special facilities, and is therefore limited to a small patient population.[23]

References

1   Fibrinolytic Therapy Trialists' (FTT) Collaborative Group. Indications for fibrinolytic therapy in suspected acute myocardial infarction: collaborative overview of early mortality and major morbidity results from all randomised trials of more than 1000 patients. *Lancet* 1994; **343**: 311–22.

2   ISIS-2 (Second International Study of Infarct Survival) Collaborative Group. Randomised trial of intravenous streptokinase, oral aspirin, both, or neither among 17 187 cases of suspected acute myocardial infarction: ISIS-2. *Lancet* 1988; **2**: 349–60.

3   Gruppo Italiano per Studio della Sopravvivenza nell'Infarto Miocardico. GISSI-2: a factorial randomised trial of alteplase versus streptokinase and heparin versus no heparin among 12 490 patients with acute myocardial infarction. *Lancet* 1990; **336**: 65–71.

4   ISIS-3 (Third International Study of Infarct Survival) Collaborative Group. A randomised comparison of streptokinase vs. tissue plasminogen activator vs. anistreplase and of aspirin plus heparin vs. aspirin alone among 41 299 cases of suspected acute myocardial infarction: ISIS-3. *Lancet* 1990; **339**: 753–70.

5   The GUSTO investigators. An international randomized trial comparing four thrombolytic strategies for acute myocardial infarction. *N Engl J Med* 1993; **329**: 673–82.

6   The GUSTO Angiographic Investigators. The effects of tissue plasminogen activator, streptokinase, or both on coronary-artery patency, ventricular function, and survival after acute myocardial infarction. *N Engl J Med* 1993; **329**: 1615–22.

7   Ryan TJ, Anderson JL, Antman EM, et al. ACC/AHA guidelines for the management of patients with acute myocardial infarction: a report of the American College of Cardiology/American Heart Association Task Force on Practical Guidelines (Committee on Management of Acute Myocardial Infarction). *J Am Coll Cardiol* 1996; **28**: 1328–428.

8   Eckman MH, Wong JB, Salem DN, Pauker SG. Direct angioplasty for acute myocardial infarction. A review of outcomes in clinical subsets. *Ann Intern Med* 1992; **117**: 667–76.

9   O'Neill W, Timmis GC, Bourdillon PD, et al. A prospective randomized clinical trial of intracoronary streptokinase versus coronary angioplasty for acute myocardial infarction. *N Engl J Med* 1986; **31**: 812–18.

10   Zijlstra F, de Boer MJ, Hoorntje JC, Reiffers S, Reiber JH, Suryapranta H. A comparison of immediate coronary angioplasty with intravenous streptokinase in acute myocardial infarction. *N Engl J Med* 1993; **328**: 680–4.

11   Gibbons RJ, Holmes DR, Reeder GS, Bailey KR, Hopfenspringer MR, Gersh BJ. Immediate angioplasty compared with the administration of a thrombolytic agent followed by conservative treatment for myocardial infarction. The Mayo Coronary Care Unit and Catheterization Laboratory Groups. *N Engl J Med* 1993; **328**: 685–91.

12   Grines CL, Browne KF, Marco J, et al. A comparison of immediate angioplasty with thrombolytic therapy for acute myocardial infarction: the Primary Angioplasty in Myocardial Infarction Study Group. *N Engl J Med* 1993; **328**: 673–9.

13   Ribeiro EE, Silva LA, Carneiro R, et al. Randomized trial of direct coronary angioplasty versus intravenous streptokinase in acute myocardial infarction. *J Am Coll Cardiol* 1993; **22**: 376–80.

14   Michels KB, Yusuf S. Does PTCA in acute myocardial infarction affect mortality and reinfarction rates? A quantitative overview (meta-analysis) of the randomized clinical trials. *Circulation* 1995; **91**: 476–85.

15   Grines CL. Primary angioplasty—the strategy of choice. In clinical debate: should thrombolysis or primary angioplasty be the treatment of choice for acute myocardial infarction? *N Engl J Med* 1996; **335**: 1313–17.

16   Ellis SG. GUSTO II: primary PTCA versus thrombolysis substudy. Presented at the American College of Cardiology Annual Scientific Sessions: March 1996, Orlando, FL.

17   Reeder GS, Bailey KR, Gersh BJ, Holmes DR, Christianson J, Gibbons RJ. Cost comparison of immediate angioplasty versus thrombolysis followed by conservative therapy for acute myocardial infarction: a randomized prospective trial. Mayo Coronary Care Unit and Catheterization Laboratory Groups. *Mayo Clin Proc* 1994; **69**: 87–9.

18   Goldman L. Cost and quality of life: thrombolysis and primary angioplasty. *J Am Coll Cardiol* 1995; **25(7 Suppl)**: 38s–41s.

19   Every NR, Parsons LS, Hlatky M, Martin JS, Weaver WD. A comparison of thrombolytic therapy with primary angioplasty for acute myocardial infarction. *N Engl J Med* 1996; **335**: 1253–60.

20   Brodie BR. Primary angioplasty in a community hospital in the USA. *Br Heart J* 1995; **73**: 411–12.

21   Weaver WD, Lltwin PE, Martin JS, for the MITI Project Investigators. Use of direct angioplasty for treatment of patients with acute myocardial infarction in hospitals with and without on-site cardiac surgery. *Circulation* 1993; **88**: 2067–75.

22   Lange RA, Hillis LD. Thrombolysis—the preferred treatment. In clinical debate: should thrombolysis or primary angioplasty be the treatment of choice for acute myocardial infarction? *N Engl J Med* 1996; **335**: 1311–12.

23   Verheugt FW. Primary angioplasty for acute myocardial infarction: is the balloon half full or half empty? *Lancet* 1996; **347**: 1276–7.

6

Laser guidewire for recanalization of chronic total occlusions

Jaap N Hamburger and Patrick W Serruys

Introduction

Since its introduction, percutaneous transluminal coronary angioplasty (PTCA) has established itself as an important alternative to coronary artery bypass surgery (CABG) in the treatment of coronary artery disease. A continuing development of techniques and tools, has led to a considerable increase in both the number and complexity of cases performed annually.[1] Once considered to be 'a temptation to resist', the percutaneous treatment of diseased saphenous vein bypass grafts, small diameter coronary arteries, and multivessel disease is becoming the routine rather than the exception in today's angioplasty practice. The recent explosive increase in the use of intracoronary stents has played a major role in this shift of the former boundaries of PTCA.[2] One of the last remaining bastions of CABG has been the treatment of chronic total coronary occlusions. Hampered by low initial success rates[3–8] and high recurrence rates,[9–11] it was only after the introduction of improved guidewire technology[12,13] in addition to the demonstration of a positive influence of stenting on long-term vessel patency,[14] that chronic total occlusion became a more acceptable indication for percutaneous treatment. The laser guidewire is an example of such new guidewire technology.[15] It was specifically designed for the recanalization of those chronic coronary artery occlusions refractory to recanalization attempts using conventional guidewires. Earlier, our group reported on the initial clinical experience with the laser guidewire.[16] We report here on the technical aspects of laser guidewire assisted recanalization of total occlusions, a treatment modality for a potentially large group of patients.[17,18]

The laser guidewire

The Spectranetics Prima Coronary Total Occlusion System (Model 018-003) (Spectranetics, Colorado Springs CO), consists of an 0.018-inch laser guidewire and a support catheter and is designed to combine the mechanical attributes of a typical coronary guidewire with the ablative energy of the CVX-300 excimer laser in order to enable the initial crossing of total coronary occlusions (Fig. 6.1). The wire consists of optical fibers with a 45 μm diameter, encased within a 0.018-inch diameter shaft. The distal 30 cm of the wire is relatively floppy and is treated with a lubricious coating. The distal coil tip is radio-opaque for visualization under fluoroscopy. The wire tip is shapeable and, if required, re-shapeable during a procedure in order to meet specific anatomic circumstances. Furthermore, it has a torque device mounted on the proximal shaft. The support catheter, which comes with the laser guidewire is 135 cm long and has a single 0.018-inch wire compatible lumen. It has a radio-opaque marker mounted 1 mm proximal to a 2.5 F tapered tip. Finally, the system is supplied with a 15 cm long tapered 'peel-off' introducer to assist insertion of the laser guidewire into the support catheter.

The laser source for the laser guidewire is the Spectranetics CVX-300 XeCl excimer laser, emitting at a wavelength of 308 nm. The physical phenomena which occur during tissue ablation at this wavelength is described elsewhere.[19]

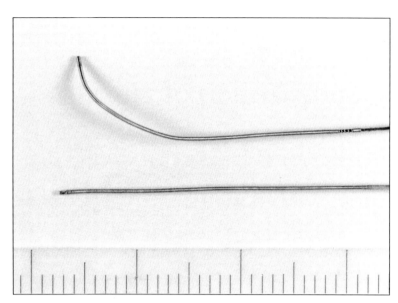

Figure 6.1
The Prima Total Occlusion System: The Prima Total Occlusion System showing the tip of the laser guidewire, shaped (top) and unshaped (bottom).

The laser guidewire procedure

The working mechanism of the laser guidewire is based on the ablation of diseased vascular tissue. Contrary to conventional guidewires that follow the path of least resistance, the laser guidewire will advance in whatever direction the wire tip is directed during activation of the laser beam. Consequently, a proper alignment of the laser guidewire is the most critical issue involved in this procedure. Therefore, to guide the steering of the wire through a missing segment, both a proximal entry point and a clear distal (anatomic) re-entry point leading to a visible true distal lumen are an absolute prerequisite for a successful procedure. As a rule, a complete distal opacification of the target vessel by collaterals (minimum: Rentrop class 2^{20}) is required to assure the visibility of the target vessel during the procedure.

Currently, at the Thoraxcentre we use the approach described below in order to optimize the chances of a successful procedure.

Puncturing of both femoral arteries with insertion of a second, smaller French-size catheter in the contralateral coronary artery is employed. By a combination of simultaneous bilateral injection of contrast medium into both coronary arteries, thus making use of the inter-coronary collateral circulation and (whenever available) biplane coronary angiography, optimal information is obtained about the anatomy of the missing segment (Fig. 6.2). A monoplane system could be used, provided multiple views from different angles are made each time prior to the advancement of the laser guidewire.

A guiding catheter, minimum 8 Fr size, that provides good coaxial alignment and back up support is chosen. An example of a guiding catheter which supplies optimal back-up support would be an Amplatz left, rather than a Judkins, guiding catheter for occlusions of either the left or right coronary artery. A large lumen Y-connector is mounted on the guiding catheter to allow for the potential introduction of a laser catheter, if crossing of the wire needs to be followed by an excimer laser coronary angioplasty (ECLA) procedure. Unless ipsilateral collaterals sufficiently supply the occluded segment, a 7 Fr diagnostic catheter introduced through the contralateral femoral artery is positioned in the ostium of the contralateral coronary artery.

To facilitate flushing of the support catheter during the procedure, a standard Y-connector with a three-way stop cock is mounted on the supplied support catheter. After flushing with a heparin solution, the support catheter is preloaded with the laser guidewire, using the peel-off introducer to avoid damage to the wire tip. Subsequently, the tip of the laser guidewire is shaped by rolling the tip gently between the first and second finger. Once positioned in the coronary artery, the tip of the wire tends to lose the imparted shape. It is therefore advisable to curve the wire tip to a larger extent than usually done with a conventional type guidewire for the same anatomical situation. After this, the laser guidewire is calibrated at a fluence of 60 mJ/mm^2 and a pulse repetition rate of 25 Hz. It should be noted that calibration of the wire

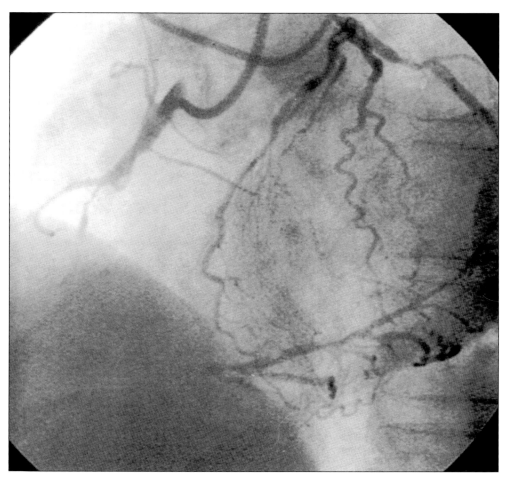

Figure 6.2
Total occlusion of a right coronary artery. A left Amplatz guiding catheter is positioned in the ostium of the RCA and a 7F Judkins left diagnostic catheter in the ostium of the left coronary artery. Bilateral simultaneous injection of contrast medium, showing the occlusion stump and the distal lumen.

is done only after shaping of the wire tip, since the tip shaping manoeuvre may damage the silica fibers inside the laser guidewire which would be manifest as a calibration failure.

Once the calibration is completed, the laser guidewire is retrieved into the support catheter and both are introduced into the guiding catheter. The support catheter is advanced toward the tip of the guiding catheter, and the wire is advanced into the stump of the occlusion. When there is a sharp bend in the artery proximal to the target occlusion (e.g. an occlusion in the circumflex artery), prior to introduction of the laser guidewire, a mechanical guidewire can be used in order to position the tip of the support catheter in the funnel of the occlusion.

In situations where there is an eccentric funnel, as an alternative to the support catheter, it may be helpful to use a balloon catheter and to inflate the balloon in the occlu-

sion stump at a low pressure, for the creation of an entry point with a central location.

Initially, advancement of the laser guidewire without activation of the laser may be attempted. In the situation where it is not possible to advance the laser guidewire mechanically, the wire is moved forward during laser activation. The fluence typically used during a laser guidewire procedure is 60 mJ/mm^2, with a pulse repetition rate of 25 Hz. The corresponding pulse energy at the tip of the wire at this fluence is approximately 1.2 mJ.

During pulse trains, with a maximum of 5 seconds, the wire is gently advanced at a rate of 0.5–1 mm per second. During advancement of the wire, continuous monitoring with biplane fluoroscopy of the position and alignment with the vessel segment to be crossed is strongly recommended. Each time the tip of the laser guidewire has

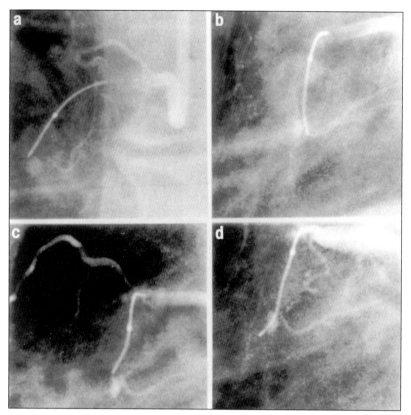

Figure 6.3
Total occlusion of the proximal right coronary artery. (A–C) The laser guidewire is steered around a calcified obstruction. (D) Angiographic confirmation of the intraluminal position of the distal tip of the laser guidewire.

reached a new position, the alignment with the distal lumen is checked by a contralateral injection of contrast medium. In case of misalignment, the advancement of the wire is discontinued and the laser guidewire is repositioned before further advancement.

If during laser activation the laser guidewire encounters intraluminal resistance which hampers its normal progression (e.g. plaque calcification), the pulse repetition rate should be increased to 40 Hz. In certain conditions, despite a pulse repetition rate of 40 Hz, wire progression can still be insufficient. This could be explained by:

- insufficient back-up support, inability of the laser guidewire to ablate the tissue it is in contact with (e.g. calcium)

- a subintimal position of the wire tip (misalignment),

- mechanical damage of the wire tip with a subsequent drop in the energy output.

In these situations the following strategy is suggested. First, advance the support catheter in order to supply additional back-up support. Although experience has taught us that nature is forgiving and staining of the occluded segment

with contrast medium (intraluminal or perivascular) should not be a reason for terminating the procedure in general, pushing of the tip of the support catheter into the occluded segment should be avoided in order to prevent dissections.

Next, especially in case of fluoroscopically visible calcifications, a slight pull-back of the tip of the wire can be tried. When readvancing the wire, the wire tip is steered around the obstruction, obviously staying within the boundaries of the arterial segment (Fig. 6.3). Another option (especially if there are indications of a subintimal position of the wire tip) would be to withdraw the tip of the laser guidewire into the proximal stump of the occlusion, in order to make a new entry point. If, despite these efforts, wire progression is negligible, the tip of the support catheter should be positioned in the stump of the occlusion and the wire removed from the support catheter. Subsequently, the tip of the laser guidewire can be examined for mechanical damage, and the energy output can be measured. In case of reduced output, the laser guidewire should be recalibrated in an attempt to restore the original output. Obviously, if the distal part of the occluded segment could not be

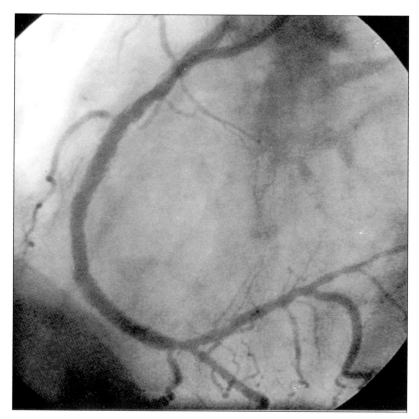

Figure 6.4
Recanalization of a chronic totally occluded right coronary artery and reconstruction of the occluded segment using multiple stents (final result of the procedure in Fig. 6.2).

crossed with the laser guidewire, the laser guidewire can be exchanged for a conventional (i.e. mechanical) guidewire, while still making use of the support catheter.

If on fluoroscopy the wire tip projects outside the boundaries of the vessel, the wire should be withdrawn into the proximal part of the coronary artery. A proximal injection is used to check for possible leakage of contrast medium into the free pericardial space. Since there is usually no perfusion pressure inside the occluded segment, especially in longer segments, leakage into the free pericardial space is not likely. Nature seems to be forgiving in this situation and a so-called 'wire exit' is not necessarily a reason to abort the procedure.

Once the laser guidewire has crossed the occlusion, the intraluminal position of the wire in the distal true lumen must be confirmed by means of a contralateral injection of contrast medium. If there is doubt regarding the wire position the support catheter should never be advanced, nor should a balloon catheter be used, since it is this impatient manoeuvre which converts a benign wire exit into a perforation with tamponade introducing unnecessarily a major, potentially life threatening complication. Thus only after the intraluminal position of the wire has been confirmed, should the laser guidewire be used as an exchange wire for the ensuing interventional procedure.

Adjunctive angioplasty

The aim of the adjunctive angioplasty is to remove as much obstructing material as possible, prior to 'dottering' of the remainder. Therefore, depending on lesion morphology and proximal reference diameter, either the 1.4 mm, 1.7 mm or 2.0 mm excimer laser catheter can be used, according to standard guidelines for the use of excimer laser equipment. Based upon the true ablation rate of the currently available multifiber catheters, the laser catheter should be advanced at a maximum speed of 0.5 mm per second, at a fluence of 50 mJ/mm^2, and a pulse repetition rate of 25 Hz, for a maximum duration of five seconds. Both prior to and during activation of the laser, it is mandatory to flush the target vessel with saline. By removing any intraluminally present contrast medium as well as clearing most of the blood interface, the deleterious side-effects on the vessel wall of shock wave formation, due to absorption of 308 nm laser energy by contrast medium and haemoglobin, are minimized. The combination of a 'slow pass' with the use of saline flush has made excimer laser related coronary dissection an unnecessary complication.[21]

Finally, the issue remains whether or not the result achieved with balloon angioplasty should be optimized by means of the placement of one or more intracoronary stents. Violaris *et al.*[22] reported on the long-term restenosis rate following successful balloon dilatation of coronary occlusions. The study population comprised 2950 patients (3549 lesions), which included 244 occlusive stenoses (6.9%). The six-month angiographic restenosis rate (>50% stenosis at follow up) was significantly higher in the occlusion group at 45% compared to 33% in the non-occlusive group. Similarly the relative loss (mm, mean ±SD) in the occlusive group, 0.17 ± 0.3, n = 244 was significantly higher than in the non-occlusive group, 0.12 ± 0.2, n = 3305, p < 0.001. However, the higher restenosis rate in the occlusion group was entirely due to increased *reocclusion*: 18% (44/244 lesions) compared to 4.7% (156/3305 lesions) for the non-occlusive group (p < 0.001). After exclusion of these reocclusions, the restenosis rate between the two groups was similar, 32.5 vs. 29.3% (p = 0.338), while the relative loss was even significantly lower in the occlusive group (0.07 ± 0.17, n = 200) than in the non-occlusive group (0.09 ± 0.16, n = 3149, p = 0.023). These results suggest that, other than what might be a population subgroup (18% early reocclusion), long-term results of successful angioplasty of total occlusions may be comparable with results of balloon angioplasty of non-occlusive coronary stenoses. Subsequent publications[14,16] have indicated that both the (early) reocclusion rate as well as the late restenosis rate after successful recanalization of total occlusions is favorably influenced by stent implantation. Therefore, is it our current policy to stent the occlusion site in all patients after successful recanalization has been achieved (Fig. 6.4). The advantage of the use of intravascular ultrasound (IVUS), especially in optimizing the stent procedure, has been reported elsewhere.[23,24]

Finally, all the patients in the Thoraxcentre are put on a medical regime with ticlopidine and aspirin for two weeks and six months, respectively, in order to reduce the possibility of subacute reocclusion.

Summary

With respect to the low success rate of PTCA for the treatment of chronic coronary total occlusions in general, and the clinical relevance of this condition to the practice of the (interventional) cardiologist, it seems justifiable to investigate new technologies aimed at increasing the opportunities of percutaneous intervention for this specific condition. Presently, the European registry with the laser guidewire, the European TOTAL Surveillance Study, has been completed.[25,26] From this experience, we have learned that following an initial failed attempt to mechanically re-establish flow, the success rate of the laser guidewire procedure is approximately 60%. Currently, the major limitation of the laser guidewire procedure is its

technical complexity, resulting in lengthy procedures with extensive use of fluoroscopic time and contrast medium. Development of alternative techniques for forward detection (e.g. ultrasound, fluorescence- or Raman spectroscopy) could prove to be essential in increasing the availability of the laser guidewire technology for general interventional practice. Although the preliminary European experience with the laser guidewire is encouraging, favorable success rates in recanalization of total coronary occlusions have been reported with new mechanical guidewires, such as the Choice PT plus wire (Scimed, BSC, Minnesota, USA), the Crosswire (Terumo, Tokyo, Japan) and the Japanese Athlete guidewire. Consequently, the ongoing European–American multicenter randomized trial comparing the laser guidewire with the best available conventional mechanical guidewires (the 'TOTAL' trial) will answer the question whether this technique will obtain a definite place in the arena of interventional cardiology.

References

1   Brand M van den. Utilization of angioplasty and cost of angioplasty disposables in 14 western European countries. *Eur Heart J* 1993; **14**: 391–7.

2   Ruygrok PN, Serruys PW. Intracoronary stenting, from concept to custom. *Circulation* 1996; **94**: 882–90.

3   Savage R, Hollman J, Gruentzig AR, Spencer King III, Douglas J, Tankersley R. Can percutaneous transluminal coronary angioplasty be performed in patients with total occlusion? *Circulation* 1982; **66**: 1319 (abstract).

4   Heyndrickx GR, Serruys PW, van den Brand M, Vandormael M, Reiber JHC. Transluminal angioplasty after mechanical recanalization in patients with chronic occlusion of coronary artery. *Circulation* 1982; **II-5**: 1319 (abstract).

5   Holmes DR, Vlietstra RE, Reeder GS, *et al.* Angioplasty in total coronary artery occlusion. *J Am Coll Cardiol* 1984; **3**: 845–9.

6   Meyer B, Gruentzig AR. Learning curve for percutaneous transluminal coronary angioplasty: skill, technology or patient selection. *Am J Cardiol* 1984; **53**: 65C–66C.

7   Kereiakes DJ, Selmon MR, McAuley BJ, McAuley DB, Sheehan DJ, Simpson JB. Angioplasty in total coronary artery occlusion: experience in 76 consecutive patients. *J Am Coll Cardiol* 1985; **6**: 526–33.

8   Stone GW, Rutherford BD, McConahay DR, *et al.* Procedural outcome of angioplasty for total coronary artery occlusion: an analysis of 971 lesions in 905 patients. *J Am Coll Cardiol* 1990; **15**: 849–65.

9   Serruys PW, Umans V, Heyndrickx GR, *et al.* Elective PTCA of totally occluded coronary arteries not associated with acute myocardial infarction; short-term and long-term results. *Eur Heart J* 1985; **6**: 2–12.

10 DiScascio G, Vetrovec GW, Cowley MJ, Wolfgang TC. Early and late outcome of percutaneous transluminal coronary angioplasty for subacute and chronic total coronary occlusion. *Am Heart J* 1986; **111**: 833–9.

11 Ivanhoe RJ, Weintraub WS, Douglas JS jr, *et al.* Percutaneous transluminal coronary angioplasty of chronic total occlusions: primary success, restenosis and long-term clinical follow-up. *Circulation* 1992; **85**: 106–15.

12 Serruys PW, Hamburger JN, de Feyter PJ, van den Brand M. Recanalization of chronic total occlusions using a laser guidewire: a preliminary experience. *Circulation* 1994; **90**: 1776 (abstract).

13 Kinoshita I, Katoh O, Nariyama J, *et al.* Coronary angioplasty of chronic total occlusions with bridging collateral vessels: immediate and follow-up outcome from a large single-center experience. *J Am Coll Cardiol* 1995; **26**: 409–15.

14 Sirnes PA, Golf S, Myreng Y, *et al.* Stenting in Chronic Coronary Occlusion (SICCO): a randomized, controlled trial of adding stent implantation after successful angioplasty. *J Am Coll Cardiol* 1996; **28**: 1444–51.

15 Hamburger JN, Serruys PW. Recanalization of chronic total occlusions using a laser guidewire. In: Sigwart U, Bertrand M, Serruys PW (eds), *Handbook of Cardiovascular Interventions* (London: WB Saunders, 1996); 493–500.

16 Hamburger JN, Airian S, Gijsbers GHM, de Feyter PJ, Serruys PW. Recanalization of chronic total coronary occlusions using a laser guidewire: a single institution experience with the initial one-hundred cases. In: Holmes DR, Serruys PW (eds), *Current Review of Interventional Cardiology*, 3rd edn (Philadelphia: Current Medicine, 1997).

17 Ruygrok PN, De Jaegere PPT, Verploegh J, van Domburg, de Feyter PJ. Immediate outcome following coronary angioplasty: a contemporary single center audit. *Eur Heart J* 1995; **16(Suppl)**: 24–9.

18 Kahn JK. Angiographic suitability for catheter revascularization of total coronary occlusions in patients from a community hospital setting. *Am Heart J* 1993; **126**: 561–4.

19 Hamburger JN, Gijsbers GHM, Verhoofstad GGAM, *et al.* Excimer laser coronary angioplasty: a physical perspective to clinical results. In: Topol E, Serruys PW (eds), *Current Review of Interventional Cardiology*, 2nd edn (Philadelphia: Current Medicine, 1995); 159–72.

20 Cohen M, Rentrop KP. Limitation of myocardial ischemia by collateral circulation during sudden controlled coronary artery occlusion in human subjects: a prospective study. *Circulation* 1986; **74**: 469–76.

21 Deckelbaum LI, Strauss BH, Bittl JA, Rohlfs K, Scott J and PELCA investigators. Effect of intra-coronary saline infusion on dissection during excimer laser coronary angioplasty: a randomized trial. *Circulation* 1994; **90**: 1774 (abstract).

22 Violaris AG, Melkert R, Serruys PW. Long-term luminal renarrowing after successful elective coronary angioplasty of total occlusions: a quantitative angiographic analysis. *Circulation* 1995; **91**: 2140–50.

23 Colombo A, Hall P, Nakamura S, *et al.* Intracoronary stenting without anticoagulation accomplished with intravascular ultrasound guidance. *Circulation* 1995; **91**: 1676–88.

24 Prati F, Di Mario C, Hamburger JN, Gil R, von Birgelen C, Serruys PW. Guidance of multiple stent deployment in a chronic totally occluded coronary artery using three-dimensional reconstruction of intra-coronary ultrasound. *Am Heart J* 1995; **130**: 1286–9.

25 Hamburger JN, Gomes R, Simon R, *et al.* Recanalization of chronic total coronary occlusions using a laser guidewire: the European TOTAL multicenter surveillance study. *J Am Coll Cardiol* 1997; **29(A)** *in press.*

26 Serruys PW, Hamburger JN, de Feyter PJ, *et al.* Recanalization of total coronary occlusions using a laser guide wire: The European TOTAL surveillance study. *Submitted for publication.*

II

Stents, Current Practice and Future Directions

7

The current practice of coronary stenting

Antonio Colombo

Introduction

The practice of coronary stenting involves a process of decision-making at three levels: to stent or not to stent, which stent to use and how to stent. The patient clinical outcome can be successful only if all three aspects of this process are done optimally. This chapter discusses in detail, each of these three topics.

To stent or not to stent

The decision to implant an endoluminal metallic prosthesis as a treatment for an obstructive coronary stenosis needs to be supported by the assumption that the stent implantation will give superior clinical outcome compared to other current treatment modalities.

Most of the scientific evidence supporting the usage of stents comes from two well-known randomized studies, the STRESS[1] and the BENESTENT[2] trials, showing superiority of stent over coronary angioplasty in terms of primary success and restenosis rate for a selected group of patients. The stenting technique used in 1994 has, since, improved, and the results of the stent arm would improve if these trials were repeated today. The preliminary results of the BENESTENT II trial[3] and other observational studies[4] are showing that coronary stenting applied to classic BENESTENT–STRESS lesions is associated with an angiographic restenosis less than 15% and with an incidence of vascular and bleeding complications similar to percutaneous transluminal coronary angioplasty (PTCA). The high-pressure stent implantation technique, ticlopidine and the abolition of anticoagulant therapy have contributed to this achievement. Among the limitations to stent placement present in the first two randomized trials, proximal vessel tortuosity is no longer tenable. The introduction of new stent designs has virtually converted stent flexibility to that of a balloon.

However, along with improvements in the field of coronary stenting, there are also improvements in balloon angioplasty. The concepts of high-pressure balloon inflation and appropriate balloon sizing[5] are now being applied to PTCA. Therefore it is not surprising to see improved immediate and medium-term results of the PTCA arm of the BENESTENT II trial compared to the PTCA arm of BENESTENT I. Improved PTCA results will prevent the widening gap with stents, despite the improvements in the stent arm. The only difference could be the shift of this gap to a lower level.

While waiting for the final results of the BENESTENT II trial and for their critical evaluation we can assume that coronary stenting is the practice of choice for short lesions (less than 10 mm) located on vessels with an angiographic diameter larger than 3 mm.

Threatened and acute closure: a definite indication

Coronary stenting applied to threatened closure and to acute closure following PTCA most probably gives superior results compared to any other approach.[6-8] With the availability of stents which can reach small vessels, and with the knowledge that small vessel size does not significantly affect the incidence of stent thrombosis,[9] we can state that the treatment of choice for threatened closure and acute closure is coronary stenting.

The other lesions

Outside the boundaries of short lesions on a large vessel, and of situations associated with vessel closure, stenting is open to controversy. Evidence favoring the usage of stents in these situations is based mainly on the results of observational trials.[10]

Elective stenting of long lesions located in large vessels

The results of stenting long lesions (length $\geq$ 15 mm) are known mainly from abstract reports.[11–13] Except for use of the Wallstent (for the manufacturer's details see Table 7.3) to treat recanalized total coronary occlusions[14] there is no other published study reporting the follow-up results of coronary stenting applied to lesions longer than 15 mm located on vessels angiographically greater than 3 mm. We need to address this question by looking at the database in Milan. The angiographic follow-up was analyzed in 93 lesions 20 mm or longer located in vessels with a diameter greater than or equal to 3 mm, treated by elective implantation of Palmaz–Schatz stents. The immediate results (success and complications) are not different from the use of this stent in short lesions. The angiographic restenosis rate, by the 50% criterion, was 24% (CI: 15–33%).

The 9 cells NIR stent in its long design (32 mm) has been implanted in 20 lesions with the above characteristics and with angiographic follow-up. Except for a gain in the procedural aspects of the stent implantation (shorter, simpler and cheaper procedure), the long stent design does not seem to impact on restenosis rate. A variety of other stents have been utilized in this setting, but their angiographic follow-up is still limited. These preliminary data show that stenting applied to long coronary lesions located in vessels greater than or equal to 3 mm is associated with a higher restenosis rate compared to stenting a short lesion. Despite this higher recurrence rate of stenting applied to long lesions, PTCA does not perform any better, with an angiographic restenosis rate between 48% and 58%.[15,16]

The author believes that the operator should take the major elements that affect restenosis into account to make a specific decision. The three major elements in order of importance are:

- the reference vessel size;
- the length of the lesion, with particular attention to the subsets of patients with diffuse involvement of the vessel;
- the result achieved following the initial PTCA.

Elective stenting of long lesions located in small vessels

The information concerning this subgroup is obtained from the database in Milan. Palmaz–Schatz stents were implanted in 72 lesions longer than 20 mm located on vessels smaller than 3 mm, with angiographic follow-up. The angiographic restenosis rate of this group was 30% (CI: 19–41%). The 9 cells NIR stent was implanted in 23 similar lesions; the angiographic follow-up demonstrated a restenosis rate of 38% (CI: 18–58%).

Results with coil stents are not superior to these ones. The results of PTCA applied in this subset of lesions are not available. There is no good reason to assume that angioplasty will do better. Based on the current status of coronary stenting used to treat long lesions in small vessels, it is too soon to advocate for elective usage. Stenting in this subset of patients with long lesions in small vessels should be used very selectively, taking into account the facts that there would be no significant reduction in restenosis rate, and that procedural costs will be significantly higher than with a simple PTCA.[17]

Elective stenting of short lesions located in small vessels

Results in this lesion subset are superior than initially expected. The analysis of the author's database for the Palmaz–Schatz cohort shows angiographic follow-up on 171 lesions shorter than 20 mm and located on vessels smaller than 3 mm. The angiographic restenosis rate was 23% (CI: 17–30%). The 9 cells NIR stent implanted on corresponding lesions gave a similar restenosis rate. The results of PTCA in similar lesions are not known. For these reasons the following strategy is proposed. The operator should evaluate the PTCA results following optimal dilatation, with little hesitation to proceed to stenting if such a result does not appear adequate.

Ostial lesions

Ostial lesions, in particular aorto-ostial lesions, are associated with a high recurrence rate following PTCA.[18–20] The data available from one observational study from the author's center using stenting as a treatment modality for this lesion show an angiographic recurrence rate of 16%.[21] Despite the small number of patients included in the above report, the data are quite encouraging. No randomized study is available at present. Knowing the poor results obtained with PTCA in these lesions, this finding is not surprising. For this reason coronary stenting should be used electively to treat ostial lesions, provided the vessel size is appropriate for this technique.

Bifurcational lesions

Bifurcational lesions are another subset of lesions associated with a high recurrence rate following PTCA.[22,23] Coronary stenting has been applied using various techniques with good immediate results characterized by superior luminal gain.[24,25] Unfortunately the angiographic recurrence rate has been between 30 and 40% for any of the two branches involved. The author is exploring the combination of directional atherectomy and stenting as an approach to decrease the recurrence rate.

Total occlusions

The recurrence rate, after recanalization with subsequent PTCA of an occluded coronary artery, has been reported to be at least 45%.[26] Observational studies utilizing stenting applied to vessels of an appropriate size reported an angiographic recurrence rate as low as 20%.[27,28] Preliminary results from a randomized study in Japan do not show a significant benefit of PTCA compared to stenting[29] while another randomized study shows a significant benefit of stenting.[30] Particularly encouraging is the SICCO study from Sweden, reporting a recurrence rate following stenting of 35% compared to 75% obtained following PTCA.[31] The author therefore thinks that coronary stenting should be preferred to PTCA following reopening of an occluded artery.

Occluded arteries in the setting of acute myocardial infarction are a special situation.[32] From a theoretical point of view the fast re-establishment of the best forward flow (TIMI III) seems a very logical goal in this condition. Preliminary reports shows that coronary stenting can be applied in this setting without the fear of thrombosis, provided the appropriate technique and antiplatelet therapy are given. The author believes that the use of coronary stenting in acute myocardial infarction will significantly expand in the near future.

Saphenous vein graft lesions

In many cases the appearance of a stenosis on a vein graft is a sign of progressive disease of the graft itself. Problems related to the graft and/or to the distal runoff are sometimes associated. For this reason the clinical results reported in the literature following stenting of saphenous vein graft stenosis[33,34] are not encouraging. New strategies to cover the disease graft completely with a long stent, in the attempt to control disease progression at other sites not significantly narrowed, are now being explored.[35] The interventionist should be aware of this major limitation when deciding whether or not to stent a vein graft lesion.

Which stent to use

The development of stents is a rapidly evolving field. For this reason we will discuss only general concepts rather than specific stent designs. It is the author's view that the operator implants a stent for two reasons:

- to obtain vessel patency (no thrombosis);
- to maintain vessel patency over time (no restenosis).

Unless new information becomes available, these goals are accomplished with a 'mechanical rationale'. The stent is a mechanical tool which exerts its benefit by enlarging the lumen of the vessel. Within the limits set by nature (vessel size), the larger or the closer to normal the final lumen is, the more efficient the use of the device. This is opposed to the statement 'the bigger the better',[36] which had led people to think that the larger the lumen created, the better the outcome. Intravascular ultrasound (IVUS) evaluation following optimal stenting[37-44] has taught us that even with an optimal final result, frequently associated with an over-expanded segment, we never make the stent lumen larger than the proximal lumen and sometimes not even larger than the distal lumen. Therefore, the statement 'the bigger the better' should be corrected to be 'the closer the better'. This clarification is important because, most probably, the 'appropriate the better' and 'the bigger the better' are essentially saying the same thing and aiming at the same target. Returning to the goal we are looking for ('mechanical luminal optimization') we therefore choose among stents that give the best possible final lumen in comparable lesions. This need translates into more uniform gain as in a circle (best symmetry) and maintenance of the gain achieved quantified as minimal recoil (the implantation technique, an essential element in the achievement of the above goals, will be discussed later). The interventionist will evaluate among different stents designs and make the decision accordingly.

Other variables that come into play in this decision process are the availability of the appropriate stent length, possibility to reach the lesion with a specific chosen design and the amount of plaque coverage necessary. Concerning the latter, the author thinks that the tubular design is more appropriate for lesions with a large plaque mass. At what extent a specific stent design will affect outcome is not known. The author's experience has shown, through the analysis of matched lesions, that the Palmaz–Schatz stent gives a larger lumen (by IVUS) compared to the Gianturco–Roubin stent. Table 7.1 summarizes the angiographic parameters of the two matched groups of lesions; Table 7.2 summarizes the IVUS parameters. Note (Table 7.2) that the final IVUS cross-sectional area is significantly smaller for the lesions treated with the coil stent compared

to the ones treated with the slotted tubular stent. Plaque prolapse[45] and stent recoil are likely to account for this finding. At present, we do not know what is the clinical impact of this difference. In this particular series analyzed, the author found an angiographic restenosis rate of 24% for the Palmaz–Schatz group and 37% for the Gianturco–Roubin group ($p = $ ns). Despite the preliminary nature of these findings, and the fact that they originate from a retrospective observational study, we guide our current approach to 'preferentially' using a slotted tubular design in lesions with a large plaque mass where plaque prolapse and luminal optimization are the most important goals.

Table 7.1   Quantitative angiographic measurements.

Lesions	Group I n = 140	Group II n = 57	p value
Reference diameter (mm)			
Proximal	2.96 ± 0.26	3.01 ± 0.43	0.32
Mean	2.89 ± 0.27	2.87 ± 0.45	0.69
Preprocedure MLD (mm)	0.87 ± 0.39	0.87 ± 0.48	0.90
Preprocedure % stenosis	70 ± 14	69 ± 18	ns
Lesion length (mm)	9.96 ± 3.03	10.04 ± 4.71	0.88
Final balloon size (mm)	3.35 ± 0.38	3.29 ± 0.40	0.26
Final balloon/vessel ratio	1.14 ± 0.17	1.10 ± 0.14	0.12
Maximal inflation pressure (atm)	16 ± 3	16 ± 3	0.12
Poststent MLD (mm)	2.94 ± 0.40	2.76 ± 0.40	0.005
Poststent diameter stenosis (%)	−1.5 ± 14	4.4 ± 13	0.007

Notes:
Group I: Palmaz–Schatz stents; Group II: Gianturco–Roubin stents. Values are presented as means ± SD; MLD indicates minimal lumen diameter.

Table 7.2   Quantitative postprocedure IVUS measurements.

Lesions	Group I n = 105	Group II n = 47	p value
Proximal reference lumen CSA	8.02 ± 2.08	7.77 ± 2.32	0.53
Instent minimum lumen CSA	7.30 ± 1.70	6.25 ± 1.94	0.001
Distal reference lumen CSA	6.73 ± 2.33	5.97 ± 1.86	0.06

Notes:
Group I: Palmaz–Schatz stents; Group II: Gianturco–Roubin stents. Values are presented as means ± SD; CSA indicates cross-sectional area.

To summarize the author's view, the slotted tubular design is preferred in the following lesion subsets: aorto-ostial lesions, calcified lesions, chronic total occlusions, lesions with a large plaque mass and lesions located on saphenous vein grafts. The coil stent designs will be best used in lesions at bends, lesions involving the origin of multiple branches, dissections, lesions in tortuous vessels or in situations where rapid and predictable delivery is very important.

In the past few months we have seen the introduction of new designs which may outdate many statements. (Table 7.3 summarizes most of the available stents with their characteristics.) The miniCrown, a stent of the Palmaz–Schatz generation, has an improved flexibility and reaches optimal expansion around 3–3.25 mm in diameter. The 5 cells NIR stent follows the same concept of a less metal stent with optimal expansion at about 3 mm. These new designs may find a preferential application in medium to small-sized vessels where optimal radial strength is necessary at a small diameter. The GFX from AVE is a further refinement of the original Microstent design with a more flat wire design, elements 2 mm long and constituted by 6 crowns. This stent has unique flexibility, improved strength and lesion coverage compared to the previous microstent design. The former Cordis Tantalum coil stent has now been replaced by the Cordis Flex stent made of stainless steel. This stent maintains good flexibility and conformability with the addition of improved radial strength. A similar version with radial weldings is now being tested clinically. Only the future will show if these new designs will have an impact not only as friendly deliverable stents but also as stents able to guarantee a better final minimal lumen diameter (MLD). In addition, the issue of a possible lower vascular injury and a lower loss index with a specific design or metal is an interesting concept which so far has only been demonstrated in experimental models.[46,47]

How to stent

The following statement may sound simplistic but it cannot be stressed enough: stenting should be performed to gain the best possible lumen for a specific vessel.

Advantages of optimal dilatation

The achievement of a large final MLD sets a wide margin to compensate for late loss. A large final MLD improves the blood flow, decreases turbulences and limits stent occlusion.[48]

Disadvantages of optimal dilatation

Optimal dilatation is more time consuming and may require additional balloons and/or stents with an increase in cost. The increase in vessel trauma may induce more tissue proliferation.[49] This concept is mainly supported by animal research; clinical work in the field of stenting has not confirmed a higher loss index with aggressive dilatation. While it may be reasonable to assume that we will have the best loss index with no dilatation and the higher loss index with maximum dilatation, it is not practical and possibly dangerous (risk of thrombosis) to try to dilate at an intermediate level in order to minimize the trauma.

In order to provide data to clarify this issue the author analyzed experience by dividing the lesions in three groups according to different criteria:

- Group I: final dilatation at a pressure less than 16 atm with good final results by IVUS.
- Group II: final dilatation at a pressure higher than 16 atm without achievement of good final IVUS results.
- Group III: final dilatation at more than 16 atm with achievement of good final IVUS results.

Follow-up angiogram revealed a significantly higher restenosis rate in group II; groups I and III had a similar restenosis rate. The procedural data are summarized in Table 7.4. The preliminary conclusion from this retrospective evaluation is that restenosis rate is more influenced by the final results achieved than by the balloon pressure employed to achieve that result.

The role of IVUS

IVUS has opened the way to a new technique of coronary stenting.[39,41] Using IVUS on a routine basis, we have learned to look at the final angiographic result in a more critical way. The analysis of the lesion characteristics, the optimal balloon size, the final high-pressure inflation and the combined antiplatelet therapy with aspirin and ticlopidine have been the elements contributing to its final success. Large patient registries supplied data concerning the relative safety of using the above procedural approach without the need of IVUS evaluation.[50,51]

Two elements need to be kept in mind when evaluating the role of IVUS. First, the thrombosis rates in some subgroups, such as small vessels and stenting for threatened or acute closure, have been reported to be 10% and 6.67%, respectively. These values are higher than the 3% thrombosis rate found following stenting with IVUS guidance in vessels smaller than 3 mm.[5,52] Concerning stenting for acute closure and threatened closure, the authors did not find

Table 7.3   Available stents.

Name	Manufacturer	Structure	Material	Strut (wire) thickness (mm)	Metal/artery (%)	Recoil (%)	Fore-shortening (%)	Radiopacity	Markers	Lengths (mm)	Diameters (mm)
ACS multilink	ACS	Etched tube	Stainless steel	0.06	7–15	<5	3	Low	No	15	3.0: 3.25: 3.5
ACT one		Slotted tube	Nitinol	0.177	36	3–6	11	Moderate	No	7: 15	3.0–6.0
Angiostent	Angio-dynamics	Single wire, long spine	Platinum, iridium	0.127	10–1	7	12	High	No	15: 25: 35	3.0–6.0
AVE micro II	AVE	Wire crown	Stainless steel	0.15–0.20	8.5	8	Minimal	Moderate	No	6: 12: 18: 30: 39	2.5–3.0: 3.5–4.0
AVE GFX	AVE	Elliptorectangular	Stainless steel	0.127	21	4	Minimal	Moderate	No	8: 12: 18: 24: 30: 40	3.0–3.5: 4.0
BARD XT	BARD	Modular zigzag	Stainless steel	0.15	13–20	Minimal	None	Moderate	Yes	6: 11: 15: 19: 24: 30: 37	2.5–4.0
BeStent	InStent	Slotted tube	Stainless steel	0.075	12–18	Minimal	None	Low	Yes	15: 25: 35	3.0–5.5
DiVisio	Bio-compatibles	Interlocking arrowhead	Stainless steel	0.075	14	2	<2%	Low		8: 15: 28: 40	2.5–3.5*: 3.0–8.0*
COOK GR II	COOK	Coil and spine	Stainless steel	0.076	15–20	9–11	None	Low	Yes	20: 40	2.5–3.0: 3.5–4.0
Cordis	Cordis	Single sinusoidal helical coil	Tantalum	0.127	15	<10	10	High	No	15	3.0–3.5: 4.0
Cross Flex	Cordis	Single wire	Stainless steel	0.15	15	Minimal	5	Low	No	15	3.0–3.5: 4.0
Crown	J&J	Slotted tube	Stainless steel	0.069	17–20	2	5	Low	No	15: 22: 30	3.0–3.5: 4.0
Freedom	Global therapeutics	Single wire fishbone	Stainless steel	0.178	11–15	5–9	Minimal	Low	No	12: 16: 20: 24: 30: 40	2.5–4.5
NIR 7 CELL	Medinol	Cont. mult. design	Stainless steel			2	Minimal	Low	No	9: 16: 25: 32	2.0–3.5
NIR 9 CELL	Medinol	Cont. mult. design	Stainless steel	0.06–0.10	14–19	2	Minimal	Low	No	9: 16: 25: 32	3.0–5.0
Palmaz–Schatz	J&J	Slotted tube	Stainless steel	0.064	20	5	Minimal	Low	No	8: 9: 14: 18	3.0–5.0
PURA	DEVON	Slotted tube	Stainless steel	0.10	24	<1.9	3.14	Low	No	7: 15	3.0–5.0
PURA VARIO	DEVON	Slotted tube	Stainless steel	0.10	17–21	<2.5	3.14	Low	No	10: 16: 22: 28: 34: 40	3.0–5.0
WIKTOR	Medtronic	Single wire	Tantalum	0.13	8	9	4	High	No	16	3.0–3.5: 4.0–4.5
Wallstent	Schneider	Multiple wire braid	Elgiloy**	0.10	20	na	30	Moderate	No	15–45	4.0–6.0
TENSUM	Biotronic	Slotted tube	Tantalum	0.20	13	na	na	Good	No	14	3.0–4.0
IRIS	Uni-Cath	Slotted tube	Stainless steel	na	14	na	<10	Low	No	17: 27: 37	2.5–4.0

Notes:
*5-element structure for 2.5–3.5 mm and 6-element structure for 3.0–8.0 mm.
**Cobalt-based alloy.

Table 7.4   Analysis of lesions by group.

	≤16 atm	>16 atm (suboptimal)	>16 atm (optimal)	
Balloon diameter (mm)	3.6	3.7	3.4	$p < 0.05$
Maximum pressure (atm)	14	19	18.5	$p < 0.05$
Final angiogram (%)	26	41	29	*$p < 0.05$
IVUS CSA (mm^2)	8	5.7	7.6	*$p < 0.05$
Follow-up restenosis (%)	20	45	21	*$p < 0.005$
	692 lesions	90 lesions	399 lesions	

Note:
CSA = cross-sectional area.

this indication associated with increased risk of thrombosis when evaluating stenting in an IVUS-guided environment.[48] It may therefore be possible that the advantages of IVUS evaluation in reducing thrombosis rates may only be seen in particular subsets where the incidence of this complication is still high. Second, the restenosis rate is known to depend on the final result achieved.[36] It is therefore logical to assume that any approach which will improve the final result will have an impact in reducing the restenosis rate.

In the author's own database, the amount of further improvement obtained following IVUS subsequent to stent deployment with high-pressure optimal balloon size and visual angiographic evaluation is an increase of 33% in final cross-sectional area (CSA). According to the estimation of the risk of restenosis by the final IVUS CSA obtained from the analysis of the complete database (Fig. 7.1), we would expect a decrease in restenosis rate to the lower step in the histogram corresponding to a drop in restenosis of about 25%.

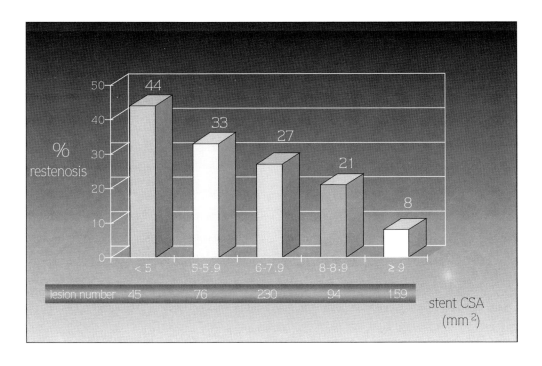

Figure 7.1
Estimated risk of angiographic restenosis by the final IVUS cross-sectional area achieved inside the stent.

It is interesting that when this concept was evaluated in two matched lesions populations (173 lesions in each group) from two institutions, we saw a cumulative restenosis rate by the traditional dichotomous 50% definition of 24% following high-pressure stent implantation without IVUS, versus 17% restenosis following stent implantation and IVUS evaluation ($p = $ ns). Due to the fact that this is a matched population of lesions it is possible that some types of lesions particularly at high risk of restenosis may have not found their match. This bias could have driven the restenosis rate in the high-pressure no-IVUS group to a lower number. Whatever the interpretation may be, the trend is presently reaching a statistical significance only by MLD analysis. By the dichotomous 50% criterion the total number of lesions should have been 800 to reach a statistical significance. IVUS evaluation maximizes the final MLD by telling us when a certain diameter has not been reached and by telling us when a vessel is bigger than its angiographic appearance. This latter situation is the one which cannot be corrected by any routine high-pressure approach.

Figure 7.2 shows a lesion in the proximal segment of a right coronary artery with an angiographic reference size of 2.78 mm. The IVUS evaluation of the corresponding reference size is 3.8–3.9 mm. We did not systematically analyze how frequent this angiographic/IVUS mismatch is present; however, this is another contributing factor which is most probably there more than expected.

We can conclude that the use of IVUS has not only led the way for adequate and optimal stenting but also continues to provide information contributing to the achievement of a larger final MLD. Appropriate questions to be asked are: is IVUS interrogation important in every lesion subset or only in some subsets? What is the role of preintervention IVUS?

The answer to this last question depends on the impact that lesion debulking will have on the long-term results of coronary stenting and, if positive, it may produce a significant change to our current practice of coronary stenting.

Full lesion coverage by the stent

The issue of full lesion coverage could end here, because no good answer has been provided so far. We initially proposed full dissection coverage and lesion coverage.[41] The major concern at that time was stent thrombosis and the main goal was blood-flow optimization. Restenosis was a secondary end-point. Now that the risk of subacute stent thrombosis has decreased, we can more quietly analyze the issue for the need of complete lesion coverage. The concept of full lesion coverage originates from two needs: 1) to avoid inflow and outflow obstruction in order to limit thrombosis; and 2) to limit edge dissections. Both these

needs act to limit stent thrombosis but not necessarily to limit restenosis. The influence of placement of a long stent to cover the entire disease segment, versus the focal treatment of the most critical segment on the restenosis rate, is unknown. The concept of focal treatment may well prove unpractical and risky. This is a major concern that has hampered the evaluation of this strategy. The question remains open and a careful study is probably needed to explore this area. Such a study will probably be possible when a truly nonthrombogenic stent becomes available. The lack of any intrinsic thrombogenicity may not require the complete elimination of any outflow and inflow restriction.

Plaque debulking prior to stenting

Appropriate stent expansion may not be achieved due to the presence of superficial vessel calcifications, limiting the dilating force of the balloon. This particular situation is, in the author's experience, present about 10% of the time. In these instances, the use of rotational atherectomy prior to stenting is important. We would like to call this type of debulking 'essential for optimal stent expansion'. Initial experience of utilizing rotational atherectomy prior to stenting calcified lesions has been quite positive. A total of 106 lesions in 75 patients have been treated with rotablator prior to stenting. What is important about this subset of lesions is that the final minimal intrastent CSA evaluated by IVUS met the criterion for adequate stent expansion (70% of the CSA of the balloon used and selected according to IVUS vessel size) in most of the lesions.

Follow-up angiography was obtained in 84% of the lesions with an angiographic restenosis rate of 22% by the dichotomous 50% criterion. The relative loss (0.34 ± 0.31) and the net gain index (0.35 ± 0.3) each accounted for approximately 50% of relative gain (0.68 ± 0.2), showing that this approach is not penalized by a greater late loss.

The initial conclusions are that debulking to allow optimal stent expansion in calcified lesions is an important adjunctive tool. It is also likely that any randomized study evaluating stenting with prior rotablation versus stenting without prior rotablation in calcified lesions will produce greater final MLD in the first strategy. It is also possible that a greater final MLD will have a positive impact on restenosis.

Another subset of lesions requiring debulking are lesions involving large bifurcations and ostial lesions, especially if the angle between the branching vessels is 90° or less. This approach is considered 'essential to prevent plaque shift'. If the lesion is not calcified, directional atherectomy is preferred because this technique will give a larger amount of plaque removal. A typical example where directional atherectomy is combined with double stenting is shown in Fig. 7.3.

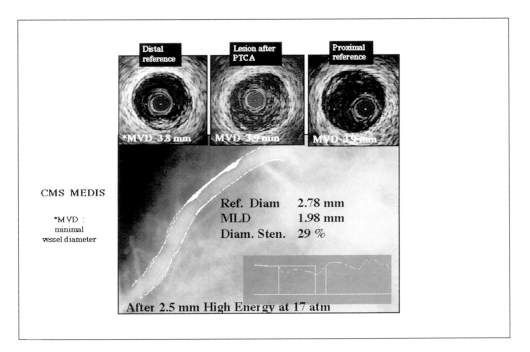

Figure 7.2
An example where the angiographic reference diameter is 2.78 mm, while the IVUS vessel diameter at the corresponding site is 3.9 mm.

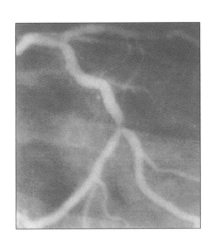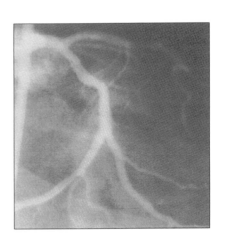

Atherectomy of both branches + NIR Medinol Scimed stents (inserted across each other)

Figure 7.3
An example of debulking prior to stenting considered important in order to minimize plaque shift.

Aside from these niche areas where debulking prior to stenting is important, the concept of the need for 'routine' debulking prior to stenting is a theoretical supposition which needs to be tested in dedicated trials (Fig. 7.4). Knowing the very good immediate and long-term results of stenting applied to focal lesions, it appears unlikely that debulking will prove to be effective in all lesion subsets. There are still a number of situations where stenting needs some help and where the evaluation of debulking prior to stenting will take place.

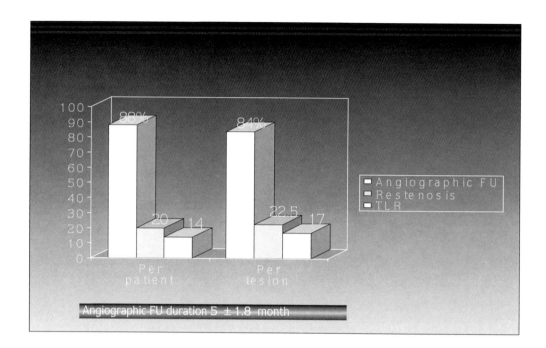

Figure 7.4
Angiographic restenosis rate and target lesion revascularization in 106 lesions in 75 consecutive patients treated with rotational atherectomy prior to stenting.

Before closing this issue on debulking it is important to clarify that debulking is not a dichotomous event. This means that minimal debulking may be as ineffective as no debulking. Any study aimed to evaluate this concept will need to quantify, probably by IVUS, the amount of plaque removal that took place.

Conclusions

The technique of optimal stenting gives the best results by combining information from lesion selection, stent selection and techniques of implantation. It would be naive to assume that good long-term clinical results could be obtained in a variety of lesion subsets without paying maximal attention to the different details in these three areas.

References

1   Fischman DL, Leon MB, Baim D, et al. A randomized comparison of coronary stent placement and balloon angioplasty in the treatment of coronary artery disease. N Engl J Med 1994; **331**: 496–501.

2   Serruys PW, de Jaegere P, Kiemeneij F, et al. A comparison of balloon expandable stent implantation with balloon angioplasty in patients with coronary artery disease. N Engl J Med 1994; **331**: 489–95.

3   Serruys PW, Emanuelsson H, van der Giessen W, et al. Heparin-coated Palmaz–Schatz stents in human coronary arteries. Early outcome of the Benestent-II Pilot Study. Circulation 1996; **93**: 412–22.

4   Colombo A, Ferraro M, Itoh A, et al. Results of coronary stenting for restenosis. J Am Coll Cardiol 1996; **28**: 830–6.

5   Stone GW, Linnemeier TJ, Frey A, et al. Incidence and implications of coronary dissection after PTCA using oversized balloons with intravascular ultrasound guidance—the CLOUT trial. Circulation 1996; **94**: I-261 (abstract).

6   Colombo A, Goldberg SL, Almagor Y, et al. A novel strategy for stent deployment in the treatment of acute or threatened closure complicating balloon coronary angioplasty. Use of short or standard (or both) single or multiple Palmaz-Schatz stents. J Am Coll Cardiol 1993; **22**: 1887–91.

7   de Feyter PJ, Ruygrok PN. Coronary intervention: risk stratification and management of abrupt coronary occlusion. Eur Heart J 1995; **16 (Suppl L)**: 97–103.

8   George B, Voorhees W, Roubin G, et al. Multicenter investigation of coronary stenting to treat acute or treated closure after percutaneous transluminal coronary angioplasty: clinical and angiographic outcomes. J Am Coll Cardiol 1993; **22**: 135–43.

9   Hall P, Colombo A, Itoh A, et al. Gianturco–Roubin implantation in small vessels without anticoagulation. Circulation 1995; **92**: I-795 (abstract).

10 Eeckhout E, Kappenberger L, Goy JJ. Stents for intracoronary placement: current status and future directions. J Am Coll Cardiol 1996; **27**: 757–65.

11   Hiroyoshi Y, Nobuyoshi M, Nosaka H, *et al*. Coronary stenting for long lesions (lesion length >20 mm) in native coronary arteries: comparison of three different types of stent. *Circulation* 1996; **94**: I-685 (abstract).

12   Pulsipher MW, Baker WA, Sawchak SR, *et al*. Outcomes in patients treated with multiple coronary stents. *Circulation* 1996; **94**: I-332 (abstract).

13   Maiello L, Hall P, Nakamura S, *et al*. Results of stent implantation for diffuse coronary disease assisted by intravascular ultrasound. *J Am Coll Cardiol* 1995; **25**: 156A (abstract).

14   Ozaki Y, Violaris AG, Hamburger J, *et al*. Short- and long-term clinical and quantitative angiographic results with the new, less shortening wallstent for vessel reconstruction in chronic total occlusion: a quantitative angiographic study. *J Am Coll Cardiol* 1996; **28**: 354–60.

15   Bourassa MG, Lesperance J, Eastwood C, *et al*. Clinical, physiologic, anatomic and procedural factors predictive of restenosis after percutaneous transluminal coronary angioplasty. *J Am Coll Cardiol* 1991; **18**: 368–76.

16   Hirshfeld JW jr, Schwartz JS, Jugo R, *et al*. Restenosis after coronary angioplasty: a multivariate statistical model to relate lesion and procedure variables to restenosis. *J Am Coll Cardiol* 1991; **18**: 647–56.

17   Cohen DJ, Breall JA, Ho KKL, *et al*. Evaluating the potential cost-effectiveness of stenting as a treatment for symptomatic single-vessel coronary disease. Use of a decision-analytic model. *Circulation* 1994; **89**: 1859–74.

18   Topol E, Ellis S, Fischman, J, *et al*. Multicenter study of percutaneous transluminal angioplasty for right coronary artery ostial stenosis. *J Am Coll Cardiol* 1987; **9**: 1214–18.

19   Mathias DW, Mooney JF, Lange HW, *et al*. Frequency of success and complications of coronary angioplasty of a stenosis at the ostium of a branch vessel. *Am J Cardiol* 1991; **67**: 491–5.

20   Rechavia E, Litvack F, Macko G, Eigler NL. Stent implantation of saphenous vein graft aorto-ostial lesions in patients with unstable ischemic syndromes: immediate angiographic results and long-term clinical outcome. *J Am Coll Cardiol* 1995; **25**: 866–70.

21   Zampieri P, Colombo A, Almagor Y, *et al*. Results of coronary stenting of ostial lesions. *Am J Cardiol* 1994; **73**: 901–3.

22   Myler RK, Shaw RE, Stertzer SH, *et al*. Lesion morphology and coronary angioplasty: current experience and analysis. *J Am Coll Cardiol* 1992; **19**: 1641–52.

23   Pan M, Medina A, Suarez de Lezo J, *et al*. Follow-up patency of side branches covered by intracoronary Palmaz–Schatz stents. *Am Heart J* 1995; **129**: 436–40.

24   Nakamura S, Hall P, Maiello L, Colombo A. Techniques for Palmaz–Schatz stent deployment in lesions with a large side branch. *Cathet Cardiovasc Diagn* 1995; **34**: 353–61.

25   Spokojny AM, Sanborn TA. The bifurcation lesion. In: Ellis SG, Holmes Dr. Jr, (eds), *Strategic Approaches in Coronary Intervention* (Baltimore, MD: Williams & Wilkins, 1996).

26   Puma JA, Sketch MH, Tcheng JE, *et al*. Percutaneous revascularization of chronic coronary occlusions: an overview. *J Am Coll Cardiol* 1995; **26**: 1–11.

27   Goldberg SL, Colombo A, Maiello L, *et al*. Intracoronary stent insertion after balloon angioplasty of chronic total occlusions. *J Am Coll Cardiol* 1995; **26**: 713–19.

28   Maiello L, Colombo A, Almagor Y, *et al*. Coronary stenting with a balloon expandable stent after the recanalization of chronic total occlusions. *Catch Cardiovasc Diagn* 1992; **25**: 293–6.

29   Sato Y, Nosaka H, Kimura T, Nobuyoshi M. Randomized comparison of balloon angioplasty versus coronary stent implantation for total occlusions. *J Am Coll Cardiol* 1996; **27**: 152A (abstract).

30   Thomas M, Hancock J, Holmberg S, Wainwright R, Jewitt D. Coronary stenting following successful angioplasty for total occlusions: preliminary results of a randomized trial. *J Am Coll Cardiol* 1996; **27**: 153A (abstract).

31   Per Simes A, Golf S, Myreng Y, *et al*. Stenting in chronic coronary occlusions (SICCO): a multicenter, randomized, controlled study. *J Am Coll Cardiol* 1996; **28**: 1444–51.

32   Rodriguez A, Fernandez M, Santaera O, *et al*. Coronary stenting in patients undergoing percutaneous transluminal coronary angioplasty during acute myocardial infarction. *Am J Cardiol* 1996; **77**: 685–9.

33   Wong SC, Baim DS, Schatz RA, *et al*. Immediate results and late outcome after stent implantation in saphenous vein graft lesions: the multicenter US Palmaz–Schatz stent experience. The Palmaz–Schatz Study Group. *J Am Coll Cardiol* 1995; **26**: 704–12.

34   de Jaegere P, van Domburg RT, de Feyter P, *et al*. Long-term clinical outcome after stent implantation in saphenous vein grafts. *J Am Coll Cardiol* 1996; **28**: 89–96.

35   Marco J, Fajadet J, Brunel P, *et al*. Anatomy reconstruction of native coronary arteries and vein grafts with the less shortening self-expandable wallstent. *J Am Coll Cardiol* 1996; **27**: 179A (abstract).

36   Kuntz R, Safian R, Carrozza J, *et al*. The importance of acute luminal diameter in determining restenosis after coronary atherectomy or stenting. *Circulation* 1992; **86**: 1827–35.

37   Tobis JM, Mallory J, Mahon D, *et al.* Intravascular ultrasound imaging of human coronary arteries *in vivo*: analysis of tissue characteristics with comparison to *in vitro* histologic specimens. *Circulation* 1991; **83**: 913–26.

38   Honye J, Mahon DJ, Jain A, *et al.* Morphological effects of coronary balloon angioplasty *in vivo* assessed by intravascular ultrasound imaging. *Circulation* 1992; **85**: 1012–25.

39   Nakamura S, Colombo A, Gaglione S, *et al.* Intracoronary ultrasound observations during stent implantation. *Circulation* 1994; **89**: 2026–34.

40   George G, Haude M, Ge J, Voegele E, *et al.* Intravascular ultrasound after low and high inflation pressure coronary artery stent implantation. *J Am Coll Cardiol* 1995; **26**: 725–30.

41   Colombo A, Hall P, Nakamura S, *et al.* Intracoronary stenting without anticoagulation accomplished with intravascular guidance. *Circulation* 1995; **91**: 1676–88.

42   Lee DY, Eigler N, Luo H, Nishioka T, *et al.* Effect of intracoronary ultrasound imaging on clinical decision making. *Am Heart J* 1995; **129**: 1084–93.

43   Hoffmann R, Mintz GS, Dussaillant GR, *et al.* Patterns and mechanisms of in-stent restenosis. A serial intravascular ultrasound study. *Circulation* 1996; **94**: 1247–54.

44   Colombo A, Hall P, Itoh A, *et al.* The optimal pressure for stent implantation. In: Sigwart U (Ed), *Endoluminal Stenting* (London: W.B. Saunders, 1996): 280–4.

45   Itoh A, Hall P, Moussa I, *et al.* Comparison of quantitative angiography and intravascular ultrasound after coronary stent implantation with 6 different stents. *Circulation* 1996; **94**: I-263 (abstract).

46   Rogers C, Edelman ER. Endovascular stent design dictates experimental restenosis and thrombosis. *Circulation* 1995; **91**: 2995–3001.

47   Sheth S, Litvach F, Dev V, *et al.* Subacute thrombosis and vascular injury resulting from slotted-tube nitinol and stainless steel stents in a rabbit carotid artery model. *Circulation* 1996; **94**: 1733–40.

48   Moussa I, Di Mario C, Di Francesco L, *et al.* Subacute stent thrombosis and the anticoagulation controversy: changes in drug therapy, operator technique, and the impact of intravascular ultrasound. *Am J Cardiol* 1996; **78 (suppl 3A)**: 13–17.

49   Schwartz RS, Murphy JG, Edwards WD, *et al.* Restenosis and the proportional neointimal response to coronary artery injury: results in a porcine model. *J Am Coll Cardiol* 1992; **19**: 267–74.

50   Goods CM, Al-Shaibi KF, Yadav SS, *et al.* Utilization of the coronary balloon-expandable coil stent without anticoagulation or intravascular ultrasound. *Circulation* 1996; **93**: 1803–8.

51   Karrillon GJ, Morice MC, Benveniste E, *et al.* Intracoronary stent implantation without ultrasound guidance and with replacement of conventional anticoagulation by antiplatelet therapy. 30-day clinical outcome of the French multicenter registry. *Circulation* 1996; **94**: 1519–27.

52   Hall P. Colombo A, Almagor Y, *et al.* Intravascular ultrasound guided coronary stenting of angiographic small vessels (< 3.0 mm). *J Am Coll Cardiol* 1994; **23**: 136A (abstract).

8

Functional design characteristics and clinical results with balloon-expandable and self-expanding stents

Rafael Beyar and Martin B Leon

Introduction: clinical trends with stents over a decade

The first coronary stents were implanted in patients in 1986 by Jacques Puel (Toulouse) and Ulrich Sigwart (Lausanne).[1,2] In these early cases stents were implanted for prevention of restenosis, despite the absence of animal studies indicating an anti-restenosis action. The first 5 years of stenting should be considered the 'learning curve' of the medical community in using the proper technique of stent deployment and administering the proper adjunct pharmacologic therapies. The first clinical experiences with the self-expanding Wallstent (Schneider [Europe] AG, Bülach, Switzerland) were under suboptimal anticoagulation treatment conditions and the complication rate of subacute thrombosis was as high as 20%.[3,4] Later, with more intense anticoagulation and the use of the Palmaz–Schatz (Cordis, a Johnson & Johnson Co, Warren NJ, USA)[5,6] and Gianturco–Roubin (Cook Inc, Bloomington IN, USA)[7] stents, the subacute thrombosis rate was reduced to 3–5%. An important boost to stenting came with the published evidence that the Gianturco–Roubin coil stent can be used effectively to treat acute and threatened occlusion and thus prevent the need for emergency surgery with associated high mortality and morbidity.[7] In addition, two major randomized trials[5,6] comparing primary stenting to balloon angioplasty in short lesions in native arteries, using the balloon expandable slotted-tube stent, showed a clear benefit in restenosis rate and late revascularization events at 6 months, thus establishing the concept of primary stenting for prevention of restenosis.

Two other recent factors have led to a dramatic progress in the field. First, intravascular ultrasound (IVUS) techniques have shown that the pressures routinely used to expand the Palmaz–Schatz stent (6–8 atm) were insufficient to appose completely the stent struts against the wall, and much higher pressures of 14–20 atm were required to result in complete apposition and full expansion of the stent.[8] This was recognized by Antonio Colombo and his colleagues as an important parameter in reducing subacute thrombosis, thereby obviating the need for anticoagulation.[9] The other major finding has been the introduction of a more potent antiplatelet agent, ticlopidine, as a short-term treatment (2–4 weeks) after stenting.[10,11] The use of ticlopidine in combination with aspirin, and without the use of anticoagulation, resulted in a reduction of the subacute thrombosis rate to 1.3% in the multicenter French registry.[10] Recently, randomized trials[12,13] confirmed this observation, showing that ticlopidine with aspirin is the most efficient treatment in preventing subacute thrombosis within stents. Today, the combination of high pressure dilatation within the stent, and the use of ticlopidine for 1 month or less have become the standard treatment after stenting, maintaining the subacute thrombosis rate as low as 1% and reducing the restenosis rate to 15–20% in the latest series of clinical stent trials.[14]

With the field of stenting rapidly growing—reaching 25–50% in most clinical interventional programs and even higher at some leading centers[15]—the spirited race for better stent designs has ensued. It is clear that none of the original stents were optimal under all clinical circumstances. The optimal stent should be delivered easily and safely to various locations in the coronary circulation; therefore, it should be flexible, low profile, and with smooth contours on the delivery system. In addition, the stent must sustain sufficient radial hoop stress in order to resist the external force by a hard calcified plaque that compresses centrally towards the lumen. Since the metal surface of the stent is in contact with the blood for the first 2–4 weeks after stenting and is in contact with the growing intimal proliferative tissue afterwards, blood and tissue compatibility are required. To some extent, each of the metal stents used today is thrombogenic and provokes some inflammatory response in the tissue. While it is clear that some metals (copper) provoke an intense proliferative response, it is not yet clear which metals may have the best biocompatibility in the clinical setting. The question as to whether or not there is an optimal surface treatment to make the stent more compatible with both blood and tissue is a major subject of research today. The purpose of this chapter is to address the fundamental characteristics of the many different stent designs that are in use today, and to introduce some of the more important clinical stent trials.

Mechanical principals of balloon-expandable stents

The family of balloon-expandable stents utilizes a balloon as the delivery system. The stent is either crimped on a dedicated balloon by the manufacturer or on a standard balloon by the operator. The stent is deployed by inflating the balloon which plastically deforms the metal stent. The metal has to be 'annealed' for that purpose, minimizing the elastic 'spring back' properties of the stent. Various metals have been used to construct such stents, such as stainless steel (316L), tantalum, platinum, nitinol in its martensite form, and others. All these stents have some level of 'spring back' (defined as free stent recoil) which ranges from 2–8%. This means that if the stent is dilated to a certain dimension, upon balloon deflation it will recoil from its maximum diameter by 2–8%. While this stent property, which depends on the individual metal properties and stent design, is defined independent of the vessel wall, it is clear that in diseased coronary arteries, stent recoil is also affected by the elastic properties of the vessel wall. Therefore, the recoil of the stent–artery complex is somewhat larger than the recoil of the free stent.

The family of balloon expandable stents can be further sub-classified into two other types:

- tubular, or multicellular stents which are primarily constructed in a tubular configuration with a pre-specified geometry allowing expansion from a compressed to an open pattern;
- coil stents, which are designed as a single wire or a combination of wires, looped or formed to create an endoluminal scaffold.

Mechanical principles of self-expanding stents

Self-expanding stents are composed of metals that are in the elastic or pseudoelastic range of deformation. Today, there are only a few stents in this family and they are comprised mainly of stainless steel or nitinol. These stents are withheld on a delivery system by a special restraining mechanism that is released as the stent is positioned across the lesion. Once the restraining mechanism is released, the stent self-expands using its spring-like properties towards its free diameter. As the stent touches the arterial wall, it reaches a balance of forces where its dimension is usually smaller than the free dimension. Since the metal is in its 'spring' form or pseudoelastic form for nitinol, it will continue to apply radial force on the wall after the stent has been deployed.

Current balloon-expandable stents in clinical use

Tables 8.1 and 8.2 detail the balloon-expandable stents in clinical use today. Table 8.1 lists the tubular, or multicellular, stents. These stents are usually constructed from a metal tube cut into a special design, which allows it to expand on the balloon. Note that a similar design to the slotted tube, initially introduced with the Palmaz stent series,[3] has also been adopted in the ACT-One nitinol stent (Progressive Angioplasty Systems Inc, Menlo Park CA, USA),[18] as well as the Tensum stent (Biotronik, Berlin, Germany).[19] While this design provides adequate scaffolding and radial strength, it is limited in its longitudinal flexibility, therefore, mandating the use of relatively short segments combined by flexible articulations. Spiral articulations have replaced the single articulation in the PS-153 (Cordis, a Johnson & Johnson Co) design in order to improve the scaffolding properties at the center of the stent.[16] The Crown stent (Cordis, a Johnson & Johnson Co)[16] is the recent version of the slotted tube design in which the slots are designed in a wavy pattern, therefore improving the longitudinal flexibility of the stent without impeding its scaffolding properties.

More recent designs such as the Multilink stent (Guidant/Advanced Cardiovascular Systems, Santa Clara CA, USA),[17] the NIR stent (Boston Scientific, Maple Grove MN, USA)[20] and the beStent (Medtronic InStent, Minneapolis MN, USA)[21] provide higher longitudinal flexibility than the standard tube design, with high scaffolding properties. A multicellular design is a common concept to all

Table 8.1 Balloon-expandable stents with tubular, multicellular designs

Stent	Manufacturer	Metal	Design	Radio-opacity	Coverage	Strut thickness	Lengths
PS-153[3]	J&J	SS 316L	slotted tube	+	<20%	0.065 mm	15 mm
Spiral art. (12 rows[16])	J&J	SS 316L	slotted tube	+ +	<20%	0.095 mm	8, 14, 18 mm
Crown[16]	J&J	SS 316L	wavy slots	+ +	<20%	0.07 mm	15, 19, 31 mm
Multilink[17]	ACS	SS 316 L	linked tubular wavy rings	+	<15%	0.05 mm	15, 25, 35 mm
GFX Micro III	AVE	SS 316L	linked 2 mm wavy segments	+ + +	<15%	0.13 mm	8–40 mm
ACT-One[18]	PAS	nitinol	slotted tube	+ + +	23%	0.18 mm	8, 17 mm
Tensum[19]	Biotronik	tantalum/ si-carbide	slotted tube	+ + + +	13%	0.08 mm	8.9–18.5 mm
NIR[20]	Medinol-Boston-Scientific	SS 316L	uniform multicellular	+ + + + + + (Gold plated)	11–18%	0.1 mm	9, 16, 32 mm
beStent[21]	InStent-Medtronic	SS 316L	serpentine, rotating junctions	+ + + + + (Gold markers)	11–18%	0.075 mm	8, 15, 25 mm

Table 8.2 Balloon-expandable stents with primary coil like design or zig-zag elements.

Stent	Manufacturer	Metal	Design	Radio-opacity	Coverage	Strut thickness	Lengths
GRI (GRII)[7,22]	Cook	SS 316L	single flat wire clamshell (longitudinal spine)	+ + (+ + + + Gold marker)	16%	round (flat) 0.13 mm	10, 20, 40 mm
Wiktor GX[23]	Medtronic	tantalum	single wire semi-helical coil	+ + + +	7–9%	0.127 mm	16 mm
Wiktor-i[24]	Medtronic	tantalum	dense weave	+ + + +	8–9.5%	0.127 mm	10, 20, 30 mm
Micro II[25]	AVE	SS 316L	linked repeated sinusoidal ring	+ +	8.4%	0.2 mm	12–29 mm
Cordis[26] (Crossflex)	Cordis, J&J	tantalum (SS 316L)	waved wire waved wire	+ + + + + +	15–18% 15–18%	0.127 mm 0.127 mm	18 mm 18 mm
AngioStent[27]	AngioDynamics	platinum-iridium	single helical wire with longitudinal spine	+ + + +	9.4–12.5%	0.127 mm	15, 25, 35 mm
Freedom[28]	Global	SS 316LVM	zig-zag fishscale	+ +	10.7–15.4%	0.177 mm	12–40 mm
STS[29]	Catholic University Leuven	SS 316L	single wire sinusoidal coil	+ +	5–15%	0.15–0.25 mm	12–60 mm
XT[30]	BARD	SS 316LVM	zig-zag modules on a spine	+ + +	–	0.15 mm (round)	6–37 mm

these stents. Upon expansion, some stents (NIR) become stiffer longitudinally due to their unique design.[20] The beStent gains its radial force from an orthogonal locking principle after the rotational junctions dissipate stress concentrations along the stent struts.[21] End markers delineate this stent allowing better X-ray visibility. In general, the multicellular designs combine the features of excellent scaffold-ing and longitudinal flexibility and enables the introduction of relatively long stents that were more difficult with the classical slotted tubular design. These features have expanded the horizons of stenting beyond simple and short lesions toward treatment of complex diffuse coronary diseases. The major tubular or multicellular stents are shown in Fig. 8.1.

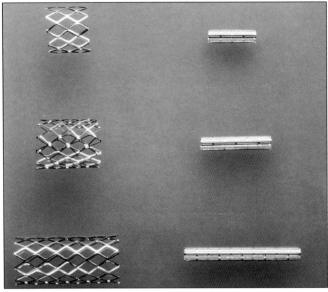

a

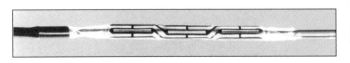

b

c

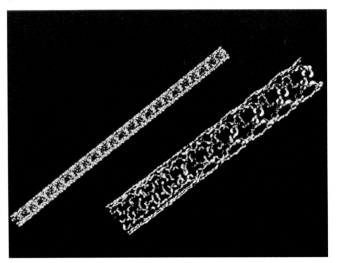

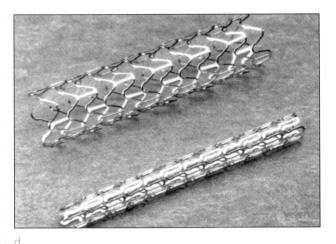

d

Figure 8.1

The common balloon-expandable stents with primarily tubular design. (a) The slotted tube, Palmaz stents. (b) The mounted Palmaz–Schatz stent with three elements connected with two spiral articulations. (c) The Crown stent. (d) The ACS Multilink stent before and after expansion. (e) The Biotronik Tensum stent, before and after expansion. (f) The expanded Act-One nitinol stent. (g) The mounted NIR stent. (h) The beStent at its unexpanded and balloon-expanded states.

e

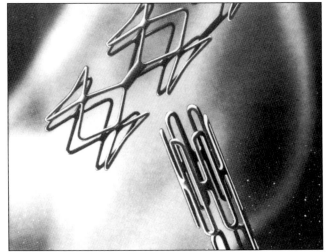

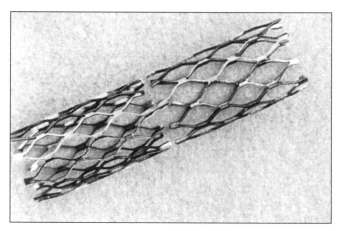

f

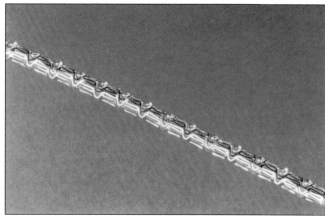

g

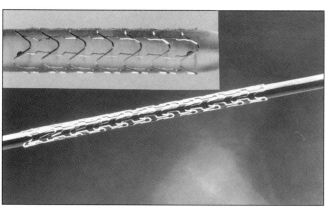

h

The major coil-like balloon-expandable stents are listed in Table 8.2 and are shown in Fig. 8.2. The GRII[22] is a flat wire version of the classical GRI with better scaffolding properties. A longitudinal backbone has been added to prevent stent deformation and end-markers were introduced to allow visibility of the stent margins. One of the perceived advantages of the coil stents over the tubular stents have been their longitudinal flexibility and better side branch patency. Other coil stents are made of wavy tantalum (Wiktor-GX) (Medtronic Interventional Vascular–Europe, Kerkrade, The Netherlands)[23] and its more dense version (Wiktor-i)[24] and the Cordis stent.[26] The different versions of the Microstent (Arterial Vascular Engineering Inc, Santa Rosa CA, USA)[25] which are made of welded zig-zag segments provide a highly flexible stent with scaffolding properties intermediate between the coil stents and the tubular multicellular stents. The Angiostent (Angio-Dynamics, Glen Falls NY, USA),[27] which is similar to the GRII stent with a longitudinal spine, is densely radio-opaque owing to its platinum–iridium composition. Single wire stents such as the Freedom (Global Therapeutics Inc, Broomfield CO, USA)[28] and the STS (Catholic University, Leuven, Belgium)[29] stents can be made in variable lengths because of their high flexibility. Finally, a unique design with a spine connected to wire segments characterizes the newly introduced XT stent (Bard Ireland Ltd, Galway, Ireland).

Current self-expanding stents in clinical use

The self-expanding stents in clinical trails are detailed in Table 8.3 and are shown in Fig. 8.3. The Wallstent[1] was the first stent implanted in humans and has undergone extensive modification over the past decade. The initial version, released by pulling a rolling membrane, has been

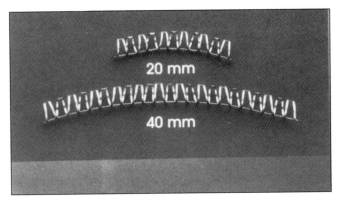

a

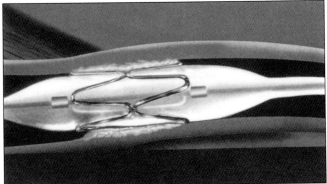

c

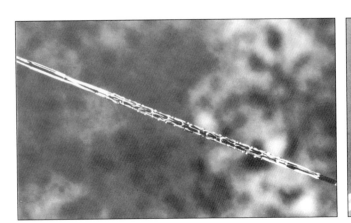

b

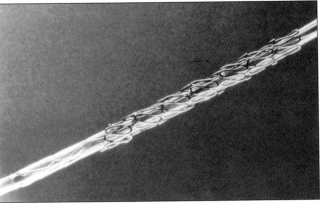

d

Figure 8.2
Balloon expandable stents with primarily coil or coil like design or zig-zag elements. (a) The Gianturco–Roubin II stent.
(b) The mounted Wiktor stent. (c) The AVE microstent with two connected zig-zag units. Multiple units can form long flexible stents.
(d) The AngioStent mounted on balloon.

Table 8.3 The self-expanding stents.

Stent	Manufacturer	Metal	Design	Radio-opacity	Coverage	Strut thickness	Lengths
Wallstent[1]	Schneider	SS 316L	double helical wire mesh	+ +	14%	0.08–0.1 mm	15–50 mm
Magic Wallstent[31]	Schneider	platinum with outer Cobalt alloy	double helical mesh	+ + +	14%	0.08–0.1 mm	15–50 mm
Radius[32]	SciMED	nitinol	linked zig-zag	+ +	20%	0.11 mm	14, 20, 30 mm
Cardiocoil[33]	InStent-Medtronic	nitinol	continuous coil	+ +	12–15%	0.12–0.18 mm	15, 20 mm

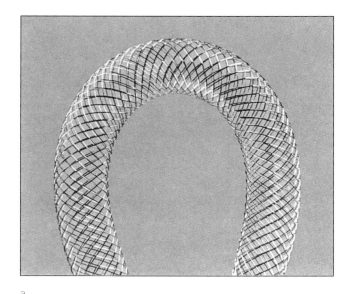

a

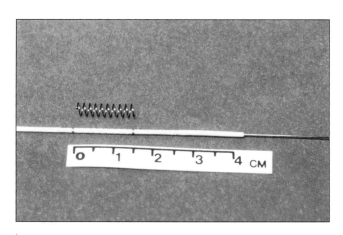

b

Figure 8.3
Self expanding stents. (a) The Wallstent. Note the extreme flexibility of this stent which is made of opposite interwoven helican stainless steel wires. (b) The Cardiocoil by InStent. The nitinol coil in its expanded configuration is shown adjacent to the delivery system with the two radio-opaque markers.

characterized by marked and sometimes unpredictable shortening of the stent, making it more difficult to position precisely. The latest versions, such as the Magic Wallstent,[31] have been made more radio-opaque by changing the metal and have been integrated with a better delivery system using a retracting sheath rather than a rolling membrane. This retracting sheath has the important property of recapturing the stent after partial deployment if the position requires further adjustment. In addition, the most recent

version of the Wallstent has been modified so that it shortens less upon expansion, a feature that improves the user-friendly aspects of the stent by allowing more accurate deployment to cover the lesion.

The Radius stent (SciMed Live Systems, Maple Grove MN, USA)[32] is a nitinol zig-zag linked design that is restrained by a plastic sheath and expands in units upon expansion. The Cardiocoil (Medtronic InStent, Minneapolis MN, USA)[33] is a nitinol continuous coil restrained on a delivery system by a release wire. Upon release of the wire the stent self-expands to its open configuration utilizing the pseudoelastic feature of nitinol, where martensite is transformed to austenite over a large strain range of up to 8%.

All of the self-expanding stents require a restraining system which is part of the stent delivery system. The restraining system is in the shape of a membrane or a plastic sheath in three of the stents, and in the form of a release wire for the Cardiocoil. The self-expanding stents are generally oversized relative to the reference artery size and will continue to apply chronic outward force against the wall over time.

Design parameters affecting short- and long-term performance

The exact relationship between stent design and clinical performance is currently under investigation. While mechanical aspects of stent design such as stent flexibility, ability to resist radial force, and scaffolding properties, are relatively easy to assess, the long-term performance of different stents in their ability to prevent restenosis is more difficult to study. The acute clinical performance of a stent is strictly dependent on its ability to be delivered to the lesion site (which depends on its profile, flexibility and the surface smoothness) and its ability to scaffold plaque effectively against the vessel wall, even in situations of excessive plaque bulk and calcified non-compliant lesions. With these properties there is a tradeoff between stent length and the ability to deliver. Delivery is affected by stent length; thus longer stents (especially tubular) are in general more difficult to deliver in tortuous arteries. Although, in general, coil stents are more flexible than tubular stents owing to inherent design differences, their scaffolding properties are inferior and the possibility of plaque herniation between the coils is more likely, which may influence late restenosis rates. This feature, including more 'open space', may be an advantage in the case when a vessel needs to be stented over a major side-branch. In this situation, coil stents are less likely to 'jail' the side-branch than tubular stents. Stent deformation has been attributed to some of the coil stents;

this problem has been partially solved by providing the stent with a longitudinal 'backbone' structure such as in the Angiostent, the GRII and the XT stent. The Microstent II has been recognized as one of the more flexible stents of the coil-like family, but provides angiographic results which are somewhat smoother and less corrugated than the classical coil stents.

The older slotted tubular design[3] required an articulating joint to provide the stent with reasonable flexibility over the two-segment 15-mm length. This articulating joint is a site of possible plaque herniation within the stent and may also be a common site for restenosis.[34] This problem is reduced in the newer multicellular, second generation designs such as the NIR, Crown, Multilink and beStent stents. Another important aspect of stent deliverability is the availability of a protecting membrane. The flexible Wallstent is capable of reaching tortuous locations, which is in part due to the presence of the smooth restraining sheath. The overall smoothness of the stent delivery system surface is sometimes more important than its profile in determining its ultimate delivery to the lesion site.

Stent thrombogenicity is an important feature of the stent that appears within hours and days after stent implantation. It is well-known that all current stent metals used are thrombogenic. It has not been shown that among the classical metals used for stenting, a particular metal is more or less thrombogenic than other metals in a clinical environment. However, it has been shown that the degree of smoothness of the stent surface (achieved by electropolishing) determines the amount of thrombus adhering to the stent,[35] which may in turn effect the intimal proliferative response.[36] In addition, it has been shown in an animal model that stent design may influence stent thrombogenicity.[37] By comparing the slotted tube design to the tubular corrugated ring flexible design in an animal model, it was shown that the latter leads to lower injury to the wall,[37,38] lower platelet accumulation[37] and less restenosis at three months.[38] This worthwhile study, together with another study[39] comparing the Palmaz, Strecker and Wallstent designs in canine iliac arteries, showed for the first time that stent design may determine the short- and long-term outcomes after stenting. The Strecker stent had the lowest mechanical strength resulting in greater immediate recoil and higher intimal growth than the other stents at four months. The slotted tube design had the least early recoil and the lowest late loss of these designs. The properties of wire crossing points and increasing stent profile were suggested as mechanisms of differing proliferative responses.

Since restenosis is multifactorial, it is not clear whether the above observations in animal models translate to similar differences in patients. Stent thrombogenicity may depend on multiple factors including stent surface characteristics, the amount of wall injury caused by stent deployment, as well as physical or mechanical interference with the flow field within the artery. It has been well-recognized[8,9] that in order to minimize thrombogenicity of a stent in patients, the single most important parameter is its adherence to the wall, which for the Palmaz–Schatz stent has been shown to occur at implantation pressures of 16 atm or higher.

The issue of optimal pressure for stent deployment remains controversial. The general rule of high pressure adjunct balloon dilatation, first appreciated by intravascular ultrasound (IVUS) examinations with the Palmaz–Schatz stent, has been considered the optimal method of deployment.[8,9] However, extrapolating this concept to all stent designs is problematic. It has been suggested for some of the new stents in the laboratory that optimal stent deployment may be achieved at much lower pressures, thus minimizing the risk of vessel trauma and distal dissections. Nevertheless, the optimal deployment pressure for each stent is as yet an unresolved issue, that will have to be answered in the future with well controlled clinical trials.

Stent visibility is another important factor, as the more visible the stent, the easier the procedure and the more accurate is stent placement. However, a very radio-opaque stent may interfere with the qualitative and quantitative measurements of stenting by angiography, both during inflation and during long-term assessment. Intermediate solutions have been considered to overcome this problem, such as thicker (more radio-opaque) metal for the AVE and ACT stent, stent markers for the GRII[22] and the beStent,[21] and gold-plating for the NIR-Royal stent.

Cross-sectional area metal coverage of a stent is another variable that ranges between values as low as 8% and as high as 23%. It has been felt that high metal content may be associated with high subacute thrombosis rates and possibly high restenosis rates. However, there are no clinical data either to support or to reject this hypothesis and it is currently thought that as long as the metal content is below a certain threshold, its effect is minor. The percent metal coverage by a stent is related to some extent to its scaffolding properties. Yet, the long-term proliferative response may also be determined by the metal coverage. In one study where a coil stent with different gap sizes was implanted in animal models, it was shown that the proliferative response is enhanced when no gaps are left between the coils.[40]

Comparative late clinical response of different stent designs is unknown. However, long-term data (3 and 5 years) in patients treated with Palmaz–Schatz and Wallstent stents have shown no tendency toward late deleterious pathobiologic responses.[41] It is possible that current studies in progress—randomly comparing different stent designs in patients—will show a difference in 6-month restenosis rates. Current data are inconclusive since different stents were tested in different lesion subsets. For example, the Wallstent was studied in longer lesions than the classical BENESTENT lesions and has shown a much higher proliferative response.[42] Current observations show

Table 8.4 Published and on-going studies with stents.

Topic	Acronym	Clinical subset	Design	Stent
CABG vs. stenting	ARTS	multivessel disease	randomized	Crown
	SOS	multivessel disease	randomized	various stents
Native, *de novo* lesions	STRESS[6]	stent vs. balloon; large vessels, short lesions	randomized	PS-153
	BENESTENT I[5]	stent vs. balloon; large vessels, short lesions	randomized	PS-153
	BENESTENT II[14,44]	stent vs. balloon; large vessels, short lesions	pilot registry/ randomized	heparin-coated PS-153
	START[52]	stent vs. balloon	randomized	PS-153
	WIDEST[53]	stent vs. balloon	randomized	Wiktor
	WISE	low vs. high pressure	randomized	Wiktor
	Tensum	stent vs. balloon	randomized	Tensum
Acute and threatened closure	GRACE[54]	acute closure	randomized	GRI
	TASC II[55]	stent vs. prolonged inflation	randomized	PS-153
	STENT-BY[56]	stent vs. balloon	randomized	PS-153
SVG disease	RAVES[46]	stent with reduced anticoagulation	registry	PS-153
	SAVED	stent vs. balloon	randomized	PS-153
	TECBEST	stent vs. TEC	randomized	PS-153
Chronic total occlusion	SPACTO	stent vs. balloon for total occlusions	randomized	Wiktor
	SICCO	stent vs. balloon	randomized	PS-153
	STOP	stent vs. balloon	randomized	AVE Microstent II/GRX
Restenosis after PTCA	REST[51]	stent vs. balloon	randomized	
	WIN	stent vs. balloon	randomized	Wallstent
In-stent restenosis	LARS	laser for stent restenosis	registry	any stent
Stent comparisons	GRII	native, *de novo* <30 mm	randomized	GRII vs. PS-153
	ASCENT	native, *de novo* vessels	randomized	Multilink vs. PS-153
	Wiktor	abrupt/threatened closure	registry	Wiktor
	Goy *et al.*[57]	abrupt closure	randomized	Wiktor vs. PS-153
	SMART	native, *de novo* <30 mm	randomized	Microstent vs. PS-153
	ACT-ONE	*de novo* lesions	randomized	ACT-I vs. PS-153
	SCORES	native, *de novo*/restenosis	randomized	Radius stent vs. PS-153
	NIRVANA	native, *de novo*/restenosis	randomized <30 mm	NIR stent vs. PS-153
	WINS	SVG disease	randomized	Wallstent vs. PS-153
New and old stent registries	ESSEX	European experience	open registry	Radius
	WEST I, II	short, *de novo* native arteries	registries	Multilink
	FINESS I, II	variable/short *de novo* in native arteries	registries	NIR
	LOBSTER		registry	Freedom/Global
	Cardiocoil/Pilot	suboptimal results	open registry	Cardiocoil
	ACT-UP	short, *de novo* in native arteries	registry	ACT-One
	ROSE	short, *de novo* in native arteries	registry	beStent

that long lesions are associated with higher restenosis rates, which are probably due to an increased proliferative response.[43] Therefore, some of the studies with the newer generation stents that allowed treatment of more complex lesions than with the older stent designs, paradoxically show higher restenosis rates. This is probably due to the longer and more complex lesion subsets.

The importance of surface characteristics

Surface characteristics of a stent have been shown to be a factor affecting the rate of platelet deposition on the wall and may have an important effect on late outcome after stenting.[36] Therefore, it is recognized that metallic surface modification may have an effect on two interrelated components of thrombosis, platelet adhesion and aggregation, and factor XII activation. Any method which inhibits absorption of protein on the stent should interact with the process of thrombosis by one or both of the above mechanisms. Surface modification of the mechanical aspects of the stent surface involves various processes of stent polishing to reduce the surface inhomogeneities, and therefore platelet adhesion. Other interactions with the physical properties of the surface may involve modification of the ionic charge, or coating of the stent with a thin film of a biocompatible material. Various modalities of stent coatings, including covalently bound heparin,[44] and polymer coatings which can be used for drug delivery are reviewed in other chapters of this book.[45]

Major clinical trials

Stent studies have formed the basis for the clinical use of stenting today. The landmark studies that had major impact on the current practice of stenting are those that have shown that stents reduce restenosis rate as compared to balloon angioplasty in native vessels larger than 3 mm with short *de novo* lesions.[5,6] Multiple other studies addressing different clinical questions are now underway. Although final conclusions will be derived after completion of these randomized clinical trials, it can also be suggested that stents are effective in the treatment of vein graft disease,[46,47] chronic total occlusions,[48] restenosis lesions, ostial disease, and possibly in revascularization during acute MI.[49-51] Many new stents that have been recently introduced are being used to test some other important questions such as the use of stents in long lesions and in small vessels. The US Food & Drug Administration (FDA) has triggered stent-to-stent comparisons that will answer an important unresolved question: are some stents different than others in their anti-restenosis or other effects?

The major clinical trials that have been completed or are in progress are summarized in Table 8.4. Important clinical trials in progress compare stenting vs. surgery for multivessel disease and relate to the question as to whether the aggressive use of stents for multivessel disease will be comparable to or better than surgery. These critical issues, together with new developments in modification of the biological response to stenting, may dramatically change our attitudes toward the treatment of ischemic heart disease over the coming years.

Conclusions

Stents are a breakthrough technology[58] that has emerged explosively over the last four years after an initial five years of uncertainty and learning experiences. Following the initial experience with the Wallstent, the pioneering stent studies using the Palmaz–Schatz stents and the Gianturco–Roubin stents have opened the field of stenting for innovative new designs, aimed at improving delivery, scaffolding and biocompatibility. This huge step forward, together with numerous studies and constant improvement in stent technology will continue to expand the scope of our ability to treat coronary artery disease in the catheterization laboratory. A necessary step forward is the modification of the biological response to stenting, which can be achieved by multiple methods including stent coatings,[4] adjunctive drug treatment,[10-13] molecular biology techniques[58] and, finally, radiation.[59-61] The latter has proven to be a very effective method in limiting intra-stent intimal proliferation in animals and humans, although long-term clinical studies must be conducted before definite conclusions can be drawn.

The breakthrough of stenting has made angioplasty predictable even for highly complex lesions, resulting in reduced restenosis and reduced early and late adverse clinical events. The proliferative response to stenting is still the Achilles heel, leading to restenosis in 15–25% of short lesions, and probably to higher values approaching 40–50% for long diffuse lesions. An effective and safe prevention of this proliferative response may be the next 'breakthrough' in this dynamic field of percutaneous revascularization.

References

1   Sigwart U, Puel J, Mirkovitch V, Joffre F, Kappenberger L. Intravascular stents to prevent occlusion and restenosis after transluminal angioplasty. *N Engl J Med* 1987; **316**: 701–706.

2   Puel J, Joffre F, Rousseau H, *et al.* Endo-protheses coronariennes and auto-expansives dans la preventions des

restenoses après angioplastie transluminale. *Arch Mal Coeur* 1987; **8**: 131–2.

3   Schatz RA, Baim DS, Leon M, *et al.* Clinical experience with the Palmaz–Schatz coronary stent. Initial results of a multicenter study. *Circulation* 1991; **83**: 148–61.

4   Serruys PW, Stauss BN, Beatt KJ, *et al.* Angiographic follow up after placement of a self expanding coronary artery stent. *N Engl J Med* 1991; **324**: 13–17.

5   Serruys PW, de Jagere P, Kiemeneij F, *et al.* for the Benestent Study Group. A comparison of balloon expandable stent implantation with balloon angioplasty in patients with coronary artery disease. *N Engl J Med* 1994; **331**: 489–95.

6   Fishman DL, Leon MB, Baim DS, *et al.* for the Stent Restenosis Study Investigators. A randomized comparison of coronary stent placement and balloon angioplasty in the treatment of coronary artery disease. *N Engl J Med* 1994; **331**: 496–501.

7   Roubin GS, Cannon AD, Agrawal SK, *et al.* Intracoronary stenting for acute or threatened closure complicating PTCA. *Circulation* 1992; **85**: 916–27.

8   Goldberg SL, Colombo A, Nakamura S, Almagor Y, Maiello L, Tobis JM. Benefit of intracoronary ultrasound in the development of the Palmaz–Schatz stents. *J Am Coll Cardiol* 1994; **24**: 996–1003.

9   Colombo A, Hall P, Nakamura S, *et al.* Intracoronary stenting without anticoagulation accomplished with intravascular ultrasound guidance. *Circulation* 1995; **91**: 1676–88.

10   Morice MC, Zemour G, Benveniste E, *et al.* Intracoronary stenting without coumadin: one month results of a French multicenter study. *Cath Cardiovasc Diag* 1995; **35**: 1–7.

11   Van Belle E, McFadden EP, Lablanche JM, Bauters C, Hamon M, Bertrand ME. Two-pronged antiplatelet therapy with aspirin and ticlopidine without systemic anticoagulation: an alternative therapeutic strategy after bailout stent implantation. *Coron Artery Dis* 1995; **6**: 341–5.

12   Hall P, Nakamura S, Maiello L, *et al.* A randomized comparison of combined ticlopidine and aspirin therapy versus aspirin therapy alone after successful intravascular stent implantation. *Circulation* 1996; **93**: 215–22.

13   Schomig A, Neumann FJ, Kastrati A. A randomized comparison of antiplatelet and anticoagulant therapy after the placement of coronary artery stents. *N Engl J Med* 1996; **334**: 1084–9.

14   Serruys PW, Emanuelsson H, van der Giessen W, *et al.* Heparin-coated Palmaz–Schatz stents in human coronary arteries. Early outcome of the Benestent-II pilot study. *Circulation* 1996; **93**: 412–22.

15   Meyer BJ, Meyar B, Bonzel T, *et al.* Interventional cardiology in Europe 1994. *Eur Heart J* 1996; **17**: 1318–28.

16   Schatz RA, Firth BG. The Palmaz–Schatz coronary stent: new developments. In: Serruys P (ed.). *Handbook of Coronary Stents* (London: Martin Dunitz, 1997): 23–34.

17   Priestley KA, Clague JR, Buller NP, Sigwart U. First clinical experience with a new, flexible low profile metallic stent and delivery system. *Eur Heart J* 1996; **17**: 434–44.

18   Litvack F, Mahrer K, Dev V, *et al.* Current status and potential applications of the HARTS removable stent. *J Interven Cardiol* 1994; **7**: 165–75.

19   Bonnier H, Koolen J, Schaldach M. The Tensum Biotronik coronary stent: In: Serruys P (ed.). *Handbook of Coronary Stents* (London: Martin Dunitz, 1997): 131–8.

20   Richter K, Almagor Y, Leon M. NIR stent, transforming geometry. In: Serruys P (ed.). *Handbook of Coronary Stents* (London: Martin Dunitz, 1997): 139–46.

21   Beyar R. The beStent. In: Serruys P (ed.). *Handbook of Coronary Stents* (London: Martin Dunitz, 1997): 153–63.

22   Roubin JS, Yadav JS. The Gianturco Roubin II (GRII) stent. In: Serruys P (ed.). *Handbook of Coronary Stents* (London: Martin Dunitz, 1997): 17–22.

23   White CJ, Ramee SR, Banks AK, *et al.* A new balloon-expandable tantalum coil stent: Angiographic patency and histology in an atherogenic swine model. *J Am Coll Cardiol* 1992; **19**: 870–6.

24   White CJ. The Wiktor-GX and Wiktor-i stents. In: Serruys P (ed.). *Handbook of Coronary Stents* (London: Martin Dunitz, 1997): 35–42.

25   Stertzer SH, Pomerantsev E. AVE Microstent-II. In: Serruys P (ed.). *Handbook of Coronary Stents* (London: Martin Dunitz, 1997): 43–51.

26   Ozaki Y, Keane D, Nobuyoshi M, Hamasaki N, Popma JJ, Serruys PW. Coronary lumen at six-month follow-up of a new radio-opaque Cordis tantalum stent using quantitative angiography and intracoronary ultrasound. *Am J Cardiol* 1995; **76**: 1135–43.

27   Hijazi ZM, Aronovitz MJ, Marx GR, Fulton DR. Successful placement and reexpansion of a new balloon expandable stent to maintain patency of the ductus arteriosus in a newborn and animal mode. *J Invas Cardiol* 1993; **5**: 351–7.

28   Chevalier B, Glatt B, Royer T. Coronary artery reconstruction with the Freedom™ stent. *Eur J Cardiol* 1997; in press.

29   De Scheerder I, Wilczek K, Wang K, Van Humbeek J, Piessens J. Experimental results and initial clinical experience with a home-made coronary stent. In: Sigwart U

(ed.). *Endoluminal Stenting* (London: WB Saunders, 1996): 238–42.

30 Rickards AF. The Bard XT coronary stent. In: Serruys P (ed.). *Handbook of Coronary Stents* (London: Martin Dunitz, 1997): 147–53.

31 Ruygrok P, de Feyter P. The coronary Wallstent. In: Serruys P (ed.). *Handbook of Coronary Stents* (London: Martin Dunitz, 1997): 3–16.

32 Gregoire J, van der Giessen WJ, Holmes DR jr, Schwartz RS. The SciMED self-expanding stent. In: Serruys P (ed.). *Handbook of Coronary Stents* (London: Martin Dunitz, 1997): 73–9.

33 Beyar R, Shofti R, Grenadier E, Henry M, Globerman O, Beyar M. Self expandable nitinol stent for cardiovascular applications: canine and human experience. *Cathet Cardiovasc Diagn* 1994; **32**: 162–70.

34 Dussaillant GR, Mintz GS, Pichard AD, *et al.* Small stent size and intimal hyperplasia contribute to restenosis: a volumetric intravascular ultrasound analysis. *J Am Coll Cardiol* 1995; **26**: 720–4

35 De Scheerder IK. Stent coating. *XVIII Congress of the Eur Soc Cardiology*, Birmingham, UK, August 25–29, 1996.

36 De Scheerder IK, Wilczek KL, Verbeken EV, *et al.* Biocompatibility of polymer-coated oversized metallic stents implanted in normal porcine coronary arteries. *Atherosclerosis* 1995; **114**: 105–14.

37 Rogers C, Karnovsky MJ, Edelman ER. Inhibition of experimental neointimal hyperplasia and thrombosis depends on the type of vascular injury and the site of drug administration. *Circulation* 1993; **88**: 1215–21.

38 Rogers C, Edelman ER. Endovascular stent design dictates experimental restenosis and thrombosis. *Circulation* 1995; **91**: 2995–3001.

39 Barth KH, Virmani R, Froelich J, *et al.* Paired comparison of vascular wall reactions to Palmaz stents, Strecker tantalum stents, and Wallstents in canine iliac and femoral arteries. *Circulation* 1996; **93**: 2161–9.

40 Tominaga R, Kambic HE, Emoto H, Harasaki H, Sutton C, Hollman J. Effects of design geometry of endovascular prostheses on stenosis rate in normal rabbits. *Am Heart J* 1992; **123**: 21–8.

41 Kimura T, Yokoi H, Nakagawa Y, *et al.* Three-year follow-up after implantation of metallic coronary artery stents. *N Engl J Med* 1996; **334**: 561–6.

42 Ozaki Y, Keane D, Ruygrok P, van der Giessen WJ, de Feyter P, Serruys PW. Six-month clinical and angiographic outcome of the new, less shortening Wallstent in native coronary arteries. *Circulation* 1996; **93**: 2114–20.

43 Lablanche J-M, Danchin N, Grollier G, *et al.* Factors predictive of restenosis after stent implantation managed by ticlopidine and aspirin. *Circulation* 1996; **94 (Suppl I)**: 1–256 (abstract).

44 Serruys PW, Emannuelson H, van der Giessen W, *et al.* Heparin coated Palmaz–Schatz stents in human coronary arteries. Early outcome of the Benestent II pilot study. *Circulation* 1996; **93**: 412–22.

45 Kostopoulos KG, Wang K, De Scheerder I. Local drug delivery with stents. In: Beyar R, Keren G, Serruys PW, Leon MB (eds). *Frontiers in Interventional Cardiology* (London: Martin Dunitz, 1997): 183–192.

46 Douglas JS, Savage MP, Bailey ST, *et al.* Randomized trial of coronary stent and balloon angioplasty in the treatment of saphenous vein graft stenosis. *J Am Coll Cardiol* 1996; in press.

47 Wong SC, Baim DS, Schatz RA, *et al.* Acute results and late outcomes after stent implantation in saphenous vein graft lesions: the multicenter USA Palmaz–Schatz stent experience. *J Am Coll Cardiol* 1995; **26**: 704–12.

48 Medina A, Melian F, Suarez de Lezo J, *et al.* Effectiveness of coronary stenting for the treatment of chronic total occlusion in angina pectoris. *Am J Cardiol* 1994; **73**: 1222–6.

49 Ahmad T, Webb JB, Carere RR, Dodek A. Coronary stenting for acute myocardial infarction. *Am J Cardiol* 1995; **76**: 70–73.

50 Tanvir A, Webb J, Carere R, Dodek A. Coronary stenting for acute myocardial infarction. *Am J Cardiol* 1995; **76**: 77–80.

51 Erbel R, Haude M, Höpp HW, *et al.* Restenosis Stent (REST)-study: randomised trial comparing stenting and balloon angioplasty for treatment of restenosis after balloon angioplasty. *J Am Coll Cardiol* 1996; **27**: 732–4 (abstract)

52 Masotti M, Serra, A, Fernández-Avilés F, *et al.* Stent versus angioplasty restenosis trail (START). Angiographic results at six-months follow-up. *Eur Heart J* 1996; **17**: 712 (abstract).

53 Foley JB, Brown RI, Penn RM. Thrombosis and restenosis after stenting in failed angioplasty: comparison with elective stenting. *Am Heart J* 1994; **128**: 12–20.

54 Keane DK, Roubin GS, Marco J, Fearnot N, Serruys PW. GRACE Gianturco–Roubin stent acute closure evaluation: substrate, challenges, and design of a randomized trial of bailout management. *J Interven Cardiol* 1994; **7**: 333–9.

55 Penn IM, Ricci DR, Brown RI, *et al.* Randomised study of stenting versus prolonged balloon dilatation in failed angio-

plasty: preliminary data from the trial of angioplasty and stents in Canada (TASC II). *Circulation* 1993; **88**: I-601 (abstract).

56   Haude M, Erbel R, Höpp HW, Heublein B, Sigmund M, Meyer J. STENT-BY study: a prospective randomised trial comparing immediate stenting versus conservative treatment strategies in abrupt vessel closure or symptomatic dissections during coronary balloon angioplasty. *Eur Heart J* 1996; **17**: 172–P965 (abstract).

57   Goy JJ, Eeckhout E, Vogt P, Stauffer JC, Kappenberger L. Emergency endoluminal stenting for abrupt closure following coronary angioplasty: a randomized comparison of the Wiktor and Palmaz–Schatz stents. *Cathet Cardiovasc Diagn* 1995; **34**: 128–32.

58   Dichek DA, Neville RF, Zweibel JA, Freeman SM, Leon MB, Anderson WF. Seeding of intravascular stents with genetically engineered endothelial cells. *Circulation* 1989; **80**: 1347–53.

59   Hehrlein C, Gollan C, Donges K, *et al.* Low-dose radioactive endovascular stents prevents smooth muscle cell proliferation and neointimal hyperplasia in rabbits. *Circulation* 1995; **92**: 1570–5.

60   King SB III. Radiation for restenosis: an overview. In: Beyar R, Keren G, Serruys PW, Leon MB (eds). *Frontiers in Interventional Cardiology* (London: Martin Dunitz, 1997): 135–39.

61   Waksman R. Intracoronary radiation: does it really work? In: Beyar R, Keren G, Serruys PW, Leon MB (eds). *Frontiers in Interventional Cardiology* (London: Martin Dunitz, 1997): 141–50.

9

Seven years of coronary stenting: evolution of therapeutics, techniques and results

Jean Marco and Jean Fajadet

Introduction

Dotter and Judkins were the first, in 1964, to propose stenting as a new technique for transluminal treatment of an arteriosclerotic obstruction.[1] Since the first implantation of a coronary stent, performed by Puel in 1986,[2] stenting has been proposed for the treatment of coronary dissections,[3,4] acute or threatened closure[5] and prevention of restenosis after coronary angioplasty.[6–8] Promising results were reported using different stents: Palmaz–Schatz stents,[6,7] Wallstent,[2,3] Gianturco–Roubin Flex stent[5] and the Wiktor stent,[8] each with its own particular design. Despite aggressive anticoagulation therapy, leading to bleeding and vascular access complications, subacute stent thrombosis emerged as a serious complication with a wide variation, from 4.3 to 27.5%, related to different stent indications.[9–13] Predicting factors of subacute stent thrombosis have been reported to be multiple stents, proximal or distal dissections uncovered by the stent, poor inflow or outflow, arterial diameter of less than 3.0 mm, bail-out implantation, and impaired left ventricular ejection fraction.[14–17] Despite more careful selection of patients and more closely controlled anticoagulation,[13] the rate of subacute thrombosis remained unacceptable, suggesting that coumadin and aspirin were ineffective in preventing thrombus formation at the site of stent implantation.

Colombo et al.[18] pointed out that the key issue in the prevention of subacute thrombosis was the optimization of stent deployment, in order to ensure a normal rheology inside the stent as well as its inflow and outflow, and not aggressive anticoagulation therapy. Intravascular imaging showed that incomplete stent apposition, persistence of residual luminal narrowing and the presence of significant disease of the proximal and distal reference segment could not be detected with angiography.[19] These observations prompted Colombo et al.[18] to propose a strategy based on high-pressure dilatation in order to obtain optimal stent deployment.

In parallel, a new anticoagulation protocol was initiated in France by Morice et al.[20] In a prospective multicenter study, patients receiving coronary stents were treated with ticlopidine-aspirin-heparin for 2–3 days and low molecular weight heparin for 1 month, without coumadin; this new treatment resulted in a 1.3% subacute thrombosis rate.

In Clinic Pasteur, we implanted the first Palmaz–Schatz coronary stent in March 1989 and, between March 1989 and 1 December 1996, stents were implanted in 3509 patients. During this 7-year period, anticoagulation, antiplatelet therapy, implantation techniques, optimization of stent deployment and type of stents implanted have progressively and prospectively developed over four different stages. We report this experience and the influence of different changes in preventive treatment and techniques on the major complications occurring during the first month following stent implantation.

Methods and patients
Methods

The four stages of therapy, techniques and stent used are detailed below.

Stage I: 752 patients – March 1989 to July 1993

This period included the learning curve in coronary stenting (four interventional cardiologists) with mistakes in patients' selection and techniques.

The anticoagulation and antiplatelet regimen consisted of the following:

- Aspirin 250 mg/day at least 2 days before stenting.

- A bolus of 15 000 units of heparin and a dextran drop (100 cc/hr) during the procedure.

- Immediately after the procedure, aspirin 250 mg/day + dipyridamole 75 mg t.i.d. and dextran 100 cc/hr for 24 hr; a heparin infusion for 5 days, with a drip adapted in order to maintain activated partial thromboplastin time (PTT) between 60 to 90 sec, followed by subcutaneous heparin 12 500 units b.i.d., and coumadin started on Day-1 (dose adapted to obtain international normalized ratio (INR) between 3.5 and 4.5 before discharge).

- At discharge, aspirin 250 mg/days + dipyridamole 75 mg t.i.d., subcutaneous heparin 12 500 units b.i.d. for 7 days, and coumadin for 2 months.

Of the 6125 percutaneous transluminal coronary angioplasty (PTCA) procedures performed, stents were implanted in 752 patients (12.3%). Palmaz–Schatz stents (Cordis, a Johnson & Johnson Co, Warren NJ, USA), manually crimped on the balloon or premounted with the sheath delivery systems were implanted in 645 patients, and Gianturco–Roubin Flex stents (Cook Inc, Bloomington IN, USA) were implanted in 107 patients. Stents were delivered with a balloon using an inflation pressure of 6–10 atm.

Stage II: 553 patients – July 1993 to December 1994

In order to achieve optimal stent deployment in all patients, high-pressure balloon inflations were performed using a noncompliant or semicompliant balloon, inflated up to 16 atm, with a ratio of balloon diameter/vessel diameter of 1.1/1.

Ticlopidine was introduced and subacute thrombosis preventive treatment was as follows:

- At least 2 days before coronary stenting, aspirin 250 mg/day and, if planned, ticlopidine 250 mg b.i.d.

- During the procedure, a bolus of 15 000 units of heparin.

- After the procedure, aspirin 250 mg/day—ticlopidine 250 mg b.i.d., heparin infusion with a drip adapted in order to maintain PTT between 60 to 90 sec for 2 days, low molecular weight heparin (100 UI/kg antiXa b.i.d.).

- At discharge, aspirin (250 mg/day) + ticlopidine (250 mg b.i.d.) for 1 month, and low molecular weight heparin (LMWH 100 UI/kg b.i.d.) for 15 days.

Of the 2545 PTCA procedures performed, stents were implanted in 553 (20%): 383 patients received at least one Palmaz–Schatz stent (Cordis, a Johnson & Johnson Co.) manually crimped on the balloon and 107 patients received Gianturco–Roubin Flex stents (Cook Inc.). The transfemoral approach was most frequently used (8–9F), removing the sheath 6–8 hours after the bolus of heparin (PTT less than 90 seconds). We started the transradial approach in February 1994.

Stage III: 1087 patients – January 1995 to December 1995

The prospective changes were as follows: for all the procedures, we validated the delineation of the angiographic contours and final results with the digital angiographic system and quantitative coronary angiography (QCA) on-line (Phillips Medical Systems, Best, The Netherlands). Automated edge detection in multiple view after stenting was used to detect the persistence of residual stenosis. We tried to achieve a final vessel lumen of uniform caliber in the stented segments with repeated high-pressure inflation of a non- or semicompliant balloon, matching the size of an angiographically normal segment to obtain a final result as perfect as possible, with residual stenosis lower than 5%. Low molecular weight heparin (LMWH) was only used in patients considered as 'high-risk', i.e. long dissection not correctly covered by the stents, reconstruction of the left main and long degenerated saphenous vein grafts.

The anticoagulation and antiplatelet regimen consisted of the following:

- At least 2 days before coronary stenting, aspirin 250 mg/day and ticlopidine 250 mg b.i.d. (except in case of emergency or nonplanned PTCA).

- A bolus of 10 000 units of heparin during the procedure.

- After the procedure, aspirin 250 mg/day and ticlopidine 250 mg b.i.d. (500 mg administered immediately after the procedure in case of emergency or nonplanned PTCA), and LMWH (100 UI/kg antiXa b.i.d. for 5 days) only in 'high risk' patients.

Patients were discharged on Day-2 with aspirin 100 mg/day and ticlopidine 250 mg b.i.d. for 1 month.

Of the 2014 PTCA procedures performed, stents were implanted in 1087 (54%). The stents used were Palmaz–Schatz stents manually crimped on the balloon in 556 patients, Gianturco–Roubin Flex stents in 430 patients, and Less-Shortening Wallstent (Schneider [Europe] AG, Bülach, Switzerland) in 101 patients.

QCA on-line was determined before and after stenting in all patients. Whatever the type of stent, we recrossed the stent with a semicompliant balloon catheter inflated up to 15 atm with a final ratio balloon diameter/maximum vessel diameter of 1.1.

The transfemoral approach was used in 64% of the cases and the transradial (6F) in 34%.

Stage IV: 1117 patients – January 1996 to December 1996

We adapted the dose of heparin during the procedure according to body weight (100 units/kg) and used a new generation of stents, with lesion-specific selection of the type of stents.

The anticoagulation and antiplatelet regimen consisted of the following:

- At least three days before coronary stenting: 250 mg/day and ticlopidine 250 mg b.i.d. (except in case of emergency or nonplanned PTCA).

- Immediately before the procedure, an initial bolus of Heparin (100 units/kg of weight), with activated clotting time (ACT) controlled during the procedure (Hemocron, Medtronic, California, USA), maintained between 250 and 300 sec, with adjunctive bolus (2500 units) if needed.

- After the procedure: aspirin 250 mg/day, ticlopidine 250 mg b.i.d. (500 mg administered immediately after the procedure in case of emergency or nonplanned PTCA).

Low molecular weight heparin (100 UI/kg antiXa b.i.d. for 3 days) was used only in 'high risk' patients.

Of the 2077 PTCA procedures, 1477 stents were implanted in 1117 patients (54%): Gianturco–Roubin I and II Flex stents = 583, NIR = 386, Palmaz–Schatz stents = 238 stents (manually crimped = 121, Power Grip = 117), Less-Shortening Wallstent = 116, ACS = 81 and other stents (Wiktor: 45, In-stents: 25, AVE: 17) = 87.

The high-pressure technique after stent deployment and optimization of the final stent deployment by on-line QCA in order to obtain a final result with near 0% residual stenosis was applied for all types of stent. The transfemoral approach was used in 46% of the cases and the transradial in 54%.

Data collection

All demographic, clinical, angiographic, procedural and post-procedural data were collected prospectively on standard forms and entered into a computerized database. Data were summarized as mean ± SD value as continuous variables and frequencies for the categorical variables. One month follow-up information has been obtained by the referring physician or patient phone calls.

We analyzed the in-hospital major adverse cardiac events, bleeding and vascular access complications, and subacute thrombosis rate occurring during the first 28 days following stent implantation, period of time considered as required for re-endothelization, formation of new intima and disappearance of initial platelet and fibrin thrombi that cover the struts of the stent.

Successful stenting was defined by correct placement of the stent, TIMI III flow and residual stenosis of less than 10%, with no distal embolism, no major side-branch occlusion and no other major complications.

Major adverse cardiac events after stenting included deaths (all deaths irrespective of cause), acute myocardial infarction (MI) with or without Q-waves and coronary artery bypass grafting (CABG). MI was defined as the development of new pathological Q-waves (>30 msec) and/or creatine kinase (CK) elevation twice the upper normal limit, with elevated MB fraction.

Proven or suspected subacute thrombotic occlusion was defined as angiographically proven or clinically suspected occlusion occurring during the first month after stent implantation. For complicated cases in whom angiographic control of the stented artery could not be performed, subacute occlusion was defined as sudden death, clinical symptoms of prolonged chest pain with ST elevation and new Q-waves, with or without CK elevation.

Vascular access and bleeding complications included major hematoma requiring transfusion or surgical repair, pseudoaneurysm larger than 1 cm or arteriovenous fistula diagnosed by echo-Doppler, gastrointestinal bleeding, hematuria or any other significant bleeding requiring transfusion.

Clinical and angiographic data of the patients and stents implanted

The ratio of stent implantation to PTCA procedure progressively increased from 12.3% during stage I of our experience to 54% during stage IV (Table 9.1).

The clinical and angiographic data of the patients according to the different stage and type of stent are summarized in Tables 9.2–9.5. There were no differences in demographic and clinical presentations of the patients treated; the rate of patients with three-vessel disease increased from stage I to III–IV and type-C lesions were more frequent in the Gianturco–Roubin Flex stent subgroup in stage I and II, but more frequent in the Wallstent and Gianturco–Roubin subgroup in stage IV.

The distribution of attempted vessels was similar (Table 9.4) except for an increase of left main coronary stenting. Diseased saphenous vein grafts represents 30% and 28% of Wallstent implantation in stages III and IV, respectively.

Table 9.1 Ratio of stenting to total PTCA procedures.

	Stage I	Stage II	Stage III	Stage IV
PTCA	6125	2545	2014	2077
Stenting	752	553	1087	1117
Ratio	12.3%	20%	54%	54%

Table 9.2 Clinical characteristics.

| | Stage I | | Stage II | | Stage III | | | Stage IV | | | |
	PS n=645	GR n=107	PS n=383	GR n=170	PS n=556	GR n=430	WS n=101	GR n=583	PS n=238	NTR n=386	WS n=116
Age (years)	59.5±9.3	57.0±10.6	61.8±10.5	61.6±10.6	61.8±10	64.6±10	64.4±10	64.7±11.4	61.8±10	62.7±11.2	64.0±96
	(30–82)	(27–83)	(29–83)	(35–90)	(39–84)	(33–88)	(34–85)				
Stable angina	28%	25%	23%	16%	24%	24%	26%	40%	47%	38%	34%
Unstable angina	65%	58%	64%	65%	60%	60%	59%	45%	33%	46%	46%
Recent MI (<15d)	9%	12%	13%	14%	16%	16%	15%	15%	20%	18%	20%

Notes:

PS = Palmaz–Schatz, GR = Gianturco–Roubin, WS = Wallstent, NIR = NIR stent.

Table 9.3 Angiographic data (%).

| | Stage I | | Stage II | | Stage III | | | Stage IV | | | |
	PS	GR	PS	GR	PS	GR	WS	GR	PS	NTR	WS
LVEF	57.0±9.6	56.0±8.8	59.2±12.4	57.5±11	57.1±11	61.2±12.1	56.9±12.6	56.0±8.8	57.0±9.6	57.5±11	59.2±12.4
	(20–88)	(25–70)	(15–85)	(17–85)	(30–80)	(35–80)	(20–85)				
Type											
A	26%	8%	29%	5%	6%	2%	2%	1%	62%	13%	2%
B	58%	49%	46%	46%	47%	44%	12%	70%	4%	66%	62%
C	18%	43%	25%	49%	47%	54%	86%	29%	34%	21%	36%
1VD	46%	37%	31%	27%	22%	23%	23%	24%	30%	35%	16%
2VD	31%	36%	29%	34%	20%	24%	21%	32%	35%	36%	28%
3VD	23%	27%	40%	39%	48%	53%	56%	44%	35%	29%	56%

Notes:

$p = 0.006$ (GR); $p < 0.0001$ (PS).

PS = Palmaz–Schatz, GR = Gianturco–Roubin, WS = Wallstent, NIR = NIR stent, VD = vessel disease.

Table 9.4 Attempted stenting of vessels (%).

		Stage I		*Stage II*		*Stage III*		*Stage IV*			
PS	*GR*	*PS*	*GR*	*PS*	*GR*	*WS*	*GR*	*PS*	*NIR*	*WS*	
LAD	41	47	36	46	41	55	21	53	36	40	12
Lcx	15	16	15	20	16	15	13	20	18	17	12
RCA	32	34	35	31	33	21	41	23	38	40	48
LM	1	3	3	1	4	9	0	4	2	10	
SVG	11	0.0	11	2	6	0	34	0.5	6	2	28

Notes
LAD=left anterior descending;
Lcx=left circumflex
RCA=right coronary artery;
LM=left main;
SVG=saphenous vein graft.

Table 9.5 Stenting indications (%).

	Stage I	*Stage II*	*Stage III*	*Stage IV*
Bail-out	9	4	1	0.3
Planned	6	28	33	38

Table 9.6 Angiographic AHA/ACC classification and characteristics of the lesions treated in stage IV.

	GR n = 583	*PS* n = 121	*NIR* n = 386	*WS* n = 116
Type A lesion	1%	62%	13%	2%
Type C lesion	29%	34%	21%	36%
Chronic occlusion	7%	7%	6%	6%
Long lesion	33%	6%	8%	41%
Bend >45°	39%	30%	18%	19%
Bifurcation	45%	16%	28%	8%
Ostial lesion	3%	29%	4%	9%
SVG	0.4%	1%	24%	40%

Notes:
PS = Palmaz–Schatz, GR = Gianturco–Roubin, WS = Wallstent, NIR = NIR stent.

The implantation of stents in bail-out situations was 9% during stage I, and decreased to less than 0.5% during stage III–IV. The incidence of planned procedures increased from 6 to 38% (Table 9.5).

During stage IV (1996), the ability to use a new generation of stent allowed us to select preferentially different types of stents, according to the type of lesion treated.

Table 9.6 summarizes AHA/ACC classification and major angiographic characteristics of the lesions treated and the number of different types of stents implanted.

Considering the different sizes of each stent subgroup (Gianturco–Roubin: 583, NIR: 386, Palmaz–Schatz: 121, Wallstent: 116), we have expressed the number of stents implanted according to the anatomy of the lesions treated.

Type A lesions represent 62% of Palmaz–Schatz indications and type-C lesions 36% of Wallstent indications. Gianturco–Roubin Flex stents were implanted in 33% of long lesions, in 45% of bifurcations and 39% of lesions located in the bed. The structure of the coil-stent allows access to large side-branches and to perform bifurcation reconstruction. Ostial lesions were treated with Palmaz–Schatz in 29%, and old saphenous vein grafts lesions represent 40% of Wallstent indications. There was no predilection of stents for chronic total occlusions.

Table 9.7 Mean final stent diameter (mm).

| | Stage I | | Stage II | | Stage III | | | | Stage IV | | |
	PS	GR	PS	GR	PS	GR	WS	GR	PS	NIR	WS
Final diameter	3.54 ± 0.4	3.04 ± 0.5	3.62 ± 0.5	3.32 ± 0.4	3.52 ± 0.5	3.36 ± 0.4	3.84 ± 0.5	3.61 ± 0.6	3.44 ± 0.5	4.0 ± 0.7	3.42 ± 0.4

Notes:
PS = Palmaz–Schatz, GR = Gianturco–Roubin, WS = Wallstent, NIR = NIR stent.

Results

Immediate results

Primary success was achieved in 93.5% of the procedures performed in stage I, 97% in stage II, 98.5% in stage III and 98.5% in stage IV.

The mean final diameter (Table 9.7) was stable for the Palmaz–Schatz stent subgroup (3.54 ± 0.4 mm, 3.62 ± 0.5 mm, 3.52 ± 0.5 mm, 3.61 ± 0.6 mm in stages I, II, III and IV, respectively) and increased progressively for the Gianturco–Roubin Flex stent subgroup (3.04 ± 0.5 mm, 3.32 ± 0.4 mm, 3.36 ± 0.4 mm, 3.44 ± 0.5 mm, in stages I, II, III and IV, respectively). In the Wallstent group, the mean final stent diameter was 3.84 ± 0.54 mm and 4.0 ± 0.7 mm in stages III and IV, respectively. The NIR stent, used only in 1996, gave a mean final stent diameter of 3.42 ± 0.4 mm.

In-hospital major adverse cardiac events (MACE) and stent thrombosis (Tables 9.8 and 9.9)

Major in-hospital adverse cardiac events significantly decreased from 6.4% during stage I to 1.5% in stage IV. There was a significant decrease in the subacute thrombosis rate between stage I (PS = 6.6%, GR = 5.6%), stage II (PS = 0.8%, GR = 0.6%; $p < 0.001$) and Stage IV (GR = 0.3%, PS = 0.4%; $p < 0.01$).

Stage I

Major cardiac events occurred in 48 patients (6.4%) and were related to subacute thrombosis in 46 (6.1%). In the Palmaz–Schatz stent subgroup, subacute thrombotic occlusion occurred in 42 patients (6.6%) from 1 to 21 days (mean 6.2 ± 4.6 days; 1–20 days) after stenting. Only one patient had an occlusion within the first 24 hours postprocedure, related to underdeployment of the stent in a calcified artery.

Subacute thrombosis occurred in 23 patients (3.6%) during the in-hospital phase and in 19 patients (3%) after discharge. Five patients could be recanalized without MI or need for CABG and the 37 other patients (5.8%) suffered

Table 9.8 In-hospital major adverse cardiac events (%).

	Stage I n = 752	Stage II n = 553	Stage III n = 1087	Stage IV n = 1117
Non Q MI	2 (0.3%)	1 (0.2%)	7 (0.6%)	4 (0.3%)
Q-wave MI	26 (3.5%)	3 (0.5%)	4 (0.4%)	2 (0.2%)
CABG	9 (1.2%)	3 (0.5%)	2 (0.2%)	1 (0.1%)
Death	10 (1.3%)	5 (0.9%)	4 (0.4%)	11 (1%)
Total	48 (6.4%)	12 (2.2%)	17 (1.6%)	18 (1.6%)

Table 9.9 Subacute thrombosis rate.

	Stage I		Stage II		Stage III			Stage IV			
	PS	GR	PS	GR	PS	GR	WS	GR	PS	NIR	WS
%	6.6	5.6	0.8	0.6	0.7	0.7	1	0.3	0.4	0	0

Notes:
PS: $p < 0.0001$ Stage I vs. II GR: $p = 0.02$ Stage I vs. II NS   Stage II vs. III   NS   Stage II vs. III
PS = Palmaz–Schatz. GR = Gianturco–Roubin. WS = Wallstent. NIR = NIR stent.

a major ischemic complication. Two additional patients had a significantly increased CK-MB after a bail-out stenting procedure but the stent was patent at angiography control. These two non-Q-wave MI were attributed to prolonged ischemia or occlusion of the side-branches during the bail-out procedure.

In the Gianturco–Roubin Flex stent subgroup, 6 patients (5.6%) had a subacute thrombosis, two of which resulted in death (one after ventricular fibrillation and one despite CABG surgery for unsatisfactory results at the left anterior descending artery (LAD) with extended thrombus from LAD stent to left main, 15 days after surgery). The four other patients underwent successful recanalization and angioplasty.

Stage II

Major cardiac events were reduced to 2.2% (12/553 patients). These events were related to subacute thrombosis in 5 (0.7%) patients. In the Palmaz–Schatz stent subgroup, three patients died. One patient with severe three-vessel disease, left ventricular ejection fraction (LVEF) = 25%, history of frequent ventricular tachycardia and incomplete revascularization of LAD died on Day-3. On Day-6 two other patients with unsatisfactory stent deployment in the major vessel died. In the Gianturco–Roubin stent subgroup, two patients died (one of a fatal stroke on Day-4 and the other, a female with severe depressed left ventricular function (EF = 17%) and cardiac failure presented with refractory ventricular fibrillation 5 days after the procedure).

Stage III

Major cardiac events occurred in 17 patients (1.6%) and were related to subacute thrombosis in 8 (0.7%). In the Palmaz–Schatz stent subgroup, one patient with a previously occluded saphenous vein graft and severely depressed ejection fraction (25%) died suddenly 8 days after the procedure. Another patient with LVEF = 24% died consequently of cardiac heart failure after unprotected left main stenting. One patient in the Gianturco–Roubin subgroup died. This patient, with previous bypass surgery, had three occluded bypasses and a critical stenosis of the left circumflex, the only patent vessel. A stent was implanted in the circumflex and high-pressure inflation with an oversized balloon resulted in rupture of the vessel. It was impossible to correct this complication, and the patient died 24 hours later. Another patient died from severe gastrointestinal bleeding 4 days after stenting of an unprotected left main artery. Two other patients underwent inadequate stent implantation, with dissection not completely covered by the stent, and suffered subacute occlusion of the stented vessel.

Only one patient had a subacute thrombosis after Wall-stent implantation during stage III. Due to side-effects, this patient discontinued ticlopidine 8 days after stent placement and suffered an acute MI on day 17, which was treated with IV thrombolysis. Angiography control 24 hours after lytic therapy showed normal stent patency without residual thrombosis.

Stage IV

Despite widespread use of stenting (54% of the PTCA procedures) and implantation of stents in patients with more complex lesions, only three patients (0.3%) suffered

Table 9.10 Bleeding complications (%).

	Stage I		Stage II		Stage III			Stage IV			
	PS	GR	PS	GR	PS	GR	WS	GR	PS	NIR	WS
Vascular access	6.5	9.3	2.2	1.8	0.9	2.3	2	0.4	0.5	0.6	0.8
Other	1.3	1.9	1.0	1.2	0.5	0.5	0	0.2	0.1	0.1	0.2

Notes:
PS = Palmaz–Schatz, GR = Gianturco–Roubin, WS = Wallstent, NIR = NIR stent.

evidence of subacute thrombosis (one following Palmaz–Schatz stent implantation after recanalization of the right coronary artery (RCA) during primary PTCA of inferior MI, and incomplete coverage of a long dissection with a Palmaz–Schatz stent, two after Gianturco–Roubin stent implantation and a distal dissection not fully covered by the strut of the stent). These three patients were successfully recanalized, with implantation of additive stents to treat the distal dissection flap. Major adverse cardiac events were denoted in 18 patients (1.6%), including these three previous patients. Eleven patients (1%) died. Three patients died during the procedure. In one patient, following reconstruction of the RCA with a Wallstent and a Gianturco–Roubin Flex stent, a left main stenosis was treated with a NIR stent and a distal lesion on the LAD could not be dilated and stented. Acute occlusion of the LAD occurred with refractory ventricular fibrillation. Two other patients who were not candidates for surgery died during emergency recanalization and stenting of left main stenosis or LAD. Four patients, older than 75 years, presented a stroke following complex procedures (with administration of ReoPro in 2). Two patients suffered multifocal cholesterol emboli with acute renal insufficiency and two others died after no reflow phenomenon in SVG (1) or occlusion of a large diagonal (1).

Q-wave (0.4%) or non-Q-wave MIs (0.3%) were related, after angiographic control, to occlusion of a non-stented side-branch in five patients, and to occlusion of the vessel beyond the patent stent in three patients, related to distal dissection not fully covered by the stent, which was successfully recanalized.

Bleeding and vascular access complications (Table 9.10)

Stage I

Severe vascular access complication occurred in 6.5% in the Palmaz–Schatz subgroup and 9.3% after implantation of Gianturco–Roubin Flex stent using a 9F guiding catheter.

Stage II

We introduced the use of a Femostop device, a gradual ambulation protocol, the transradial approach and a 6F guiding catheter to implant a Palmaz–Schatz stent. Vascular access complications occurred in 2.2% in the Palmaz–Schatz subgroup and 1.8% after implantation of Gianturco–Roubin Flex stent using an 8F guiding catheter.

Stage III

Fifty-five percent of the stenting procedures with the Palmaz–Schatz stent were performed using the transradial approach with no severe vascular complications. The vascular access complication was 0.9% in this subgroup, versus 2.3 and 2.2%, respectively, after Gianturco–Roubin Flex stent or Wallstent implantation, requiring an 8F guiding catheter and transfemoral approach.

Stage IV

The transradial approach was used in 54% of procedures and vascular complication was lower than 0.5%. Other bleeding complication rate decreased from 1.9% to less than 0.5%.

Comments

All the coronary stents implanted were metallic and thrombogenic. From the experience acquired with mechanical prosthetic heart valves, it was presumed that chronic anticoagulation with coumadin was sufficient to prevent stent thrombosis.[2-6] The use of aggressive anticoagulation therapy did not prevent the risk of subacute occlusion which occurred in 6.7% of the patients in our series during stage I. In another series reported during the same period of time, the incidence of subacute stent thrombosis varied between 9 and 28% in bail-out stenting and 2–6% after elective stenting procedures.[21-27] Bail-out procedures, multiple stent implantation, final stent diameter less than 3.0 mm and left ventricular ejection fraction (LVEF) below 45% were identified as factors associated with subacute thrombosis.[15,22,23] Subacute thrombosis, which occurs with a peak incidence between day 5 and day 7 after stent implantation, was the primary determining major adverse cardiac event during hospitalization or after discharge.

The aggressive anticoagulation regimen used in the first period exposed the patients to an increased risk of serious bleeding complications and a prolonged hospital stay. The groin hemorrhagic complication rate was initially reported from 3.5 to 16%.[10-17] Bleeding was not only an independent complication but interruption or reduction in anticoagulation could precede stent thrombosis.

In the BENESTENT[26] study, the incidence of bleeding and vascular complications was significantly higher in the stent group compared to the balloon group (13.5% vs. 3.1%; $p < 0.001$) and the mean hospital stay was longer (8.5 days vs. 3.1 days; $p < 0.001$).

In order to simplify medication protocol and to decrease the incidence of bleeding, several French[20] teams decided to replace coumadin by LMWH. This change was based on the assumption that the switch from heparin to coumadin was responsible for the increased incidence of subacute thromboses. Despite this therapeutic change, subacute thromboses occurred in 10.3% (4% in the elective patients group and 30% for the bail-out group), suggesting that both coumadin and LMWH were ineffective in preventing thrombus formation at the site of stent implantation, with a peak occurrence of subocclusion between day 5 and day 8, corresponding to platelet half-life.

A co-operative inhibitor effect of ticlopidine and aspirin in disrupting platelet adhesion and inhibiting the resultant thrombosis was reported.[28] Ticlopidine is a potent inhibitor of ADP-induced platelet aggregation, whereas inhibitory effects of acetylsalicylic acid are directed against thromboxane A2.[29] This aggressive antiplatelet therapy based on ticlopidine/aspirin added to LMWH was introduced in the French multicenter study[30] with a significant reduction in the rate of major adverse cardiac events (2.9%) and overall mortality (0.6%).

This protocol was experimentally introduced in our institution in July 1993 and the incidence of subacute thrombosis decreased dramatically from 6.6% during stage I to less than 1% during stage II, despite an increased rate of patients treated with type-C lesions or/and three-vessel disease and the widespread use of stenting. In a randomized comparative study, Schoming et al.[30] clearly demonstrated the reduction of subacute occlusion and bleeding complications with the substitution of ticlopidine for poststent heparin and coumadin.

In our experience, during stages II–IV, the reduction of subacute thrombosis was probably the result of two additional factors: high-pressure balloon inflations performed routinely after stenting in order to achieve optimal deployment of the stent, and the combination of ticlopidine-aspirin.

More adequate stent deployment and the normalization of the rheology inside the stented vessel have been shown to be effective in subacute thrombosis rate reduction by Colombo et al.,[18] who focused on the modalities of unsatisfactory stent deployment despite satisfactory angiographic results.[19] Intravascular imaging showed that incomplete stent apposition, persistence of residual luminal narrowing and the presence of significant disease of the proximal and distal reference segment could not be detected with angiography.[19] These observations prompted the authors to propose a strategy based on high-pressure dilatation in order to obtain adequate stent expansion.

It was proposed that the adequacy of stent deployment cannot be appreciated by QCA and in some reported cases, optimal stent deployment was not achieved despite apparently satisfactory angiographic results.[19] In our experience, intravascular ultrasound was not used to ascertain adequacy of stent deployment. In day-to-day practice we carefully validated the delineation of the angiographic contours, and the final results with the digital angiographic system and online QCA. Automated edge detection in multiple views after stenting allows the detection of the persistence of residual stenosis. After stent implantation, further dilatations performed with high-pressure of up to 16 atm, carefully matching the size of the balloon to the diameter of the presumed angiographically normal coronary segment, achieved a near zero angiographic residual stenosis, and the preventive treatment of added ticlopidine-aspirin seemed effective to resolve the problem of subacute thrombosis. Retrospectively, in the three patients with subacute thrombosis during stage IV, the final angiographic results were inadequate, with a dissection flap not completely covered by stents struts. Higher accuracy in the assessment of final angiographic results and the use of additional stents to cover distal dissections can allow a decrease in the rate of stent thrombosis to near zero.

The use of intracoronary ultrasound (IVUS) is time-consuming and costly. The concept that IVUS guidance is necessary to perform optimal stenting and to prevent sub-acute thrombosis must be addressed.

Hall et al.[32] reported a result of 2.9% of stent thrombosis patients treated with aspirin only versus 0.8% in the aspirin-ticlopidine group in a randomized study comparing aspirin alone with the combination of aspirin and ticlopidine, following intravascular-guided stenting. Goods et al.[33] compared a group of patients managed with aspirin alone to a group of patients managed with the combination of aspirin and ticlopidine after Gianturco–Roubin Flex stent implantation in native coronary arteries in a prospective nonrandomized study. The incidence of stent thrombosis was 6.5% in patients treated with aspirin only versus 0.9% in the aspirin and ticlopidine group. In this study, high-pressure balloon inflations were performed after stenting and adequacy of stent placement was assessed angiographically without IVUS. The 0.9% subacute thrombosis rate in the ticlopidine group in these two studies is similar to our results. In the French multicenter study,[30] IVUS was not used, and major cardiac events are similar to those reported by Hall et al.[32]

It has been demonstrated, in vivo, that ticlopidine added to aspirin and heparin reduces the generation of thrombin and platelet activation in patients undergoing balloon angioplasty or stenting.[34,35] The replacement of aggressive anticoagulant therapy by ticlopidine-aspirin has also dramatically reduced the rate of bleeding and vascular access complications, from 10 to 1.5%.

Many factors could be involved in the reduced complication rate: sheath removal when the PTT was less than 60 sec, manual compression followed by a mechanical compression using the Femostop (Radi Medical Systems, Sweden) for 3 hours, a gradual ambulation protocol, a transradial approach for coronary stenting[36] and/or a small-sized guiding catheter.

In the French multicenter study,[30] predisposing factors for local vascular complications were identified. These factors include female gender, bail-out procedures, subcutaneous LMWH, therapy duration and sheath size. Adjunctive LMWH treatment does not appear to be useful in prevention of stent thrombosis, but significantly increases the risk of bleeding and vascular complications. In stage IV, LMWH probably played a role in three of the fatal strokes occurring poststenting. Following an optimal final result, with adequate stent placement after high-pressure inflation as assessed angiographically, ticlopidine-aspirin treatment appears to be sufficient, and additional subcutaneous LMWH can be restricted to patients with stenting during acute MI, or for a thrombus-containing lesion.

Conclusion

More appropriate selection of stented vessels, high-pressure balloon inflation for optimal stent deployment, careful assessment of final angiographic results with near zero residual stenosis, full covering of dissections by the distal struts of the stent, and the association of ticlopidine-aspirin allow the effective resolution, in day-to-day practice, of the problem of stent thrombosis. Therefore, the widespread use of stenting seems 'justified'. However, two problems remain to be solved: the additional cost of stenting procedures and the unpredictable within-stent restenosis.

References

1 Dotter CT, Judkins MP. Transluminal treatment of arteriosclerotic obstruction: description of a new technique and a preliminary report of its application. Circulation 1964; **30**: 654–70.

2 Sigwart U, Puel J, Mirkovitch V, et al. Intravascular stents to prevent occlusion and restenosis after transluminal angioplasty. N Engl J Med 1987; **316**: 701–6.

3 Sigwart U, Urban P, Golf S, et al. Emergency stenting for acute occlusion after coronary balloon angioplasty. Circulation 1988; **78**: 1121–7.

4 De Feyter PJ, de Scheerder I, van den Brand M, et al. Emergency stenting for refractory acute coronary artery occlusion during coronary angioplasty. Am J Cardiol 1990; **66**: 1147–50.

5 Roubin GS, King SB, Douglas JS, et al. Intracoronary stenting during percutaneous coronary angioplasty. Circulation 1990; **81**: IV-92–IV-100.

6 Schatz RA. A view of vascular stents. Circulation 1989; **79**: 445–7.

7 Schatz RA, Baim D, Leon M, et al. Clinical experience with the Palmaz–Schatz coronary stent. Initial results of a multicenter study. Circulation 1991; **83**: 148–61.

8 De Jaegere PP, Serruys PW, Bertrand M, et al. Wiktor stent implantation in patients with restenosis following balloon angioplasty of a native coronary artery. Am J Cardiol 1992; **69**: 598–602.

9 Colombo A, Maiello L, Almagor Y, et al. Coronary stenting single institution experience with the initial 100 cases using the Palmaz–Schatz stent. Cath Cardiovasc Diagn 1992; **26**: 171–6

10 Haude M, Erbel R, Straub U, et al. Results of intracoronary stenting for management of coronary dissection after balloon angioplasty. Am J Cardiol 1991; **77**: 691–6.

11 Roubin GS, Cannon AC, Agrawal SK, *et al.* Intracoronary stenting for acute and threatened closure complicating percutaneous transluminal coronary angioplasty. *Circulation* 1992; **85**: 916–27.

12 Fajadet J, Marco J, Cassagneau B, *et al.* Emergency coronary stenting for acute dissection during PTCA. *J Am Coll Cardiol* 1991; **17**: 53A.

13 Erbel R, Swars H, Hofner G, *et al.* Reduction of subacute thrombotic stent occlusion by improved anticoagulation monitoring. *Circulation* 1991; **84**: II-558.

14 Kimura T, Nosaka H, Yokoi H, *et al.* Emergency coronary stenting for abrupt closure and dissection after balloon angioplasty. *J Am Coll Cardiol* 1992; **19**: 198.

15 Doucet S, Fajadet J, Cassagneau B, *et al.* Early thrombotic occlusion following coronary Palmaz–Schatz stent implantation: frequency and clinical or angiographic predictors. *Eur Heart J* 1992; **13**: 159.

16 Haude M, Erbel R, Straub U, *et al.* Short- and long-term results after intracoronary stenting in human coronary arteries: monocentre experience with the balloon expandable Palmaz–Schatz stent. *Br Heart J* 1991; **66**: 337–46.

17 Nath FC, Muller DWM, Ellis SG, *et al.* Early thrombotic occlusion of coronary stents: frequency, predictors, therapy and clinical outcome. *Circulation* 1991; **84**: II-587.

18 Colombo A, Hall P, Nakamura S, *et al.* Intracoronary stenting without anticoagulation accomplished with intravascular ultrasound guidance. *Circulation* 1995; **21**: 15–25.

19 Nakamura S, Colombo A, Gaglione A, *et al.* Intracoronary ultrasound observation during stent implantation. *Circulation* 1994; **89**: 2030–5.

20 Morice MC. Advances in post stenting medication protocol. *J Inv Cardiol* 1995; **7**: 32A.

21 Herman HC, Hirshfeld JW jr, Buchbinder M, *et al.* Emergent coronary artery stenting for failed PTCA. *Circulation* 1991; **84**: II-590.

22 Fishman DL, Savage MP, Leon MB, *et al.* Angiographic predictors of subacute thrombosis following coronary artery stenting. *Circulation* 1991; **84**: II-558.

23 Fajadet J, Marco J, Cassagneau B, *et al.* Coronary stenting with the Palmaz–Schatz stent: the Clinic Pasteur interventional cardiology unit experience. In: Sigwart U, Frank GI (eds). *Coronary Stents* (Berlin and Heidelberg: Springer-Verlag, 1992): 57–77.

24 Carrozza JP, Kuntz RE, Levine MJ, *et al.* Angiographic and clinical outcome of intracoronary stenting: immediate and long-term results from a large single center experience. *J Am Coll Cardiol* 1992; **20**: 328–37.

25 Fischman DL, Savage MP, Leon M, *et al.* Angiographic predictors of subacute thrombosis following coronary artery stenting. *Circulation* 1991; **84**: II-558.

26 Serruys PW, de Jaegere P, Kiemeneij F, *et al.* for the Benestent Study Group. A comparison of balloon-expandable-stent implantation with balloon angioplasty in patients with coronary artery disease. *N Engl J Med* 1994; **331**: 489–95.

27 Sutton JM, Ellis SG, Roubin GS, *et al.* for the Gianturco–Roubin Intracoronary Stent Investigator Group. Major clinical events after coronary stenting: the multicenter registry of acute and elective Gianturco–Roubin stent placement. *Circulation* 1994; **89**: 1126–37.

28 De Caterina R, Sicari R, Bernini W, *et al.* Benefit/risk profile of combined antiplatelet therapy with ticlopidine and aspirin. *Thromb Haemost* 1991; **65**: 504–10.

29 Cattaneo M, Akkawat B, Lecchi A, *et al.* Ticlopidine selectively inhibits human platelet response to adenosine diphosphate. *Thromb Haemost* 1991; **66**: 694–9.

30 Karillon GJ, Morice MC, Benveniste E, *et al.* Intracoronary stent implantation without ultrasound guidance and with replacement of conventional anticoagulation by antiplatelet therapy. *Circulation* 1996; **94**: 1519–27.

31 Schoming A, Schuhien H, Blasini R, *et al.* Anticoagulation versus antiplatelet therapy after intracoronary Palmaz–Schatz stent placement. *Circulation* 1995; **92 (Suppl I)**: I-280.

32 Hall P, Nakamura S, Maiello L, *et al.* A randomized comparison of combined ticlopidine and aspirin therapy versus aspirin therapy alone after successful intravascular-guided stent implantation. *Circulation* 1996; **93**: 215–22.

33 Goods C, Al-Shaibi K, Liu M, *et al.* Comparison of aspirin alone versus aspirin plus ticlopidine after coronary stenting. *Am J Cardiol* 1996; **78**: 1042–4.

34 Gregorini L, Marco J, Fajadet J, *et al.* Reduction of hemostasis activation with a new anticoagulation protocol during PTCA and stent implantation. *J Invasive Cardiol* 1995; **7**: 14A (abstract).

35 Gregorini L, Marco J, Fajadet J, *et al.* Ticlopidine and aspirin pretreatment reduces coagulation and platelet activation during coronary dilatation procedures. *J Am Coll Cardiol* 1997; **29**: 13–20.

36 Marco J, Fajadet J, Cassagneau B, *et al.* Transradial coronary stenting: A passing fad or widespread use in the future? *J Inv Cardiol* 1996; **8 (Suppl E)**: 16–21 (abstract).

10

Stent design and the biologic response

Joseph Garasic, Campbell Rogers and Elazer R Edelman

Introduction

A fundamental question in interventional cardiology is whether the improved patency and reduced rates of restenosis seen with endovascular stents compared to balloon angioplasty[1,2] vary with stent design, or are a result of acute gains in lumen size alone.[3–5] If lumen size predominates, then there will be a limit to what stents can achieve clinically, and restenosis, though reduced, will still occur in 15–30% of stented arteries. On the other hand, if novel stent designs can produce better results, there may be great promise for extended applications and reduced complications. Elucidating the biologic response to vascular injury and the chronic response to an indwelling vascular implant is essential to obtaining an answer to this question.

Clinical evidence suggests that the immediate postprocedural result is a primary determinant of late luminal diameter regardless of the intervention—angioplasty, stent or atherectomy.[3–5] On the other hand, experimental data from animal models show that the biologic response which follows endovascular stent implantation differs fundamentally from that which follows simple balloon angioplasty.[6–8] Stent struts impose a far deeper injury than the balloon alone, and because they are left in place, impose chronic strain upon the vessel wall. They also possess the potential to elicit a foreign body reaction that includes a brisk inflammatory response. Only by understanding the intricacies of these biologic processes can one hope to make rational alterations in future stent design in an effort to attenuate restenosis.

The goals of this chapter are threefold: 1) to characterize the time course of stent-induced biologic responses; 2)

to review experimental data that illustrate how alterations in stent design may modify these responses; and 3) to suggest future directions for investigation in this field.

Biologic response: overview

As the use of stents is in its infancy, there is a dearth of data from human pathologic specimens.[9,10] Stents cannot be extracted except at surgery or autopsy, and what few specimens are available reflect the extremes of adverse outcomes including acute thrombosis or pronounced restenosis. Histologic examination of arteries from the great majority of stents with less severe outcomes is lacking. As a result, the majority of data detailing the biologic response to intravascular stenting have been extrapolated from studies in animal models. Stents have been placed in normal or hypercholesterolemic rabbit, porcine or canine, peripheral, carotid or coronary arteries, with and without predilatation and endothelial denudation. Though no animal model perfectly recapitulates the human coronary artery response, striking similarities in the biologic processes between different species may shed light on the pathology of human restenosis. In general, the biologic response to endovascular stent implantation can be divided into four temporally continuous and interdependent stages: thrombosis, inflammation, neointimal cell proliferation/thickening and vascular remodeling (Fig. 10.1).

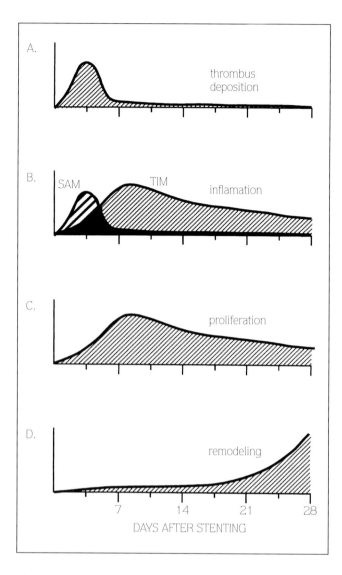

Figure 10.1

Schematic representation of four phases of vascular repair after stent-induced arterial injury. (a) Early after stent implantation, platelet-rich thrombus accumulates at sites of deep stent strut injury. Thrombus burden peaks 3–4 days after stent deployment and causes the majority of early luminal loss. Within 10 days of stent placement, the occurrence of stent thrombosis and thrombus burden have decreased considerably. Coincident with early thrombus deposition, inflammatory cells (b), in particular surface adherent monocytes (SAM), are recruited to the arterial lumen both adjacent to struts as well as in interstrut regions. Between 3 and 7 days after stenting, these cells migrate into the neointima as tissue infiltrating macrophages (TIM). Large numbers of these cells persist within the neointima weeks after stent deployment. Proliferation of smooth muscle cells and monocyte/macrophages within the neointima (c) peaks 7 days after stent implantation, and continues above baseline levels for weeks thereafter. In the final phase of vascular repair after stent-induced injury (d), collagen deposition in the adventitia and throughout the tunica media and neointima leads to arterial shrinkage, or remodeling. This causes the artery to be compressed upon the struts of the stent from without.

Biologic response: stage 1—thrombosis

The thrombotic phase of stent-induced vascular injury begins in the first 3 days after stent deployment (Fig. 10.1(a)), and is characterized by aggregation of platelets, fibrin and trapped erythrocytes.[11,12] Prevention of occlusive intravascular thrombosis after coronary stenting, and its attendant morbidity and mortality,[13] has required the use of high-dose systemic anticoagulant and antiplatelet therapy. Aspirin, heparin, warfarin, ticlopidine, dextran, urokinase and other such agents have been variably effective in reducing early thrombotic events at the cost of a 7–13% risk of hemorrhagic complications.[14,15] These complications have driven attempts to reduce thrombosis after vascular intervention via local or stent-based drug delivery.

Stent thrombosis is pathophysiologically and temporally distinct from abrupt closure after balloon angioplasty. While the latter typically occurs within 24 hours of percutaneous transluminal coronary angioplasty (PTCA), stent thrombosis is most common 3–10 days after implantation. Following stent deployment, there is significant endothelial denudation and fibrin-rich thrombus formation most marked at sites where stent struts induce severe vascular trauma. Studies in porcine coronary arteries have led Schwartz et al.[16] to describe a graded measure of the severity of vessel wall damage, from minimal injury with an intact internal elastic lamina, to laceration of the internal elastic lamina, media and external elastic lamina and associated early thrombosis. Human pathologic data confirm the presence of heavy platelet deposition on the luminal surface of stented segments, but with little extension beyond the site of dilatation.[9,10] Furthermore, mural thrombus and marked platelet deposition were only seen in vessels that suffered medial tears. Thrombus formation, then, seems to represent a response to violating the endovascular continuity and to the addition of a metal stent to the vascular milieu.

Several distinct biologic variables including arterial injury, stent surface properties and stent geometry determine the rate of stent thrombosis in animal studies. Modification of these variables, as well as local and systemic drug delivery, can affect thrombosis in animal models.[8,17,18] For example, changing stent configuration alone from a slotted-tube design to a more flexible corrugated-ring design with 29% fewer strut–strut intersections, while holding surface area, mass and material constant, reduced the complete thrombosis rate from 42 to 15%. The arterial injury score was also 42% lower. Surface properties of intravascular stents may likewise affect the thrombotic response. For example, application of a heparin coating to Palmaz–Schatz slotted-tube stents may have reduced thrombosis in porcine coronary arteries.[19] Furthermore, coating both slotted-tube and corrugated-ring stents with an inert polymer or with ionically bound heparin has been shown virtually to eliminate complete thrombosis.[8,17] This suggests that bare metal itself has thrombogenic properties, perhaps related to platelet adhesion and aggregation, which can be attenuated by such coatings. These experimental findings are supported by clinical data from the Benestent II pilot study showing no subacute stent thrombosis in slotted-tube stents coated with polyamine and endpoint-attached heparin.[20] Thus, the biologic response of subacute stent thrombosis can be modulated by variations in stent design, material and coating.

Biologic response: stage 2—inflammation

The next temporal pathologic state of stent-induced vascular injury is the marked accumulation of inflammatory cells (Fig. 10.1(b)). Scanning-electron micrographs of stented human saphenous vein grafts demonstrate large deposits of leukocytes and platelets adherent to the luminal aspect of stent struts at 3 days after implantation.[9,10] Similarly, reactive inflammatory infiltrates including lymphocytes, eosinophils and histiocytes can be seen extending from the luminal surface of stented coronary or peripheral vessels, through the wall and into the adventitia.[21] Multinucleated giant cells are frequently observed around stent wires suggesting the induction of a protracted foreign body reaction.[12] Such cellular infiltrates can be seen as early as 15 minutes or as late as 56 days after implantation in animal models. In contrast, early inflammatory infiltrates are virtually absent in the same arteries subject to balloon injury alone.[22]

The presence of inflammatory infiltrates at sites of deep vascular injury has been well documented. Of particular interest is the possible role of mononuclear cells in the pathogenesis of neointimal hyperplasia. Tissue monocyte number rises commensurate with proliferative indices after intravascular stenting, and is most pronounced 7 days after implantation.[12] In an experimental model, treatments which reduce adherent and tissue monocytes produced reductions in intimal cell proliferation and intimal thickening.[12] Besides providing a substantial portion of the mass of neointima after stenting, monocytes release cytokines, mitogens and tissue growth factors which may play an important role in later stages of stent-induced vascular injury and repair.

Alterations in stent material, coating and design have also been shown to impact upon the recruitment of inflammatory cells. The metallic alloys used in most currently available stents do not appear to be absolutely biologically inert, and even surgical steel provokes a foreign body response. However, not all metallic alloys are equivalent, as stent struts fabricated from copper,[23] for example, elicit a particularly aggressive response. Because protracted foreign body-type reactions and vessel wall strain imposed by stent geometry have been implicated in the pathogenesis of restenosis, the use of biodegradable polymeric stents has been proposed to avoid the potential problems associated with chronic indwelling devices, and to limit long-term vessel wall strain. Polyethylene terephthalate polymeric stents implanted in porcine coronary arteries have been found to evoke a profound degree of inflammation.[24] It may be that the hydrolysis and lysosome-dependent degradation of polymeric materials produces a brisk, local inflammatory response. Synthetic polymer coatings have been examined for use with stents both as surface modifiers to reduce thrombosis and as a potential reservoir for local drug delivery. In one recent study, portions of metal stents were coated with an array of biodegradable and nonbiodegradable polymer materials and then implanted in porcine coronary arteries.[25] In all animals, the inflammatory response and neointimal thickening were significantly greater in the coated segments than in uncoated portions of the same stents, and though observed with all materials, certain polymers induced greater inflammatory and proliferative reactions than others. Thus, synthetic materials thought to be inert can still evoke brisk, protracted and material-specific inflammatory infiltrates when implanted into the blood vessel wall. Alterations in stent design and geometry have also been shown to affect the host inflammatory response. Work from the authors' laboratory has compared the effects of differing stent geometries on biologic endpoints. In particular, as discussed above, comparison of the slotted-tube design to a corrugated-ring stent of similar mass showed monocyte accumulation to be markedly reduced in arterial segments containing the latter.[17]

Biologic response: stage 3—proliferation

Restenosis after vascular intervention is driven by proliferation of vascular smooth muscle cells in the media and neointima (Fig. 10.1(c)). In stented vessels, a link between the inflammation described above and proliferative events has been reported. Moreover, experimental and clinical data have shown stent-induced neointimal thickening to be both more extensive and protracted than that provoked by balloon angioplasty alone.[6–8] Alterations in stent material, coating and design have all been found to have an impact upon the degree of subsequent neointimal thickening. As discussed above, although initial stent designs utilized the plastic properties of surgical steel to achieve adequate hoop strength and counteract elastic vessel recoil, other materials have been examined in an effort to eliminate chronic mechanical strain and inflammatory reaction. Not only do polymeric stents constructed of such materials as polyethylene terphthalate induce marked inflammatory aggregates but they are also associated with an intense proliferative response and resultant luminal obliteration within 4–6 weeks of implantation.[24] This response is accompanied by only minimal vascular injury, suggesting that polymeric stent-induced restenosis is attributable to factors beyond mechanical vessel wall damage. Thus, though the bioabsorbable and drug-carrying properties of some polymer materials may be attractive to vascular biologists, their adverse inflammatory and proliferative effects may prove insurmountable. Copper alloys have likewise been shown to evoke a profound proliferative response in stented vessels,[23] raising further questions regarding the optimal choice of stent materials.

While various coatings applied to metallic stents have succeeded in modulating thrombosis, similar efforts to reduce proliferation and restenosis have been far less successful. For example, although clinical data from the Benestent II trial have suggested a reduction in subacute thrombotic events among patients given heparin-coated stents, no clear reduction in late events or in restenosis has been demonstrated.[20] Experimentally, heparin and inert polymer material stent coatings have shown antithrombotic, though not antiproliferative, effects.[8,17,26,27]

Alterations in stent geometry, strut morphology and postprocedural luminal diameter have all been suggested as factors which may affect cellular proliferation and thereby the eventual restenosis response. The severity of strut-induced injury to the various anatomic structures of the vessel wall has been shown to correlate strongly with neointimal thickness 4 weeks after stent deployment.[16] Comparison of two endovascular devices of differing geometry (slotted tube vs. corrugated ring), but similar mass and surface area, has demonstrated that reducing the number of strut–strut intersections by 29% in the corrugated-ring configuration reduced disruption of vessel wall structures by 42% and neointimal volume by 38% at 14 days (Fig. 10.2).

In another report, Palmaz–Schatz slotted-tube stents were compared to both the Strecker and Wallstent devices.[18] The Strecker stent had the lowest mechanical hoop strength of the three designs and, though highly flexible, showed significantly greater immediate loss of stent diameter (recoil) as well as greater 4-month neointimal growth. Slotted-tube stents demonstrated the least early and late luminal loss of the three designs. Both the Strecker and Wallstent devices have crossing struts that increase stent profile. Since both these designs had comparable neointimal thickening, it may be that the ultimate luminal contour is determined principally by the extent to which struts protrude into the vessel lumen, with the neointima thickening until a smooth endovascular profile is achieved. This process, in concert with early elastic recoil in the Strecker stent, may account for the high degree of late restenosis with this design.

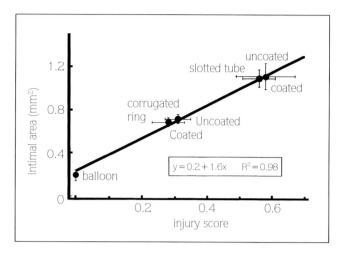

Figure 10.2
Line graph shows the relationship between design-dependent deep arterial injury and resultant neointimal hyperplasia (adapted from reference 17). Stainless-steel balloon-expandable stents of the same mass, surface area and diameter were constructed as slotted tubes or a more flexible series of corrugated rings. Some stents of each design were then coated with a thin layer of an inert polymer material. Fourteen days after implantation into denuded rabbit iliac arteries the degree of neointimal hyperplasia differed two-fold between stents of different design. The difference in intimal growth was directly commensurate with the degree of deep injury caused by stent struts. The addition of the inert polymer material had no effect upon neointimal hyperplasia. Balloon injury alone provoked minimal deep vessel wall injury and correspondingly less neointimal hyperplasia. (Adapted from Rogers et al,[17] with permission.)

In another study using two coiled-wire stents of identical material that differed only in the presence or absence of gaps in the design,[28] it was hypothesized that stents without gaps would block smooth muscle 'invasion' from the media, and potentially lessen neointimal hyperplasia. In addition, coils without gaps were postulated to possess stronger radial force at the hypothetical cost of delayed endothelialization and reduced side-branch patency. As predicted, side-branch patency was preserved in stents with gaps. However, significantly greater hyperplasia was noted in arterial segments with gap-free stents. These experimental data show that stent geometry, coatings and materials all serve as important determinants of stent-induced cellular proliferation and neointimal hyperplasia.

Biologic response: stage 4—remodeling

Vascular remodeling is the final and least well defined stage of the arterial response to endoluminal stenting.[29,30] It has been argued that stented vessels do not recoil, and that once embedded within the wall, stents become quiescent and inert. Although the number of luminal and tissue polymorphonuclear cells drops significantly 3 months after implantation, tissue macrophages and multinucleated giant cells persist, suggesting a prolonged foreign body reaction. There is experimental evidence that initial vessel injury and protracted inflammation are later met with adventitial cicatrixation as collagen accumulates around the outer surface of the vessel.[31] Vessel injury scores determined by the Schwartz schema have been found to increase between 3 days and 28 days after stenting, while stent diameter remains constant.[31] It has, then, been hypothesized that stent-induced vessel injury, foreign body reaction and collagen deposition elicit the formation of a fibrocellular adventitial cicatrix. Contracture of this element against the fixed metallic scaffolding of a stent may impale vessel structures on each strut, while the tunica media protrudes through the interstrut spaces. Alternatively, a stent with limited hoop strength may actually recoil under this external compressive force, further adding to late luminal loss.

Clinically, restenosis has been proposed as the net outcome of acute gain and late loss in luminal area.[4] In fact, postprocedural vessel diameter has proved to be an important determinant of long-term patency. The reduced rate of restenosis seen with endovascular stents compared to balloon angioplasty most likely results, in part, from the augmented acute result at the cost of greater late loss. Even in stented arteries, however, the effects of vascular remodeling may play a role in the eventual size of the arterial lumen following vascular stenting.

Conclusions

To date, a variety of pathologic and experimental evidence has shown that elements of stent design have an impact upon the biologic responses to these devices. As clinical use continues, additional specimens acquired at autopsy or via surgically harvested bypass grafts will allow more thorough examination of the human response. The widespread use of endovascular devices mandates further elucidation of their pathobiology. Only by expanding this knowledge base may we apply optimal therapy to a variety of lesions and clinical scenarios, including the genesis of effective strategies against in-stent restenosis. The application of principles derived from experimental data in a number of ongoing clinical stent trials is encouraging. Clearly, the future of endovascular stenting is bright, especially as basic scientific principles are applied to this complex clinical scenario.

References

1   Serruys PW, de Jaegere P, Kiemeneij F, et al. A comparison of balloon-expendable-stent implantation with balloon angioplasty in patients with coronary artery disease. N Engl J Med 1994; **331**: 489–95.

2   Fischman DL, Leon MB, Baim DS, et al. A randomized comparison of coronary artery-stent placement and balloon angioplasty in the treatment of coronary artery disease. N Engl J Med 1994; **331**: 496–501.

3   Kuntz RE, Safian RD, Levine MJ, Reis GJ, Diver DJ, Baim DS. Novel approach to the analysis of restenosis after the use of three new coronary devices. J Am Coll Cardiol 1992; **19**: 1493–9.

4   Kuntz RE, Safian RD, Carrozza JP, Fishman RF, Mansour M, Baim DS. The importance of acute luminal diameter in determining restenosis after coronary atherectomy or stenting. Circulation 1992; **86**: 1827–35.

5   Kuntz RE, Gibson CM, Nobuyoshi M, Baim DS. Generalized model of restenosis after conventional balloon angioplasty, stenting, and directional atherectomy. J Am Coll Cardiol 1993; **21**: 15–25.

6   Hanke H, Kamenz J, Hassenstein S, et al. Prolonged proliferative response of smooth muscle cells after experimental intravascular stenting. Eur Heart J 1995; **16**: 785–93.

7   Karas SP, Gravanis MB, Santoian EC, Robinson KA, Anderberg KA, King SB III. Coronary intimal proliferation after balloon injury and stenting in swine: an animal model of restenosis. J Am Coll Cardiol 1992; **20**: 467–74.

8   Rogers C, Karnovsky MJ, Edelman ER. Inhibition of experimental neointimal hyperplasia and thrombosis depends on the type of vascular injury and the site of drug administration. Circulation 1993; **88**: 1215–21.

9   Anderson PG, Bajaj RK, Baxley WA, Roubin GS. Vascular pathology of balloon-expandible flexible coil stents in humans. J Am Coll Cardiol 1992; **19**: 372–81.

10   van Beusekom HMM, van der Giessen WJ, van Suylen RJ, Bos E, Bosman FT, Serruys PW. Histology after stenting of human saphenous vein bypass grafts: observations from surgically excised grafts 3 to 320 days after stent implantation. J Am Coll Cardiol 1993; **2**: 45–54.

11   Schwartz RS, Holmes DH, Topol EJ. The restenosis paradigm revisited: an alternative proposal for cellular mechanisms. J Am Coll Cardiol 1992; **20**: 1284–93.

12   Rogers C, Welt FGP, Karnovsky MJ, Edelman ER. Monocyte recruitment and neointimal hyperplasia in rabbits: coupled inhibitory effects of heparin. *Arterio, Thromb and Vas Biol* 1996; **16**: 1312–18.

13   Hasdai D, Garratt KN, Holmes DRJ, Berger PB, Schwartz RS, Bell MR. Coronary angioplasty and intracoronary thrombolysis are of limited efficacy in resolving early intracoronary stent thrombosis. *J Am Coll Cardiol* 1996; **28**: 361–7.

14   Sutton JM, Ellis SG, Roubin GS, *et al*. Major clinical events after coronary stenting: the multicenter registry of acute and elective Gianturco–Roubin stent placement. *Circulation* 1994; **89**: 1126–37.

15   Levine MJ, Leonard BM, Burke JA, *et al*. Clinical and angiographic results of balloon-expandable intracoronary stents in right coronary arteries. *J Am Coll Cardiol* 1990; **16**: 332–9.

16   Schwartz RS, Huber KC, Murphy JG, *et al*. Restenosis and proportional neointimal response to coronary artery injury: results in a porcine model. *J Am Coll Cardiol* 1992; **19**: 267–74.

17   Rogers C, Edelman ER. Endovascular stent design dictates experimental restenosis and thrombosis. *Circulation* 1995; **91**: 2995–3001.

18   Barth KH, Virmani R, Froelich J, *et al*. Paired comparison of vascular wall reactions to Palmaz stents, Strecker tantalum stents, and Wallstents in canine iliac and femoral arteries. *Circulation* 1996; **93**: 2161–9.

19   Hardhammar PA, van Beusekom HM, Emanuelsson HU, *et al*. Reduction in thrombotic events with heparin-coated Palmaz–Schatz stents in normal porcine coronary arteries. *Circulation* 1996; **93**: 423–30.

20   Serruys PW, Emanuelsson H, van der Giessen W, *et al*. Heparin-coated Palmaz–Schatz stents in human coronary arteries. Early outcome of the Benestent-II Pilot Study. *Circulation* 1996; **93**: 412–22.

21   Carter AJ, Laird JR, Farb A, Kufs W, Wortham DC, Virmani R. Morphologic characteristics of lesion formation and time course of smooth muscle cell proliferation in a porcine proliferative restenosis model. *J Am Coll Cardiol* 1994; **24**: 1398–405.

22   Kamenz J, Hanke H, Hassenstein S, *et al*. Time course of accumulation of macrophages and intimal cell proliferation following experimental stenting. *Circulation* 1993; **88**: I-652.

23   Tanigawa N, Sawada S, Koyama T, *et al*. An animal experiment on the arterial wall reaction to stents coated with gold, silver, and copper. *Nippon Igaku Hoshasen Gakki Zasshi* 1991; **51**: 1195–200.

24   Murphy JG, Schwarts RS, Edwards WD, Camrud AR, Vlietstra RE, Holmes DRJ. Percutaneous polymeric stents in porcine coronary arteries. *Circulation* 1992; **86**: 1596–604.

25   van der Giessen WJ, Lincoff M, Schwartz RS, *et al*. Marked inflammatory sequelae to implantation of biodegradable and nonbiodegradable polymers in porcine coronary arteries. *Circulation* 1996; **94**: 1690–7.

26   Bailey SR, Guy DM, Garcia OJ, Paige S, Palmaz JC, Miller DD. Polymer coating of Palmaz–Schatz stent attenuates vascular spasm after stent placement. *Circulation* 1990; **82**: III-541 (abstract).

27   Bailey SR, Paige S, Lunn A, Palmaz J. Heparin coating of endovascular stents decreases subacute thrombosis in a rabbit model. *Circulation* 1992; **86**: I-186 (abstract).

28   Tominaga R, Kambic HE, Emoto H, Harasaki H, Sutton C, Hollman J. Effects of design geometry of endovascular prostheses on stenosis rate in normal rabbits. *Am Heart J* 1992; **123**: 21–8.

29   Isner JM. Vascular remodelling. Honey, I think I shrunk the artery. *Circulation* 1994; **89**: 2937–41.

30   Anderson HR, Maeng M, Thorwest M, Falk E. Remodeling rather than neointimal formation explains luminal narrowing after deep vessel wall injury. *Circulation* 1996; **93**: 1716–24.

31   Rogers C, Parikh S, Edelman ER. A unified model of vascular repair after mechanical injury. *Circulation* 1995; **92**: I-300.

11

Belief and bias: insights from comparative trials of whether to stent or not

Anoop Chauhan and Ian M Penn

Introduction

The 1990s have witnessed the development of a variety of new angioplasty devices driven by the need to address the two major limitations of percutaneous transluminal coronary angioplasty (PTCA): abrupt vessel closure and restenosis. One of the more successful of these is the intracoronary stent. Sigwart et al.[1] implanted the first stent in a human coronary artery in 1986 using the self-expanding Wallstent. Since then, more than a million stents of differing design have been implanted for an increasingly broad range of indications. Despite this proliferation of use, establishing a clearly defined and justifiable role of stenting in the routine practice of angioplasty is only now beginning to emerge. To define the role of intracoronary stents, a num-ber of randomized trials have been completed comparing stent implantation with balloon angioplasty for a number of indications (Table 11.1). The purpose of this chapter is to summarize critically the experience of these randomized trials and attempt to determine the basis for how far these studies support the growth of stenting.

De novo lesions

Two landmark large international studies, the Belgium–Netherlands Stent Trial (BENESTENT)[2] and the Stent Restenosis Study (STRESS),[3] were performed independently of each other to test the hypothesis that stent

Table 11.1 Randomized studies comparing intracoronary stenting with balloon angioplasty.

De novo lesions	Restenotic lesions	Failed PTCA	Saphenous vein graft disease	Total occlusions
BENESTENT Trial[2] STRESS Trial[3] START	TASC I REST	TASC II STENT-BY	SAVED	SICCO Thomas et al.[47] Sato et al.[48]

implantation reduces the angiographic restenosis rate. In both studies the study design was open, multicenter and randomized. Both commenced patient recruitment in 1991 and patients were randomized to receive conventional balloon angioplasty (with stenting available as bail-out therapy) or Palmaz–Schatz stent implantation in a primary lesion of a native coronary artery. The target lesion was discrete, less than 15 mm long in a large vessel with the reference diameter being 3 mm or greater. Exclusion criteria for the studies were broad including the presence of thrombus, ostial lesions, bifurcation lesions, diffuse disease, severe proximal tortuosity, abnormally functioning myocardium subtended by the lesions, the presence of contraindications to anticoagulation and ineligibility for coronary artery bypass surgery (CABG).

The BENESTENT study recruited 516 patients (257 balloon and 259 stents) in 28 centers across Europe. The primary end-point of this trial was freedom from death, stroke, myocardial infarction (MI) or repeat target vessel percutaneous revascularization between the time of the initial procedure and follow-up angiography performed at 6 months (±4 weeks). The primary angiographic end-point

was a minimal luminal diameter (MLD) at follow-up. The secondary end-points included an angiographic success rate (reduction in stenosis to 50% or less by visual estimate), a procedural success rate, the functional angina class and the results of exercise test at follow-up, and the restenosis rate (stenosis ≥50%) at follow-up.

The STRESS study recruited 407 patients (202 balloon and 205 stents) in 20 centers across North America. The primary end-point of the trial was angiographic evidence of restenosis, defined as at least 50% stenosis on follow-up angiogram. Secondary angiographic end-points included angiographic evidence of procedural success (reduction in stenosis to 50% or less by quantitative analysis) and absolute MLD at follow-up. The secondary clinical end-point was a composite end-point, defined as whichever of the following occurred first: death, MI, CABG or the need for repeated angioplasty within the first 6 months (±60 days) after the initial revascularization.

The angiographic results of the BENESTENT and STRESS trials are summarized in Table 11.2. There was no significant difference in the MLD at baseline between the two groups in both trials. The lumen diameter was larger

Table 11.2 Angiographic results of the BENESTENT and STRESS trials.

Variable	Stent (n = 237)	BENESTENT PTCA (n = 240)	p value	Stent (n = 205)	STRESS PTCA (n = 202)	p value
Reference diameter (mm)						
Before	2.99 ± 0.45	3.01 ± 0.46	NS	3.03 ± 0.42	2.99 ± 0.50	NS
After	3.16 ± 0.43	3.09 ± 0.44	0.045	3.05 ± 0.40	2.99 ± 0.47	NS
Follow-up	2.96 ± 0.48	3.05 ± 0.49	0.04	3.00 ± 0.41	2.98 ± 0.49	NS
MLD (mm)						
Before	1.07 ± 0.33	1.08 ± 0.31	NS	0.77 ± 0.27	0.75 ± 0.25	NS
After	2.48 ± 0.39	2.05 ± 0.33	<0.001	2.49 ± 0.43	1.99 ± 0.47	<0.001
Follow-up	1.82 ± 0.64	1.73 ± 0.55	0.09	1.74 ± 0.60	1.56 ± 0.65	0.007
Stenosis (%)						
Before	64 ± 10	64 ± 10	NS	75 ± 9	75 ± 8	NS
After	22 ± 8	33 ± 8	<0.001	19 ± 11	35 ± 14	<0.001
Follow-up	38 ± 18	43 ± 16	0.003	42 ± 18	49 ± 19	0.001
Elastic recoil (%)	NR	NR		15 ± 11	24 ± 15	<0.001
Restenosis rate	22	32	0.02	31.6	42.1	0.046
Change in MLD						
Immediate gain (mm)	1.40 ± 0.44	0.97 ± 0.39	<0.001	1.72 ± 0.46	1.23 ± 0.48	<0.001
Late loss (mm)	0.65 ± 0.57	0.32 ± 0.47	<0.001	0.74 ± 0.58	0.38 ± 0.66	<0.001
Net gain (mm)	0.75 ± 0.66	0.65 ± 0.59	0.09	0.98 ± 0.62	0.80 ± 0.63	0.01

MLD, Minimum Lumen Diameter; NR, not reported. NS, not significant.

Table 11.3 Clinical outcome in the BENESTENT and STRESS trials.

| Variable | BENESTENT | | | STRESS | | |
	Stent (n = 259)	PTCA (n = 257)	p value	Stent (n = 205)	PTCA (n = 202)	p value
Angiographic success %	96.9	98.1	NS	99.5	96.5	0.04
Procedural success %	92.7	91.1	NS	96.1	89.6	0.01
Death %	0.8	0.4	NS	1.5	1.5	NS
CVA	0.0	0.8	NS	1.0	0.5	NS
MI %	3.4	4.6	NS	6.3	6.9	NS
Q-wave	2.7	1.9		3.4	3.5	
Non-Q-wave	1.5	2.7		NR	NR	
CABG %	6.2	4.2	NS	4.9	8.4	NS
Repeat PTCA %	13.5	23.3	0.02	11.2	12.4	NS
Any event %	20.1	29.6	<0.05	19.5	23.8	NS
Vascular complications %	13.5	3.1	<0.05	7.4	5.0	<0.05
Hospital stay (days)	8.5	3.1	<0.05	5.8	2.8	<0.05

Notes:
CABG = coronary artery bypass surgery; CVA = cerebrovascular accident; MI = myocardial infarction; PTCA = percutaneous transluminal coronary angioplasty; NR = not reported; NS = not significant.

immediately after the procedure in the stent group as compared to patients assigned to PTCA (2.48 vs. 2.05 mm for BENESTENT, 2.49 vs. 1.99 mm for STRESS). Both trials reported a larger MLD at follow-up in the stent group as compared to patients assigned to PTCA. The incidence of restenosis was significantly lower in the patients treated with stents as compared to patients treated with PTCA in both studies (22% vs. 32% in Benestent, 32% vs. 42% in STRESS).

The clinical outcome in the BENESTENT and STRESS trials is summarized in Table 11.3. The stent and the balloon angioplasty groups were well matched with respect to the risk factors for coronary artery disease in the two trials. There was a significant difference in successful clinical procedural outcome in favor of stenting in the STRESS trial (96.1% vs. 89.6%; $p = 0.01$) but no significant difference in the BENESTENT trial (92.7% vs. 91.9%). The reduction in restenosis in the BENESTENT trial was associated with a reduction in the need for re-PTCA and also the overall primary clinical events. In the STRESS trial there was no significant difference in the overall composite clinical end-point between the two groups and there was no significant difference in the overall need for re-PTCA and CABG in the stent and PTCA groups. However, there was a trend towards a reduced need for target lesion revascularization on late follow-up in patients treated with stents (10.2% vs. 15.4%; $p = 0.06$).

The re-PTCA rate in the stent groups was similar in both studies. The angiographic and clinical success rates in the PTCA arm of BENESTENT were much higher and the restenosis rate was lower than that in STRESS. However, the need for re-PTCA in the PTCA group was higher in BENESTENT (20.6%) as compared to STRESS (12.4%). It is of note that in the majority of patients in the BENESTENT trial the need for re-PTCA was driven predominantly by symptoms of angina, and objective evidence of ischemia was available only in 24% of patients. The difference in MLD at follow-up between the stent and PTCA groups was lower in the BENESTENT trial as compared to the STRESS trial and yet there was a greater need for re-PTCA in the angioplasty group. The clinical benefits of stents in BENESTENT was due mostly to the increased re-PTCA rate in the balloon angioplasty group. These differences in results between the two studies may be due to differences in trial design.

There was no significant difference in the rate of acute vessel closure or stent thrombosis between the stent and balloon angioplasty groups in both studies. There was an increased incidence of bleeding and vascular complications in the group treated with stents in both studies. The STRESS trial showed a nonsignificant trend for an increase in access site complications with stenting (7.3% vs. 4.0%; $p = 0.14$), but in the BENESTENT trial this trend was significant (13.5% vs. 3.1%; $p < 0.001$). The hospital stay was also significantly longer in the stent group in both studies.

Late follow-up at one year has been reported for the BENESTENT trial.[4] The relative benefits of stenting over balloon angioplasty were preserved at one year. Although there was no significant difference in mortality (1.25% vs. 0.8%), stroke (0.0% vs. 0.8%), MI (5.0% vs. 4.2%) or CABG (6.9% vs. 5.1%) between the stent and balloon angioplasty groups, the need for target lesion revascularization was significantly reduced in the stent group (10%) as compared to the PTCA group (21%, $p = 0.001$). The overall primary end-points were also less frequently reached by the stent group of patients (23.2%) than those in the balloon group (31.5%, $p = 0.04$).

The preliminary results from the Stents vs. Angioplasty Restenosis Trial (START), a multicenter randomized Spanish trial, have also been presented recently.[5] The aim of this study was to compare elective balloon angioplasty (PTCA) and Palmaz–Schatz coronary stenting in de novo coronary artery lesions. The primary end-point of the study was angiographic restenosis at 6 months. From June 1992 to December 1995, a total of 452 consecutive patients were entered in the study: 229 patients were randomized to the stent arm and 223 to PTCA. Over 70% of the patients in the study had unstable angina. The procedural success rate (<50% residual stenosis in the absence of major complications) was significantly higher in the stent group (94% vs. 86%; $p < 0.01$) as compared to the PTCA group. There were 11% crossovers to stent in the PTCA group.

Angiographic follow-up was available at 6.8 ± 2 months. Stenting was associated with a greater initial gain (2.06 ± 0.6 vs. 1.49 ± 0.6 mm; $p < 0.0001$) and late loss (0.87 ± 0.6 vs. 0.63 ± 0.7 mm; $p < 0.01$) as compared to PTCA. However, the net gain was significantly greater in the stent group (1.20 ± 0.8 vs. 0.85 ± 0.7 mm; $p < 0.0001$). The stent group had a significantly lower restenosis rate (22%) as compared to the PTCA group (37%, $p < 0.01$). The angiographic outcome has also been analyzed in terms of reference vessel size. Vessel size was 3.0 mm and larger in 240 patients and larger than 2.5 but smaller than 3.0 mm in the remaining 212 patients. Regardless of reference vessel size the net gain was greater with stenting in all vessels. The restenosis rate was 21% after stenting as compared to 32% ($p = 0.12$) in vessels 3.0 mm in diameter or more. The restenosis rate was 24% after stenting as compared to 43% ($p < 0.02$) in vessels under 3.0 mm. The clinical outcome data from the trial are awaited.

De novo lesions: impressions

In summary, selective reading of these studies suggests primary coronary stenting with the Palmaz–Schatz stent for de novo native coronary artery lesions improves the angiographic outcome and reduces restenosis rate. The acute and intermediate clinical outcome also appears to be improved after stenting. However, this applies to highly selected lesions (<15 mm long, reference diameter ≥3 mm) stented in the highly selected patient populations. Moreover these studies are not consistently in support of these conclusions. In STRESS there was no overall clinical benefit of stenting, although there was an improved procedural success, less angiographic restenosis and late revascularization in the stent group. In BENESTENT, the only benefit was less late re-PTCA in the stent group, reducing late and overall clinical events. There was no demonstrated angiographic benefit. These discordant results in the two major trials underpinning the approval of stents in the USA are of concern. Moreover, these devices need to be tested in more complex clinical and angiographic scenarios, prior to extrapolating a benefit to all patient and lesion situations (e.g. long lesions, use of multiple stents, smaller vessels). For example, the benefit of stenting in non-LAD territories has yet to be demonstrated. In many interventional practices these lesion subsets may represent less than 10% of all procedures. Bias and belief may expand the conclusion that stents are a 'standard of care' for all de novo lesions, but this is not yet supported by randomized trials.

Restenotic lesions

Restenosis after PTCA and other coronary interventional procedures occurs in 30–50% of cases.[2,3,6–9] Restenotic lesions have been anecdotally characterized as 'easier' lesions, with a more benign procedural course and worse late outcome. Repeat PTCA can be performed with a high success rate (>95%) and low complication rates (<3–5%).[10–12] There is some evidence from observational studies that patients with restenotic lesions are at a higher risk of recurrence of restenosis after repeat coronary angioplasty.[11–16] Early registry data reported higher restenosis rates after stenting of restenotic lesions compared to de novo lesions.[17] More recently, however, a study of 139 restenotic lesions treated with Palmaz–Schatz stents reported a restenosis rate of only 25%.[18] Two multicenter, randomized studies have compared the strategy of stenting vs. PTCA in restenotic lesions (Table 11.1) and are discussed below.

The Trial of Angioplasty and Stents in Canada (TASC I) compared the strategy of elective coronary artery stenting to elective balloon angioplasty with stents available as bail-out measures in both de novo and restenotic lesions.[19] This study was not powered to look at subgroup differences between the de novo and restenotic lesions. However, this was the first randomized study to include restenotic lesions, allowing the examination of the potential benefit of coronary stents in this subset of patients. Patients undergoing elective PTCA for *de novo* or restenotic lesion were eligible for the study if they were over the age of 18 years, had no contraindication to anticoagulation or antiplatelet therapy, the lesion was less than 15 mm in length, lesion stenosis was greater than 70% and there was objective evidence of reversible ischemia by abnormal exercise test, an abnormal thallium stress test or reversible electrocardiographic changes with pain. Patients were excluded from the study if they had a recent MI (less than 48 hours), had contraindications for anticoagulation, multilesion disease (a 70% stenosis 1 cm beyond or proximal to the target lesion), multivessel coronary artery disease with lesions more than 70% stenosed in another dilatable nontarget artery, patients with stenosis greater than 30% of the unprotected left main coronary artery, coronary ostial disease 50% severity or more, lesions at the site of coronary bifurcation with a nonstented vessel that was greater than 2.5 mm in caliber, a large nondiseased side-branch within 5 mm of the lesion, and patients with diffuse distal disease and poor coronary outflow. A total of 270 patients were randomly assigned to receive a Palmaz–Schatz stent (137 patients) or standard balloon angioplasty (133 patients) electively in single coronary artery lesions. There were 148 patients (75 randomized to stent and 73 to balloon angioplasty) with *de novo* lesions and 122 patients with

restenotic lesions (62 randomized to stent and 60 to balloon angioplasty). The primary end-point of the study was angiographic restenosis. Coronary angiography was performed at baseline, immediately after the procedure, and 6 months later. One hundred and twenty-two patients with *de novo* lesions in this study were included in the STRESS trial.[3] The *de novo* results from TASC I will not be discussed here independently but are included for comparison between *de novo* and restenotic lesions.

The angiographic data are summarized in Table 11.4 and the clinical outcome at 6 months is summarized in Table 11.5. There was no significant difference in the rate of procedural success between the two groups. There was a significantly larger immediate increase in the luminal diameter, and a larger luminal diameter immediately after the procedure in both the *de novo* and restenotic lesions treated by stenting as compared to angioplasty. The angiographic restenosis rate was significantly lower in the *de novo* group treated with stents (29% vs. 50%; $p = 0.01$) as compared to patients treated with PTCA but there was no significant difference in the restenosis rate between the stent and angioplasty groups in the restenotic lesions (33% vs. 42%). Repeat late target lesion revascularization (8.1% vs. 21.7%; $p = 0.03$) and the need for overall target lesion revascularization (9.7% vs. 21.7%; $p = 0.07$) were reduced with stenting as compared to angioplasty in restenotic

---

Table 11.4 Angiographic results in TASC I trial.

Variable	TASC I restenosis		TASC I de novo	
	Stent (n = 62)	*PTCA* (n = 60)	*Stent* (n = 75)	*PTCA* (n = 73)
Angiographic success %	100	93*	100	92**
MLD (mm)				
Before	0.74 ± 0.36	0.76 ± 0.35	0.72 ± 0.31	0.73 ± 0.27
After	2.27 ± 0.43	1.92 ± 0.45***	2.46 ± 0.38	1.93 ± 0.41***
Follow-up	1.71 ± 0.78	1.50 ± 0.63	1.70 ± 0.55	1.51 ± 0.59
Stenosis (%)				
Before	75 ± 11	73 ± 11	76 ± 10	76 ± 9
After	21 ± 12	32 ± 13	21 ± 10	36 ± 11
Follow-up	42 ± 22	48 ± 19	42 ± 17	50 ± 18
Lesion length	10.31 ± 3.32	10.96 ± 3.77	9.54 ± 2.89	9.25 ± 2.91
Elastic recoil (%)	16 ± 9	28 ± 12***	13 ± 11	26 ± 12***
Restenosis rate %	33	42	29	50**

Notes:

Values are given as mean ± SD unless otherwise indicated. MLD = minimum lumen diameter.

*$p = 0.04$; **$p = 0.01$; ***$p = <0.0001$.

Table 11.5 Clinical outcome in TASC I trial.

Variable	TASC I restenosis			TASC I de novo		
	Stent (n = 62)	PTCA (n = 60)	p value	Stent (n = 75)	PTCA (n = 73)	p value
Procedural success %	95	88	NS	93	89	NS
Death %	0	1.7	NS	1.3	1.4	NS
CVA %	0	0	NS	0	0	NS
MI %	4.8	0	NS	9.3	2.7	NS
CABG %	0	6.7	0.06	8.0	2.7	NS
Re-PTCA %	9.7	20.0	NS	10.7	8.2	NS
Re-PTCA or CABG %	9.7	21.7	0.07	14.7	11.0	NS
Late† CABG or re-PTCA %	8.1	21.7	0.03	7.0	7.0	NS
Any event %	11.3	21.7	NS	16	12.3	NS
Stent thrombosis/abrupt closure %	3	0	NS	8	3	NS
Significant vascular complications %	1.6	1.7	NS	1.3	1.4	NS
Hospital stay (days, mean ± SD)	5.7 ± 1.7	2.8 ± 1.5	$p < 0.001$	6.1 ± 3.2	3.2 ± 2.1	$p < 0.001$

Notes:
†Late, 44 days to 6-month follow-up; CABG = coronary artery bypass surgery; CVA = cerebrovascular accident; MI = myocardial infarction; PTCA = percutaneous transluminal coronary angioplasty.

lesions. However, there was no significant difference between the stent and angioplasty groups in *de novo* lesions. Event-free survival favored those patients assigned to stenting in the restenotic lesions (88.7% vs. 78.3%; $p = 0.18$) but there was no significant difference in the *de novo* lesions (84% vs. 88%; $p =$ NS). The peripheral vascular complications requiring surgical repair, blood transfusion or both were similar with stenting and angioplasty in both the *de novo* and restenotic groups. The mean hospital stay was significantly longer in the patients assigned stent placement in both *de novo* and restenotic lesions.

The effects of stenting in comparison with repeat balloon angioplasty to treat restenotic lesions in native coronary arteries have also been evaluated in the multicenter, randomized, Restenosis Stent (REST) study.[20] Patient enrollment was completed in May 1995 and a total of 400 patients were recruited. Only patients with angina or documented ischemia and a restenotic lesion 10 mm long or less, 6 months after a previous PTCA in a vessel, suitable to receive a 3.0-mm Palmaz–Schatz stent, were included in the study. The primary end-point was 6 months angiographic patency and restenosis rate. The secondary clinical end-point was the clinical outcome. The preliminary data from this study show an improved MLD at 6 months after stenting as compared to balloon angioplasty (2.04 ± 0.66 vs. 1.85 ± 0.56; $p < 0.01$). The binary restenosis rate was reduced after stenting (18%) as compared to balloon

angioplasty (32%). The need for target lesion revascularization was significantly lower in the patients treated with stents (10% vs. 27%; $p = 0.006$). The 6-month event-free survival also favored patients treated with stents (84% vs. 72%; $p < 0.05$). Complete data with detailed information regarding functional class, stress testing and clinical outcome in different lesion types are not yet available.

Restenotic lesions: impression

The above trials provide the only current data available from controlled studies. TASC I failed to show a benefit of stenting in terms of angiographic restenosis but the study was small and was not powered to look at subgroup differences. Stenting in TASC I resulted in a decrease in the need for late target lesion revascularization. The complete data from the REST trial are awaited. In this larger study, coronary stenting reduced the rate of restenosis and also improved the 6-month clinical outcome. We would recommend primary stenting of restenotic lesions based on the above data. However, once again, lesion characteristics have to be selected carefully until further data are available on the outcome of stenting in more complex restenotic lesions. Both studies are outdated, using 'classical anticoagulation', and with higher than currently acceptable early stent complications, in restenosis lesions affecting the overall clinical outcome. Similarly, the role of stenting in recalcitrant lesions which have renarrowed several times post-PTCA, stenting longer bulkier lesions and what to do with the restenosed stents have yet to be subjected to 'clarifying' trials.

Total occlusion

Conventional PTCA is applied commonly to coronary occlusions in the subacute and chronic setting. PTCA of chronic total occlusion represents 10–20% of all angioplasty procedures, and inability to revascularize these lesions is one of the most common reasons for referring patients for CABG. The most common causes of failed intervention include the inability to cross the occlusion with a guidewire (80%), failure to cross the occlusion with a balloon (15%) and failure to dilate the stenosis (5%).

Compared to PTCA of nontotal occlusions, where the successful revascularization rates exceed 90%, successful PTCA is achieved in only 47–81% of total occlusions.[21–31] The overall incidence of major complications occurs with equal frequency after PTCA of total occlusions as compared to nontotal occlusions.[21–31] Major complications include acute closure rates of 5–10%, MI rates of 0–2%, emergency CABG rates of 0–3% and death rates of 0–1%. The long-term angiographic results are poor and are characterized by excessive restenosis and reocclusion. Late outcome after balloon angioplasty has been reported by several studies.[22,23,25,28,31–34] Up to 76% of patients are asymptomatic at one year after a successful PTCA.[22] However, absence of symptoms does not exclude restenosis as up to 40% of patients with angiographic restenosis may be free of angina.[35] Although successful PTCA of chronic total occlusion reduces the need for CABG by 50–75%, the overall survival or the incidence of late MI is not reduced.[22–25,31–34] Restenosis rates of 45–71% have been reported after successful PTCA of chronic total occlusion.[22,23,27,31,32,36]

The presence of a chronic total occlusion was once a relative contraindication to stenting. However, there have been several small observational studies of stenting in chronic total occlusion.[37–42] Almagor et al.[43] reported their experience of stenting in 65 chronic total occlusions. The stents were successfully deployed in 97% of lesions. The major complication rate was 3% and the restenosis rate was 24%. Two other smaller studies have reported 3- and 6-month restenosis rates of only 5%.[37,38] Ooka et al.[44] reported their experience in an observational study of stenting (n = 47) and PTCA (n = 65) in chronic total occlusions. Stenting reduced the reocclusion rate (10% vs. 35%) and restenosis rate (44% vs. 68%) compared to

balloon angioplasty alone. Early post-PTCA angiography demonstrates a large degree of recoil and unexpected dissection, which are likely the precursors of poor late results.[45] Stents provide a theoretical ideal solution to these mechanical problems. However, the milieu of total occlusions may be more thrombotic than that seen in nonocclusive lesions and the mechanical advantage offered by stents may be substantially undermined by the prothrombotic nature of the stents. This has prompted randomized trials to address these concerns and to confirm the favorable outcome after primary stenting of chronic total occlusions.

Stenting in Chronic Coronary Occlusion (SICCO) was a randomized, controlled trial in four Scandinavian centers which has been published recently.[46] The aim of the study was to assess the potential benefit of additional stent implantation after successful angioplasty of a chronic coronary occlusion. The study randomized 119 patients with a satisfactory result after successful recanalization by PTCA of a chronic coronary occlusion to 1) a control (PTCA) group with no other intervention; or 2) a group in which PTCA was followed by implantation of Palmaz–Schatz stents with full anticoagulation. Both total and functional occlusions were included and occlusions less than 2 weeks old were excluded. Follow-up angiography was performed before randomization, after-stent implantation and at 6-month follow-up.

The primary end-point of the study was the rate of restenosis (≥50% diameter stenosis). Secondary angiographic end-points were the rate of reocclusion and changes in MLD and diameter stenosis. The primary clinical end-point was the occurrence of major clinical adverse events (cardiac death, cerebrovascular accident, MI, target lesion revascularization). A secondary clinical end-point was the functional angina class.

The patients were recruited between March 1994 and May 1995. Two patients were excluded after randomization. Thus, the study group consisted of 117 patients (59 in the PTCA group and 58 in the stent group). Angiographic follow-up data were available in 114 patients and are summarized in Table 11.6. MLD at follow-up was significantly greater after stenting (1.92 ± 0.95 mm) as compared to PTCA (1.11 ± 0.78 mm; $p < 0.001$). Correspondingly, the percent diameter stenosis was significantly smaller in patients with stenting than in the patients treated with PTCA alone (45.1 ± 26.1 vs. 66.4 ± 24.5%; $p < 0.001$). Restenosis developed in 32% of patients with stenting and in 74% of patients with PTCA only ($p < 0.001$).

Clinical outcome is summarized in Table 11.7. Reocclusion was found in 12.3% of patients in the stent group and in 26.3% of patients in the PTCA group ($p = 0.058$) at follow-up angiography. However, this excluded vessel closures within the first 2 weeks, which occurred in 6.9% of patients in the stent group and 5.1% of patients in the PTCA group ($p = NS$). This rate of subacute stent thrombosis (6.9%) is higher than those reported in the STRESS

Table 11.6 Angiographic results in the SICCO trial.

	Stent (n = 57)	PTCA (n = 57)	p value
Reference diameter (mm)			
At randomization	3.16 ± 0.49	3.17 ± 0.53	NS
At follow-up	3.44 ± 0.70	3.30 ± 0.59	NS
DS (%)			
At randomization	29.8 ± 12.4	33.5 ± 10.4	NS
At follow-up	44.6 ± 26.1	66.4 ± 24.3	<0.001
MLD (mm)			
At randomization	2.21 ± 0.50	2.13 ± 0.27	NS
At follow-up	1.92 ± 0.95	1.11 ± 0.78	<0.001
Late loss from randomization to follow-up	0.30 ± 0.90	1.02 ± 0.96	0.001
Late loss from/after procedure to follow-up	0.85 ± 0.92	1.02 ± 0.96	NS
Reocclusion	12.3%	26.3%	0.06
Restenosis			
Defined as ≥50% DS	31.6%	73.7%	<0.001
Defined as ≥70% DS	15.8%	42.1%	0.002
Defined as <1.5 mm MLD	24.6%	66.7%	<0.001

Notes:

DS = diameter stenosis; MLD = minimal luminal diameter; NS = not significant.

Table 11.7 Clinical outcome in the SICCO trial.

Variable	Stent (n = 58)	PTCA (n = 59)
Death %	0	0
CVA %	0	0
AMI %	1.7	0
CABG %	5.2	1.7
Re-PTCA %	2.9	6.8
TLR within 300 days %	22.4	42.4*
Acute closure <2 weeks %	6.9	5.1
Major vascular complication %	6.9	0
Duration of hospital stay (days, mean ± SD)	5.3 ± 1.3	1.9 ± 0.9**
Patients free of angina %	57	24*

Notes:

*p = 0.025, **p < 0.001. CABG = coronary artery bypass surgery; CVA = cerebrovascular accident; AMI = acute myocardial infarction; PTCA = percutaneous transluminal coronary angioplasty; TLR = target lesion revascularization.

(3.4%) and the BENESTENT (3.5%) trials,[2,3] although the same anticoagulation regimen was used in all three studies. This may suggest a greater tendency towards stent thrombosis in recanalized occlusions than in simple lesions. This may be particularly relevant as the number of early reocclusions may have ben underestimated due to silent reocclusions within the first 24 hours.[30,45]

At follow-up, 57% of patients with stenting were free from angina compared with 24% of patients with PTCA only ($p < 0.001$). There were no deaths in the study and there was no significant difference in the rates of MI, CABG or re-PTCA between the two groups. However, the increased frequency of restenosis and angina in the PTCA group was reflected in an increased rate of target lesion revascularization within 300 days (42.4% PTCA group vs. 22.4% stent group; $p = 0.025$).

This is the first randomized study to report an improved long-term angiographic and clinical outcome after stenting of chronic coronary occlusion following successful recanalization with PTCA. The authors concluded that stenting is recommended in all successfully recanalized chronic coronary occlusions regardless of the result after PTCA alone.

The preliminary results of two other randomized studies have been presented. Thomas et al.[47] randomized 30 patients to 'stent' and 30 patients to 'no stent' groups following successful PTCA of a total occlusion. The time of occlusion was similar in both groups (14 ± 17 vs. 9 ± 10 weeks). There was no significant difference in the baseline left ventricular ejection fraction (59.6% vs. 53.1%; $p = NS$). The postprocedure angiographic result was significantly better in the stent group with a greater MLD (3.3 vs. 2.8 mm; $p < 0.01$) and a lower residual stenosis (-1.1% vs. 19.1%; $p < 0.001$). There was no clinical in-hospital vessel closure in either group. Six-month angiographic follow-up data was available in 20 patients in each group. Coronary patency (95% vs. 70%; $p < 0.05$), percent stenosis (37.8% vs. 60.0%; $p < 0.05$) and left ventricular ejection fraction (70.1% vs. 58.0%; $p < 0.05$) were significantly better in the stent group. There was no significant difference, however, in the MLD (2.0 ± 1.0 vs. 1.5 ± 1.3 mm; $p = NS$) and the restenosis rate (20% vs. 30%; $p = NS$). The clinical events at a mean follow-up to 37 weeks were similar in both groups, with a target lesion revascularization rate of 10% vs. 20% ($p = NS$).

Sato et al.[48] have reported the preliminary results in 60 lesions; 30 lesions were randomized to 'stent' and 30 lesions to 'balloon angioplasty' groups following successful PTCA of a total occlusion. Follow-up angiography was performed at 24 hours, and at 3 and 6 months. All procedures in the stent group were successful with no subacute stent thrombosis. Nine (30%) lesions in the balloon angioplasty group required 'bail-out' stenting for delayed distal flow (2 lesions) and residual stenosis ≥50% (7 lesions). Two (9%) lesions in the angioplasty group required coronary stenting for reocclusion at 24 hours. MLD immediately after the procedure (2.29 ± 0.47 vs. 1.87 ± 0.40 mm; $p < 0.001$) and at 24 hours (2.23 ± 0.41 vs. 1.63 ± 0.64 mm; $p < 0.001$) was significantly greater in the stent group. However, there was no significant difference in MLD at follow-up (1.57 ± 0.60 vs. 1.60 ± 0.72; $p = NS$) between the two groups. The binary restenosis rate was 36% in the stent group and 33% in the balloon angioplasty group ($p = NS$). The target lesion revascularization rate was 32% in the stent group and 29% in the balloon angioplasty group ($p = NS$). Thus, although coronary stenting was effective in preventing early reocclusion and was associated with a larger postprocedure and 24-hour MLD, the favorable luminal outcome was not sustained at follow-up and balloon angioplasty supported by bail-out stenting was equally effective as elective stenting in the management of total occlusions.

A large multicenter, randomized, international study is also currently underway and is expected to complete recruitment by May 1997. The Total Occlusion Study of Canada (TOSCA) is a randomized, multicenter study of stents versus PTCA for occluded coronary arteries. The aim of the study is to test the hypothesis that primary coronary stenting of total coronary occlusions will stabilize the postintervention lumen by preventing early recoil and sealing established dissection planes in the arterial wall and would result in a clinically significant reduction in target segment reocclusion, restenosis and adverse clinical events. A total of 382 patients will be randomized after successful crossing of the occlusion with a guidewire to receive PTCA only (with stent available as backup) or to stenting with a heparin-bonded Palmaz–Schatz stent. High-pressure stent optimization and treatment with aspirin and ticlopidine after stenting are a standard part of the protocol. The primary end-point of the study is failure of sustained patency (defined as TIMI <3 flow with target lesion stenosis ≥70% at follow-up angiography) with clinical outcome as a secondary end-point.

Total occlusion: impression

The data from published randomized studies of coronary stenting in total occlusions, at present, are based on small patient populations. The results of larger studies using improved stenting techniques and reduced anticoagulation therapy are awaited. Confirmation of favorable acute and long-term results from larger studies, such as TOSCA, is required before primary stenting of chronic total occlusions can be recommended. Subacute thrombosis of 6.9% and reocclusion in 12% of the patients are hardly acceptable; the time course and mechanism must be investigated and better understood to direct our treatment prior to acceptance of this therapy as a standard of care. Although it is logical that stenting, by reducing acute recoil and early closure, will result in greater late patency, this has yet to be confirmed in a major study. More importantly the role of patency *per se* on symptoms and left ventricular (LV) function at rest and exercise has to be clarified. Unless there is an improvement in functional outcome, the role of recanalization with stenting or PTCA must remain in the realm of belief and bias.

Stenting for failed angioplasty

Abrupt or threatened vessel closure is a serious complication of PTCA and results in a marked increase in morbidity and mortality.[49-52] Acute coronary occlusion developing during or early after PTCA has been reported in 3–9% of recent series.[49-54] The National Heart, Lung and Blood Institute 1985–86 PTCA Registry reported that 20% of all deaths, 40% of MIs and 25% of CABG recorded at 1-year follow-up study occurred in the 6.8% of patients who had periprocedural coronary occlusion.[49,55] One of the most powerful predictors of acute closure is the occurrence of coronary wall dissection after PTCA.[56,57] When multiple repeat inflations fail to rectify the vessel closure, patients have conventionally undergone emergency CABG which carries a significantly higher perioperative risk than elective surgery.[58-61] Several new percutaneous techniques have been advocated as an alternative ('bail-out') to emergency CABG including standard,[62] perfusion[63,64] and laser balloon angioplasty,[65] atherectomy[66] and intracoronary stenting.[67-73]

Intracoronary stent placement has become a widely accepted procedure for the management of abrupt or threatened occlusion during PTCA. There is a large body of evidence confirming the dramatic effectiveness of stent placement for improving the immediate angiographic outcome in these situations.[67-75] Despite the practical difficulties of precise stent placement in dissected vessels, angiographically successful stent deployment with restoration of Thrombolysis in Myocardial Infarction (TIMI) Grade III flow is possible in over 90% of the cases. In the Hirulog Angioplasty Trial,[76] abrupt vessel closure occurred in 9.2% (378) of the patients enrolled. Bail-out stenting was performed in 40% and 60% were treated with repeat PTCA. Patients treated with stents had a lower incidence of emergency CABG (10% vs. 19%; *p* < 0.05) and a lower incidence of recurrent ischemic events at 6 months (54% vs. 71%; *p* < 0.001) compared to patients treated with repeat PTCA. Nonetheless, data on the effectiveness of bail-out stenting are either a purely noncomparative observational series using historical and matched case controls, or nonrandomized prospective data with different definitions of threatened closure, different case selection and end-point definitions. Data from two randomized studies comparing stenting with the use of prolonged inflations with a perfusion balloon (PB) have been presented (Table

11.1). PB have been reported to be successful in 67–95% of cases and have the advantage of rapid deployment, having a minimal learning curve, and a relatively low cost.[77-80] Such randomized comparisons are important, because the use of stents in bail-out situations may be trading off an initially excellent cosmetic result for a higher risk of vascular and cardiac complications than for elective use, with stent thrombosis rate of up to 23%.[67-70,81-83] Moreover, there is no evidence that emergency stenting improves medium-term outcome after failed PTCA.

The Trial of Angioplasty and Stents in Canada II (TASC II) was a multicenter study recruiting from four centers across Canada between August 1991 and December 1993.[84] The primary end-points of the trial were immediate angiographic success (<50% residual stenosis with TIMI grade III flow and reduction in dissection grade to A or B) and procedural success (angiographic success in the absence of major cardiac complications or the need for emergency CABG) at 24 hours after the procedure. The first major event occurring in a given patient was taken as the end-point. Major events were defined in rank order as death, stroke, acute MI, CABG and repeat target vessel PTCA. Secondary end-points were bleeding complications requiring transfusion or surgical intervention, duration of hospital stay, 6-week freedom from major cardiovascular events, 6-month restenosis rates, functional status at 6 weeks and 5 months, and clinical outcome at 6 months.

Failed PTCA was defined as the presence of one of the following, associated with persistent ischemia:

1   Stenosis larger than 50% after a minimum of three inflations for 60 sec with an appropriately sized balloon (balloon artery ratio 0.9–1.1 by visual estimate).

2   Reduction in thrombolysis in myocardial infarction (TIMI) flow by one grade after PTCA.

3   Stenosis larger than 30% with less than 3 cm dissection of National Heart, Lung and Blood Institute (NHLBI) classification grade C–F.[85]

In the event of the failure of randomized treatment (a primary end-point) the patient could be treated at the operator's discretion. For failed perfusion balloon inflations, the preferred treatment was coronary stenting. Treatment failure was defined as persistent ischemia in association with 1) inability to transform dissection grade to A or B; 2) residual stenosis 50% or more; and 3) inability to obtain TIMI grade III flow.

Forty-four patients were randomized in the trial with 22 patients randomized to each treatment arm. There was no difference in baseline clinical and angiographic characteristics between the randomized groups. The angiographic results and clinical outcome are summarized in Tables 11.8 and 11.9, respectively. Immediate angiographic success was achieved in 20 of the 22 patients (91%) randomized to stenting as compared to 10 of the 22 patients (46%,

Table 11.8 Angiographic results in the TASC II study.

	Stent (n = 22)	PTCA (n = 22)
De novo lesions %	86	86
Restenosis lesions %	14	14
Lesion length (mm)	12.8 ± 4.6	9.9 ± 4.1
Percent diameter stenosis		
Baseline	78 ± 14	73 ± 14
Post-PTCA	58 ± 18	61 ± 17
Postrandomized procedure	20 ± 11	48 ± 20*
Follow-up	45 ± 20	46 ± 24
Minimal lumen diameter (mm)		
Baseline	0.62 ± 0.39	0.78 ± 0.43
Post-PTCA	1.16 ± 0.55	1.16 ± 0.53
Postrandomized procedure	2.18 ± 0.42	1.50 ± 0.52*
Follow-up	1.52 ± 0.68	1.58 ± 0.69
Recoil postrandomized procedure (mm)	0.33 ± 0.35	0.98 ± 0.51*
Restenosis rate %	26.3	31.3

Notes:
Data are presented as mean ± SD unless otherwise indicated. *$p < 0.001$.

Table 11.9 Clinical outcome in the TASC II study.

	Stent (n = 22)	PTCA (n = 22)
Angiographic success %	91	46*
Procedural success %	87	46**
Crossover treatment %	0	50***
Procedural MI %	0	4.6
24-hour TLR %	14	9
Any event in-hospital %	14	14
Hospital stay (days, mean ± SD)	7.4 ± 2.5	8.0 ± 7.7
Total MI at 6 weeks %	4.6	13.6
Total re-PTCA at 6 weeks %	4.6	0
Total CABG at 6 weeks %	9.1	9.1
Any event %	18.2	22.7
Vascular complications %	0	18.2

Notes:
*$p = 0.001$; **$p = 0.004$; ***$p < 0.001$. CABG = coronary artery bypass surgery; MI = myocardial infarction; PTCA = percutaneous transluminal coronary angioplasty; TLR = target lesion revascularization.

$p = 0.001$) randomized to perfusion balloon (PB). The procedural success rate was also significantly higher in the stent group (87% vs. 46%; $p = 0.004$).

Baseline angiographic analysis was available on all 44 patients. Preprocedural lesion characteristics were similar in both randomized groups. Results of the initial PTCA were also similar. The major difference in angiographic parameters after randomized treatments was the significant reduction in recoil with stent placement ($p < 0.001$), with a resulting increase in MLD ($p < 0.001$) and reduction in residual stenosis ($p < 0.001$). Stenting was also more efficient in obliterating complex dissections. Twelve patients randomized to stenting had a complex dissection (grade C–F) following the initial PTCA. Following stent placement eight of these had been obliterated, three improved to a minor dissection (grade A or B) with no flow limitation, and in one there was no change. Eight of the patients randomized to PB had a complex dissection following the initial procedure. Of these, one was obliterated, three improved and in four there was no change. In one patient, dissection grade worsened from A to D following PB treatment. Dissections were completely eradicated in all 9 patients who crossed successfully to stenting following failed PB treatment. Follow-up angiography was performed in 35 patients, 19 in the stent group and 16 in the PB group. There were no significant differences between the groups in the percent stenosis, minimal luminal diameter or the restenosis rate.

The total number of patients with in-hospital events was identical in both groups and there were no deaths in either group. All three patients requiring femoral vascular repair before hospital discharge were failed perfusion balloon patients who crossed over to stenting. Hospital stay for the initial procedure was 7.4 ± 2.5 days in the stent group and 8.0 ± 7.7 days in the PB group ($p = NS$). Stay for a successful PB procedure was 3.2 ± 1.3 days ($p < 0.001$ compared to stent group) compared with 12.8 ± 8.4 days for those crossing over to stenting ($p = 0.001$).

At 6 weeks, 18 (81.8%) of the patients in each group remained free of major events. Data on functional status according to the classification of the Canadian Cardiovascular Society were available in all 36 patients with no major events at 6 weeks. Fourteen (78%) patients were asymptomatic in the stent group as compared to 11 (66%) in the PB group ($p = NS$). There was no significant difference in the results of the exercise test between the two groups. Seventeen patients in each randomized group (77%) remained event-free at 6 months. Data on functional status and exercise tests were available in 32 of the 34 patients free of major cardiac events at 5 months. Nine (60%) patients were asymptomatic in the stent group as compared to 12 (70.6%) in the PB group ($p = NS$). There was no significant difference in the results of the exercise test between the two groups.

TASC II is the first randomized study to show that stenting is more successful than prolonged PB dilatation, as primary therapy for failed PTCA. The use of PB dilatation as primary therapy for failed PTCA does not jeopardize a successful result with a secondary stent and the combined approach can prevent emergency CABG for failed PTCA in over 90% of the cases. The immediate angiographic results and 24-hour procedural success rate of the strategy of primary stenting for failed PTCA were superior to PB. The mechanism of superiority of stent over PB is a reduction of acute recoil and elimination of complex dissections. The restenosis rate at 6 months was similar in patients receiving PB for failed PTCA (with stents available as backup) to those receiving a primary stent. The restenosis rate in both groups at 6 months is also similar to that reported in patients receiving an elective stent in *de novo* lesions.[2,3]

The preliminary data from the STENT-BY study have also been presented recently.[86] The study randomized 100 patients with TIMI 0 or TIMI 1 flow with angina and/or ischemia to Palmaz–Schatz stent implantation or 'conservative therapy' including prolonged balloon inflation and bypass surgery. The lesions included were larger than 15 mm in vessels less than 2.5 mm in diameter. The lesion had to be suitable to receive a single stent of 3.0 mm in diameter. The patients were treated with warfarin for 3 months after successful stenting. The crossover rate was 6% in the stent arm as compared to 16% in the conservative arm. Stabilization (TIMI 3 flow, no angina and no ischemia) was achieved in 93% of patients treated with stents as compared to 77% in the conservative therapy ($p = 0.05$). The restenosis rate was 26% after stenting as compared to 52% after PTCA ($p = 0.01$). The occurrence of death, acute MI, CABG and target lesion revascularization at 6 months after stent implantation and conservative treatment was 2% vs. 2%, 8% vs. 16%, 0% vs. 4% and 24% vs. 65%, respectively. The event-free survival was significantly better after stenting (29% vs. 69%; $p < 0.05$).

Acute closure: impression

Randomized trials in acute closure are difficult to perform. The number of patients studied in the above trials has been necessarily small. Despite this, bail-out stenting for acute or threatened closure complicating PTCA is of established value and can prevent emergency CABG in the majority of cases. Surgery may still be required in patients with failure of stent therapy (e.g. due to difficulties in crossing the lesion or inability to seal complex dissections) or in patients with left main coronary dissections. Registry data for stents allowing side-branch patency and bifurcation stents in acute closure may confirm their benefit in more complex scenarios.

Stenting in saphenous vein grafts

The management of patients with recurrent ischemia after CABG poses a difficult problem. The rate of saphenous vein graft failure after CABG is 8% at 1 year, 38% at 5 years and 75% at 10 years.[87] Furthermore, progression of coronary artery disease occurs in approximately 5% of the patients per year.[88] Repeat CABG is associated with a 2- to 4-fold higher risk than the initial operation with a periprocedural MI rate of 2–8% and mortality of 2–5%.[89–93] Moreover, the likelihood of complete relief of symptoms is less compared with a first operation. The 5-year event-free survival- and angina-free survival are only 64% and 50% respectively.[94,95] Other treatment modalities such as percutaneous revascularization techniques are therefore being proposed as an alternative to repeat CABG.

In selected cases, PTCA of vein grafts can be performed with a high procedural success rate varying from 78 to 97%.[88,96,97] The major complication rate is low with a mortality of 0–5%, an MI rate of 0–8% and a need for urgent surgery of less than 3.5%. However, the major limitation of PTCA in saphenous vein grafts is restenosis, which occurs in 23–73% of patients within 6 months.[88,96,97]

Several observational studies have reported that a variety of stents can be deployed in saphenous vein grafts with a high procedural success rate (93–100%), a low incidence of stent thrombosis (0–10%) and major clinical complications (0–4%).[98–102] The restenosis rates also appear to be lower. However, these favorable results are offset by poor late clinical outcome. Event-free survival was 75% at 6 months, 67% at 12 months and only 55% at 2 years.[103] This was mostly due to progressive disease in nonstented vessels. In a recent observational study, the mean ± SD estimated survival at 5 years after stent implantation was 83 ± 5%, survival free from MI at 5 years was 61% ± 6% and event-free survival at 5 years (from MI, CABG and angioplasty) was 30 ± 7%.[104] Laham et al.[105] have reported that patients who had been treated with a stent for vein graft disease had a lower 5-year survival rate (70.5% vs. 93.4%) and event-free survival (21.1% vs. 63.3%) compared to those treated with a stent for native coronary disease.

The multicenter, prospective, randomized Study of Stent vs. Angioplasty for Vein Graft Disease (SAVED) trial has now been completed and the preliminary results have been presented.[106] Patients who were symptomatic, or had objective evidence of ischemia, with significant disease in a single vein graft, were randomized to elective Palmaz–Schatz stent implantation or standard balloon angioplasty, with stent crossover for failed PTCA, between January 1993 to June 1995. Eligible patients included those with stenoses larger than 60% by visual estimate in vessels 3.0–5.0 mm in diameter. Clinical and angiographic exclusion criteria included a recent MI, evidence of thrombus, diffuse disease (>2 stents required) and evidence of poor distal runoff.

The trial randomized 220 patients with 242 new saphenous vein graft lesions to PTCA (n = 110) or stenting (n = 110). Angiographic follow-up at 6 months was performed in 86% (166/193) of eligible patients. The angiographic data is summarized in Table 11.10. The overall restenosis rate in the study was 41% (78/189 lesions). Restenosis occurred in 47% of lesions treated by PTCA as compared to 36% of lesions treated by stenting (p = 0.11). Restenosis was associated with a higher incidence of diabetes mellitus (39% vs. 26%; p = 0.07). Other significant predictors of restenosis were smaller reference vessel diameter (3.02 ± 0.57 vs. 3.23 ± 0.56 mm; p < 0.05), complex ulcerated lesion morphology (48% vs. 30%; p = 0.02), smaller baseline MLD (0.85 ± 0.41 vs. 0.97 ± 0.40 mm; p < 0.05) and smaller postprocedural MLD (2.27 ± 0.59 vs. 2.61 ± 0.55 mm; p < 0.0001).

The clinical outcome is summarized in Table 11.11. Both the angiographic success (<50% stenosis by quantitative angiography) and the procedural success (angiographic success in the absence of major in-hospital complication) were superior in patients treated with stenting. There was a trend towards a decreased rate of target lesion revascularization in the group treated with stents. There was a significant reduction in the composite clinical end-point of patients with major cardiac adverse events in the stent group (25.9% vs. 39.3%; p = 0.04). Classical anticoagulation with warfarin was used in the study, after stenting, and the incidence of vascular complications and the duration of hospital stay in the stent group were significantly higher. Kaplan-Meir estimates that at 1 year, the occurrence of death, Q-wave MI, repeat CABG and target lesion revascularization were 90, 94, 96 and 76% after stent implantation and 85, 94, 85 and 70% after balloon angioplasty, respectively. The composite analysis of all clinical events at one year after stent implantation and balloon angioplasty was 72 and 56%, respectively.[107]

Clinical documentation of early stent thrombosis (0–30 days) was only reported in one patient (1%).[108] Late angiographic follow-up revealed target vessel occlusion in 9% of stent patients and 6% of PTCA patients (p = NS). However, only 3 of the 9 (33%) stented patients with complete graft occlusion, demonstrated by late angiography, had a major cardiac event (death or MI).[108] This would suggest that vein graft occlusion within 6 months occurs frequently after intervention and may be inherent to the biology of this circulation. Because total occlusion of bypass grafts following coronary intervention is infrequently accompanied by major clinical events, the true incidence of stent thrombosis in saphenous vein bypass grafts may have been underestimated by previous studies.

During the course of the SAVED study the use of high-pressure stent deployment evolved into routine clinical practice. The use of high-pressure inflations (≥16 atm)

Table 11.10 Angiographic results in the SAVED study.

	Stent (n = 108)	PTCA (n = 107)
Graft age (years)	10.1 ± 4.2	9.4 ± 4.3
Number of lesions treated %		
1	82	83
2	14	10
≥3	4	7
Lesion length (mm)	9.6 ± 5.4	9.8 ± 5.2
Percent diameter stenosis		
Baseline	72 ± 12	71 ± 12
Postprocedure	12 ± 13	32 ± 17*
Follow-up	46 ± 30	51 ± 26
Minimal lumen diameter (mm)		
Baseline	0.90 ± 0.42	0.94 ± 0.44
Postprocedure	2.81 ± 0.49	2.16 ± 0.57*
Follow-up	1.73 ± 1.02	1.49 ± 0.88**
Net gain in minimal lumen diameter (mm)	0.85 ± 0.96	0.54 ± 0.91***
Restenosis rate %		
By lesion	35.7	47.3
By patient	37.2	46.3

Notes:
Data are presented as mean ± SD unless otherwise indicated. *$p < 0.001$; **$p = 0.05$; ***$p = 0.03$

Table 11.11 Clinical outcome (0–240 days) in the SAVED study.

	Stent (n = 108)	PTCA (n = 107)
Angiographic success %	97	86*
Procedural success %	92	69**
Death %	6.5	9.3
CVA	0	0
Q-wave MI %	4.6	3.7
Non-Q-wave MI %	5.6	11.2
CABG %	7.4	12.1
re-PTCA	13.0	15.9
TLR %	16.7	26.2
Any event %	25.9	39.3***
Vascular complications %	16.7	4.7*
Hospital stay (days, mean ± SD)	7.1 ± 6.1	3.8 ± 6.7**

Notes:
*$p < 0.01$; **$p < 0.001$; ***$p = 0.04$. CABG = coronary artery bypass surgery; CVA = cerebrovascular accident; MI = myocardial infarction; PTCA = percutaneous transluminal coronary angioplasty; TLR = target lesion revascularization.

significantly increased during the later stages of the trial ($p < 0.001$). A subset analysis compared the 6-month angiographic results of stented vein graft lesions treated with high-pressure (≥ 16 atm, $n = 31$ lesions) and lower (≥ 15 atm. $n = 88$ lesions) pressure deployment.[109] Stented lesions treated with high-pressure inflations demonstrated significantly smaller MLD at follow-up as compared to those lesions treated with lower-pressure inflations (1.26 mm vs. 1.91 mm; $p < 0.01$). The suboptimal 6-month outcome with high-pressure inflations was due to the significantly greater late loss (1.47 mm vs. 0.91 mm; $p < 0.01$). These results suggest that deployment of stents with 16 atm or more inflation pressures has a deleterious effect on late lumen loss and 6-month angiographic outcome in vein grafts. Further studies are required to confirm this observation and to investigate the process underlying this increased late loss.

Saphenous vein grafts: impression

In summary, stenting appears to be superior to angioplasty in selected short, nonostial, *de novo* saphenous vein graft lesions in patients without acute MI, thrombus or poor left ventricular function. These are of questionable clinical relevance, being uncommon as compared to the progressive aggressive disease affecting 'end of life' grafts. In this latter, more common scenario, it may be more appropriate to 'regraft' the entire vessel internally with long graft stents or denser-weave devices. Certainly, further trials including different lesion subsets and longer follow-up are required to establish definitively the value of stenting in saphenous vein graft lesions.

The future

Several studies have suggested that patients treated with stenting do well with reduced anticoagulation regimen that excludes intravenous dextran, oral coumadin and prolonged heparin, when high-pressure balloons result in full stent apposition with the vessel wall.[110–112] Antiplatelet therapy with aspirin and ticlopidine as compared to anticoagulation therapy with heparin, phenprocoumon and aspirin has been shown to be associated with a significant risk reduction for MI, reduced need for a repeat intervention, decreased peripheral vascular events and a reduction in occlusion of the stented vessel.[113] It has also been recently shown using intravascular ultrasound that high-pressure balloon inflations to 18 or 20 atm are more effective in achieving ideal apposition of the stent to the vessel wall as compared to standard-pressure balloons of larger than

stent size.[110] The adoption of these techniques may significantly reduce the incidence of subacute stent thrombosis and may result in improved clinical outcome after coronary stenting. Currently a number of ongoing randomized studies will address the role of high-pressure stent optimization, the use of heparin-bonded stents, and the safety and efficacy of reduced anticoagulation with aspirin or aspirin and ticlopidine. The use of abciximab in patients with an increased risk of PTCA has been shown to reduce the occurrence of ischemic events immediately after PTCA and during the 6-month follow-up period significantly, and is associated with a significant reduction in repeat revascularization (22% vs. 16%).[114] This has prompted the hypothesis that the combined use of a stent and abciximab will further reduce the restenosis rate and improve the long-term clinical outcome. This will be studied in the Epilog Stent Study, in which 1500 patients will be randomized to either PTCA with abciximab, Palmaz–Schatz stent implantation with placebo or Palmaz–Schatz stent implantation with abciximab. The safety and efficacy of stenting, as compared to balloon angioplasty in multilesion or multivessel disease, has been investigated in the BENESTENT II study, which has now been completed. It will be apparent to the most casual reader that there is a major difference between clinical practice and randomized trials. We do not propose that only randomized controlled trials should establish the role of a new device. Certainly, the careful review of registry data may provide insightful support to these. However, belief and bias, balanced precariously on a narrow set of studies, must be challenged. Stents have been rigorously tested in a narrow subset of our practice; the authors, rather than decry the use of stents, support the broadening of these studies to link academic well controlled data to the 'real world' of belief and bias.

References

1   Sigwart U, Puel J, Mirkovitch V, *et al.* Intravascular stents to prevent occlusion and restenosis after transluminal angioplasty. *N Engl J Med* 1987; **316**: 701–6.

2   Serruys PW, de Jaegere P, Kiemeneij F, *et al.* A comparison of balloon expandable stent implantation with balloon angioplasty in patients with coronary artery disease. *N Engl J Med* 1994; **331**: 489–95.

3   Fischman DL, Leon MB, Baim D, *et al.* A randomized comparison of coronary stent placement and balloon angioplasty in the treatment of coronary artery disease. *N Engl J Med* 1994; **331**: 496–501.

4   Macaya C, Serruys P, Ruygrok P, *et al.* Continued benefit of coronary stenting versus balloon angioplasty: one-year clinical follow-up of Benestent Trial. *J Am Coll Cardiol* 1996; **27**: 255–61.

5   Masotti M, Serra A, Fernandez-Aviles F, *et al.* Stent vs. Angioplasty Restenosis Trial (START). Angiographic results at six month follow-up. *Circulation* 1996; **94**: 1-685.

6   Nobuyoshi M, Kimura T, Nosaka H, *et al.* Restenosis after successful percutaneous transluminal coronary angioplasty: serial angiographic follow-up of 229 patients. *J Am Coll Cardiol* 1988; **12**: 616–23.

7   Holmes DR jr, Vlietstra RE, Smith HC, *et al.* Restenosis after percutaneous transluminal coronary angioplasty (PTCA): a report from the PTCA Registry of the National Heart, Lung, and Blood Institute. *Am J Cardiol* 1984; **53**: 77C–81C.

8   Gruentzig AR, King SB III, Schlumpf M, Siegenthaler W. Long-term follow-up after percutaneous transluminal coronary angioplasty: the early Zurich experience. *N Engl J Med* 1987; **316**: 1127–32.

9   Hirshfeld JW jr, Schwartz JS, Jugo R, *et al.* Restenosis after coronary angioplasty: a multivariate statistical model to relate lesion and procedural variables to restenosis. *J Am Coll Cardiol* 1991; **18**: 647–56.

10 Meier B, King SBI, Gruentzig AR. Repeat coronary angioplasty. *J Am Coll Cardiol* 1984; **4**: 463–6.

11 Williams DO, Gruentzig A, Kent K, Detre K, Kelsey S, To T. Efficacy of repeat percutaneous transluminal coronary angioplasty for coronary restenosis. *Am J Cardiol* 1984; **53**: 32C–35C.

12 Dimas AP, Gringera F, Arora RR, *et al.* Repeat coronary angioplasty as treatment for restenosis. *J Am Coll Cardiol* 1992; **19**: 1310–14.

13 Savage MP, Fischman DL, Schatz RA, *et al.* Long-term angiographic and clinical outcome after implantation of a balloon-expandable stent in the native coronary circulation. *J Am Coll Cardiol* 1994; **24**: 1207–12.

14 Black A, Anderson V, Roubin G, *et al.* Repeat coronary angioplasty: correlates of a second restenosis. *J Am Coll Cardiol* 1988; **11**: 714–18.

15 Teirstein P, Hoover C, Ligon R, *et al.* Repeat coronary angioplasty: efficacy of a third angioplasty for a second restenosis. *J Am Coll Cardiol* 1989; **13**: 291–6.

16 Mittal S, Weiss DL, Hirshfeld JW, Kolansky DM, Herrman HC. Restenotic lesions have a worse outcome after stenting. *Circulation* 1996; **94**: 1-331 (abstract).

17 Ellis SG, Savage M, Fischman D, *et al.* Restenosis after placement of Palmaz–Schatz stents in native coronary arteries. Initial results of a multicentre experience. *Circulation* 1992; **86**: 1836–44.

18 Beatt KJ, Serruys PW, Luijten HE, *et al.* Restenosis after coronary angioplasty: the paradox of increased lumen diameter and restenosis. *J Am Coll Cardiol* 1992; **19**: 258–66.

19 Penn IM, Ricci DR, Almond DG, *et al.* Coronary artery stenting reduces restenosis: final results from the Trial of Angioplasty and Stents in Canada (TASC) I. *Circulation* 1995; **92 (Suppl)**: 1-279.

20 Erbel R, Haude M, Hopp WH, *et al.* Restenosis Stent (REST) study: randomized trial comparing stenting and balloon angioplasty for treatment of stenosis after angioplasty. *J Am Coll Cardiol* 1996; **27**: 139A.

21 Stone GW, Rutherford BD, McConahay DR, *et al.* Procedural outcome of angioplasty for total coronary artery occlusion; an analysis of 971 lesions in 905 patients. *J Am Coll Cardiol* 1990; **15**: 849–56.

22 Bell MR, Berger PB, Bresnahan JF, Reeder GS. Initial and longterm outcome of 354 patients after coronary balloon angioplasty of total coronary artery occlusion. *Circulation* 1992; **85**: 1003–11.

23 Ivanhoe RJ, Weintraub WAS, Douglas JS jr, *et al.* Percutaneous transluminal coronary angioplasty of chronic total occlusions. Primary success, restenosis and longterm clinical follow up. *Circulation* 1992; **85**: 106–15.

24 Maiello L, Colombo A, Gianrossi R, *et al.* Coronary angioplasty of chronic occlusions: factors predictive of procedural success. *Am Heart J* 1992; **124**: 581–4.

25 Stewart J, Denne L, Bowker T, *et al.* Percutaneous transluminal coronary angioplasty in chronic coronary artery occlusion. *J Am Coll Cardiol* 1993; **21**: 1371–6.

26 Ishizaka N, Issiki T, Saeki F, *et al.* Angiographic follow up after successful percutaneous coronary angioplasty for chronic total occlusion: experience in 110 consecutive patients. *Am Heart J* 1994; **127**: 8.

27 Kinoshitaw I, Katoh O, Nariyama J, *et al.* Coronary angioplasty of chronic total occlusions with bridging collateral vessels: immediate and follow up outcome from a large single center experience. *J Am Coll Cardiol* 1995; **26**: 490–515.

28 Ruocco NA jr, Ring ME, Holubkov R, *et al.* Results of coronary angioplasty of chronic total occlusions (the National Heart, Lung and Blood Institute 1985–1986 Percutaneous Transluminal Angioplasty Registry). *Am J Cardiol* 1992; **69**: 69–76.

29 Tan K, Sulke N, Taub N, Sowton E. Clinical and lesion morphology determinants of coronary angioplasty success and complications: current experience. *J Am Coll Cardiol* 1995; **25**: 855–65.

30 Favereaux X, Corcos T, Guerin Y, *et al.* Early re-occlusion

after successful coronary angioplasty success and complications. Current experience. *J Am Coll Cardiol* 1995; **25**: 139A.

31 Berger PB, Holmes DR, Ohman M, *et al.* Restenosis, reocclusion and adverse cardiovascular events after successful balloon angioplasty of occluded versus nonoccluded coronary arteries. Results from the Multicentre American Research Trial with Cilazapril after Angioplasty to Prevent Transluminal Coronary Obstruction and Restenosis (MARCATOR). *J Am Coll Cardiol* 1996; **27**: 1–7.

32 Violaris A, Melkert R, Serruys P. Longterm luminal renarrowing after successful elective coronary angioplasty of total occlusions. A quantitative angiographic analysis. *Circulation* 1995; **91**: 2140–50.

33 Safian RD, McCabe CH, Sapperly ME, *et al.* Initial success and longterm follow up of percutaneous transluminal coronary angioplasty in chronic total occlusions versus conventional stenoses. *Am J Cardiol* 1988; **61**: 23G–28G.

34 Finci L, Meier B, Fayre J, *et al.* Longterm results of successful and failed angioplasty for chronic total coronary arterial occlusion. *Am J Cardiol* 1990; **66**: 660.

35 Haerer W, Schmidt A, Eggeling T, *et al.* Angioplasty of chronic total coronary occlusions. Results of a controlled randomized trial. *J Am Coll Cardiol* 1991; **17**: 113A.

36 Anderson TJ, Knudtson ML, Roth DL, *et al.* Improvement in left ventricular function following PTCA of chronic totally occluded arteries. *Circulation* 1991; **84**: II-519.

37 Hsu Y-S, Tamai H, Ueda K, *et al.* Clinical efficacy of coronary stenting in chronic total occlusions. *Circulation* 1994; **90**: I-613.

38 Ooka M, Suzuki T, Kosokawa H, Kukkutomi T, Yamashita K, Hayase M. Stenting vs. non-stenting after revascularization of chronic total occlusion. *Circulation* 1994; **90**: I-613.

39 Maiello L, Hall P, Shigeru N, *et al.* Results of stent implantation for diffuse coronary disease assisted by intravascular ultrasound. *J Am Coll Cardiol* 1995; **25**: 156A.

40 Reimers B, Di Mario C, Nierop P, Paquetto G, Camenzind E, Ruygrok P. Longterm restenosis after multiple stent implantation. A quantitative angiographic study. *Circulation* 1995; **92**: I-327.

41 Ooka M, Suzuki T, Yokoya K, *et al.* Stenting after revascularization of chronic total occlusion. *Circulation* 1995; **92**: I-94.

42 Goldberg SL, Colombo A, Maiello L, *et al.* Intracoronary stent insertion after balloon angioplasty of chronic total occlusion. *J Am Coll Cardiol* 1995; **25**: 713–19.

43 Almagor Y, Borrione M, Maiello L, Khalt B, Finci L, Colombo A. Coronary stenting after recanalization of chronic total coronary occlusions. *Circulation* 1993; **88**: I-504.

44 Ooka M, Suzuki T, Yokoya K, *et al.* Stenting after revascularization of chronic total occlusion. *Circulation* 1995; **92**: I-94.

45 Buller CE, Penn IM, Ricci DR, Ray S, Fox R, Mancini GBJ. Recoil, dissection, and reocclusion early following PTCA of total coronary occlusions. *Can J Cardiol* 1994; **10**: 135C.

46 Sirnes PA, Golf S, Myreng Y, *et al.* Stenting in chronic coronary occlusion (SICCO): a randomized, controlled trial of adding stent implantation after successful angioplasty. *J Am Coll Cardiol* 1996; **28**: 1444–51.

47 Thomas M, Hancock J, Holmberg S, Wainwright R, Jewitt D. Coronary stenting following successful angioplasty for total occlusions: preliminary results of a randomized trial. *J Am Coll Cardiol* 1996; **27**: 153A.

48 Sato Y, Nosaka H, Kimura T, Nobuyoshi M. Randomized comparison of balloon angioplasty versus coronary stent implantation for total occlusion. *J Am Coll Cardiol* 1996; **27**: 152A.

49 Detre KM, Holmes DR, Holubkov R, *et al.* Incidence and consequences of periprocedural occlusion: the 1985–1986 National Heart, Lung, and Blood Institute Percutaneous Transluminal Coronary Angioplasty Registry. *Circulation* 1990; **82**: 739–50.

50 De Feyter PJ, van der Brand M, Laarman GJ, van Domburg R, Serruys PW, Suryapranata H. Acute coronary artery occlusion during and after percutaneous coronary angiography: frequency, prediction, clinical course, management, and follow-up. *Circulation* 1991; **83**: 927–36.

51 Lincoff AM, Popma JJ, Ellis SG, Hacker JA, Topol EJ. Abrupt vessel closure complicating coronary angioplasty: clinical, angiographic and therapeutic profile. *J Am Coll Cardiol* 1992; **19**: 926–35.

52 Ellis SG, Roubin GS, King SB III, *et al.* In-hospital cardiac mortality after acute closure after angioplasty: analysis of risk factors from 8,027 procedures. *J Am Coll Cardiol* 1988; **11**: 211–16.

53 Ellis SG, Roubin GS, King SB, *et al.* Angiographic and clinical predictors of acute closure after native vessel coronary angioplasty. *Circulation* 1988; **77**: 372–9.

54 Tenaglia AN, Fortin DF, Califf RM, *et al.* Predicting the risk of abrupt closure after angioplasty in an individual patient. *J Am Coll Cardiol* 1994; **24**: 1004–11.

55 Detre K, Holubkov R, Kelsey S, *et al.* One-year follow-up results of the 1985–1986 National Heart, Lung, and Blood

Institute's Percutaneous Transluminal Coronary Angioplasty Registry. *Circulation* 1989; **80**: 421–8.

56   Praysons RA, Ratliff NB. An analysis of outcome following percutaneous transluminal coronary angioplasty: an autopsy study. *Arch Pathol Lab Med* 1990; **114**: 1211–17.

57   Herrmann WRM, Foley DP, Rensing BJ, *et al.* Usefulness of quantitative and qualitative angiographic lesion morphology, and clinical characteristics in predicting major adverse cardiac events during and after native coronary balloon angioplasty. *Am J Cardiol* 1993; **72**: 14–20.

58   Stark KS, Satler LF, Krucoff MW, Rackley CE, Kent KM. Myocardial salvage after failed coronary angioplasty. *J Am Coll Cardiol* 1990; **15**: 78–82.

59   Talley JD, Weintraub WS, Roubin GS, *et al.* Failed elective percutaneous transluminal coronary angioplasty requiring coronary artery bypass surgery: in-hospital and late clinical outcome at 5 years. *Circulation* 1990; **82**: 1203–13.

60   Buffet P, Danchin N, Villemot JP, *et al.* Early and long-term outcome after emergency coronary artery bypass surgery after failed coronary angioplasty. *Circulation* 1991; **84 (Suppl III)**: III-254–III-259.

61   Craver JM, Weintraub WS, Jones EL, Guyton RA, Hatcher CR jr. Emergency coronary artery bypass surgery for failed percutaneous coronary angioplasty: a 10-year experience. *Ann Surg* 1992; **215**: 425–33.

62   Marquis J-F, Schwartz L, Aldridge H, Majid P, Henderson M, Matushinsky E. Acute coronary artery occlusion during percutaneous transluminal coronary angioplasty treated by redilation of the occluded segment. *J Am Coll Cardiol* 1984; **4**: 1268–71.

63   Leitschuh ML, Mills RM, Jacobs AK, Ruocco NA, LaRosa D, Faxon D. Outcome after major dissection during coronary angioplasty using the perfusion balloon catheter. *Am J Cardiol* 1991; **67**: 1056–60.

64   Foley JB, Sridhar K, Dawdy J, Konstantinou C, Brown FRIG, Penn IM. Pros and cons of perfusion balloons in failed angioplasty. *Cathet Cardiovasc Diagn* 1994; **31**: 264–9.

65   Jenkins RD, Spears JR. Laser balloon angioplasty. A new approach to abrupt coronary occlusion and chronic restenosis. *Circulation* 1990; **81 (Suppl IV)**: IV-101–8.

66   Lee TC, Hartzler GO, Rutherford BD, McConahay DR. Removal of an occlusive coronary dissection flap by using an atherectomy catheter. *Cathet Cardiovasc Diagn* 1990; **20**: 185–8.

67   Sigwart U, Urban P, Golf S, *et al.* Emergency stenting for acute occlusion after coronary balloon angioplasty. *Circulation* 1988; **78**: 1121–7.

68   Herrman HC, Buchbinder M, Clemen MW, *et al.* Emergent use of balloon-expandable coronary artery stenting for failed percutaneous transluminal coronary angioplasty. *Circulation* 1992; **86**: 812–19.

69   Roubin GS, Cannon AD, Agarawal SK, *et al.* Intracoronary stenting for acute and threatened closure complicating percutaneous transluminal coronary angioplasty. *Circulation* 1992; **85**: 916–27.

70   Schomig A, Kastrati A, Mudra H, *et al.* Four-year experience with Palmaz–Schatz stenting in coronary angioplasty complicated by dissection with threatened or present vessel closure. *Circulation* 1994; **90**: 2716–24.

71   Hearn JA, King SB III, Douglas JS, *et al.* Clinical and angiographic outcomes after coronary artery stenting for acute or threatened closure after percutaneous transluminal angioplasty: initial results with a balloon-expandable stainless steel design. *Circulation* 1993; **88**: 2086–96.

72   Haude M, Erbel R, Straub U, Dietz U, Schatz R, Meyer J. Results of intracoronary stents for management of coronary dissection after balloon angioplasty. *Am J Cardiol* 1991; **67**: 691–6.

73   Foley JB, Brown RIG, Penn IM. Thrombosis and restenosis after stenting in failed angioplasty: comparison with elective stenting. *Am Heart J* 1994; **128**: 12–20.

74   George BS, Voorhees WD, Roubin GS, *et al.* Multicentre investigation of coronary stenting to treat acute or threatened closure after percutaneous transluminal coronary angioplasty: clinical and angiographic outcomes. *J Am Coll Cardiol* 1993; **22**: 135–43.

75   Sutton JM, Ellis SG, Roubin GS, *et al.* Major clinical events after coronary stenting. *Circulation* 1994; **89**: 1126–37.

76   Meckel C, Kjelsberg M, Ahmed W, *et al.* Bailout stenting for abrupt closure during coronary angioplasty. *Circulation* 1995; **92**: 1-688.

77   Saenz CR, Schwartz KM, Slysh SJ, Palanca K, Curry RC. Experience with the use of coronary autoperfusion catheter during complicated angioplasty. *Cathet Cardiovasc Diagn* 1990; **20**: 276–8.

78   Leitschuh ML, Mills RM, Jacobs AK, Ruocco NA, LaRosa D, Faxon D. Outcome after major dissection during coronary angioplasty using the perfusion balloon catheter. *Am J Cardiol* 1991; **67**: 1056–60.

79   Jackman JD, Zidar JP, Tcheng JE, Overman AB, Phillips HR, Stacks RS. Outcome after prolonged balloon inflations of >20 minutes for initially unsuccessful percutaneous transluminal coronary angioplasty. *Am J Cardiol* 1992; **69**: 1417–21.

80   Van Lierde JM, Glazier JJ, Stammen FJ, *et al.* Use of an

autoperfusion catheter in the treatment of acute refractory vessel closure after coronary balloon angioplasty: immediate and six month follow-up results. *Br Heart J* 1992; **68**: 51–4.

81 Kastrati A, Schomig A, Dietz R, Neumann F-J, Richardt D. Time course of restenosis during the first year after emergency coronary stenting. *Circulation* 1993; **87**: 1498–505.

82 Maiello L, Colombo A, Gianrossi R, McCanny R, Finci L. Coronary stenting for treatment of acute or threatened closure following dissection after coronary balloon angioplasty. *Am Heart J* 1993; **125**: 1570–5.

83 Kiemeneij F, Laarman GJ, van der Wieken R, Suwarganda J. Emergency coronary stenting with the Palmaz–Schatz stent for failed transluminal coronary angioplasty: results of a learning curve. *Am Heart J* 1993; **126**: 23–31.

84 Ricci DR, Ray S, Buller CE, *et al.* Six month followup of patients randomized to prolonged inflation or stent for abrupt occlusion during PTCA—clinical and angiographic data: TASC II. *Circulation* 1995; **92**: I-475.

85 Coronary artery angiographic changes after PTCA: Manual of operations NHLBI PTCA Registry, 1985–6; Baseline form: 9.

86 Haude M. Third Thoraxcenter course on coronary stenting, Rotterdam, The Netherlands, December 1996.

87 Campeau L, Enjalbert M, Lesperance J, *et al.* The relation of risk factors to the development of atherosclerosis in saphenous vein bypass grafts and the progression of disease in the native circulation. *N Engl J Med* 1984; **311**: 1329–32.

88 De Feyter P, van Suylen RJ, de Jaegere P, *et al.* Balloon angioplasty for the treatment of lesions in saphenous venous bypass grafts. *J Am Coll Cardiol* 1993; **21**: 1539–49.

89 Reul GJ, Cooley DA, Ott DA, *et al.* Reoperation for recurrent coronary artery disease. *Arch Surg* 1979; **114**: 1269–75.

90 Foster ED, Fisher LD, Kaiser GC, *et al.* Comparison of operative mortality and morbidity for initial and repeat coronary artery bypass grafting: the Coronary Artery Surgery Study (CASS) Registry experience. *Ann of Thoracic Surg* 1984; **38**: 563–70.

91 Pidgeon J, Brooks N, Magee P, *et al.* Reoperation for angina after previous aortocoronary bypass surgery. *Br Heart J* 1985; **53**: 269–75.

92 Laird-Meeter K, VanDomBurg R, Vanden Brand MJBM, *et al.* Incidence, risk and outcome for reintervention after aortocoronary bypass surgery. *Br Heart J* 1987; **57**: 427–35.

93 Verheul HA, Moulign AC, Hondema S, *et al.* Late results of 200 repeat coronary artery bypass operations. *Am J Cardiol* 1991; **57**: 24–30.

94 Verheul H, Moulijn A, Hondema S, Schouwink M. Late results of 200 repeat coronary artery bypass operations. *Am J Cardiol* 1991; **57**: 24–30.

95 Lytle B, Loop F, Cosgrove D, Taylor P. Fifteen hundred coronary reoperations. *J Thorac Cardiovasc Surg* 1987; **93**: 847–59.

96 Tan K, Henderson R, Sulke N, Cooke R. Percutaneous transluminal coronary angioplasty in patients with prior coronary artery bypass grafting: ten years' experience. *Cath Cardiovasc Diagn* 194; **31**: 11–17.

97 Morrison D, Crowley S, Veerakul G, Barbire C, Grover F, Sacks J. Percutaneous transluminal angioplasty of saphenous vein grafts for medically refractory unstable angina. *J Am Coll Cardiol* 1994; **23**: 1066–70.

98 Wong SC, Baim D, Schatz R, *et al.* Immediate results and late outcomes after stent implantation in saphenous vein graft lesions: the multicentre US Palmaz–Schatz stent experience. *J Am Coll Cardiol* 1995; **26**: 704–12.

99 Rechavía E, Litvack F, Macko G, Eigler N. Stent implantation of saphenous vein graft aorto-ostial lesions in patients with unstable ischemic syndromes: immediate angiographic results and longterm clinical outcome. *J Am Coll Cardiol* 1995; **25**: 855–70.

100 Wong SC, Popma J, Pichard A, Kent K. Comparison of clinical and angiographic outcomes after saphenous vein grafts angioplasty using coronary versus 'biliary' tubular slotted stents. *Circulation* 1995; **91**: 339–50.

101 Piana R, Moscucci M, Cohen D, *et al.* Palmaz–Schatz stenting for treatment of focal vein graft stenosis: immediate results and longterm outcome. *J Am Coll Cardiol* 1994; **23**: 1296–304.

102 Leon MB, Wong SC, Pichard A. Balloon expandable stent implantation in saphenous vein grafts. In: Hermann HC, Hirschfeld JW (eds). *Clinical Use of the Palmaz–Schatz Intracoronary Stent* (Future Publishing, 1993): 111–21.

103 Sketch M, Wong C, Chuang Y, *et al.* Progressive deterioration in late (2-year) clinical outcomes after stent implantation in saphenous vein grafts: the Multicenter JJIS experience. *J Am Coll Cardiol* 1995; **25**: 79A.

104 de Jaegere P, Domburg RT, de Feyter PJ, *et al.* Long-term clinical outcome stent implantation in saphenous vein grafts. *J Am Coll Cardiol* 1996; **28**: 89–96.

105 Laham RJ, Carrozza JB, Berger C, *et al.* Longterm (4–6 year) outcome of Palmaz–Schatz stenting: paucity of late clinical stent related problems. *J Am Coll Cardiol* 1996; **28**: 820–6.

106   Fischman DL, Savage MP, Bailey S, *et al.* Predictors of restenosis after saphenous vein graft interventions. *Circulation* 1996; **94**: I-62I.

107   de Jaegere P, Serruys P. Clinical trials on intracoronary stenting. *The Thoraxcenter Journal* 1996; **8/4**: 40–4.

108   Fischman DL, Bailey S, Goldberg S, *et al.* Total occlusion of saphenous vein bypass grafts following transcatheter intervention: six month angiographic findings from the SAVED trial. *J Am Coll Cardiol* 1997 (in press).

109   Savage MP, Fischman DL, Douglas JS jr, *et al.* The dark side of high pressure stent deployment. *J Am Coll Cardiol* 1997 (in press).

110   Colombo A, Hall P, Nakamura S, *et al.* Intracoronary stenting without anticoagulation accomplished with intravascular ultrasound guidance. *Circulation* 1995; **91**: 1676–88.

111   Serruys PW, Di Mario C. Who was thrombogenic, the stent or the doctor? *Circulation* 1995; **91**: 1891–93.

112   Morice MC, Zemour G, Benveniste E, *et al.* Intracoronary stenting without coumadin: one month results of a French multicenter study. *Cathet Cardiovasc Diag* 1995; **35**: 1–7.

113   Schomig A, Neumann F-J, Kastrati A, *et al.* A randomized comparison of antiplatelet and anticoagulant therapy after the placement of coronary artery stents. *N Engl J Med* 1996; **334**: 1084–9.

114   The EPIC Investigators. Use of a monoclonal antibody directed against the platelet glycoprotein IIb/IIIa receptor in high risk coronary angioplasty. *N Engl J Med* 1994; **330**: 956–61.

12

Anticoagulation strategies after stenting

Alexandra J Lansky, Jeffrey J Popma, John R Laird and Martin B Leon

Introduction

The use of intracoronary stents for the treatment of coronary artery disease has increased dramatically over the past several years, with stent use comprising as many as 25–70% of interventional procedures at some high-volume institutions.[1] Many questions remain, however, about the optimal post-procedural management of patients undergoing stent implantation, particularly with respect to the method and duration of anticoagulant therapy that should be given. Traditional regimens, which included the use of aspirin, dipyridamole, dextran, prolonged intravenous heparin, and coumadin, have largely been replaced with 'reduced' anticoagulation strategies. These reduced anticoagulation methods have used aspirin alone, or in combination with ticlopidine after successful stent placement. In patients at 'high-risk' for subacute stent thrombosis, other agents, such as low molecular weight heparin and the novel platelet glycoprotein IIb-IIIa receptor inhibitors (e.g. c7E3), have also been used with reported success.[2] Further refinements in anticoagulation recommendations may be needed as stent use expands to patients with acute myocardial infarction and other thrombus-mediated acute ischemic syndromes.[3,4]

The purposes of this chapter are three-fold:

- the clinical studies evaluating antithrombotic regimens after stent placement will be summarized;
- the criteria used to identify high- and low-risk patients for subacute thrombosis after stent deployment will be discussed;
- the alternative antithrombotic agents used after stent placement in 'high-risk' patients will be reviewed.

Randomized studies of stent use versus balloon angioplasty

At least four randomized clinical trials comparing balloon angioplasty and stent placement have shown that intracoronary stent placement results in an improved early and late clinical outcome in selected patients with symptomatic coronary stenosis.[5-7] In the STent REStenosis Study (STRESS-I), 410 patients with focal (≤15 mm), *de novo* stenoses were randomly assigned to Palmaz–Schatz (Cordis, a Johnson & Johnson Co) stent placement or balloon angioplasty.[5] Using quantitative angiographic methods, the residual percentage diameter stenosis was lower in stent-treated patients (19% versus 35% in balloon-treated patients; $p < 0.001$),[5] resulting in a reduction in angiographic restenosis in stent-treated patients (32% versus 42% in balloon-treated patients; $p = 0.046$). An extended analysis of the STRESS-I study included an additional 189 patients randomly assigned to stent placement or balloon angioplasty after STRESS-I enrollment had been completed (STRESS-II); the combined STRESS I + II analysis, comprising 596 patients, demonstrated that stent-treated patients had improved procedural success (89.4% versus 82.6% in balloon-treated patients; $p = 0.02$), reduced 6-month angiographic restenosis (30.4% versus 45.4% in balloon-treated patients; $p = 0.0001$), lower rates of symptom-driven target lesion revascularization (9.8% versus 18.2% in balloon-treated patients; $p = 0.003$) and better 12-month event-free survival (80.3% versus 71.5% in balloon-treated patients; $p = 0.008$).[8]

In the BElgium NEtherlands STENT (BENESTENT)

Study, 520 patients with focal, *de novo* native coronary lesions were randomly assigned to Palmaz–Schatz stent placement or balloon angioplasty. Angiographic restenosis (≥50% follow-up diameter stenosis) occurred less often in stent-treated patients (22% versus 32% in balloon-treated patients; $p = 0.02$); target lesion revascularization (coronary bypass operation or repeat angioplasty) also occurred less frequently in stent-treated patients (20% versus 30% of balloon-treated patients: $p = 0.02$).[6]

In a third study, the Trial of Angioplasty and Stents in Canada (TASC-I), 270 elective patients with *de novo* ($n = 148$) or restenotic ($n = 122$) lesions were assigned to Palmaz–Schatz stent placement or balloon angioplasty.[7] In patients with *de novo* lesions, there was a significant reduction in angiographic restenosis in stent-treated patients (29% versus 49% in balloon-treated patients; $p = 0.02$).[7] In patients undergoing treatment of restonic lesions, stenting did not offer a statistical advantage over balloon angioplasty (33% versus 43% in balloon-treated patients; $p = NS$),[7] but based on the apparent absolute reduction in restenosis rates associated with stenting in this subset of patients, it is reasonable to assume that stent use may also be beneficial for the treatment of patients with restenosis after conventional angioplasty. Preliminary results from the Restenosis Stent (REST)-Study, a trial of 383 patients randomized to Palmaz–Schatz stenting or balloon angioplasty, also suggest a beneficial effect of stenting on early and late outcome in patients with restenotic lesions.[9]

In aggregate, these four randomized studies, comprising nearly 1800 patients, convincingly demonstrate the clinical advantage of stent use over balloon angioplasty in patients with focal lesions in native coronary arteries. The overwhelming factor influencing the clinical and angiographic benefit after stenting has been the very low (19–21%) residual percentage diameter stenosis achieved with stent placement.

Fewer randomized stent studies have been performed in patients with saphenous vein graft (SVG) stenoses. This is due to the fact that the clinical acceptance of stenting in patients with SVG stenosis based on the early registry series[10] has made it difficult to recruit patients for these randomized studies. To date, one randomized study has been performed which included 220 patients randomly assigned to balloon angioplasty or stenting for *de novo* lesions in saphenous vein grafts.[11] Preliminary results in this study suggested a trend toward lower restenosis rates in patients treated with stents (36% versus 47% in balloon treated patients; $p = 0.11$);[12] a significant reduction in late clinical events was also shown in stent-treated patients.[11]

Complications in the early stent experience

Despite the benefits associated with native vessel and saphenous vein graft stenting in these and other[13,14] clinical studies, early enthusiasm for stent use was tempered by the occurrence of two major complications. Subacute stent thrombosis developed in 3.5–8.6% of patients,[5,6,13–15] often delayed 2–14 days (average, 6 days) after stent placement.[5] Subacute thrombosis was virtually always associated with major clinical events, such as death, transmural myocardial infarction, or emergency revascularization. The clinical impact of subacute thrombosis was evaluated in a single center series of 2849 patients undergoing stent implantation; subacute thrombosis occurred in 46 (1.6%) patients. Patients with subacute thrombosis had a 15% in-hospital mortality rate; 30% of patients developed a Q-wave myocardial infarction and 54% of patients experienced in-hospital death, Q-wave myocardial infarction, and or revascularization.[16] It is clear from this study that the occurrence of subacute thrombosis has been a major contributor to morbidity and mortality after coronary stenting.

The second major limitation of early stenting was the frequent occurrence of bleeding complications. Aggressive anticoagulation regimens were given in these early studies to avert the occurrence of subacute thrombosis; most patients were given aspirin (325 mg daily), dipyridamole (75 mg three times daily), intravenous low molecular weight dextran-40 and heparin until therapeutic systemic anticoagulation had been achieved with coumadin (INR between 2.0–3.5). It is not surprising that major bleeding complications and vascular events (>13%) were extremely common in stent-treated patients.[5,6] Similarly, the length of hospitalization was also longer in stent-treated patients.[5,6]

Intravascular ultrasound (IVUS)-detected incomplete stent expansion

It is now apparent that anatomic factors, such as under-dilatation of the stent, proximal and distal dissections, poor inflow or outflow obstruction, of less than 3 mm diameter vessels, rather than suboptimal anticoagulation regimens contributed to the development of subacute thrombosis in the early stent series.[17,18] IVUS studies showed that incomplete apposition of the stent struts against the vessel wall, asymmetric expansion, and incomplete stent dilatation, in comparison to the proximal and distal reference segments, frequently occurred with stent deployment in the absence of high-pressure balloon inflation.[19–22] In one study, complete and symmetric stent expansion occurred in less than

30% of cases after initial deployment; after high pressure (>12 atm) balloon inflation, complete and symmetric stent expansion was found in nearly 70% of cases.[22] It seems reasonable to assume that the relatively high (3.5–5.0%) rates of subacute thrombosis were triggered by platelet and fibrin deposition in the regions of incomplete stent strut expansion. IVUS-guided stent deployment studies have shown that high pressure (12–20 atm) balloon dilatations and minimally oversized balloons (balloon:artery ratios 1.1–1.2:1) are required for consistent stent strut apposition and expansion.[21] With the widespread acceptance of high-pressure post-deployment dilatation methods, lower (<2%) frequencies of subacute stent thrombosis have been achieved. This has allowed a progressive reduction in the intensity of anticoagulation after stent deployment.[19–21]

Given the clinical acceptance of high-pressure balloon dilatation, it is not clear whether IVUS guidance can further reduce the occurrence of subacute thrombosis after stent placement, although randomized studies with IVUS-guidance and angiographic guidance are currently underway. One of these studies, the Strategy of ICUS-guided PTCA and Stenting (SIPS) trial, is a randomized evaluation of angiography- versus intracoronary ultrasound-guided stent implantation strategy.[23] Early results suggest that IVUS-guided stent deployment results in greater acute lumen gains than obtained without IVUS.[23] Whether these immediate improvements in lumen diameter will impact on early and late clinical outcome justify the systematic use of IVUS guidance for stent placement has not yet been demonstrated.

Reduced anticoagulation series

More than 20 single and multicenter series have since reported the use of less aggressive anticoagulation regimens after stent placement (Table 12.1).[2,21,24–51] While each of the regimens included aspirin and post-deployment stent dilatation using high-pressure (≥10–17 atm) balloons, they have varied with respect to:

- the type of stent used,
- the procedure priority (elective versus failed angioplasty),
- the concomitant use of intravascular ultrasound,
- ticlopidine,
- post-procedural heparin,
- low molecular weight heparin,
- warfarin.

Despite these differences, subacute thrombosis with these less aggressive anticoagulation regimens has ranged

from 0–3.6% and vascular complications have decreased from 0–4.4% (Table 12.1).

In a single center experience, 221 patients undergoing successful IVUS-guided stent deployment in either native vessels (n = 152) or saphenous vein grafts (n = 97) received post-procedural aspirin (325 mg) + ticlopidine (250 mg twice daily for 2 weeks followed by 250 mg daily for 2 weeks), but no post-procedural heparin or coumadin. High pressure (≥12 atm) balloon inflation was performed in all patients after stent deployment. Criteria for successful IVUS-guided stent deployment included the attainment of full stent strut apposition against the vessel wall, stent symmetry with the minor to major axis ratio greater than 0.7 in the most eccentric portion of the stent, and maximum expansion with the minimal stent cross-sectional area greater than 80% of the smaller of the proximal or distal reference diameter. Vascular complications were infrequent, and occurred in 8 (3.6%) patients. Two (1%) deaths occurred within 30 days in this series: one of these was unrelated to the stent placement procedure and one was sudden 3 days following the stent procedure, presumably due to subacute thrombosis.[2] There were no additional episodes of subacute thrombosis, lending support to the safety of a reduced anticoagulation regimen when combined with an aggressive stent deployment strategy.

Virtually all reduced anticoagulation regimens have included peri-procedural aspirin as part of the anticoagulation regimen, however, a number of series have evaluated the effectiveness of aspirin *alone* after stenting with reported subacute thrombosis rates below 2%.[52,53] In one retrospective series of 801 patients comparing the combined use of aspirin and ticlopidine to aspirin alone, the 30-day subacute thrombosis rate was similar in both groups (1.9% for aspirin, and 1.3% for aspirin + ticlopidine; $p = 0.5$); however, the aspirin alone treated group tended to have fewer risk factors for subacute thrombosis than the group treated with the combination of aspirin + ticlopidine.[52] These findings underscore the importance of randomized clinical trials to evaluate the comparative efficacy of the various anticoagulation regimens after coronary stenting.

There is little question that the use of the potent antiplatelet agent, ticlopidine, has had an important influence on the subacute thrombosis rate after stent placement. In an attempt to more closely characterize the clinical events associated with reduced anticoagulation regimens that included ticlopidine, two registry studies were performed. The European MUlticenter Stent with Ticlopidine (MUST) study was an open-label, prospective 260-patient observational study that evaluated the use of aspirin (100 mg daily) and ticlopidine (250–500 mg daily) after planned stent deployment performed with high-pressure balloon dilatation. The acute complications were low, and included no deaths, emergency bypass surgery in 1 (0.4%) patient, myocardial infarction in 6 (2.1%) patients, subacute

Table 12.1 Antithrombotic regimens in patients undergoing stent placement

Author	Patients (n)	Stent Type	Priority	IVUS Criteria	Aspirin	Ticlop	Heparin	LMWH	Coumadin	Death (%)	MI (%)	CABG (%)	SAT (%)	V-Comp (%)
Haase[37]														
Phase 1	174	PS	C	–	100 mg daily**	–	+	–	+	8	7	6.3	22.5	12
Phase 2	67	PS	C	–	100 mg daily**	–	+	–	+	3	4	7.5	7	6
Phase 3	46	PS	C	–	100 mg daily**	500 mg	IP	–	–	0	0	0	0	0
Hall[38]	62	GR	C. 22% EI. 78%	88%	325 mg	500 mg	IP	–	–	1	NR	NR	1	0
Wong[39]	221			+	325 mg	500 mg ×1 m	IP	–	–	0.9	0	0	1	3.6
Goods[40]	152	GR	C. 10 EI. 90	–	+	+	IP	–	–	0	0	0.7	0.7	2
Belli[36]	88			66%	+	+	IP	–	–	0	0	0	0	4.5
Russo[19]	83	PS	EI	+	325 mg	500 mg ×1 m	IP	–	–	0	NR	NR	0	NR
Bunel[41]														
Phase 1	752	NR	NR	–	+	–	+	–	+	NR	NR	NR	6.5	6.9
Phase 2	553	NR	NR	–	+	+	IP	+	–	NR	NR	NR	0.7	2
Phase 3	263	NR	NR	–	100 mg	250 mg	IP	–	–	NR	NR	NR	1.1	1.1
Morice[31]	1156	PS 71% AVE 22% GR 3.6% WK 1.6%	C. 3 EI. 97	–	100 mg	250 mg or 500 mg if >50 kg	IP	–	–	0.26	2.7	0.34	1.6	0.6
Fernandez-Aviles[16]	52	PS	EI	–	+	–	IP	EN 40 mg until INR = 2–3	+	0	0	0	0	0
Blasini[17]	60	PS	C	+	300 mg	750 mg	× 24 h	–	–	0	0	0	0	1.6
Van Belle[21]	53	WK 75% PS 10% GR 15%	C. 94% EI. 6%	–	200 mg	500 mg × 3 m	× 48 h	–	–	0	0	2.4	0	0
Colombo[18]	78	GR	C. 28% EI. 72%	83%	+	+	IP	–	–	1.0	0	4	0	0
Colombo[20]	59	WK	C. 27% EI. 73%	+	+	+	IP	–	–	1.7	NR	3.4	1.7	1.7
Lablanche[22]	334	WK 70% PS 23% GR 7%	C. 78% EI. 22%	–	200 mg	500 mg × 3 m	IP	–	–	0.2	0.01	0	2.1	1.8
Barragan[23]	208	PS 90% GR 10%	C. 30% EI. 70%	–	NR	500 mg	NR	–	–	1.0	1.0	0.5	0.5	0.5
Buszman[24]	100	PS	C	–	75 mg	–	NR	5000 U SQ × 7 d	INR 2.5– 3.5 × 30 d	1.0	0	0	1.0	2.0

Table 12.1 (Continued): Antithrombotic regimens in patients undergoing stent placement

Author	Patients (n)	Stent Type	Priority	IVUS Criteria	Aspirin	Ticlop	Heparin	LMWH	Coumadin	Death (%)	MI (%)	CABG (%)	SAT (%)	V-Comp (%)
Carvalho[25]	87	GR	NR	—	250 mg	500 mg	IP	+	—	0	0	0	1.1	2.3††
	107				250 mg	—	IP+	—	+	2	1	1	5.6	9.3
Elias[26]	79	WK	C. 63% EI. 37%	—	250 mg	500 mg	×48 h	0.1 mg per 10 kg	—	0	1.3	0	1.3	1.3
Barragan[27]	238	PS 94% Str 5% GR 1%	C. 63% EI. 37%	—	—	500 mg	×20 h	PTT adjusted ×7 d	—	2	1.2	0	4.2	4.6
Colombo[14]	359*	PS	C. 21% EI. 79%	+	325 mg	500 mg	IP	—	—	1.1	4.2	3.9	1.4	0.3
Blengino[28]	41	PS 66% WK 25% GR 9%	NR	+	325 mg	—	IP	—	—	NR	NR	NR	0	NR
	33				—	500 mg	IP	—	—	NR	NR	NR	0	NR
Jordan[29]	748	PS	C. 54% EI. 46%	—	250 mg	—	+	—	+	NR	NR	NR	6.3	NR
	219				250 mg	500 mg	IP	—	—	NR	NR	NR	0.5†	NR
Morice[30]														
Phase I	145	PS	C. 54%		250 mg	—	×48 h	×2 m	NR	NR	NR	NR	10.4	NR
Phase II	237		E. 46%		100 mg	250 mg	×48 h	×2 m	NR	NR	NR	NR	1.3	NR
Phase III	523				100 mg	250 mg	×48 h	×2 weeks	NR	NR	NR	NR	1.7	NR
Phase IV	491				100 mg	250 mg	×48 h	1 week	NR	NR	NR	NR	1.8	NR
Stenting in acute myocardial infarction														
Saito[74]	32	PS	AMI	—	+	+	IP	—	—	NR	NR	NR	0	NR
Monassier[88]	109	NR	AMI <24 hrs		100 mg	250 mg ×1 mo	×72	×7–14 d	—	4	—	1	1.9	2.7
	202	NR	AMI >24 hrs		100 mg	250 mg ×1 mo	×72	×7–14 d	—	2	—	0.5	1.4	2

C = unplanned use including dissections, occlusion, and suboptimal results; CABG = coronary bypass surgery; d = days; EI = elective; EN = enoxaparin; IP = intraprocedural heparin; IVUS = intravascular ultrasound; GR = Gianturco–Roubin stent; h = hours; LMWH = low molecular weight heparin; m = months; MI = Q-wave myocardial infarction; NR = not reported; PS = Palmaz–Schatz stent; PTT = partial thromboplastin time; QD = daily; SAT = subacute thrombosis; SQ = subcutaneous; Str = Strecker stent; SVG = saphenous vein graft; Ticlop = ticlopidine; WK = Wiktor stent; V-Comp = vascular or bleeding complications: †p < 0.01; ††p = 0.002.
*321 of these patients had successful IVUS guided stent deployment and received reduced anticoagulation regimen without coumadin. **1000 mg aspirin given at the time of the procedure.
Reproduced from Popma JJ, Lansky AJ, Mintz GS, Hong MK, Brahimi A, Burwell N, Leon, MB. Antithrombotic therapy after stent deployment. *J Invasive Cardiology* 1996; 8: 34B–42B.

thromboses in 3 (1.15%) patients, and repeat angioplasty procedures in 5 (1.9%) patients. Target lesion revascularization was required in fewer than 10% of cases, with coronary bypass surgery performed in 4 (1.5%) patients and repeat percutaneous revascularization in 15 (5.8%) patients. There were no late deaths or myocardial infarctions.[54]

The STRESS-III trial, a 250-patient study with inclusion criteria similar to those used in the STRESS I + II trial, was designed to evaluate the early and late clinical outcome in patients undergoing optimal stent deployment followed, by a reduced anticoagulation regimen of aspirin + ticlopidine therapy. Compared with STRESS, STRESS III patients had similar success rates (96.1% vs. 96.7%), fewer stent thromboses (3.4% vs. 1.2%, $p = 0.12$), and fewer bleeding and vascular complications (7.3% vs. 0.6%, $p = 0.003$).[55]

Potential adverse effects of conventional and reduced anticoagulation regimens

The safety of conventional and reduced anticoagulation regimens is related to the occurrence of both untoward bleeding complications and adverse drug effects related to the drug regimens themselves. Although the minimum effective aspirin dosage and the requisite pretreatment duration remain unclear, aspirin has been an integral component of all anticoagulation regimens after stent deployment. Because gastrointestinal side effects can occur in up to 35% of patients treated with high doses of aspirin (990 mg daily)[56] and data concerning the clinical efficacy of low dose aspirin (80 mg daily) in the setting of coronary stenting are rather limited, an empiric dosage of aspirin ($\geq$100 mg) given at least 2 hours before the stent procedure has been recommended. Further studies are needed to determine whether an aspirin dosage of 80 mg is as effective as higher doses in patients undergoing coronary stent placement.

Peri-procedural dextran and dipyridamole has largely been abandoned in the reduced anticoagulation regimens as these agents have provided no incremental benefit over aspirin alone. It is well known that dextran-40 can cause serious adverse reactions, including anaphylactoid reactions and life-threatening allergic reactions in 0.6% and 0.2% of patients, respectively[57–59] and there appears to be no current indication for its use.

Most reduced anticoagulation regimens after stent deployment have added ticlopidine (250–750 mg daily for 1–3 months) to aspirin. It is now thought that because both aspirin (via cyclo-oxygenase inhibition) and ticlopidine (via ADP-mediated inhibition of platelet-fibrinogen binding) have independent mechanisms of action, the combination of aspirin + ticlopidine may result in a synergistic

antiplatelet effect. Lower markers of thrombin generation (thrombin antithrombin complexes and prothrombin fragment 1 + 2) have been seen in patients treated with aspirin (200 mg daily) + ticlopidine (500 mg daily begun three days before angioplasty) than in patients treated with aspirin alone (200 mg daily) after coronary intervention.[60] Combined use of aspirin (200 mg daily) + ticlopidine (500 mg daily) after stent implantation also reduced monocyte-dependent procoagulant effects when compared to treatment with heparin + coumadin.[61] Without question, the major limitations of ticlopidine are its side effects and toxicities. Gastrointestinal symptoms (20%),[62] cutaneous rashes (4.8–15%),[62] and biochemical abnormalities in liver function tests[62] may occur with ticlopidine. In addition to these somewhat minor adverse reactions, the major side effect associated with ticlopidine use is the unpredictable occurrence of severe leukopenia (granulocyte count <450/µl), developing in approximately 1% of patients.[62,63] The leukopenia is reversible after discontinuation of ticlopidine in most cases,[64] but episodes of sepsis and death have occurred.

With the exception of 'high risk' patients undergoing stent implantation, the use of coumadin, an inhibitor of vitamin K dependent coagulation factors, has largely been abandoned; this is due to increased bleeding complications, extended hospitalizations required to reach therapeutic dosing, and the general inconvenience and cost associated with maintaining therapy. One recent single-center series has even suggested that use of prolonged intravenous heparin and coumadin may be associated with an increased risk of subacute thrombosis and other untoward events after stent deployment.[65] In a series of 517 patients randomly assigned to an intensive (intravenous heparin for 5–10 days, a warfarin derivative for 30 days, and aspirin, 200 mg daily; $n = 260$) or reduced (intravenous heparin for 12 hours, ticlopidine, 500 mg daily for 30 days, and aspirin, 200 mg daily, $n = 257$) anticoagulation, a substantial reduction in 30-day cardiac events (death, myocardial infarction, and reintervention) was noted in the reduced anticoagulation group. Subacute thrombosis occurred in none of the reduced anticoagulation group compared with 5% of those in the intensive anticoagulation group. Bleeding and vascular complications were also significantly less common in the reduced anticoagulation group.[66]

Randomized anticoagulation studies in patients undergoing stent placement

Several randomized studies have been performed to assess the optimal anticoagulation strategies in patients undergoing stent placement. An open-label, randomized study of 226 patients was performed to compare clinical event rates after IVUS-guided stent implantation in patients treated with aspirin (325 mg daily) + ticlopidine (500 mg daily for one month) or aspirin alone (325 mg daily).[67] Although there were no significant differences in the 30-day occurrence of subacute stent thrombosis (0.8% in ticlopidine + aspirin-treated patients versus 2.9% in aspirin alone-treated patients), because of the limited number of patients included in this study, a trend toward a better outcome in ticlopidine + aspirin-treated patients may not have reached statistical significance.[67]

The Enoxaparin and Ticlid for Elective Stenting Study (ENTICES) randomly assigned 120 patients after stent replacement to low molecular weight heparin (weight-adjusted enoxaparin 30–50 mg subcutaneously twice daily), aspirin, and ticlopidine or to aspirin, ticlopidine, dextran, and coumadin (Principal Investigator: James P Zidar, MD). Analysis of the primary hemostatic endpoints of the study is forthcoming, and a second larger, 2000 patient clinical trial evaluating the incremental clinical benefit of low molecular weight heparin in patients at high-risk for subacute thrombosis after stent placement is currently underway (Principal Investigator: James P Zidar, MD).

Recent randomized comparisons of antiplatelet regimens to full anticoagulation regimens have confirmed the benefits of antiplatelet therapy with aspirin and ticlopidine alone.[66] A comparison of antiplatelet and anticoagulant therapy after successful placement of Palmaz–Schatz coronary stents was performed where 257 patients were randomized to aspirin and ticlopidine therapy and 260 patients to heparin, coumadin, and aspirin therapy. Coumadin-treated patients had significantly higher cardiac event (death, myocardial infarction, repeat angioplasty, or coronary bypass surgery) (6.2% vs. 1.6% in aspirin + ticlopidine treated patients) and subacute thrombosis (5.4% vs. 0.8% in aspirin + ticlopidine treated patients) rates. Aspirin and ticlopidine-treated patients had an 82% lower risk of myocardial infarction, a 78% lower need for repeat interventions, and an 87% reduction in vascular complications.[66]

The STent Antithrombotic Regimen Study (STARS) included 1650 patients undergoing successful intracoronary stent placement, randomly assigned to treatment with aspirin alone (325 mg), aspirin (325 mg) + ticlopidine (250 mg twice daily for 1 month), or aspirin (325 mg) + coumadin (target INR 2.0–2.5 for 1 month).[68] Patients were excluded from STARS if they had a myocardial infarction within the past seven days, a suboptimal (>10% residual stenosis) angiographic result, more than two stents per lesion or four stents per patient, a proximal or distal dissection, angiographic thrombus, or persistently reduced anterograde perfusion. Preliminary data from STARS suggests that the 30-day major adverse cardiac event and subacute thrombosis rates were significantly lower in the aspirin + ticlopidine treated group compared to the aspirin alone or aspirin and coumadin groups.[69]

Defining patients at 'high risk' for subacute thrombosis and restenosis after stent placement

Reduced anticoagulation regimens (i.e. aspirin + ticlopidine) have been primarily recommended in patients at 'low-risk' for subacute thrombosis after stent placement (i.e. residual stenosis less than 20%, no thrombus, recent myocardial infarction, or significant peri-procedural dissection or outflow limitation). It is less clear whether additional antithrombotic therapy is indicated in patients at 'high-risk' for subacute thrombosis, such as those with a residual proximal or distal dissection[50,70] or angiographic thrombus,[71,72] abrupt closure,[73] multiple (≥3) stents,[50] smaller (<3.0 mm) vessels,[38,70] total occlusions, or those with recent (<1 week) myocardial infarction.[74] In a series of 606 high risk patients undergoing bailout stenting, and stenting for suboptimal results treated with aspirin and ticlopidine alone, stent-related ischemic events occurred in 5.7% of patients after 'bail out' stenting, 2.1% of patients after stenting for suboptimal results and 0.9% of patients after elective stenting.[50] Until more information is available from randomized clinical trials, empiric use of conventional antithrombotic agents, such as coumadin for 1 month or low molecular weight heparin for 2–4 weeks, may be useful in some 'high-risk' patients.

Recently, the use of intracoronary stents has been expanded to patients with acute ischemic syndromes, including those with acute myocardial infarction.[44,75] Acceptable rates (<2%) of subacute thrombosis have been reported with reduced aspirin + ticlopidine regimens after stent placement for acute myocardial infarction.[3,44,75–79] In the PAMI stent pilot trial, 230 of 300 (77%) patients with acute myocardial infarction underwent primary stenting; 96% were treated with aspirin and ticlopidine alone, 2% had subcutaneous heparin, and in 2% coumadin was added. In-hospital death occurred in 0.4%, re-infarction in 1.3%, repeat angioplasty in 2.1%, and coronary bypass surgery in 1.7%; these data suggest very favorable clinical outcomes associated with primary stenting compared to primary balloon angioplasty.[80] The benefit of additional antithrombotic agents, such a c7E3, low molecular weight heparin, or heparin-coated stents has not been extensively studied, although additional clinical trials are planned. For example, the Stent PAMI randomized trial will evaluate the heparin-coated Palmaz–Schatz stent compared to balloon angioplasty in 1000 patients with acute myocardial infarction (Principal Investigator: Cindy Grines, MD).

Pharmacologic adjuncts in high risk patients

Other novel antithrombotic agents may improve early clinical outcome in patients at 'high risk' for subacute thrombosis after stent placement. Glycoprotein IIb-IIIa receptor inhibition has been shown to reduce peri-procedural ischemic events by 35% in 'high-risk' patients undergoing coronary angioplasty,[81] and, although bleeding complications were twice as common in c7E3 bolus and infusion treated patients than in placebo-treated patients, the risk for bleeding was subsequently attributable to the relatively high doses of non-weight adjusted heparin used in this study.[81] Fewer bleeding complications were subsequently seen with low weight-adjusted heparin administration in a later study of 103 patients undergoing coronary angioplasty.[82]

There may be several potential uses of GP IIb-IIIa inhibitors in patients undergoing stent placement. Experimental data suggests that murine 7E3 is highly effective in inhibiting stent thrombosis,[83] and bolus and infusion c7E3 may reduce the occurrence of subacute thrombosis in high-risk patients, particularly those who have residual coronary dissections or intraluminal thrombus after intervention. Administration of c7E3 may also reduce the occurrence of 'no reflow' during saphenous vein graft stent placement, particularly when adjunct new devices such as extraction atherectomy, excimer laser angioplasty, or rheolytic thrombectomy are used. Similar reductions in non-Q-wave myocardial infarction rates may also be seen when stents are used in conjunction with plaque ablative device (e.g. rotational atherectomy). Although the empiric adjunct use of c7E3 in patients treated with stents seems attractive based on the reduction in death and myocardial infarction observed after conventional coronary intervention,[81] additional clinical studies are required before the routine use of c7E3 in patients undergoing stent placement can be recommended. Moreover, little data is currently available about the combined use of ticlopidine and c7E3 in patients after stent placement.

Other approaches for the prevention of thrombosis and restenosis have included coating stents with thromboresistant agents, such as heparin, glycoprotein IIb-IIIa antibody,[84] hirudin[85] or phosphorylcholine.[86] The safety and early clinical efficacy of the heparin coated Palmaz–Schatz stent was evaluated in the second BElgium NEtherlands STENT (BENESTENT-II) Pilot Study; this study used a four-phase reduction in the anticoagulation regimen through its enrollment, with the fourth phase including patients treated with aspirin and ticlopidine only.[87] There were no episodes of subacute stent thrombosis in the 202 patients enrolled in the BENESTENT-II pilot study. High pressure (>12 atm) post-stent dilatation without IVUS guidance was performed in the majority of cases. Bleeding complications were reduced from 7.9% in phase I to 0% in phase IV; hospital stay was also reduced from 7.4 days in phase I to 3.1 days in phase IV. The BENESTENT-II randomized trial, a study of 827 patients randomly assigned to heparin-coated Palmaz–Schatz stent placement or balloon angioplasty, has recently been completed; evaluation of the early and late clinical benefit of the heparin-coated stent over balloon angioplasty is currently underway.[88]

There is little question that anticoagulation regimens after stent placement will continue to evolve over the next several years. The Stent Antithrombotic Regimen Study (STARS) has definitively demonstrated the incremental value of ticlopidine and aspirin over aspirin alone in patients at 'low-risk' for subacute thrombosis after stent placement. Clinical acceptance of 'reduced anticoagulation' regimens which have eliminated dextran, dipyridamole, and coumadin has resulted in low rates (1%) of subacute thrombosis and significantly reduced lengths of stay and hospitalization costs.[89]

In patients at higher risk for complications, other novel agents, such as low molecular weight heparin, can also be added to the standard coagulation regimen as an alternative to coumadin. Inhibition of the GP IIb-IIIa receptor has been used in the setting of stent placement to reduce the risk of subacute thrombosis, myocardial infarction, and periprocedural embolic events, such as no reflow; however, the optimal timing, case selection, and therapeutic benefit will require further evaluation.

References

1   Peterson ED, Lansky AJ, Muhlbaier LH, et al. Evolving trends in angioplasty device selection: A National Cardiovascular Network (NCN) Database Report. *J Am Coll Cardiol* 1997; **29**: 495A (abstract).

2   Wong SC, Hong MK, Chuang YC, et al. The antiplatelet treatment after intravascular ultrasound guided optimal stent expansion (APLAUSE) trial. *Circulation* 1995; **92**: I-795.

3   Ahmad T, Webb JB, Carere RR, Dodek A. Coronary stenting for acute myocardial infarction. *Am J Cardiol* 1995; **76**: 77–80.

4   Wong PH, Wong CM. Intracoronary stenting in acute myocardial infarction. *Cathet Cardiovasc Diagn* 1994; **33**: 39–45.

5   Fischman DL, Leon MB, Baim DS, et al. A randomized comparison of coronary-stent placement and balloon angioplasty in the treatment of coronary artery disease. Stent Restenosis Study Investigators. *N Engl J Med* 1994; **331**: 496–501.

6   Serruys PW, de Jaegere P, Kiemeneij F, *et al*. A comparison of balloon-expandable-stent implantation with balloon angioplasty in patients with coronary artery disease. Benestent Study Group. *N Engl J Med* 1994; **331**: 489–95.

7   Penn IM, Ricci DR, Almond DG, *et al*. Coronary artery stenting reduces restenosis: Final results from the trial of angioplasty and stents in Canada (TASC) I. *Circulation* 1995; **92**: I-279.

8   Wong SC, Zidar JP, Chuang YC, *et al*. Stents improve late clinical outcomes: Results from the combined (I + II) STent REStenosis Study. *Circulation* 1995; **92**: I-282 (abstract).

9   Erbel R, Haude M, Hopp HW, *et al*. REstenosis STent (REST)-Study: Randomized Trial comparing stenting and balloon angioplasty for treatment of restenosis after balloon angioplasty. *J Am Coll Cardiol* 1996; **27**: 139A (abstract).

10 Wong SC, Baim DS, Schatz RA, *et al*. Immediate results and late outcomes after stent implantation in saphenous vein graft lesions: the multicenter U.S. Palmaz–Schatz stent experience. The Palmaz–Schatz Stent Study Group. *J Am Coll Cardiol* 1995; **26**: 704–12.

11 Douglas JS, Savage MP, Bailey SR, *et al*. Randomized trial of coronary stent and balloon angioplasty in the treatment of saphenous vein graft stenoses. *J Am Coll Cardiol* 1996; **27**: 178A (abstract).

12 Fischman DL, Savage MP, Bailey S, Werner JA, Rake R, Goldberg S. Predictors of restenosis after saphenous vein graft interventions. *Circulation* 1996; **94**: I-621 (abstract).

13 Roubin GS, Cannon AD, Agrawal SK, *et al*. Intracoronary stenting for acute and threatened closure complicating percutaneous transluminal coronary angioplasty. *Circulation* 1992; **85**: 916–27.

14 Hearn JA, King SB III, Douglas JS jr, Carlin SF, Lembo NJ, Ghazzal ZM. Clinical and angiographic outcomes after coronary artery stenting for acute or threatened closure after percutaneous transluminal coronary angioplasty. Initial results with a balloon-expandable, stainless steel design. *Circulation* 1993; **88**: 2455–7.

15 Schomig A, Kastrati A, Mudra H, *et al*. Four-year experience with Palmaz–Schatz stenting in coronary angioplasty complicated by dissection with threatened or present vessel closure. *Circulation* 1994; **90**: 2716–24.

16 Yokoi H, Nosaka H, Kimura T, *et al*. Coronary stent thrombosis: management and long term follow-up results. *J Am Coll Cardiol* 1997; **29**: 171A (abstract).

17 Schatz RA. New challenges in coronary stenting. *J Invas Cardiol* 1995; **7**: 43A.

18 Serruys PW, Di Mario C. Who was thrombogenic: the stent or the doctor? [editorial; comment]. *Circulation* 1995; **91**: 1891–3.

19 Goldberg SL, Colombo A, Nakamura S, Almagor Y, Maiello L, Tobis JM. Benefit of intracoronary ultrasound in the deployment of Palmaz–Schatz stents. *J Am Coll Cardiol* 1994; **24**: 996–1003.

20 Hall, P, Colombo A, Almagor Y. Preliminary experience with intravascular ultrasound-guided Palmaz–Schatz coronary stenting: the acute and short-term results on a consecutive series of patients. *J Interv Cardiol* 1994; **7**: 141–59.

21 Colombo A, Hall P, Nakamura S, *et al*. Intracoronary stenting with anticoagulation accomplished with intravascular guidance [see comments]. *Circulation* 1995; **91**: 1676–88.

22 Kiemeneij F, Laarman G, Slagboom T. Mode of deployment of coronary Palmaz–Schatz stents after implantation with the stent delivery system: an intravascular ultrasound study. *Am Heart J* 1995; **129**: 638–44.

23 Hodgson JM, Muller C, Roskamm H, Frey AW. Ultrasound (ICUS)-guided PTCA and stenting improves acute angiographic results: acute analysis of the Strategy of ICUS-guided PTCA and stenting (SIPS) trial. *J Am Coll Cardiol* 1997; **29**: 96A.

24 Fernandez-Aviles F, Alonso J, Duran JM, *et al*. Absence of bleeding and subacute occlusion after Palmaz–Schatz coronary stenting using a new antithrombotic regimen. *J Am Coll Cardiol* 1995; **25**: 196A (abstract).

25 Blasini R, Mudra H, Schuhlen H, *et al*. Intravascular ultrasound guided optimized emergency coronary Palmaz–Schatz stent placement without post-procedural systemic anticoagulation. *J Am Coll Cardiol* 1995; **25**: 197A (abstract).

26 Colombo A, Nakamura S, Hall P, *et al*. A prospective study of Gianturco-Roubin coronary stent implantation without anticoagulation. *J Am Coll Cardiol* 1995; **25**: 50A (abstract).

27 Russo R, Schatz RA, Sklar MA, Johnson AD, Tobis JM, Teirstein PS. Ultrasound guided coronary stent placement without prolonged systemic anticoagulation. *J Am Coll Cardiol* 1995; **25**: 50A (abstract).

28 Colombo A, Nakamura S, Hall P, Maiello L, Finci L, Martini G. A prospective study of Wiktor coronary stent implantation without anticoagulation. *J Am Coll Cardiol* 1995; **25**: 239A (abstract).

29 Van Belle E, McFadden EP, Bauters C, Hamon M, Bertrand ME, Lablanche J-M. Combined antiplatelet therapy without anticoagulation. An effective alternative to prevent subacute thrombosis after coronary stenting. *J Am Coll Cardiol* 1995; **25**: 197A (abstract).

30 Lablanche JM, Grollier G, Bonnet JL, *et al.* Ticlopidine aspirin stent evaluation (TASTE); a French multicenter study. *Circulation* 1995; **92**: I-476 (abstract).

31 Barragan P, Silverstri M, Sainsous J, *et al.* Prevention of sub-acute occlusion after coronary stenting with ticlopidine regimen without intravascular ultrasound guided stenting. *J Am Coll Cardiol* 1995; **25**: 182A (abstract).

32 Buszman P, Clague J, Gibbs S, *et al.* Improved post stent management: high gain and low risk. *J Am Coll Cardiol* 1995; **25**: 182A (abstract).

33 Carvalho H, Fajadet J, Jordan C, Cassagneau B, Robert G, Marco J. A lower rate of complications after Gianturco–Roubin stenting using a new antiplatelet and anticoagulation protocol. *Circulation* 1994; **90**: I-25 (abstract).

34 Elias J, Monassier JP, Puel J, *et al.* Medtronic–Wiktor implantation without coumadin: hospital outcome. *Circulation* 1994; **90**: I-124 (abstract).

35 Barragan P, Sainsous J, Silvestri M, *et al.* Ticlopidine and subcutaneous heparin as an alternative regimen following coronary stenting. *Cathet Cardiovasc Diagn* 1994; **32**: 133–8.

36 Blengino S, Maiello L, Hall P, Nakamura S, Martini G, Colombo A. Randomized trial of coronary stent implantation without anticoagulation: aspirin versus ticlopidine. *Circulation* 1994; **90**: I-124 (abstract).

37 Jordan C, Carvalho H, Fajadet J, Cassagneau B, Robert G, Marco J. Reduction of subacute thrombosis after stenting using a new anticoagulation protocol. *Circulation* 1994; **90**: I-125 (abstract).

38 Morice MC, Amor M, Benveniste E, *et al.* Coronary stenting without coumadin phase II, III, IV, V. Predictors of major complications. *Circulation* 1995; **92**: I-795.

39 Morice MC, Breton C, Bunouf P, *et al.* Coronary stenting without anticoagulant, without intravascular ultrasound. Result of the French registry. *Circulation* 1995; **92**: I-796.

40 Morice MC, Zemour G, Benveniste E, *et al.* Intracoronary stenting without coumadin: one month results of a French multicenter study [see comments]. *Cathet Cardiovasc Diagn* 1995; **35**: 1–7.

41 Wong SC, Popma J, Mintz G, *et al.* Preliminary results from the Reduced Anticoagulation in Saphenous Vein Graft (RAVES) Trial. *Circulation* 1994; **90**: I-125 (abstract).

42 Van Belle E, McFadden EP, Lablanche JM, Bauters C, Hamon M, Bertrand ME. Two-pronged antiplatelet therapy with aspirin and ticlopidine without systemic anticoagulation: an alternative therapeutic strategy after bailout implantation. *Coron Artery Dis* 1995; **6**: 341–5.

43 Belli G, Whitlow PL, Franco I, *et al.* Intracoronary stenting without oral anticoagulation: The Cleveland Clinic Registry. *Circulation* 1995; **92**: I-796.

44 Saito S, Kim K, Hosokawa G, Hatano K, Tanaka S. Primary Palmaz–Schatz stent implantation without coumadin in acute myocardial infarction. *Circulation* 1995; **92**: I-796 (abstract).

45 Haase J, Reifart N, Baier T, *et al.* Bail-out stenting (Palmaz–Schatz) without anticoagulation. *Circulation* 1995; **92**: I-795.

46 Hall P, Colombo A, Itoh A, *et al.* Gianturco–Roubin stent implantation in small vessels without anticoagulation. *Circulation* 1995; **92**: I-795.

47 Goods CM, Al-Shaibi KF, Lyer SS, *et al.* Flexible coil coronary stenting without anticoagulation or intravascular ultrasound: a prospective observational study. *Circulation* 1995; **92**: I-795.

48 Brunel P, Jordan C, Fajadet J, Cassagneau B, Marco J. Successive steps in the management of coronary stenting. *Circulation* 1995; **92**: I-87.

49 Saito S, Nobuyoshi M, Oohata K. Ticlopidine without coumadin is enough for the prevention of stent thrombosis after elective intracoronary Palmaz–Schatz stent implantation-results of no-PAIN trial. *J Am Coll Cardiol* 1997; **29**: 95A (abstract).

50 Lablanche JM, Bonnet JL, Grollier G, *et al.* Combined antiplatelet therapy without anticoagulation after stent implantation: the ticlopidine aspirin stent evaluation (TASTE) study. *J Am Coll Cardiol* 1997; **29**: 95A.

51 Goods CM, Al-Shaibi KF, Yadav SS, *et al.* Utilization of the coronary balloon-expandable coil stent without anticoagulation or intravascular ultrasound. *Circulation* 1996; **93**: 1803–8.

52 Albeiro R, Hall P, Itoh A, *et al.* Effectiveness of aspirin alone compared with a combination of ticlopidine and aspirin for the prevention of subacute stent thrombosis after successful optimized stent implantation. *J Am Coll Cardiol* 1997; **29**: 95A.

53 Calver AL, Dawkins KD, Haywood GA, Gray HH, Morgan JM, Simpson IA. Multilink stenting, a 'minimalist' approach using aspirin alone. No ticlopidine, no coumadin, no IVUS and no QCA. *J Am Coll Cardiol* 1997; **29**: 95A.

54 Morice MC, Dumas P, Voudris V, *et al.* The MUST Trial. In-hospital and clinical events at six months. Final results. *J Am Coll Cardiol* 1997; **29**: 93A (abstract).

55 Fishman DL, Savage MP, Penn I, *et al.* High pressure inflation in conjunction with ticlopidine and aspirin following

coronary stent placement: results of the STRESS III results. *J Am Coll Cardiol* 1997; **29**: 171A (abstract).

56 Schwartz L, Bourassa MG, Lesperance J, *et al.* Aspirin and dipyridamole in the prevention of restenosis after percutaneous transluminal coronary angioplasty. *N Engl J Med* 1988; **318**: 1714–19.

57 Brown RI, Aldridge HE, Schwartz L, Henderson M, Brooks E, Coutanche M. The use of dextran-40 during percutaneous transluminal coronary angioplasty: a report of three cases of anaphylactoid reactions – one near fatal. *Cathet Cardiovasc Diagn* 1985; **11**: 591–5.

58 Klugmann S, Salvi A, Valente M, Zanei P, Maiolino P, Camercini F. Coronary artery spasm after administration of dextran 40: implications concerning percutaneous transluminal coronary angioplasty. *Am Heart J* 1986; **111**: 1202–4.

59 Taylor MA, Di Blasi SL, Bender RM, Santoian EC, Cha SD, Dennis CA. Adult respiratory distress syndrome complicating intravenous infusion of low-molecular weight dextran. *Cathet Cardiovasc Diagn* 1994; **32**: 249–53.

60 Gregorini L, Marco J, Fajadet J, Brunel P, Cassagneau B, Bossi I. Ticlopidine attenuates post-angioplasty thrombin generation. *Circulation* 1995; **92**: I-609.

61 May A, Neumann FJ, Gawaz M, Ott I. Monocyte function after coronary stent implantation. Effect of two different antithrombotic regimens. *Circulation* 1995; **92**: I-86.

62 Hass WK, Easton JD, Adams HP, *et al.* A randomized trial comparing ticlopidine hydrochloride with aspirin for the prevention of stroke in high-risk patients. Ticlopidine Aspirin Stroke Study Group. *N Engl J Med* 1989; **321**: 501–7.

63 Rodriquez JN, Fernandez-Jurado A, Dieguez JC, Amian A, Prados D. Ticlopidine and severe aplastic anemia. *Am J Hematol* 1994; **47**: 332.

64 Bellavance A. Efficacy of ticlopidine and aspirin for prevention of reversible cerebrovascular events. The Ticlopidine Aspirin Stroke Study. *Stroke* 1994; **25**: 1452–7.

65 Shomig A, Schuhlen H, Blasini R, *et al.* Anticoagulation versus antiplatelet therapy after intracoronary Palmaz–Schatz stent placement. *Circulation* 1995; **92**: I-280.

66 Schomig A, Neumann FJ, Kastrati A, *et al.* A randomized comparison of antiplatelet and anticoagulant therapy after the placement of coronary-artery stents. *N Engl J Med* 1996; **334**: 1084–9.

67 Hall, P, Nakamura S, Maiello L, *et al.* A randomized comparison of combined ticlopidine and aspirin therapy versus aspirin therapy alone after successful intravascular ultrasound-guided stent implantation. *Circulation* 1996; **93**: 215–22.

68 Leon MB, Wong SC. Intracoronary stents. A breakthrough technology or just another small step? [editorial; comment]. *Circulation* 1994; **89**: 1323–7.

69 Leon MB, Baim DS, Gordon P, *et al.* Clinical and angiographic results from the Stent Antithrombotic Regimen Study (STARS). *Circulation* 1996; **94**: I-4002 (abstract).

70 Liu MW, Voorhees WD 3rd, Agrawal S, Dean LS, Roubin GS. Stratification of the risk of thrombosis after intracoronary stenting for threatened or acute closure complicating coronary balloon angioplasty: a Cook registry study. *Am Heart J* 1995; **130**: 8–13.

71 Schomig A, Kastrati A, Dietz R, *et al.* Emergency coronary stenting for dissection during percutaneous transluminal coronary angioplasty: angiographic follow-up after stenting and after repeat angioplasty of the stented segment. *J Am Coll Cardiol* 1994; **23**: 1053–60.

72 Herrmann HC, Buchbinder M, Clemen MW, *et al.* Emergent use of balloon-expandable coronary artery stenting for failed percutaneous transluminal coronary angioplasty. *Circulation* 1992; **86**: 812–19.

73 Benzuly KH, O'Neil WW, Gangadharan V, *et al.* Stenting in acute myocardial infarction (STAMI): bailout, conditional and planned stents. *J Am Coll Cardiol* 1997; **29**: 456A (abstract).

74 Moussa I, Di Mario C, Di Francesco L, Reimers B, Blengino S, Colombo A. Subacute stent thrombosis and the anticoagulation controversy: changes in drug therapy, operator technique, and the impact of intravascular ultrasound. *Am J Cardiol* 1996; **78**: 13–17.

75 Saito S, Hosokawa FG, Kim K, Tanaka S, Miyake S. Primary stent implantation without coumadin in acute myocardial infarction. *J Am Coll Cardiol* 1996; **28**: 74–81.

76 Monassier JP, Elias J, Raynaud P, Joly P. Results of early (<24 hr) and late (>24 hr) implantation of coronary stents in acute myocardial infarction. *Circulation* 1995; **92**: I-609.

77 Neumann FJ, Walter H, Schmitt C, Alt E, Schomig A. Coronary stenting as an adjunct to direct balloon angioplasty in acute myocardial infarction. *Circulation* 1995; **92**: I-609.

78 Alfonso F, Rodriguez P, Phillips P, *et al.* Clinical and angiographic implications of coronary stenting in thrombus-containing lesions. *J Am Coll Cardiol* 1997; **29**: 96A.

79 Neumann FJ, Walter H, Richardt G, Schmitt C, Schomig A. Coronary Palmaz–Schatz stent implantation in acute myocardial infarction. *Heart* 1996; **75**: 121–6.

80 Stone GW, Brodie B, Griffin J, *et al.* Safety and feasibility of primary stenting in acute myocardial infarction. In hospital

and 30 day results of the PAMI stent pilot trial. *J Am Coll Cardiol* 1997; **29**: 389A.

81   Investigators The EPIC. Use of a monoclonal antibody directed against the platelet glycoprotein IIb/IIIa receptor in high-risk coronary angioplasty. *New Engl J Med* 1994; **330**: 956–61.

82   Lincoff AM, Tcheng JE, Bass TA, *et al.* A multicenter, randomized, double-blind pilot trial of standard versus low dose weight-adjusted heparin in patients treated with the platelet GP IIb/IIIa receptor antibody c7E3 during percutaneous coronary angioplasty. *J Am Coll Cardiol* 1995; **25**: 80–81A (abstract).

83   Makkar RR, Eigler NL, Nakamura M, *et al.* Monoclonal antibody to IIb-IIIa receptor (m7E3) is highly effective in inhibiting acute stent thrombosis. *Circulation* 1995; **92**: I-685.

84   Aggarwal RK, Ireland DC, Azrin MA, Ezekowitz MD, deBono DP, Gershlick AH. Antithrombotic properties of stents eluting platelet glycoprotein IIb/IIIa antibody. *Circulation* 1995; **92**: I-488.

85   Schmidmaier G, Stemberger A, Alt E, Gawaz M, Schomig A. Time release characteristics of a biodegradable stent coating with polyactic acid releasing PEG-Hirudin and PG12-Analog. *J Am Coll Cardiol* 1997; **29**: 94A (abstract).

86   Chronos NAF, Robinson KA, Kelly AB, *et al.* Thrombo-resistant phosphorylcholine coating for coronary stents. *Circulation* 1995; **92**: I-685.

87   Serruys PW, Emanuelsson H, van der Giessen W, *et al.* Heparin-coated Palmaz–Schatz stents in human coronary arteries. Early outcome of the Benestent-II Pilot Study. *Circulation* 1996; **93**: 412–22.

88   Legrand V, Serruys PW, Emanuelsson H, *et al.* BENE-STENT-II Trial—Final results of visit I: A 15-day follow-up. *J Am Coll Cardiol* 1997; **29**: 170A (abstract).

89   Goods CM, Liu MW, Iyer SS, *et al.* A cost analysis of coronary stenting without anticoagulation versus stenting with anticoagulation using warfarin. *Am J Cardiol* 1996; **78**: 334–6.

III

Restenosis and Arterial Remodeling

13

Radiation for restenosis: an overview

Spencer B King III

Introduction: mechanisms of restenosis

Restenosis following coronary interventions remains its most significant problem. From Gruentzig's first experience[1] through the collection of the early NHLBI registry,[2] the restenosis rate for relatively ideal lesions has been judged to be about 30%. This restenosis rate has finally been influenced by intracoronary stenting. The STRESS and Benestent trials[3,4] demonstrated a $\frac{1}{4}$ to $\frac{1}{3}$ reduction in angiographically demonstrated coronary restenosis at 6 months. The recently completed Benestent II trial with optimal stenting is reported to show restenosis in the 13% range, again for ideally suited lesions with optimal stenting technique. Nonetheless, many lesions, particularly those previously dilated or in diffusely diseased segments, small vessels, bifurcations, ostial locations, vein grafts, etc., carry a higher restenosis rate as pointed out recently by Nobuyoshi and colleagues.[5] Stenting in these subsets carried a 27–40% rate of restenosis. The Emory Angioplasty vs. Surgery Trial of multivessel disease had an angiographic follow-up arm which looked at restenosis at one year. Among patients undergoing angioplasty, 44% of all lesions dilated exhibited angiographic restenosis within one year. Many of these lesions would not have been suitable for intracoronary stenting, or if stented would not have fit the criteria utilized in the most optimistic stenting trials.[6]

The recent advent of IIb/IIIa blockade gave promise for a reduction in restenosis as the EPIC trial showed.[7] Subsequent IIb/IIIa trials using different compounds such as the IMPACT II and RESTORE trials did not show any sugges-

tion of reduction of late restenosis and the subsequent EPILOG trial of the 7E3 monoclonal antibody IIb/IIIa receptors also did not show any suggestion that clinical restenosis or angiographic restenosis was modified by this approach.

For many years the mechanism of restenosis has been felt to be due largely to intimal proliferation resulting from vascular injury. It has also been known that some recoil occurs immediately after the procedure and this recoil can be totally opposed by intracoronary stenting. The third component of restenosis, chronic vascular contraction or remodeling, has been reported to contribute to the restenotic process.[8] Ultrasonic observations have suggested as much as 50–75% of the cross-sectional area loss may be due to chronic remodeling while histopathologic reports suggest that this contribution may be approximately one third. In any case, there is no argument that neointimal proliferation remains an important component of restenosis and this is the prime target of endovascular radiation therapy.

The animal model most akin to human coronary arteries is the pig coronary artery system with balloon overstretch injury. This model is not perfect in that it is not an atherosclerotic model but it does provide an opportunity to simulate the type of injury occurring in balloon angioplasty and stenting. Scott and Wilcox[9] at Emory have investigated the cellular mechanism for restenosis in this model and have suggested that a significant amount of injury occurs to the periadventitial tissues. There is early cellular proliferation in these tissues and the possibility exists that that response contributes to the neointimal proliferation or at least to the perivascular scarring which may contribute to vascular remodeling. Subsequent studies from the author's laboratory with more specific staining[10] suggest the cells responsible for the neointimal proliferation in this model are the cells of the vessel media rather than the periadventitial tissues. In any case, the cells of the vessel wall and surrounding tissues can contribute to early injury and proliferation and they are the targets of endovascular radiation therapy. Wilcox and Waksman[11] have shown that BRDU staining for proliferating cells common 3 days following balloon overstretch injury can be markedly suppressed by endovascular radiation delivered at the time of the injury.

Rationale for local endovascular radiation therapy

Radiation therapy has long been known to be a potent inhibitor of cell replication.[12-14] Other forms of injury resulting in exhuberant scar formation such as keloids on the skin and pterygium on the sclera have been suppressed by low-dose radiation applied after their surgical removal. This principle was applied by Liermann and associates.[15] In their studies patients with prior restenosis following femoral popliteal angioplasty have been redilated and stented and had local endovascular radiation applied. Long-term follow-up of those patients has been encouraging in terms of absence of clinical restenosis or flow studies to suggest significant restenosis.

Animal investigation

Based on these encouraging findings a program of endovascular radiation in the overstretch porcine coronary model was undertaken at Emory.[16] The initial animal experimentation involved the use of an ^{192}Ir-containing ribbon with an activity of up to 135 millicuries placed in the coronary artery for approximately 30 min in order to achieve a dose of 7–14 Gy at a depth of 2 mm. The findings in those studies were very impressive with dramatic reduction in neointimal proliferation in a dose-dependent manner.[16] The suppression was seen in the animal sacrificed at 2 weeks and additional experiments were carried out in miniswine with survival of the animals to 6 months. These 6-month animals also had significant suppression of neointima formation well after the coronary endothelium had been re-established.

The dosimetry curve of gamma radiation reflects its high degree of penetrability. In order to utilize gamma radiation systems, it would be necessary to shield the patient from the operators with equipment not currently available in cardiac catheterization suites. The sensitive tissues of the body would also receive higher radiation dosing from gamma irradiation. Because of these concerns and the impractability of prolonged indwelling coronary catheters, an isotope with more favorable characteristics was sought. This has been found in the form of ^{90}Sr/Y, a pure beta-emitting source. The dosimetry curve of this isotope is quite suitable for treatment of coronary arteries with the vast majority of the radiation delivery within 2–3 mm of the source. Novoste Corporation has developed a hydraulic catheter-based system which is quite suitable for catheterization laboratory use.

The catheter system consists of a transfer mechanism to house a train of very small cannisters containing ^{90}Sr. This transfer system is connected to and loaded into the delivery device. The catheter itself is composed of a double lumen hydraulic system which is entirely closed from the patient's circulation. A third lumen carries the guidewire for placement of the catheter in the desired location. At the completion of the angioplasty procedure, the beta-radiation delivery catheter is positioned over the guidewire in a way to span the segment of interest. Radio-opaque markers clearly identify the effective area to be irradiated. The delivery device is connected to the catheter and by hydraulic means the source train is delivered down the catheter to the prescribed site. Dosimetry is determined by the dwell time of the isotope within the artery. At the completion of the desired dosing, the radioactive seed train is delivered to the delivery device again by reversed hydraulic pressure. The catheter itself is highly flexible and measures almost 1.5 mm in diameter. This size in the post-dilated artery usually leaves enough room for antegrade flow in the typical postangioplasty 2-mm lumen but little room for eccentric positioning. In other words, centering is largely accomplished by the size of the delivery catheter device. Following completion of the radiation dosing, which usually lasts between 2 and 4 min, the isotope train is returned to the delivery device and the catheter is removed from the coronary circulation over the guidewire. A final angiographic examination completes the study.

First utilizing gamma radiation and later the beta-radiation catheter, studies were carried out in the porcine overstretch coronary model delivering doses of 7, 14, 28 or 56 Gy. At 2 weeks following administration of the radiation, there was a dose-dependent suppression of neointima formation. Importantly there was no paradoxical increase in hyperplasia seen at any dose. Maximal intimal thickness was reduced from 0.47 mm in the control animals to 0.34 mm at 14 Gy. A more consistent measure of the effect of neointimal proliferation related to the amount of injury incurred is the intimal area over the length of the fracture produced. This ratio is reduced from 0.47 in the control animals to 0.19 in the 14 Gy treated animals. The animals were also examined for evidence of re-endothelialization and injury to other tissues. There was no significant difference in the appearance of the endothelium by scanning electron microscopy or in the histologic appearance of other tissues such as myocardium, pericardium or adjacent coronary vessels.[16,17] Chronic studies were also carried out using the miniswine coronary model. Effects shown at 2 weeks were also sustained at 6 months in this model.[17]

Other systems, such as radioactive stents,[18,19] have been developed in an effort to control the restenosis process. These stents have shown promise in the rabbit model by inhibiting denudation injury-induced neointimal proliferation. These systems utilize short half-life radioactive materials which may be effective during the desired time for radiation activity. Some drawbacks of those systems include the short shelf life of such stents, the limitation to certain types of stents and the potential effect of the radiation on re-endothelialization of the vessel and the stent material. There is also a rapid dropoff in radiation dosing at the ends of the stent, a site where proliferative responses are not uncommonly seen.

Clinical trials of the beta-radiation catheter system

The US Food and Drug Administration has given approval for a feasibility trial to be conducted using the previously described catheter system. At present the 23 proscribed patients have undergone balloon angioplasty followed by endovascular irradiation. The 30-day safety endpoint examination has been completed with no adverse events noted; the patients are being followed with angiographic examinations at 6 months to document the degree of neointimal formation, the late lumen loss and loss index, the restenosis rate, and any other effects that might be observed angiographically. Although there is no control group for this study, the patients were selected by the criteria of the Lovastatin restenosis trial[20] and the quantitative angiographic assessment is being performed by the same core laboratory that performed that trial. It is hoped that adequate information may be obtained to assist in the power calculations for the multicenter randomized trial (Table 13.1).

Other studies of endovascular radiation

Two recent studies have provided encouragement regarding the proof of principle of endovascular radiation for restenosis prevention. One gamma radiation study from Venezuela[21] showed that a significant suppression of late lumen loss was achieved by the majority of the 21 patients treated. Another study, a randomized trial of gamma radiation from Scripps Clinic,[22] showed a dramatic reduction in restenosis in previously restenotic patients. In that study of 54 patients, the angiographic restenosis rate among patients in the control group was 54% and the rate among patients treated with endovascular radiation was 17%. These patients all had previous restenosis and most of them had in-stent restenosis. The procedures preceding radiation therapy were either placement of a primary stent or dilatation of the previously stented segment. Although the radiation source used in both these trials was ^{192}Ir (a gamma source), and therefore required evacuation of the laboratory by the personnel and long dwell times in the artery, this system is very similar to the one used in the early animal experiments in the author's institution. We felt, therefore, that since identical findings were seen with beta and gamma radiation in the pig coronary arteries, we can also anticipate similar encouraging findings with the more practical beta-irradiation systems in human experiments.

Table 13.1 Beta-radiation feasibility trial (baseline data: $n = 23$).

	Percent stenosis	MLD (mm)	Reference artery (mm)
Pre-PTCA	73	0.79	2.95
Post-PTCA and radiation	23	2.19	2.87

Notes:
MLD = minimum lumen diameter
PTCA = percutaneous transluminal coronary angioplasty.

Plans for randomized trials

At present, a large multicenter randomized trial is being planned for the beta-catheter radiation system to test the effectiveness of radiation in patients undergoing angioplasty for primary and restenotic lesions and in those patients undergoing stenting for primary and restenotic lesions. The possibility exists that there may be a differential effect on patients undergoing balloon angioplasty and patients undergoing stenting. Since in-stent restenosis is virtually 100% neointimal proliferation, there is the possibility that the system will be more effective when stents are used. On the other hand, since stents produce a continuing stimulus to intimal proliferation by their presence, the single exposure to radiation achieved may be more effective for the single injury balloon angioplasty model. Tierstein's findings of important effects of one-dose radiation in stented patients, however, speak to the potential that these therapies will be effective for both balloon angioplasty and stented patients. The planned multicenter randomized trial will allow, for the first time, a blinded trial of a coronary device. This is of great interest, not only to those working with the radiation systems but also for trialists at large. If the early feasibility trials are any indication, the randomized comparisons should be extremely interesting.

References

1   Gruentzig AR, Senning A, Seigenthaler WE. Nonoperative dilatation of coronary artery stenosis: percutaneous transluminal coronary angioplasty. *N Engl J Med* 1979; **301**: 61–8.

2   Holmes DR jr, Vlietstra RE, Smith HC, *et al.* Restenosis after percutaneous transluminal coronary angioplasty (PTCA): a report from the PTCA registry of the National Heart, Lung and Blood Institute. *Am J Cardiol* 1984; **53**: 77C–81C.

3   Fischman DL, Leon MB, Baim DS. A randomized comparison of coronary stent placement and balloon angioplasty in the treatment of coronary artery disease. *N Engl J Med* 1994; **331**: 496–501.

4   Serruys PW, de Jaegere P, Kiemeneij F, *et al.* A comparison of balloon-expandable stent implantation with balloon angioplasty in patients with coronary artery disease. *N Engl J Med* 1994; **331**: 489–95.

5   Sawada Y, Kimura I, Nobuyoshi M. Initial and six months outcome of Palmaz-Schatz stent implantation: STRESS/Benestent equivalent vs nonequivalent lesions. *J Am Coll Cardiol* 1996; **27 (Suppl A)**: 252 (abstract).

6   Zhao X-Q, Brown BG, Stewart DK, *et al.* Effectiveness of revascularization in the Emory Angioplasty versus Surgery Trial. A randomized comparison of coronary angioplasty with bypass surgery. *Circulation* 1996; **93**: 1954–62.

7   The EPIC Investigators. Use of a monoclonal antibody directed against the platelet glycoprotein IIb/IIIa receptor in high-risk coronary angioplasty. *N Engl J Med* 1994; **330**: 956–61.

8   Mintz GS, Popma JJ, Pichard AD, *et al.* Arterial remodeling after coronary angioplasty: a serial intravascular ultrasound study. *Circulation* 1996; **94**: 35–43.

9   Scott NA, Cipolla GD, Ross CE, *et al.* Identification of a potential role for the adventitia in vascular lesion formation after balloon overstretch injury of porcine coronary arteries. *Circulation* 1996; **93**: 2178–87.

10   Robinson KA. Pig coronary artery model of post angioplasty restenosis. In: *Vascular Brachytherapy* (Nucleotron-Oldeft, Waksman R, King SB, Crocker IR, eds, in press.

11   Wilcox JN, Waksman R, King SB, Scott NA. Role of the adventitia in the arterial response to angioplasty. In: Waksman R, King SB, Crocker IR, Mould RF, eds, *Vascular Brachytherapy* (Nuclestron-Oldeft, The Netherlands, 1996) 17–29

12   Puck TT, Morkovin D, Marcus PI. Action of x-rays on mammalian cells. II. Survival curves of cells from normal human tissues. *J Exp Med* 1957; **106**: 485–500.

13   Sinclair WK. Cyclic x-ray response in mammalian cells *in vitro. Radiat Res* 1968; **63**: 620–43.

14   Fischer-Dzoga K, Dimitrievich GS, Griem ML. Differential radiosensitivity of aortic cells *in vitro. Radiat Res* 1984; **99**: 536–46.

15   Liermann DD, d Bottcher HD, Kollath J, *et al.* Prophylactic endovascular radiotherapy to prevent intimal hyperplasia after stent implantation in femoro-popliteal arteries. *Cardiovasc Interven Radiol* 1994; **17**: 12–16.

16   Waksman R, Robinson KA, Crocker IR, *et al.* Endovascular low dose irradiation inhibits neointima formation after coronary artery balloon injury in swine: a possible role for radiation therapy in restenosis prevention. *Circulation* 1995; **91**: 1533–9.

17   Waksman R, Robinson KA, Crocker IR, *et al.* Intracoronary low-dose B-irradiation inhibits neointima formation after coronary artery balloon injury in the swine restenosis model. *Circulation* 1995; **92**: 3025–31.

18   Hehrlein C, Zimmerman M, Metz J, *et al.* Radioactive stent implantation inhibits neointimal proliferation in nonatherosclerotic rabbits. *Circulation* 1993; **88 (Suppl I)**: I-65 (abstract).

19 Fischell TA, Kharma BK, Fuschell DR, et al. Low dose B-particle emission from stent wire results in complete, localized inhibition of smooth muscle cell proliferation. Circulation 1994; **90**: 2956–63.

20 Weintraub WS, Boccuzzi SJ, Klein JL, et al. Lack of effect of Lovastatin on restenosis after coronary angioplasty. Lovastatin Restenosis Trial Study. N Engl J Med 1994; **331**: 1331–7.

21 Condado JA, Gurdiel G, Espinosa R, et al. Long-term angiographic and clinical outcome following balloon angioplasty and intracoronary radiation therapy in humans. Circulation 1996; **94 (Suppl I)**: I-209 (abstract).

22 Teirstein PS, Massullo V, Jani S, et al. Radiation therapy following coronary stenting—6 month followup of a randomized clinical trial. Circulation 1996; **94 (Suppl I)**: I-210 (abstract).

14

Intracoronary radiation: does it really work?

Ron Waksman

Introduction

Twenty years ago the first coronary balloon angioplasty by Andres R Gruentzig introduced a new dimension to the field of interventional cardiology. The main concept was that atherosclerotic plaque can be physically removed or ablated from within the vessel. However, it was learnt very early that subsequent to the intervention, a wound healing process known as restenosis significantly limits the success of this new novelty. Restenosis rates of 40–60% modified the initial enthusiasm of balloon angioplasty and challenged scientists and clinicians to find a solution for this significant medical problem. Several therapeutic approaches have been suggested: pharmaceutical agents, new devices and gene therapy. However, the problem of overexuberant cell proliferation after intervention leading to restenosis, although better understood, still remains the Achilles heel of this field. Ionizing radiation is well known as an antiproliferative agent for benign and malignant disorders since the discovery of radium by Madame Curie in 1898. It is also known that dividing cells and proliferative cells are radiosensitive to low doses of radiation. Since the major components of restenosis are felt to be due to an exuberant cellular proliferation migration and matrix synthesis in addition to early recoil and vascular remodeling,[1–6] it was hypothesized that a low-dose of ionizing radiation will result in inhibition of smooth muscle proliferation and, by that, may reduce the restenosis rate. Results from animal studies[16–30] supported the hypothesis and led to the initiation of feasibility clinical trials utilizing low-dose radiation delivered into coronary arteries following balloon angioplasty. This chapter reviews the results from these animal studies and the initial clinical trials which are currently underway in an attempt to determine whether intracoronary radiation really works for prevention of restenosis.

What have we learnt from the animal studies?

Animal models of a variety of forms of mechanical arterial injury were initially developed to study the smooth muscle cell (SMC) proliferative component of restenosis and the atherosclerotic plaque.[7,8] Several of these models were adopted to test the efficacy of endovascular radiation as an antirestenotic therapeutic strategy.

Prior to the angioplasty and the restenosis era in 1965, Freidman et al.[9] reported that exposure of radiation (using 192-iridium, a dose of approximately 14 Gy delivered intraluminally) to an injured aorta of cholesterol-fed rabbits resulted in inhibition of subsequent development of atherosclerosis by inhibition of SMC proliferation and intimal hyperplasia. This report was an early indication that restenosis may be prevented by radiation therapy.

Radiation therapy can be delivered to the coronary arteries by external radiation or by brachytherapy methods either by catheter-based systems or by radioactive stents. Catheter-based systems can use both gamma and beta emitters, which can deliver the prescribed dose in either a high or low-dose rate, manually or automatically, while radioactive stents will utilize primarily pure beta emitters in a very low-dose rate. Among the planned animal studies performed to examine the effect of radiation for prevention of restenosis, it appears that the brachytherapy approach demonstrated favorable results over external radiation. These animal results are summarized in Tables 14.1, 14.2 and 14.3.

External radiation

Several investigators have suggested that external radiation could reduce the amount of cell proliferation after balloon angioplasty.[10–12] However, the data from studies utilizing external radiation therapy for prevention of restenosis in animal models are not conclusive. Schwartz et al.[13] administered radiation (4–8 Gy) with an orthovoltage X-ray unit to porcine coronary vessels following stent placement. One month after the external radiation treatment, morphometric analysis demonstrated accentuated neointimal hyperplasia in the irradiated stented arteries versus control (nonirradiated stented arteries). These negative findings were corroborated by Hehrlien et al.[14] using 8 Gy as a single dose and 16 Gy in fractionation (2 × 8 Gy) in stented rabbit iliac artery, resulting in excess of neointimal thickening. Gellman et al.[15] used external orthovoltage X-rays (doses of 3 and 9 Gy) in a rabbit iliac postballoon angioplasty model and showed more neointimal hyperplasia in the irradiated group. Unpublished results from recent studies held at Emory using external radiation (single-dose 8 Gy), following balloon overstretch balloon injury in porcine coronary arteries, demonstrated a deleterious effect compared to control. Interestingly, similar doses, when administered intraluminally via a catheter into the coronary artery, demonstrated reduction of neointima formation. In addition, some damage to the vasa vasorum and to the myocytes was noted with external radiation. In contrast to these studies,[16,17] other investigators have reported a benefit with external radiotherapy postballoon angioplasty. Among the reports of inhibitory effect on intimal hyperplasia are those of Shimatokahara and Mayberg,[16] who have shown reduction of neointimal hyperplasia in injured rat carotid arteries using external radiation with doses of 7.5, 15 or 22.5 Gy with 137 Cs source. Other studies using external radiation corroborated these findings.[10–12,17] The variability results with external radiation in animal models and other reports of advanced atherosclerosis in coronary arteries of patients who were previously exposed to radiation suggest that external radiation should not be the treatment of choice for prevention of coronary restenosis, unless supported strongly by new animal studies.

Brachytherapy in animal models

More consistent evidence of the efficacy of radiotherapy came from groups using brachytherapy techniques (Table

Table 14.1 Preclinical studies performed using teletherapy

Author	Animal/vessel	Radiation source	Result
Abbas et al.[11]	Rabbit/iliac	Linac	6 Gy no benefit: 12 Gy benefit at 5 days postangioplasty
Schwartz et al.[13]	Pig/stented coronaries	Orthovoltage	Neointima significantly accentuated with radiation (4–8 Gy) poststent implantation
Gellman et al.[15]	Rabbit/iliacs	Orthovoltage	Increased neointima with 3 and 9 Gy postangioplasty
Hirai et al.[10]	Rabbit/femoral arteries	Orthovoltage	2 and 5 Gy no benefit; 10 and 20 Gy reduced neointimal postinjury by air drying
Shimatokahara et al.[16]	Rats/carotids	TeleCesium	Reduced neointima following balloon angioplasty
Hehrlein et al.[14]	Rabbits/stented iliacs	Orthovoltage	No beneficial effect with external radiation of stented arteries

Table 14.2 Studies with catheter-based therapy.

Author	Animal/vessel	Radiation source	Result
Waksman[18]	Pig/coronaries	192-ir	Decreased neointima with 3.5–14 Gy; sustained benefit at 6 months with 7–14 Gy
Wiedermann[22]	Pig/coronaries	192-ir	Decreased neointima with 15--20 Gy; worse with 10 Gy; benefit at 6 months with 20 Gy
Mazur et al.[21]	Pig/coronaries	192-ir-HDR	Decreased neointima with 10, 15 and 25 Gy following stent and angioplasty
Waksman	Pig/coronaries	90-Sr/Y	Benefit with 7 and 14 Gy postangioplasty; similar results to 192-ir
Verin et al.[24]	Rabbit/carotid and iliacs	90-Y	Decreased neointima with 18 Gy; no benefit with 6 and 12 Gy
Waksman[23]	Pig/coronaries; repeat injury model	192-ir	Decreased neointima only after the second injury; no effect on established neointima from initial injury
Raizner[30]	Pig/coronaries post-PTCA and stent injury	32-P HDR	Decreased neointima formation in arteries postballoon injury and in stented arteries only with a dose of 32 Gy
Waksman	Pig stented coronaries	90-Sr/Y and 192-ir	Radiation prior to stenting reduced neointima formation at 30 days

Table 14.3 Results of radioactive stents.

Author	Animal/vessel	Radiation source	Result
Laird et al.[35]	Pig/iliac	32-P stent	Decreased neointima at 6 weeks
Hehrlein[33]	Rabbit/iliac	Radioactive steel stent (Palmaz–Schatz)	Decreased neointima at 12 weeks with 35 µCi stent
Hehrlein[34]	Rabbit/iliac	32-P stent	Decreased neointima at 12 weeks with 13 µCi stent
Carter et al.[36]	Pig coronaries	32-P stent	Decreased neointima with 0.5 µCi and 3–23 µCi but increased neointima with 1 µCi at 28 days
Carter et al.[36] (personal communication)	Pig coronaries	32-P stent	No effect on neointima formation reduction with 0.5 µCi at 6 months.

14.2). Waksman et al.[18] and Wiedermann et al.[19,20] have evaluated the potential benefit of intraluminal 192-iridium with doses between 14 and 20 Gy, using hand-loading sources via a perfusion delivery catheter with a dwelling time of 30–60 min. Raizner et al.[21] also evaluated the effect of 192-Ir using a high-dose rate afterloader to deliver doses between 15 and 25 Gy within 5–10 min. All three investigators have shown the benefits of endovascular brachytherapy in the porcine model of restenosis. Some discrepancies exist among the groups regarding dose–response relationships, but all have shown that doses in the range of 14–25 Gy delivered following balloon angioplasty significantly diminished the amount of neointimal hyperplasia in the short term (2–4 weeks). Waksman[18] and Wiedermann[20] have both shown that the radiation effect was maintained at 6 months without any excess of fibrosis or other adverse effects in the treated arteries and the adjacent segments. Waksman[18] has also shown that delaying the radiation by 2 days results in a better response when compared to giving the radiation immediately postangioplasty.

Some controversies exist and remain to be resolved: Raizner[21] found in his study that radiation was not effective in the right coronary artery (RCA) in contrast to the work of others. Weidermann[22] reported that low doses of 10 Gy can stimulate intimal hyperplasia, in contrast to the work of Waksman[18] who demonstrated partial response using even lower doses such as 3.5 and 7 Gy after balloon injury in the same model. One common finding is the specific histologic pattern after radiation, showing nearly no neointima formation in the irradiated segments (Fig. 14.1).

Several groups have developed brachytherapy systems based on beta emitters and conducted a series of preclinical studies in animal models. The beta emitters which underwent preliminary evaluation are 90-yttrium as a wire, 90-strontium/yttrium in radioactive seeds delivered manually by hydraulic system to the treatment site, and P-32 in liquid or wire line source delivered by a high-dose rate afterloader.

Verin and Popowski[24,25] have used 90-Y emitter on a wire delivered via a centering balloon catheter in an atherosclerotic rabbit iliac and carotid arteries to treat with doses of 6, 12 and 18 Gy. At 6 weeks, the percent area stenosis and the number of neointimal cell layers were both significantly reduced in the group of arteries exposed to 18 Gy compared to the control group. However, there was no significant reduction of the histological indices in the 6 Gy and the 12 Gy groups. The authors concluded that 18 Gy may be sufficient for long-term inhibition of neointima formation after balloon injury, and selected this dose for their clinical study.

Waksman et al.[26,27] conducted a series of studies utilizing a catheter-based beta radiation system using 90-Sr/Y, a pure beta emitter, as the radioactive source. 90-Sr/Y has favorable characteristics in terms of permitting delivery of

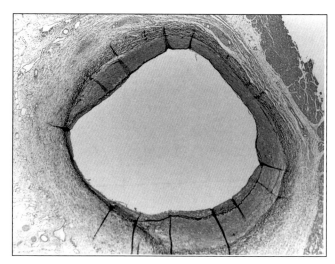

a

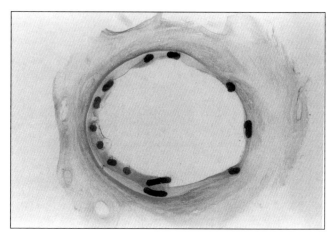

b

Figure 14.1

Representative micrographs at 40× instrument magnification of thick sections stained with Verhoeff–Van Gieson's elastin, from injured pig coronary arteries. Healing responses at (a) 2 weeks from treated group with 192-ir–14 Gy postballoon angioplasty. (b) 4 weeks from treated group with 90-Sr/Y dose of 14 Gy delivered prior to stenting.

dose to the required depth in tissue (2–3 mm) with little dose measured beyond 1 cm from the source. It has a half time of approximately 29 years, which does not require a day-to-day activity and dwelling time calculation. The source train of 90-Sr/Y isotope is delivered manually via a low-profile 4.5F noncentered catheter requiring a short treatment time of less than 4 min, to deliver doses of

14 Gy. The preclinical studies for this system were designed to determine the efficacy of this isotope and to find if 90-Sr/Y could inhibit neointima formation after balloon over-stretch injury as well as 192-Ir. Doses of 7, 14, 28 and 56 Gy were delivered following balloon angioplasty in porcine coronary arteries, and tissue examination was performed at 14 days after treatment. Morphometric indices of maximal intimal thickness and intimal area corrected for the extent of injury of irradiated vessels by beta and gamma radioisotopes were compared and found to be similar. Higher doses of 28 Gy and 56 Gy showed a more consistent effect in reduction of neointimal hyperplasia without excess of adverse effects to the treated vessel and the surrounding area. It appears that despite the different properties among the isotopes used for this application, if the right dose reached the target area, a similar effect of the radiation in reduction of the neointima will be obtained. An interesting example to support this concept was demonstrated by the group from Baylor,[30] which required a dose of 32 Gy using 32-P in order to have a reduction in neointima formation similar to that achieved with 20 Gy of 192-Ir following balloon or stent implantation in porcine coronary arteries.

Intracoronary radiation and stenting

Intracoronary radiation using a catheter-based system prior to intracoronary stenting has been examined by several investigators and proven to be effective both with gamma 192-Ir and beta 90-Sr/Y emitters in reduction of neointima formation using a dose of 14 Gy. The effect of radiation was limited when a dose of 14 Gy of 90-Sr/Y was delivered immediately poststent implantation[28–29] and when aggressive oversize stenting with high injury score was performed using 192-Ir.[31]

An attractive alternative to the use of catheter-based radiation systems for stented arteries is to couple the technology in the form of a radioactive stent. This coupled technology was suggested to address two mechanisms of restenosis: acute recoil and proliferation. Several technologies have been utilized to make the stent radioactive, among them, activation in a cyclotron, ion implantation and proton bombardment. The potential of this approach was supported initially from *in vitro* studies on cultured human, animal SMCs and endothelial cells by Fischell et al.,[32] who demonstrated that a stent impregnated with a low concentration of 32-P has a dose response effect on the inhibition of SMCs. Hehrlein et al.[32] activated Palmaz–Schatz stents in a cyclotron by which beta and x-radiation as well as high-energy gamma emitters were incorporated into the stent. The radioactive stents were placed into rabbit iliac arteries.

Morphometric analysis at 4, 12 and 52 weeks demonstrated reduction of neointima formation compared to conventional stents which were placed in the contralateral arteries. Although the study by Hehrlein et al.[34] demonstrated that stents made radioactive in a cyclotron effectively inhibit SMC proliferation and neointimal hyperplasia in rabbits, their technique has some potential drawbacks, one of which is having gamma irradiation and multiple radioisotopes including some with half-lives as long as 2.7 years. In another study, Hehrlein[39] reported that stents emitting 32-P also inhibit neointima formation, although only higher doses of 13 µCi demonstrated longevity of the inhibitory effect at 12 weeks. Laird et al.[35] and Carter et al.[36] stressed the advantages of beta emitters over the gamma irradiation such as the short half-life (14.3 days) and limited range of the beta particles in tissue (3–4 mm). Furthermore, they emphasized that by using beta-emitting radioactive stents, they essentially eliminated the risk to catheterization laboratory personnel and have minimized the exposure of surrounding cardiac and pulmonary tissues to ionizing radiation. In their studies they used a 32-P impregnated Strecker stent with a very low level of radioactivity (0.14 µCi) in a porcine iliac model. At 28 days they reported a 37% reduction in neointimal area and a 32% reduction in percent area stenosis for beta-particle-emitting stent compared with control stents.[34] Scanning electron microscopy revealed re-endothelialization of the radioactive stents at 4 weeks after implantation and no evidence of thrombosis. In another study,[36] 32-P Palmaz–Schatz stents with different activity levels of 23.0, 14.0, 6.0, 3.0, 1.0, 0.5 and 0.15 µCi were placed in porcine coronary arteries. At 28 days the neointima within the stent was examined. The investigators showed that in activities between 3.0 and 23.0 µCi the neointima and the medial density were inversely related to increases in stent activity. However, in the 1.0-µCi group the neointima was expanded and consisted of SMCs and matrix formation significantly higher compared with the nonradioactive stent. In addition, at 6 months' follow-up, 32-P stents with 0.5-µCi level of activity showed no benefit in terms of reduction of neointima over nonradioactive stents in porcine coronary arteries. Studies with a higher level of radioactive active stents at 6 months' follow-up are on their way. Indeed, several concerns have been voiced in regard to the implantation of radioactive stents. These include possible thrombosis on the stent wire due to delayed re-endothelialization of the stent struts, the area at the edges of the stent and beyond which is vulnerable to develop restenosis and will not be exposed to a sufficient dose of radiation, and the low dose rate of the radioactive stent which may not be enough in prevention of proliferation and migration of SMCs. However, fractionation of the treatment to 48 and 72 hours after the injury, when the proliferation markers and cytokines are at their peak, are supportive of this concept. It appears that radioactive implants, as for cancer therapy, will work for restenosis if a safe and efficacious dose is found and the above limitations are resolved. However, only long-term efficacy and absence of late effects on the normal vessel in humans will determine the future of the radioactive stents for this application.

By which mechanisms should radiation work?

The potential mechanisms by which radiation reduces restenosis were examined in a series of studies performed on pig coronary arteries by Waksman and Wilcox.[37] In these studies following overstretch injury, a flexible catheter with a pure beta emitter 90-Sr/Y was introduced to deliver 14 to 28 Gy (to a depth of 2 mm) into 14 of the injured sites. Animals were sacrificed at 3, 7 and 14 days after injury. 5-Bromo-2-deoxyuridine (BRDU) was administered 24 hours before sacrifice to label the proliferating cells. Immunohistochemistry was performed on frozen sections with monoclonal antibodies to BRDU and the number of BRDU positive cells relative to the total number of cells was determined using computer-based image analysis. Cell proliferation was significantly reduced after 3 days in the media and the adventitia of irradiated vessels compared to control arteries. However, there were no significant differences at the adventitia and the media by 7 days in the irradiated arteries compared to control. Alpha-actin staining for SMCs, which was used as an index for remodeling by 2 weeks after the injury, was lower in the adventitia of the irradiated vessels. A larger vessel perimeter was found in irradiated vessels: 11.3 mm (28 Gy) and 9.0 mm (14 Gy) than 8.3 mm (control) ($p < 0.0001$). Tunnel labeling detected apoptosis at 3 and 7 days in injured arteries and irradiated injured segments with no significant difference in the degree of apoptosis between these two groups. These studies suggest that endovascular radiation reduces restenosis-like response by inhibiting the first wave of cell proliferation in the adventitia and the media, and by a favorable effect on late remodeling.

What have we learnt from the feasibility clinical trials?

If the encouraging results from the brachytherapy studies in the animal models translate into success in the coming clinical trials, we will be able to conclude that intracoronary radiation works. The feasibility clinical trials which have been performed to date provide some information regarding the acute-term safety issues involving this technology, an indication of the efficacy and a clue as to how larger clinical trials should be designed in phase II and III.

The largest and longest study in endovascular therapy was performed by Schoppel et al.[38] in stented peripheral vessels of 29 patients who had developed restenosis after initially being treated by stenting to the superficial femoral artery (Table 14.4). The method of delivery was high-dose rate afterloader loaded with 192-Ir. The prescribed dose was 12 Gy to the vessel wall. More than 80% of patients maintained patency and no notable side-effects were attributed to irradiation after 6–71 months' follow-up time.

A feasibility study in 11 patients with recurrent narrowed AV-dialysis shunts was reported by Waksman et al.[39] This study utilized an HDR afterloader loaded with 192-Ir; the prescribed dose was 14 Gy to the vessel wall. At 44 weeks the patency rate of these grafts was only 36%.

The first human intracoronary radiation study to report long-term clinical and follow-up angiogram was performed by Condado et al.[40] who treated 21 patients for 22 lesions following angioplasty. The radiation source utilized in this study was 192-Ir manually delivered using either a 0.018- or 0.014-inch radioactive wire 3-cm in length, and a monorail 4.0F delivery noncentered delivery catheter system. Although the prescribed dose was 20–25 Gy, the actual dose was much higher (between 19 and 55 Gy). Angioplasty was successful (<50% residual stenosis) in 20 of 22 lesions. Insertion of the radioactive source wire was successful in all treated sites and free of major procedural complications. Angiographic study at 24 hours' postprocedure demonstrated the expected elastic recoil with reduction of luminal diameter from 1.92 ± 0.55 mm immediately after the procedure to 1.40 ± 0.27 mm at 24 hours. At 60 days, repeat angiography demonstrated total occlusion in two arteries and a pseudoaneurysm in one artery. Otherwise, all other arteries appeared normal and patent. At late follow-up ($\geqslant 6$ months) all remaining arteries (20) were patent with a mean luminal diameter of 1.65 ± 0.8 mm. The overall angiographic patency rate at late follow-up in this series was 90.9%. Analyzing the angiograms by quantitative computerized analysis suggested a detected late loss index of 0.19 while favorable remodeling was detected in 45% of the treated sites. Two years' angiographic follow-up of these patients did not detect late restenosis or any late adverse effects with nonsignificant changes in the lumen diameter of the angioplasty site.

A randomized double-blind trial for intracoronary radiation versus control in patients with intracoronary stenting and restenosis has been conducted by Tierstein et al.[41] In this study 55 patients were blindly randomized, 26 to radiation and 29 to control. Baseline characteristics were similar among the groups; 2/3 of the patients presented with in-stent restenosis. The source used was 192-Ir hand delivered and the doses varied from 7 to 30 Gy to the vessel wall. The procedure success rate was 96%. At 30 days one

Table 14.4 Results of endovascular radiation in clinical trials.

Author	Vessel	Radiation source	Result
Schoppel et al.[38]	Restenosed stented; superficial femoral arteries	192-ir HDR afterloader (12 Gy)	29 patients. Follow-up at 6–72 months: 80% patency of SFA
Waksman[39]	Restenosed AV-dialysis grafts postPTA	192-ir HDR afterloader (14 Gy)	11 patients; 18 treated lesions; patency rate at 44 weeks was 36%
Condado et al.[40]	Coronary arteries postballoon angioplasty	192-ir wire hand delivered actual doses of 19–55 Gy	At 6 months angiographic late loss index of 19; one pseudoaneurysm and two patients with total occlusion
Tierstein et al.[41]	In-stent restenosis and restenosis poststenting in coronary arteries	192-ir wire dose range 8–30 Gy to the vessel wall	Reduction of restenosis in treated arteries by angiography, ultrasound and TLR; free of major cardiac events
Urban et al.[42]	Coronary arteries postballoon angioplasty	90-Y wire 18 Gy centered balloon	At 6 months: angiographic restenosis rate 40% and TLR 27%
King et al.[43]	Coronary arteries postballoon angioplasty	90-Sr/Y seeds 12–16 Gy	6 months follow-up to be reported

patient from the radiation group had stent thrombosis, and there was no report on myocardial infarction, death or coronary artery bypass grafting. At 6 months, angiographic follow-up detected a late lumen loss of 1.03 mm in the control group compared to 0.38 mm in the treated radiation group; the late lumen loss index was 0.6 in placebo compared to 0.12 in the treated group.

Angiographic restenosis at 6 months at the stents at the borders of the stent was 53.6% in the control group versus 16.7% in the treated group and within itself the restenosis was 35.7 versus 8.3%, respectively. Tissue growth analyzed by intravascular ultrasound demonstrated 45 mm^2 in the control arteries versus 15 mm^2 in treated ones. Clinical follow-up at 12 months demonstrated target lesion revascularization of 44.8% in the control versus 11.5% in the treated group. Composite events free of death, myocardial infarction and target vessel revascularization were 85% in the treated group versus 52% in placebo group.

Two feasibility studies were performed utilizing pure beta emitters. The first performed and completed angiographic follow-up in 15 patients took place in Geneva, Switzerland.[42] In this study 90-yttrium source wire hand delivered was used through a segmented balloon centering catheter. The dose was 18 Gy to the balloon artery interface following balloon angioplasty. The radiation was delivered successfully to all patients with a mean exposure time

of 6.5 min. Fractionation of the dose was done in 4 patients due to ischemia, and 4/15 patients underwent stent implantation. All patients had clinical and angiographic 6 months' follow-up. At 6 months one patient experienced a fatal anterior myocardial infarction not related to the treatment artery; one patient required elective coronary artery bypass grafting for clinical restenosis and three patients underwent repeat percutaneous transluminal coronary angioplasty. Target lesion revascularization was reported in 4/15 patients (27%); one additional patient had another percutaneous transluminal coronary angioplasty to a nontarget lesion. The angiographic restenosis rate at 6 months was 40% with no aneurysms or any other angiographic adverse effects.

BERT[43] is the other feasibility trial utilizing pure beta emitter 90-Sr/Y. This study was approved by the FDA and was limited to 23 patients in two centers (Emory and Brown Universities). The study was designed to test the 90-Sr/Y system. The prescribed dose in this study was 12–16 Gy and the treatment time did not exceed 3.5 min. The actual radiation delivery was successful in 21 of 23 patients, with no major complications or adverse effects related to the treatment. Clinical and angiographic follow-up studies at 6 months indicated comparable initial results with 192-Ir. Restenosis rate (target lesion revascularization) at this cohort was 17%, with angiographic late loss of 10% and late loss index of 5%.

Conclusions

Intravascular radiation for prevention of restenosis is a new technology currently emerging from the working hypothesis supported by basic and animal experiments. The preclinical studies, although uncertain about external radiation, suggest that intracoronary radiation is working in animal models, both with gamma and beta isotopes. The initial feasibility studies suggest that, to some degree, this technology is working especially by using gamma radiation. Results from studies with beta radiation, either by using catheter-based systems or radioactive stents, will not be available before the end of 1998. Although the animal studies demonstrated that beta radiation is similar to gamma radiation in the pig model, it is not clear whether this will be the case in the human trials. Since the animal studies were performed in normal porcine coronaries, and in humans the radiation is delivered through an atherosclerotic and sometimes calcified coronary artery, it is likely that beta emitters will have difficulty in penetrating the atherosclerotic plaque and will require higher doses to be effective. Other issues remain open and require further investigation. The target tissue for treatment is not yet determined, nor are the late effects of radiation, the ideal isotope, dosimetry details, the minimum and the toxic doses of radiation which are feasible for this application. The challenge will be to find the ideal isotope, the right dose, and the most efficient and safe delivery system which will improve the effect of this modality for prevention of restenosis. Since other alternative therapies to reduce restenosis are launched every year, the value of intracoronary radiation will remain only if the restenosis rate drops to a single digit, either by radiation alone or combined with other pharmaceutical or mechanical modalities.

The importance of the current feasibility trials will be enhanced by providing long-term follow-up data on radiation effects. The preclinical and clinical studies described in this chapter are only the first step in a series of studies to come. They strongly support the pursuit of larger randomized trials which will enable a conclusion as to the efficacy of radiation for the prevention of restenosis.

References

1   Forrester JS, Fishbein M, Helfant R, Fagin J. A paradigm for restenosis based on cell biology; clues for the development of new preventive therapies. *J Am Coll Cardiol* 1991; **17**: 758–69.

2   Lee PC, Gibbons GH, Dzau VJ. Cellular and molecular mechanisms of coronary artery restenosis. *Coronary Artery Dis* 1993; **4**: 254–9.

3   Clows AW, Reidy MA, Clowes MM. Kinetics of cellular proliferation after arterial injury. I. Smooth muscle growth in the absence of endothelium. *Lab Invest* 1983; **49**: 327–33.

4   Schwartz RS, Holmes DR, Topol EJ. The restenosis paradigm revisited: an alternative proposal for cellular mechanisms. *J Am Coll Cardiol* 1992; **20**: 1284–93.

5   Post MJ, Borst C, Kuntz RE. The relative importance of arterial remodeling with intimal hyperplasia in lumen renarrowing after balloon angioplasty. A study in the normal rabbit and the hypercholesterolemic Yucatan micropig. *Circulation* 1994; **89**: 2816–21.

6   Mintz GS, Kovach JA, Javier SP, Ditrano CJ, Leon MB. Geometric remodeling is the predominant mechanism of late lumen loss after coronary angioplasty. *Circulation* 1993; **88 (Suppl I)**: I-654 (abstract).

7   Karas SP, Gravanis MB, Santoian EC, Robinson KA, Anderberg K, King SB III. Coronary intimal proliferation after balloon injury and stenting in swine: an animal model of restenosis. *J Am Coll Cardiol* 1992; **20**: 467–74.

8   Gravanis MB, Robinson KA, Santoian EC, Schneider JE, King SB. The reparative phenomena at the site of balloon angioplasty in humans and experimental models. *Cardiovasc Pathol* 1993; **2**: 263–73.

9   Freidman M, Byers SO. Effects of iridium 192 radiation on thromboatherosclerotic plaque in the rabbit aorta. *Arch Path* 1965; **80**: 281–91.

10   Hirai T, Korogi Y, Harada M, Takahashi M. Intimal hyperplasia in an atherosclerotic model: prevention with radiation therapy. *Radiology* 1994; 872–4.

11   Abbas MA, Afshari NA, Stadius ML, Kernoff RS, Fischell TA. Effect of x-ray irradiation on neointimal proliferation following balloon angioplasty. *Clinical Research* 1993; **41**: 79–80.

12   Dawson JT. Theoretical considerations regarding low-dose radiation therapy for prevention of restenosis after angioplasty. *Texas Heart Institute Journal* 199; **18**: 4–7.

13   Schwartz RS, Koval TM, Edwards WD, et al. Effect of external beam irradiation on neointimal hyperplasia after experimental coronary artery injury. *J Am Coll of Cardiol* 1992; **19**: 1106–13.

14   Hehrlein C, Kiaser S, Kollum M, Kinscherf R, Metz J, Fritz P. External beam radiation fails to inhibit neointima formation in stented rabbit arteries. *Circulation* 1996; **94**: I-210 (abstract).

15   Gellman J, Healey G, Qingsheng and Tselentakis. The effect of very low dose irradiation on restenosis following balloon angioplasty. A study in the atherosclerotic rabbit. *Circulation* 1991; **118**: 331A, I-319 (abstract).

16   Shimatokahara S, Mayberg MR. Gamma irradiation inhibits neointimal hyperplasia in rats after arterial injury. *Stroke* 1994; **25**: 424–8.

17   Shefer A, Eigler NL, Whiting JS, Litvack Fl. Suppression of intimal proliferation after balloon angioplasty with local beta irradiation in rabbits. *J Am Coll of Cardiol* 1993; **21**: 185.

18   Waksman R, Robinson KA, Crocker IR, Gravanis MB, Cipolla GD, King SB III. Endovascular low dose irradiation inhibits neointima formation after coronary artery balloon injury in swine: a possible role for radiation therapy in restenosis prevention. *Circulation* 1995; **91**: 1553–9.

19   Wiedermann JG, Marboe C, Schwartz A, Amols H, Weinberger J. Intracoronary irradiation reduces restenosis after balloon angioplasty in a porcine model. *J Am Coll Cardiol* 1994; **23**: 1491–8.

20   Wiedermann JG, Marboe C, Amols H, Schwartz A, Weinberger J. Intracoronary irradiation markedly reduces neointimal proliferation after balloon angioplasty in the swine: persistent benefit at 6-month follow-up. *J Am Coll Cardiol* 1995; **25**: 1451–6.

21   Mazur W, Ali MN, Dabaghi SF, *et al.* High dose rate intracoronary radiation suppresses neointimal proliferation in the stented and ballooned model of porcine restenosis. *Int J Radiat Oncol Biol Phys* 1996; **36**: 777–88.

22   Wiedermann JG, Marboe C, Ennis RD, Amols H, Schwartz A, Weinberger J. Intracoronary irradiation: dose response for the prevention of restenosis in swine. *Int J Radiat Oncol Biol Phys* 1996; **36**: 767–76.

23   Waksman R, Robinson KA, Crocker IR, *et al.* Intracoronary radiation decreases new additional intimal hyperplasia in a repeat balloon angioplasty swine model of restenosis. *Circulation* 1996; **94**: 8, I-147:1217 (abstract).

24   Verin V, Popowski Y, Urban P, *et al.* Intra-arterial beta irradiation prevents neointimal hyperplasia in a hypercholesterolemic rabbit restenosis model. *Circulation* 1995; **92**: 2284–90.

25   Popowski Y, Verin V, Papirov I, *et al.* High dose rate brachytherapy for prevention of restenosis after percutaneous angioplasty: preliminary dosimetric tests of a new source presentation. *Int J Radiat Oncol Biol Phys* 1995; **33**: 211–15.

26   Waksman R, Robinson K, Crocker I, *et al.* Intracoronary low dose β-irradiation inhibits neointima formation after coronary artery balloon injury in the swine restenosis model. *Circulation* 1995; **92**: 3025–31.

27   Waksman R, Robinson KA, Crocker IA, *et al.* Efficacy and safety of β versus γ radioisotopes for endovascular irradiation in prevention of intimal hyperplasia after balloon

angioplasty in swine coronaries. *Circulation* 1995; **92**: 8, I-146:0691 (abstract).

28   Waksman R, Robinson K, Crocker I, *et al.* Intracoronary radiation prior to stent implantation inhibits neointima formation in stented porcine coronary arteries. *Circulation* 1995; **92**: 1383–6.

29   Waksman R, Robinson KA, Crocker IA, Gravanis MB, Palmer SJ, Cipolla GD. Intracoronary beta radiation before versus after stent implantation for inhibition of neointima formation in the porcine model. *Circulation* 1996; **94**: 8, I-147:3626 (abstract).

30   Raisner A. Endovascular radiation the Baylor experience. Highlights in intracoronary radiation therapy. Thoraxcenter Rotterdam 10–11 December 1996.

31   Weiderman JG, Marobe C, Amols H, Schwartz A, Weinberger J. Intracoronary irradiation fails to reduce neointimal proliferation after oversized stenting in a porcine model. *Circulation* 1995; **92**: I-146 (abstract).

32   Fischell TA, Kharma BK, Fischell DR, *et al.* Low-dose, b-particle emission from 'stent' wire results in complete, localized inhibition of smooth muscle cell proliferation. *Circulation* 1994; **90**: 2956–63.

33   Hehrlein C, Gollan C, Donges K, *et al.* Low-dose radioactive endovascular stents prevent smooth muscle cell proliferation and neointimal hyperplasia in rabbits. *Circulation* 1995; **92**: 1570–5.

34   Hehrlein C, Stintz M, Kincherf R, *et al.* Pure β-emitting stents inhibit neointima formation in rabbit. *Circulation* 1996; **93**: 641–5.

35   Laird J, Carter A, Kufs W, *et al.* Inhibition of neointimal proliferation with a beta particle emitting stent. *Circulation* 1996; **93**: 529–36.

36   Carter JC, Laird RJ, Bailey LR, *et al.* Effects of endovascular radiation from a β particle-emitting stent in a porcine coronary restenosis model a dose-response study. *Circulation* 1996; **94**: 2364–8.

37   Waksman R, Robinson KA, Scott NA, *et al.* Intracoronary radiation affects restenosis in the swine model by reduction of cell proliferation and favorable remodeling. *Circulation* 1996; **94**: 8, I-147:0623

38   Schoppel D, Liermann LJ, Pohlit R, *et al.* 192-ir endovascular brachytherapy for avoidance of intimal hyperplasia after percutaneous angioplasty and stent implantation in peripheral vessels: years of experience. *Int J Radiat Oncol Biol Phys* 1996; **36**: 835–40.

39   Waksman R, Crocker IA, Kikeri D, Lumsden AB, MacDonald JM, Martin, LG. Long term results of endovascular radiation therapy for prevention of restenosis in the peripheral vascular system. *Circulation* 1996; **94**: 8, I-300:1745 (abstract).

40   Condado JA, Gurdiel O, Espinoza R, *et al.* Long-term angiographic and clinical outcome after percutaneous transluminal coronary angioplasty and intracoronary radiation therapy in humans. *Circulation* 1996; **94**: 8, I-209:1218 (abstract).

41   Teirstein PS, Massullo V, Jani S, *et al.* Radiation therapy following stenting—6 months follow-up of a randomized clinical trial. *Circulation* 1996; **94**: I-210:1222 (abstract).

42   Urban P, Verin V, Popowski Y, *et al.* Clinical feasibility and safety of intraluminal beta irradiation to prevent restenosis after balloon angioplasty. *Circulation* 1996; **94**: 8, I-221:1220 (abstract).

43   King SB, Crocker IA, Hillstead RA, Waksman R. Coronary endovascular beta radiation for restenosis using a novel catheter system: initial clinical feasibility study. *Circulation* 1996; **94**: 8,I-619:3625 (abstract).

15

Time course of geometrical remodeling after angioplasty

Masakiyo Nobuyoshi

Introduction

Coronary angioplasty has gained widespread acceptance as an effective revascularization procedure for selected patients with coronary artery disease. However, restenosis occurring in 30–50% of patients remains a major limitation of this procedure.[1,2] Studies in animals[3–5] and necropsy studies in humans[6–8] suggested that neointimal hyperplasia ensues in responses to injury by angioplasty devices, resulting in restenosis when these hyperplastic responses become excessive. However, pharmacologic strategies that had proven efficacy in preventing intimal hyperplasia in animal models have been strikingly ineffective in human clinical trials.[9] One possible explanation for the failure of the antiproliferative agents is that intimal hyperplasia is not the sole mechanism of restenosis after coronary angioplasty. Recent animal studies suggested that arterial remodeling, as measured in changes in total vessel area, might be a major contributing factor to the development of restenosis.[10–12] However, restenotic processes in most animal models occur in the absence of underlying complex atherosclerotic plaque and the conclusions derived from these animal models are not directly applicable to the process occurring in human diseased coronary arteries. Intravascular ultrasound (IVUS) allows direct area measurement of both vessel and lumen in human coronary arteries. Kovach et al.[13] first demonstrated constriction of the vessel at follow-up by serial IVUS examination of human coronary arteries undergoing angioplasty. This chapter reviews previously published reports as well as the author's own observations regarding arterial remodeling after coronary angioplasty.

Review of previously published results

Previously published results of serial IVUS studies after various coronary interventional procedures are listed in Table 15.1. Mintz et al.'s[14] report is the largest series, utilizing a motorized transducer pullback device. They demonstrated that at follow-up, 73% of the decrease in lumen area (from 6.6 ± 2.5 to 4.0 ± 3.7 mm^2, $p < 0.0001$) was due to a decrease in vessel area (from 20.1 ± 6.4 to 18.2 ± 6.4 mm^2, $p < 0.0001$); 27% was due to an increase in plaque plus media area (from 13.5 ± 5.5 to 14.2 ± 5.4 mm^2, $p < 0.0001$). Di Mario et al. demonstrated that constrictive remodeling was the main operative mechanism of late lumen loss after balloon angioplasty but not after directional coronary atherectomy.[15] In an analysis of 36 restenotic lesions (primarily after directional atherectomy), Braden et al. concluded that the predominant mechanism of late lumen loss was an increase in plaque area rather than constrictive remodeling.[16] The author's 6 months' follow-up data from the Serial Ultrasound Restenosis (SURE)[17] study (detailed later) as well as the report by Sumitsuji et al.[18] revealed a more balanced contribution of constrictive remodeling and an increase in plaque plus media area on late lumen loss.

We could not explain the reason why results from serial IVUS studies are not consistent regarding the role of constrictive remodeling on late lumen loss. However, Mintz et al.[15] also reported that remodeling was bidirectional; 22% of lesions showed an increase in vessel area at follow-up. In their report, despite a greater increase in plaque plus media

Table 15.1 Results of serial IVUS studies after coronary angioplasty.

Author	No. of lesions	Type of intervention	Restenosis rate (%)	Δ postprocedure ~follow-up		
				Vessel area	Plaque plus media area	Lumen area
Mintz et al.[15]	212	Balloon angioplasty (29) Directional atherectomy (114) Rotational atherectomy (45) Excimer laser angioplasty (24)	47	-1.9 ± 3.6 mm^2 (73%)**	0.7 ± 2.3 mm^2	-2.6 ± 3.3 mm^2
Kimura et al.[17]	61	Balloon angioplasty (35) Directional atherectomy (26)	31	-0.99 ± 2.58 mm^2 (51%)**	0.94 ± 1.91 mm^2	-1.93 ± 2.49 mm^2
Di Mario et al.[15]	34	Balloon angioplasty (18)	39*	-1.44 ± 1.66 mm^2 (68%)**	0.68 ± 2.95 mm^2	-2.12 ± 1.81 mm^2
		Directional atherectomy (16)	25*	-0.18 ± 2.02 mm^2 (8%)**	2.11 ± 1.83 mm^2	-2.29 ± 2.46 mm^2

Author	No. of lesions	Type of intervention	Restenosis rate (%)	Vessel area		Plaque plus media area	
				Postprocedure	Follow-up	Postprocedure	Follow-up
Breden et al.[16]	36	Balloon angioplasty (7) Directional atherectomy (26) Rotational atherectomy (3)	100	18.7 ± 6.3 mm^2 (39%)**	18.6 ± 6.9 mm^2	13.0 ± 6.00 mm^2	16.5 ± 6.8 mm^2
Sumitsuji et al.[18]	95	Directional atherectomy	21	19.0 ± 1.1 mm^2*** (39%)	16.3 ± 1.3 mm^2***	9.4 ± 0.9 mm^2***	13.7 ± 1.3 mm^2***

Notes:
* = clinical restenosis rate; ** = percentage of Δ vessel area relative to Δ lumen area; *** = data from 20 lesions with angiographic restenosis.

area (1.5 ± 2.5 vs. 0.5 ± 2.0 mm², $p = 0.0009$), lesions exhibiting an increase in vessel area had 1) no change in lumen area (−0.1 ± 3.3 vs. −3.6 ± 2.3 mm², $p < 0.0001$); 2) a reduced restenosis rate (26% vs. 62%, $p < 0.0001$); and 3) a 49% frequency of late lumen gain (vs. 1%, $p < 0.0001$) compared with lesions without an increase in vessel area. Considering the bidirectional nature of arterial remodeling, small sample size might be potentially misleading. Also, we do not know any consistent clinical, lesion-related or procedure-related predictors of the direction or magnitude of the change in vessel area. Therefore it is possible that differences in patient population and in procedural variables might affect the relative contribution of remodeling and tissue growth on late lumen loss. Finally, since current IVUS has some inherent limitations, well controlled methodology is critically important to draw valid conclusions.

In summary, from the available data constrictive remodeling has played a predominant role in late lumen loss, at least in some proportions of lesions undergoing balloon angioplasty or atherectomy. Adaptive remodeling (an increase in total vessel area at follow-up) also occurs in some lesions, compensating for tissue growth and contributing to occasional late lumen gain.

Results from the Serial Ultrasound Restenosis (SURE) study

The SURE study is a co-operative study in Washington Hospital Center, USA, and Kokura Memorial Hospital, Japan.[17] To understand remodeling better, serial IVUS and quantitative angiographic examination was performed pre- and postintervention, at 24 hours, 1 month and 6 months in 61 lesions undergoing balloon coronary angioplasty or directional atherectomy. Methodologic issues were detailed elsewhere.[17] In short, focal lesions without significant fluoroscopic calcification were prospectively enrolled in a follow-up study. Meticulous care was taken to control quantitative coronary angiography, thereby validating serial changes in lumen area assessed by IVUS. Identification of the same anatomic cross-section was performed by utilizing a motorized transducer pullback device, and independent cross-sectional measurement, performed at two centers, revealed excellent agreement.

Quantitative angiographic and IVUS results are shown in Table 15.2 and graphically in Fig. 15.1. At 24 hours, both vessel area (from 17.32 ± 5.35 to 17.89 ± 5.38 mm²;

Table 15.2 Quantitative angiographic and IVUS results from the Serial Ultrasound Restenosis (SURE) study.

	Before procedure	After procedure	24 hours	1 month	6 months
Angiographic					
Minimal luminal diameter (mm)	1.02 ± 0.27	2.16 ± 0.43	2.15 ± 0.47	2.29 ± 0.48	1.65 ± 0.56
Reference diameter (mm)	2.98 ± 0.53	3.07 ± 0.5	3.1 ± 0.54	3.23 ± 0.48	3.01 ± 0.55
Percent stenosis	64.9 ± 9.3	26.5 ± 9.8	26.9 ± 11.3	21.9 ± 11.8	45.1 ± 16.2
Intravascular ultrasound					
Lumen area (mm²)	2.08 ± 0.7	6.81 ± 2.24	6.93 ± 2.53	8.22 ± 2.79	4.88 ± 2.86
Vessel area (mm²)	15.45 ± 5.24	17.32 ± 5.35	17.89 ± 5.38	19.39 ± 5.33	16.33 ± 5.54
Plaque plus media area (mm²)	13.37 ± 5.04	10.51 ± 4.38	10.96 ± 4.49	11.17 ± 4.11	11.45 ± 4.45

Note:
$p < 0.05$ for the comparison between the points linked by brackets.

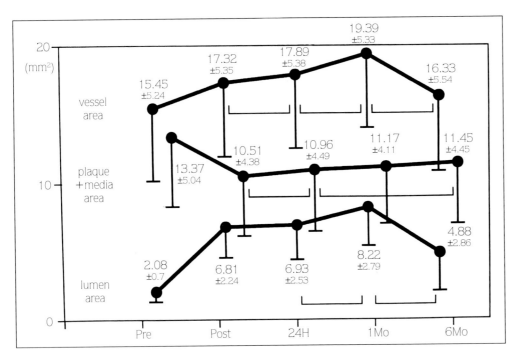

Figure 15.1
Serial changes in vessel, lumen and plaque plus media area. Serial changes in the lumen area closely paralleled those in the vessel area. Significant enlargement of the vessel was observed within 24 hours and between 24 hours and 1 month. Marked constriction of the vessel was seen between 1 and 6 months. Plaque plus media area increased significantly within 24 hours and between 24 hours and 6 months ($p < 0.05$ for the comparison between the points linked by brackets.)

$p = 0.002$) and plaque plus media area (from 10.51 ± 4.38 to 10.96 ± 4.49 mm²; $p = 0.0008$) increased significantly with no change in lumen area (from 6.81 ± 2.24 to 6.93 ± 2.53 mm²; $p = 0.37$). Between 24 hours and 1 month, vessel area increased significantly (from 17.89 ± 5.38 to 19.39 ± 5.33 mm²; $p = 0.0001$), resulting in significant improvement of lumen area (from 6.93 ± 2.53 to 8.22 ± 2.79 mm²; $p = 0.0001$). Between 1 and 6 months, vessel area decreased significantly (from 19.39 ± 5.33 to 16.33 ± 5.54 mm²; $p = 0.0001$). Constriction of the vessel resulted in marked lumen loss in this interval (from 8.22 ± 2.79 to 4.88 ± 2.86 mm²; $p = 0.0001$). Plaque plus media area increased significantly from 24 hours to 6 months (from 10.96 ± 4.49 mm² to 11.45 ± 4.45 mm²; $p = 0.03$). Early enlargement and late constriction of the vessel were similarly seen both after balloon angioplasty and directional atherectomy. Representative cases are shown in Figs 15.2 and 15.3.

In this study, remodeling after coronary angioplasty or atherectomy was characterized by early (within 24 hours, and 24 hours–1 month) enlargement of the vessel and late (1–6 months) constriction of the vessel. In addition, significant increase in the plaque plus media area was observed both within 24 hours and from 24 hours to 6 months.

Early increase in the plaque plus media area could be explained by thrombosis.[19] Alternatively, if one of the mechanisms of balloon angioplasty is axial redistribution of plaque,[20] partial reversal of this phenomenon might explain early increase in the plaque plus media area observed in a single-slice analysis. On the other hand, early enlargement of the vessel observed at 24 hours could be partly explained by release of vasospasm.

Further enlargement of the vessel at 1 month could be explained by the increase in the wall shear stress resulting from the augmented local flow after angioplasty.[21–23] Release of the cicatrizing effects of the noncompliant plaque by angioplasty might increase coronary distensibility, allowing the vessel to distend in response to arterial pressure.[24] This adaptive remodeling could also result from the response to early growth of neointimal tissue, analogous to the original observation by Glagov et al.[25] Adaptive

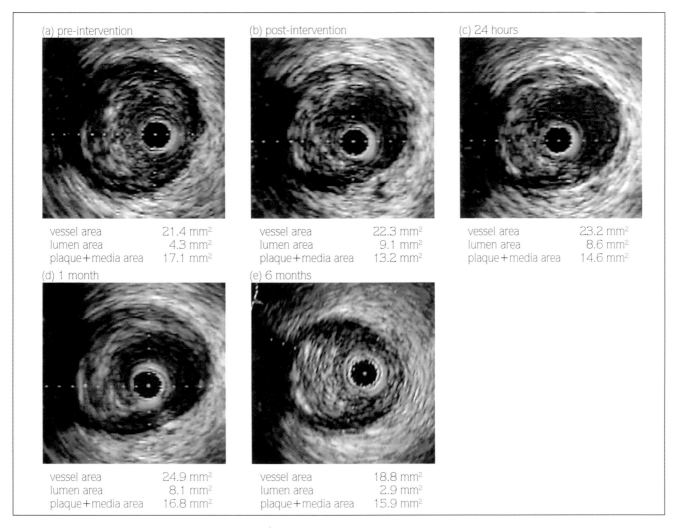

(a) pre-intervention

vessel area	21.4 mm²
lumen area	4.3 mm²
plaque+media area	17.1 mm²

(b) post-intervention

vessel area	22.3 mm²
lumen area	9.1 mm²
plaque+media area	13.2 mm²

(c) 24 hours

vessel area	23.2 mm²
lumen area	8.6 mm²
plaque+media area	14.6 mm²

(d) 1 month

vessel area	24.9 mm²
lumen area	8.1 mm²
plaque+media area	16.8 mm²

(e) 6 months

vessel area	18.8 mm²
lumen area	2.9 mm²
plaque+media area	15.9 mm²

Figure 15.2

IVUS images showing typical biphasic remodeling after directional coronary atherectomy. A proximal left anterior descending coronary artery lesion was treated by directional coronary atherectomy. Acute lumen gain was mostly related to reduction in the plaque plus media area. At 1 month, lumen area was preserved due to compensatory enlargement of the vessel, despite increase in the plaque plus media area. Between 1 and 6 months, marked lumen loss was predominantly due to constriction of the vessel from 24.9 mm² to 18.8 mm². Plaque plus media area decreased in this interval from 16.8 mm² to 15.9 mm².

remodeling explains why most patients are so stable up to 1 or 2 months after coronary angioplasty, even in the presence of extensive dissection and/or an overtly suboptimal result.

Significant increase in the plaque plus media area from 24 hours to 6 months, which would be an ultrasonographic index of intimal proliferation, substantiates the importance of intimal hyperplasia as a mechanism of restenosis. However, this study demonstrated that late constriction of the vessel is an additional important mechanism of restenosis.

Between 1 and 6 months when luminal renarrowing was most prevalent, constriction of the vessel contributed to lumen loss much more than the increase in plaque plus media area. In contrast to the serial ultrasound studies comparing postprocedure result with that at 6 months follow-up, remodeling between 1 and 6 months was demonstrated to be more consistent in direction (constrictive) and more marked in magnitude.

Several mechanisms could be proposed to explain

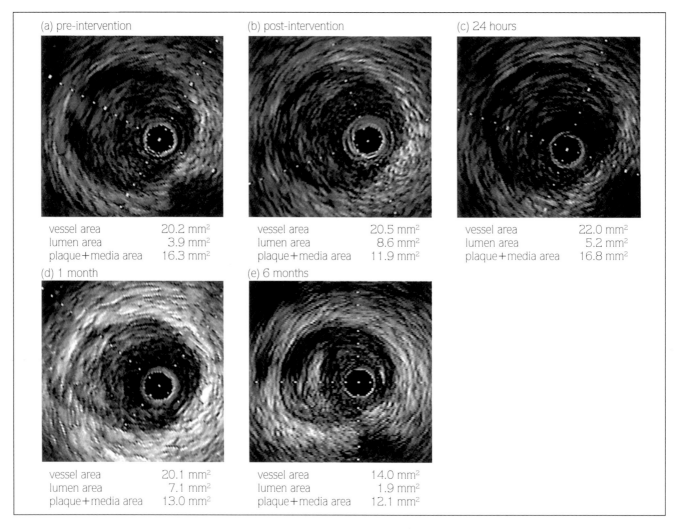

Figure 15.3

IVUS images showing marked late constrictive remodeling after balloon coronary angioplasty. A proximal left anterior descending coronary artery lesion was treated by balloon angioplasty. Acute lumen gain was predominantly related to reduction in the plaque plus media area. At 24 hours, increase in the plaque plus media area resulted in decrease in lumen area despite some increase in vessel area. In this lesion, adaptive enlargement of the vessel was not observed at 1 month and marked constriction of the vessel resulted in restenosis at 6 months. Between 1 and 6 months, plaque plus media area decreased from 13.0 mm^2 to 12.1 mm^2.

constriction of the vessel. This study clearly demonstrated that constriction of the vessel is a late event and therefore is distinct from early passive elastic recoil. Adventitial fibrosis could play an important role in constricting the vessel.[26] However, we do not believe that adventitial fibrosis can be evaluated with current IVUS technology. In this and other studies[14] using serial IVUS, extreme decrease in the vessel area was often associated with a decrease in the plaque

plus media (Fig. 15.4), suggesting the presence of plaque retraction and/or apoptosis.[27]

Comparing the postprocedure result and that at 6 months follow-up in the study, lumen area decreased from 6.81 ± 2.24 mm^2 postintervention to 4.88 ± 2.86 mm^2 at 6 months. Decrease in the vessel area $(-0.99 \pm 2.58$ mm$^2)$ and increase in the plaque plus media area $(0.94 \pm 1.91$ mm$^2)$ almost equally contributed to late

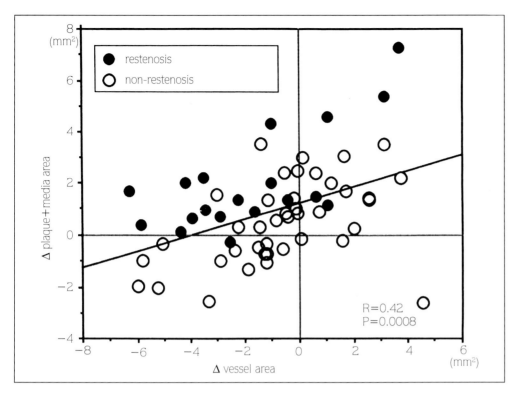

Figure 15.4

Scatterplots illustrating correlation between changes in vessel area and changes in plaque plus media area from postintervention to 6 months' follow-up. Significant positive correlation was seen between changes in the vessel area and changes in the plaque plus media area. Restenotic lesions, as compared with nonrestenotic lesions, tended to have more increase in the plaque plus media area with given changes in the vessel area. With enlargement of the vessel, moderate increase in the plaque plus media area could be tolerated, and with shrinkage of the vessel, small increase in the plaque plus media area resulted in restenosis.

lumen loss. We could not disregard the importance of intimal hyperplasia as evidenced in many human necropsy studies.[6–8] However, the changes in the vessel area and plaque plus media area were not independent but were significantly correlated ($R = 0.42$; $p = 0.0008$) (Fig. 15.4). With increase in the plaque plus media, the vessel area tended to enlarge. Restenotic lesions, as compared with nonrestenotic lesions, tended to have more increase in the plaque plus media area with given changes in the vessel area. With enlargement of the vessel, moderate increase in the plaque plus media area could be tolerated, and with shrinkage of the vessel a small increase in the plaque plus media area resulted in restenosis. Therefore, relative contributions of remodeling and increase in the plaque plus media area varied widely among individual lesions, partially

explaining the apparent inconsistency of several IVUS studies. A case of balloon angioplasty is shown in Fig. 15.5, in which restenosis resulted from marked increase in the plaque plus media area despite enlargement of the vessel.

The study demonstrated that mechanisms of late lumen loss after coronary angioplasty were heterogeneous with a variable contribution of each mechanism depending on the time after the procedure. Intracoronary stents could reduce the rate of restenosis[28,29] by eliminating early increase in the plaque plus media area and late constriction of the vessel as well as obtaining a larger lumen immediately after the procedure. However, this is at the expense of early compensatory enlargement and more prominent intimal hyperplasia.

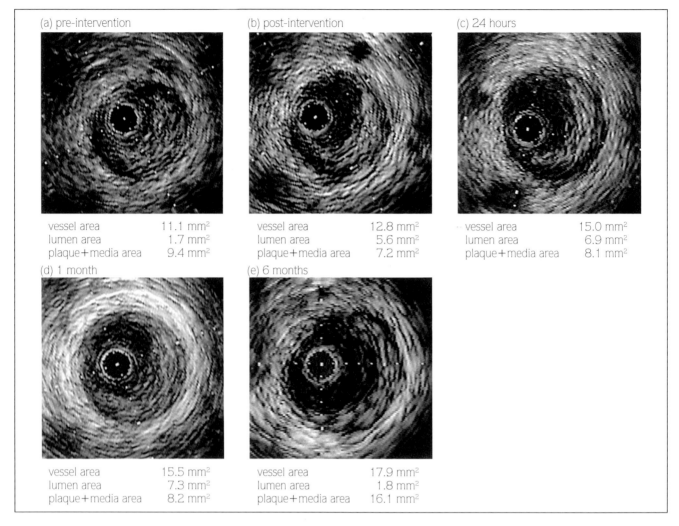

(a) pre-intervention

vessel area	11.1 mm²
lumen area	1.7 mm²
plaque+media area	9.4 mm²

(b) post-intervention

vessel area	12.8 mm²
lumen area	5.6 mm²
plaque+media area	7.2 mm²

(c) 24 hours

vessel area	15.0 mm²
lumen area	6.9 mm²
plaque+media area	8.1 mm²

(d) 1 month

vessel area	15.5 mm²
lumen area	7.3 mm²
plaque+media area	8.2 mm²

(e) 6 months

vessel area	17.9 mm²
lumen area	1.8 mm²
plaque+media area	16.1 mm²

Figure 15.5

IVUS images showing marked increase in the plaque plus media area after balloon coronary angioplasty. A proximal left interior descending coronary artery lesion was treated by balloon angioplasty. Acute lumen gain was related to a combination of vessel expansion and reduction in plaque plus media area. Restenosis at 6 months resulted from marked increase in the plaque plus media area despite increase in the vessel area. Newly proliferated tissue around the ultrasound catheter was characteristically hypoechoic.

Conclusions

Coronary arteries undergo dramatic remodeling responses within 6 months after coronary intervention. The time course of remodeling after coronary angioplasty was typically biphasic, that is early adaptive and late constrictive remodeling. The biphasic remodeling seemed not to be device specific, although current studies are unable to discriminate differences in the magnitude of remodeling between balloon angioplasty and directional atherectomy.

The bidirectional nature of remodeling demonstrated by Mintz et al.[15] could be explained by the difference in the magnitude of early adaptive and late constrictive remodeling. Remodeling after coronary angioplasty should be regarded not only as a cause of restenosis but also as a mechanism maintaining patency. Therefore, future strategies to reduce restenosis should target prevention of constrictive remodeling and enhancement of adaptive remodeling as well as suppression of intimal hyperplasia.

References

1　Holmes DR, Vlietstra RE, Smith H, *et al.* Restenosis after percutaneous transluminal coronary angioplasty (PTCA): a report from the PTCA registry of the NHLBI. *Am J Cardiol* 1984; **53**: 77C–81C.

2　Detre K, Holubkov R, Kelsey S, *et al.* Percutaneous transluminal coronary angioplasty in 1985–1986 and 1977–1984. The National Heart, Lung and Blood Institute Registry. *N Engl J Med* 1988; **318**: 265–70.

3　Califf RM, Fortin DF, Frid DJ, *et al.* Restenosis after coronary angioplasty: an overview. *J Am Coll Cardiol* 1991; **17**: 2B–13B.

4　Nobuyoshi M, Kimura T, Nosaka H, *et al.* Restenosis after successful percutaneous transluminal coronary angioplasty: serial angiographic follow-up of 229 patients. *J Am Coll Cardiol* 1988; **12**: 616–23.

5　Serruys PW, Luijten HE, Beatt KJ, *et al.* Incidence of restenosis after successful coronary angioplasty: a time-related phenomenon. *Circulation* 1988; **77**: 361–71.

6　Steele PM, Chesebro JH, Stanson AW, Holmes DR, Dewanjee MK, Badimon L. Balloon angioplasty: natural history of the pathophysiological response to injury in a pig model. *Circ Res* 1985; **57**: 105–12.

7　Schwartz RS, Huber KC, Murphy JG, *et al.* Restenosis and the proportional neointimal response to coronary artery injury: results in a porcine model. *J Am Coll Cardiol* 1992; **19**: 267–74.

8　Muller DWM, Ellis SG, Topol EJ. Experimental models of coronary artery restenosis. *J Am Coll Cardiol* 1992; **19**: 418–32.

9　Franklin SM, Faxon DP. Pharmacologic prevention of restenosis after coronary angioplasty: review of the randomized clinical trials. *Coron Art Dis* 1993; **4**: 232–42.

10　Austin GE, Ratliff NB, Hollman J, Tabei S, Phillips DF. Intimal proliferation of smooth muscle cells as an explanation for recurrent coronary artery stenosis after percutaneous transluminal coronary angioplasty. *J Am Coll Cardiol* 1985; **6**: 369–75.

11　Nobuyoshi M, Kimura T, Ohishi H, *et al.* Restenosis after percutaneous transluminal coronary angioplasty: pathologic observations in 20 patients. *J Am Coll Cardiol* 1991; **17**: 433–9.

12　Post MJ, Borst C, Kuntz RE. The relative importance of arterial remodeling compared with intimal hyperplasia in lumen renarrowing after balloon angioplasty: a study in the normal rabbit and the hypercholesterolemic Yucatan micropig. *Circulation* 1994; **89**: 2816–21.

13　Kovach JA, Mintz GS, Kent KM, *et al.* Serial intravascular ultrasound studies indicate that chronic recoil is an important mechanism of restenosis following transcatheter therapy. *J Am Coll Cardiol* 1993; **21**: 484A (abstract).

14　Lafont A, Guzman LA, Whitlow PL, Goormastic M, Cornhill JF, Chisolm GM. Restenosis after experimental angioplasty: intimal, medial, and adventitial changes associated with constrictive remodeling. *Circ Res* 1995; **76**: 996–1002.

15　Mintz GS, Popma JJ, Pichard AD, *et al.* Arterial remodeling after coronary angioplasty: a serial intravascular ultrasound study. *Circulation* 1996; **94**: 35–43.

16　Currier JW, Faxon DP. Restenosis after percutaneous transluminal coronary angioplasty: have we been aiming at the wrong target? *J Am Coll Cardiol* 1995; **25**: 516–20.

17　Kimura T, Kaburagi S, Tamura T, *et al.* Remodeling of human coronary arteries undergoing coronary angioplasty or atherectomy. *Circulation*, in press.

18　Sumitsuji S, Katoh O, Tsuchikane E, Nakagawa Y, Funamoto M, Kobayashi T. Chronic vessel remodeling as a cause of restenosis after directional coronary atherectomy. *J Am Coll Cardiol* 1996; **27 (Suppl A)**: 156A (abstract).

19　Schwartz RS, Holmes DR jr, Topol EJ. The restenosis paradigm revisited: an alternative proposal for cellular mechanisms. *J Am Coll Cardiol* 1992; **20**: 1284–93.

20　Kimura T, Yokoi H, Nakagawa Y, *et al.* Three-year follow-up after implantation of metallic coronary-artery stents. *N Engl J Med* 1996; **334**: 561–6.

21　Nishimura RA, Edwards WD, Warnes CA, *et al.* Intravascular ultrasound imaging: *in vitro* validation and pathologic correlation. *J Am Coll Cardiol* 1990; **16**: 145–54.

22　Fuessl RT, Mintz GS, Pichard AD, *et al.* In vivo validation of intravascular ultrasound length measurements using a motorized transducer pullback system. *Am J Cardiol* 1996; **77**: 1115–18.

23　Matthews DE, Farewell VT. *Using and Understanding Medical Statistics* (2nd edn) (Basel: Karger, 1988).

24　Glagov S, Weisenberg E, Zarins CK, Stankunavicius R, Kolettis GJ. Compensatory enlargement of human atherosclerotic coronary arteries. *N Engl J Med* 1987; **316**: 1371–5.

25　Gertz SD, Gimple LW, Banai S, *et al.* Geometric remodeling is not the principal pathogenetic process in restenosis after balloon angioplasty. *Circulation* 1994; **90**: 3001–8.

26　Di Mario C, Gil R, Camenzind E, *et al.* Quantitative assessment with intracoronary ultrasound of the mechanisms of restenosis after percutaneous transluminal coronary angioplasty and directional coronary atherectomy. *Am J Cardiol* 1995; **75**: 772–7.

27   Braden GA, Young TM, Utley L, Kutcher MA, Appelegate J, Herrington DM. Fibro-intimal hyperplasia is the predominant mechanism of late lumen loss in symptomatic patients with coronary restenosis. *Circulation* 1995; **92**: 1-148 (abstract).

28   Fischman DL, Leon MB, Baim BS, *et al.* A randomized comparison of coronary-stent placement and balloon angioplasty in the treatment of coronary artery disease. *N Engl J Med* 1994; **331**: 496–501.

29   Serruys PW, de Jaegere P, Kiemeneij F, *et al.* A comparison of balloon expandable-stent placement and balloon angioplasty in patients with coronary artery disease. *N Engl J Med* 1994; **331**: 489–95.

16

Arterial remodeling as a mechanism of restenosis following interventional coronary procedures: evidence from serial intravascular ultrasound studies

Gary S Mintz, Kenneth M Kent, Jeffrey J Popma, Augusto D Pichard, Lowell F Satler and Martin B Leon

Background

Restenosis occurs within the first 6 months after 30–50% of transcatheter procedures; it remains the major limitation to percutaneous coronary revascularization.[1,2] The conventional view of restenosis is as follows. Catheter-induced vascular injury causes release of factors leading to platelet aggregation, thrombus formation, inflammation and activation of macrophages and smooth muscle cells. These events induce the production and release of growth factors and cytokines. These, in turn, may promote their own synthesis and release from target cells to initiate a self-perpetuating cascade. This cascade results in the migration of smooth muscle cells from their usual location in the media to the intima where they undergo a phenotype change, produce extracellular matrix and proliferate. The restenotic lesion is, therefore, thought to be a proliferative lesion. The exaggeration of the normal reparative processes following angioplasty-induced local vessel trauma is thought to lead to proliferation of both cellular and matrix components causing an increased tissue mass and restenosis.[3–7] Attempts have been made to attack restenosis by interfering with this cascade. Although the results in animal models have been impressive, pharmacologic trials using antiproliferative agents in humans have been ineffective in humans.[8]

Conversely, recent animal and clinical studies have begun to question the predominant role of cellular proliferation. O'Brien et al.[9] used proliferating cell nuclear antigen (PCNA) immunohistochemical labeling of human directional atherectomy specimens to show that proliferation in primary and restenotic lesions occurs infrequently. (Inter-estingly, in one previous human necropsy report, 40% of restenotic lesions lacked intimal proliferation[10] while other reports found similar levels of smooth muscle cell proliferation in restenotic and nonrestenotic lesions.[11,12]) Kakuta et al.[13] examined the quantitative histologic results from hypercholesterolemic rabbits sacrificed immediately after angioplasty and 4 weeks later; total arterial cross-sectional area increased by 20% to accommodate nearly 60% of the neointimal tissue formation. Furthermore, the neointimal cross-sectional areas in the restenotic and non-restenotic lesions were virtually identical; the differences in lumen areas resulted from significant differences in total arterial cross-sectional areas. In the nonrestenotic lesions a given increase in intimal area was associated with a greater increase in arterial cross-sectional area to preserve the lumen, while in the restenotic lesions there was a lesser increase in total arterial cross-sectional area suggesting inadequate adaptive arterial remodeling. A study by Post et al.[14] showed similar results. In the Yucatan pig iliac artery angioplasty model neointimal thickening accounted for only 11% of late lumen loss in normal pigs and 49% of late lumen loss in hypercholesterolemic pigs; in the rabbit femoral artery angioplasty model neointimal thickening accounted for only 23% of late lumen loss following conventional angioplasty and 14% of late lumen loss following thermal angioplasty. Lafont et al.[15] have shown in the atherosclerotic rabbit femoral artery model that there was only a 33% increase in neointimal area following balloon injury, but a 52% decrease in lumen area as a result of a reduction in total arterial cross-sectional area compared to the reference site. Lastly, recent re-examination of original animal experiments (using different quantitative analyses) now indicates that arterial remodeling (which was once ignored) is, in fact, an important part of the restenosis process.[16]

Importantly, serial intravascular ultrasound (IVUS) studies, which in fact preceded these animal studies, showed that arterial remodeling may be the predominant mechanism of restenosis. We review the serial IVUS evidence for remodeling following coronary interventions.

IVUS allows transmural, tomographic imaging of coronary arteries in humans *in vivo*, providing unique insights into the pathology of coronary artery disease by defining vessel wall geometry in a manner not possible using any other imaging modality. The normal coronary artery architecture (intimal, media and adventitia), the major components of the atherosclerotic plaque, and the changes that occur in coronary arterial dimensions and anatomy with the atherosclerotic disease process, during transcatheter therapy, and on follow-up, can be studied *in vivo*. Initially, sequential (preintervention and postintervention) IVUS studies were used to study mechanisms of angioplasty devices including balloon angioplasty, directional coronary atherectomy, high-speed rotational atherectomy and excimer laser coronary angioplasty.[17-21] The contribution of tissue removal (or ablation) to lumen enlargement could be separated from vessel expansion. Similarly, and more recently, serial (postintervention and follow-up) IVUS studies have been used to study the mechanisms of restenosis; using serial IVUS analysis the true natural history of the restenosis process can be studied in humans *in vivo*. In particular, restenosis (or late lumen loss) can be subdivided into two distinct underlying components, tissue proliferation and arterial remodeling.

Histologic validation of cross-sectional measurements by IVUS have shown that the external elastic membrane cross-sectional area (which represents the area within the border between the hypoechoic media and the echoreflective adventitia) is a reproducible measure of total arterial cross-sectional area.[22-27] Because IVUS cannot measure media thickness accurately,[28] plaque + media cross-sectional area (calculated as external elastic membrane cross-sectional area minus lumen cross-sectional area) is used as a measure of plaque mass. Arterial remodeling, therefore, can be measured as the change in external elastic membrane cross-sectional area. Assuming that media thickness does not change significantly during the typical 6-month postangioplasty follow-up interval, tissue proliferation can be measured as the change in plaque + media cross-sectional area.

IVUS studies of arterial remodeling and restenosis

The authors have reported the serial IVUS studies in 212 nonostial native coronary artery target lesions in 209 patients.[29] Interventional procedures performed included balloon angioplasty, directional coronary atherectomy, high-speed rotational atherectomy and excimer laser angioplasty.

To facilitate comparative image analysis of the serial IVUS studies, the authors first developed a systematic approach to image acquisition and analysis. (This systematic approach was similar to the one which we used to study mechanisms of transcatheter therapy.[17-21]) We only used IVUS systems incorporating motorized transducer pullback through a stationary imaging sheath. Motorized transducer pullback through a stationary imaging sheath permitted the transducer to move at the same speed as the proximal end of the catheter; this has been validated *in vivo*.[30] Postangioplasty (as the last step in the procedure) and on follow-up (prior to any subsequent intervention), intracoronary nitroglycerin was administered; and a complete ultrasound imaging run was performed from beyond the target lesion to the aorto-ostial junction. The same anatomic image slice was analyzed postintervention and on follow-up; and the differences were compared. By using one or more reproducible axial landmarks (for example, the aorto-ostial junction, large proximal and/or distal side-branches or unusually shaped calcium deposits) and a known pullback speed, identical cross-sectional slices on serial studies could be identified for comparison. In addition, vascular and perivascular markings (e.g. small side-branches, venous structures, calcific and fibrotic deposits) were used to confirm image slice identification. If necessary, the postintervention and follow-up studies were analyzed side by side and the imaging runs studied frame by frame to insure that the same anatomic cross-section was measured. The anatomic slice selected for serial analysis had an axial location within the target lesion at the *smallest follow-up lumen cross-sectional area* (rather than at the smallest preintervention or postintervention lumen cross-sectional area) because this defined the center of the restenotic process. If the tissue was packed around the catheter, then the lumen was assumed to be the physical size of the catheter.

The results of these serial IVUS analyses were as follows (Tables 16.1 and 16.2). At follow-up, the decrease in lumen cross-sectional area (from 6.6 ± 2.5 mm^2 to 4.0 ± 3.7 mm^2; $p < 0.0001$) was due more to decrease in external elastic membrane cross-sectional area (from 20.1 ± 6.4 mm^2 to 18.2 ± 6.4 mm^2; $p < 0.0001$) than to an increase in plaque + media cross-sectional area (from 13.5 ± 5.5 mm^2 to 14.2 ± 5.4 mm^2; $p < 0.0001$). Thus, 73% of late lumen loss was explained by the decrease in external elastic membrane cross-sectional area (Figs 16.1(a) and 16.2).

Table 16.1 Serial quantitative angiographic and IVUS results in nonstented lesions.

	Preintervention	Postintervention	Follow-up	Δ (post vs. follow-up)	p (post vs. follow-up)
EEM CSA (mm²)	18.5 ± 6.3	20.1 ± 6.4	18.2 ± 6.4	−1.9 ± 3.6	< 0.0001
Lumen CSA (mm²)	1.7 ± 0.9	6.6 ± 2.5	4.0 ± 3.7	−2.6 ± 3.3	< 0.0001
P + M CSA (mm²)	16.8 ± 6.2	13.5 ± 5.5	14.2 ± 5.4	0.7 ± 2.3	< 0.0001

Notes:
CSA = cross-sectional area, EEM = external elastic membrane, IVUS = intravascular ultrasound, P + M = plaque + media.

Table 16.2 Comparison of IVUS results in restenotic vs. nonrestenotic nonstented lesions.

	Restenosis (n = 99)	No restenosis (n = 113)	p
Δ EEM CSA (mm²)	−3.1 ± 3.0	−0.8 ± 2.9	< 0.0001
Δ lumen CSA (mm²)	−4.1 ± 2.4	−1.2 ± 2.8	< 0.0001
Δ P + M CSA (mm²)	1.0 ± 2.3	0.4 ± 2.0	0.0784

Notes:
CSA = cross-sectional area, EEM = external elastic membrane, IVUS = intravascular ultrasound, P + M = plaque + media.

The change in lumen cross-sectional area correlated more strongly with the change in external elastic membrane cross-sectional area ($r = 0.751$, $p < 0.0001$) than with the change in plaque + media cross-sectional area ($r = 0.284$, $p < 0.0001$). These results are similar to those of Lafont[15] in which the histologic stenosis four weeks after angioplasty of atherosclerotic rabbit iliac arteries correlated with the chronic constriction index ($r = -0.67$, $p = 0.0001$), but not with neointimal + medial growth ($r = 0.08$, $p = 0.63$).

The change in external elastic membrane cross-sectional area was bidirectional. Twenty-two percent of the lesions showed adaptive arterial remodeling, an increase in external elastic membrane cross-sectional area. Despite a greater increase in plaque + media cross-sectional area (1.5 ± 2.5 mm² vs. 0.5 ± 2.0 mm²; $p = 0.0009$), lesions exhibiting adaptive arterial remodeling had no change in lumen cross-sectional area (-0.1 ± 3.3 mm²) compared to a decrease in lumen cross-sectional area of 3.6 ± 2.3 mm²

for lesions exhibiting pathologic arterial remodeling ($p < 0.0001$). Adaptive arterial remodeling following coronary angioplasty resulted in a decreased incidence of restenosis (26% vs. 62%; $p = 0.0009$) and an increased incidence of late lumen gain (49% vs. 1%; $p < 0.0001$) despite an increase in plaque mass, analogous to adaptive arterial remodeling and vasodilatation early in the atherosclerotic disease process. Adaptive remodeling following coronary interventions may be similar to adaptive arterial remodeling early in the coronary artery atherosclerotic disease process, as originally described by Glagov.[31] In the coronary artery atherosclerotic disease process in noninstrumented arteries, adaptive remodeling delays the development of focal stenoses despite significant plaque accumulation to prevent the reduction in lumen dimensions until plaque occupies, on average, approximately 40–50% of the cross-sectional area within the internal elastic membrane (40–50% cross-sectional narrowing or plaque burden).[31,32] Conversely, pathologic arterial remodeling (a decrease in arterial cross-

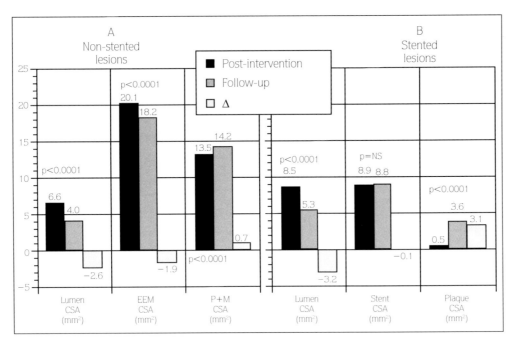

Figure 16.1
The serial (postintervention and follow-up) IVUS results are shown schematically. In nonstented lesions the decrease in lumen cross-sectional area (CSA, from 6.6 ± 2.5 mm² to 4.0 ± 3.7 mm²; $p < 0.0001$) was due more to a decrease in external elastic membrane (EEM) CSA (from 20.1 ± 6.4 mm² to 18.2 ± 6.4 mm²; $p < 0.0001$) than to an increase in plaque + media (P + M) CSA (from 13.5 ± 5.5 mm² to 14.2 ± 5.4 mm²; $p < 0.0001$). In stented lesions the decrease in lumen CSA (from 8.5 ± 3.4 mm² to 5.3 ± 3.6 mm²; $p < 0.0001$) was due almost exclusively to in-stent tissue growth (plaque CSA, from 0.5 ± 1.4 mm² to 3.6 ± 2.9 mm²; $p < 0.0001$) with essentially no change in stent CSA (from 8.9 ± 63.3 mm² to 8.8 ± 3.2 mm²; $p < 0.0001$).

sectional area, or chronic arterial constriction or shrinkage) has now been shown to contribute to lumen compromise in chronic, focal de novo stenoses in femoral and coronary arteries.[33,34] Furthermore, adaptive arterial remodeling may be the explanation for the occasional improvement in lumen dimensions seen during the follow-up period after catheter-based interventions.

OARS and the SURE trial

The occurrence of arterial remodeling following coronary angioplasty has been confirmed in at least two other studies that used similar IVUS image acquisition and analytical methodology. The Optimal Atherectomy Restenosis Study (OARS) was a multicenter study of IVUS-guided directional coronary atherectomy including angiographic and IVUS follow-up. In OARS, late lumen loss was shown to be

almost entirely the result of pathologic remodeling.[35] Lesion site remodeling accounted for 84% of late lumen loss.

The Serial Ultrasound analysis of Restenosis Trial (SURE trial) studied patients treated with balloon angioplasty and directional atherectomy pre- and immediately postintervention, 24 hours' postintervention, after 1 month of follow-up and after 6 months of follow-up. The results elucidate the time course of remodeling and help to explain the adaptive remodeling that was seen in 22% of our original patients. The SURE trial showed that there was little change in external elastic membrane cross-sectional area within the first 24 hours following intervention, *early adaptive remodeling* (an increase in external elastic membrane cross-sectional area) between 24 hours and one month, and *late pathologic remodeling* (a decrease in external elastic membrane cross-sectional area) between 1 and 6 months.[36] Thus, remodeling is typically biphasic in the same patient; and the adaptive remodeling that is seen late in *some* patients merely represents a sustaining of the

24 Nishimura RA, Edwards WD, Warnes CA, *et al.* Intravascular ultrasound imaging: *in vitro* validation and pathologic correlation. *J Am Coll Cardiol* 1990; **16**: 145–54.

25 Potkin BN, Bartorelli AL, Gessert JM, *et al.* Coronary artery imaging with intravascular high-frequency ultrasound. *Circulation* 1990; **81**: 1575–85.

26 Nissen SE, Grines CL, Gurley JC, *et al.* Application of a new phased-array ultrasound imaging catheter in the assessment of vascular dimensions. *In vivo* comparison to cineangiography. *Circulation* 1990; **81**: 660–6.

27 Tobis JM, Mallery JA, Gessert J, *et al.* Intravascular ultrasound cross-sectional arterial imaging before and after balloon angioplasty *in vitro. Circulation* 1989; **80**: 873–82.

28 Mallery JA, Tobis JM, Griffith J, *et al.* Assessment of normal and atherosclerotic arterial wall thickness with an intravascular ultrasound imaging catheter. *Am Heart J* 1990; **119**: 1392–400.

29 Mintz GS, Popma JJ, Pichard AD, *et al.* Arterial remodeling after coronary angioplasty: a serial intravascular ultrasound study. *Circulation* 1996; **94**: 35–43.

30 Fuessl RT, Mintz GS, Pichard AD, *et al. In vivo* validation of intravascular ultrasound length measurements using a motorized transducer pullback device. *Am J Cardiol* 1996; **77**: 1115–18.

31 Glagov S, Weisenberg E, Zarins CK, Stankunacicius K, Kolettis GJ. Compensatory enlargement of various human atherosclerotic arteries. *N Engl J Med* 1987; **316**: 1371–5.

32 Zarins CK, Weisenberg E, Kolettis G, Stankunavicius R, Glagov S. Differential enlargement of artery segments in response to enlarging atherosclerotic plaques. *J Vasc Surg* 1988; **7**: 386–94.

33 Pasterkamp G, Wensing PJW, Post MJ, Hillen B, Mali WPTM, Borst C. Paradoxical arterial wall shrinkage may contribute to luminal narrowing of human atherosclerotic femoral arteries. *Circulation* 1995; **91**: 1444–9.

34 Mintz GS, Griffin J, Hong MK, Bucher TA, Kehoe MK, Pichard AD. Focal arterial contraction is important in the development of coronary artery stenoses in patients with chronic stable angina. *Circulation* 1995; **92**: I-400.

35 Mintz GS, Fitzgerald PF, Kuntz RE, *et al.* Lesion site and reference segment remodeling after directional coronary atherectomy: an analysis from the optimal atherectomy restenosis study. *Circulation* 1995; **92**: I-93.

36 Kimura T, Kaburagi S, Tamura T, *et al.* Remodeling responses of human coronary arteries undergoing coronary angioplasty. *Circulation*, in press.

37 Libby P, Schwartz D, Brogi E, Tanaka H, Clinton SK. A cascade model for restenosis: a special case of atherosclerosis progression. *Circulation* 1992; **86**: III-47–III-52.

38 Glagov S. Intimal hyperplasia, vascular remodeling, and the restenosis problem. *Circulation* 1994; **89**: 2888–91.

39 Isner JM. Vascular remodeling. Honey, I think I shrunk the artery. *Circulation* 1994; **89**: 2937–41.

40 Brott BC, Labinaz M, Culp SC, *et al.* Vessel remodeling after angioplasty: comparative anatomic studies. *J Am Coll Cardiol* 1994; **23**: 138A.

41 Fischman DL, Leon MB, Baim DS, *et al.* A randomized comparison of coronary stent placement and balloon angioplasty in the treatment of coronary artery disease. *N Engl J Med* 1994; **331**: 496–501.

42 Serruys P, De Jaegere P, Kiemeneij F, *et al.* A comparison of balloon-expandable-stent implantation with balloon angioplasty in patients with coronary artery disease. *N Engl J Med* 1994; **331**: 490–5.

43 Hoffmann R, Mintz GS, Dussaillant GR, *et al.* Patterns and mechanisms of instent restenosis: a serial intravascular ultrasound study. *Circulation* 1996; **94**: 1247–54.

17

The role of the adventitia and neointima after angioplasty

Renu Virmani, Andrew Farb, Giuseppe Sangiorgi, Douglas Scott, Brigitta C Brott and Robert S Schwartz

Introduction

An initial successful revascularization rate of higher than 95% after balloon angioplasty (PTCA) has been plagued by a high rate of late restenosis that reaches 30–50%.[1,2] Early clinical and morphologic studies suggested that vascular repair from neointimal growth was the main determinant of the late high failure rate after balloon angioplasty.[3,4] It has been shown in animal models (rabbit, dog, pig and baboon) that injury to normal arteries results in neointimal growth that is proportional to the extent of injury.[5–11] However, recent clinical and animal studies have questioned the wisdom of attributing restenosis solely to neointimal growth. Human atherectomy specimens often fail to show a high rate of intimal cell proliferation that is observed in animal studies.[12,13] Studies in the baboon and pig have suggested that arterial remodeling, which is attributed to changes within the adventitia, may be the primary factor determining the final outcome after balloon angioplasty.[14,15] Clinical studies utilizing intravascular ultrasound (IVUS), which allows for better geometric definition of vessel wall than coronary angiography, have reported that restenosis appears to be determined primarily by remodeling of the external elastic membrane.[16,17] An increase in the area enclosed by external elastic lamina (EEL) at the time of PTCA is adaptive and allows for greater lumen enlargement whereas a decrease in EEL area contributes to lumen loss late after angioplasty. Insights into the role of the adventitia are provided by human pathologic studies in which the neointima, atherosclerotic plaque, media (defined at its borders by the internal elastic lamina [IEL] and [EEL]) and adventitia are more clearly delineated compared to IVUS.

Definition of neointima and adventitia

Histologic studies of human and animal arteries late (>1 month) after balloon angioplasty have defined the restenotic lesion as the accumulation of smooth muscle cells within a proteoglycan matrix that narrows the previously enlarged lumen (Fig. 17.1). In human studies, neointima forms in all arteries that have undergone traumatic injury secondary to balloon dilatation, which consists of dissection planes within the plaque that often extend into the media in eccentric lesions.[18–23] Full thickness medial rupture and extension of the arterial injury into the adventitia are not uncommon.

The adventitia is composed predominately of collagen, few fibroblasts, vasa vasorum and focal scattered lymphocytes predominately localized around the vasa vasorum (Fig. 17.1). The inner border of the area occupied by the adventitia is the EEL (which is part of the media); the outer border of the adventitia is defined by the transition from adventitial fibrous collagen to epicardial adipose tissue.

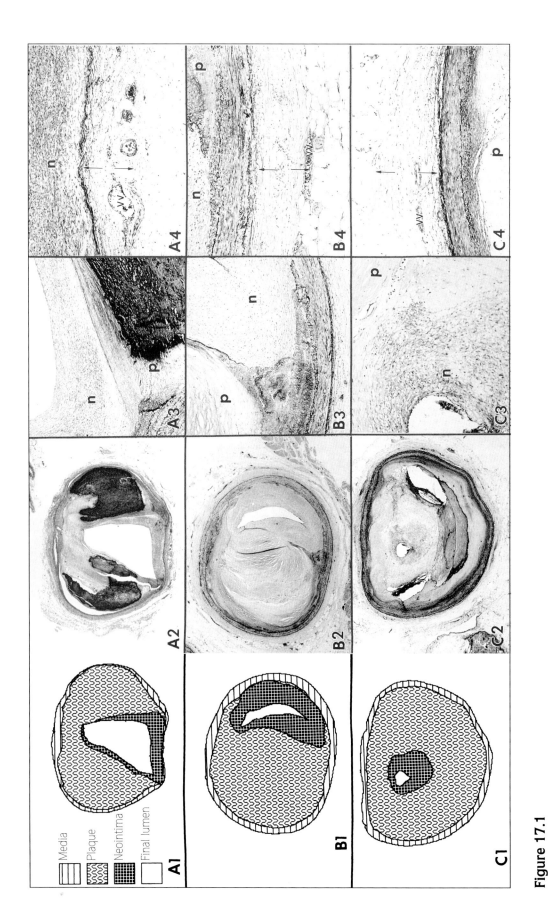

Figure 17.1

Histology with accompanying schematic diagrams of three representative coronary artery segments subjected to balloon angioplasty during life. In panel 3 of each case, the neointima (n), consisting of smooth muscle cells within a proteoglycan matrix, is shown adjacent to plaque (p). In panel 4, the adventitia containing vasa vasorum (VV) is shown. A1–4: Left anterior descending coronary artery from a 62-year-old white man who died suddenly 88 weeks following angioplasty. There is an acute and long-term histologic success in which both the acute lumen area and final lumen area are ⩾25% of the arterial area. The adventitia is shown in the area of the neointima that formed after angioplasty. Note absence of the media and a well formed EEL. B1–4: Left circumflex coronary artery from a 68-year-old white man who died postcoronary artery bypass surgery 8 weeks following angioplasty. There is an acute histologic success and long-term histologic failure ('histologic restenosis'). The acute lumen area is ⩾25% of the arterial area, and final lumen area is <25% of the arterial area. The adventitia is shown at the site of plaque rupture and neointima. Note that the media is stretched but not ruptured. C1–4: Left anterior descending coronary artery from a 41-year-old white man who died suddenly 30 weeks following angioplasty. There is an acute and long-term histologic failure in which both the acute lumen area and final lumen area are <25% of the arterial area. Note absence of medial injury and a thickened adventitia. (With permission)

Table 17.1 Morphologic data (mean ± SD) from arterial segments ($n = 85$) from 28 human coronary arteries subjected to balloon angioplasty studied at a mean of 71 weeks after PTCA.

	Long-term histologic success (n = 24)	Long-term histologic failure (n = 61)	
EEL area (mm²)	10.0 ± 4.0	11.1 ± 4.4	$p = 0.29$
IEL area (mm²)	8.9 ± 3.8	9.7 ± 3.9	$p = 0.37$
Neointima area (mm²)	1.4 ± 0.9	1.5 ± 0.9	$p = 0.49$
Final lumen area (mm²)	2.7 ± 2.1	1.1 ± 0.9	$p < 0.0001$
Acute lumen area (mm²)	4.1 ± 1.9	2.7 ± 1.4	$p < 0.001$
Neointima area/acute lumen area (%)	33 ± 12	60 ± 23	$p < 0.0001$
Final lumen area patency (%)	31 ± 7	12 ± 7	$p < 0.0001$
Acute lumen area patency (%)	46 ± 10	27 ± 11	$p < 0.0001$
Acute lumen area stenosis (%)	54 ± 10	73 ± 11	$p < 0.0001$
Acute lumen area/EEL area (%)	41 ± 9	24 ± 10	$p < 0.0001$
Plaque area (mm²)	4.8 ± 2.4	7.1 ± 3.2	$p < 0.002$

Notes:
A long-term histologic success was defined as a (Final lumen area/IEL area) × 100 of ≥25%. A long-term histologic failure was defined as a (Final lumen area/IEL area) × 100 <25%. Final lumen area patency = Final lumen area/IEL area. Acute lumen area patency = Acute lumen area/IEL area. Acute lumen area stenosis = 1 − (Acute lumen area/IEL area).

Analysis of human coronary arteries late after PTCA: histology, angiography and IVUS

We recently reported that in human coronary arteries examined 6 or more weeks after angioplasty, neointimal proliferation occurs in all dilated coronary arteries, and the amount of neointima is similar in long-term success (defined as final lumen area ≥25% of the area within the IEL) and in long-term failure (final lumen area <25% of the IEL) (Table 17.1).[23] Further morphometric examination of these vessels demonstrated that the area enclosed within the EEL was also similar and, therefore, late remodeling of the EEL did not appear to account for the success or failure after balloon angioplasty. A major difference between long-term success and failure was a smaller plaque area in long-term successes, which would indicate that the artery at the time of balloon angioplasty had less luminal narrowing in vessels that demonstrate late success. Alternatively, it is possible that the initial artery size before angioplasty was smaller in the long-term successes, and that because of the dilatation procedure, the external elastic lamina was expanded and the plaque distributed over a larger area of the expanded artery accounting for the

differences in late success and failure. We know from the work of Glagov that arteries dilate (compensatory enlargement of the IEL) with the development of atherosclerosis, and that this expansion is seen only up to 30–40% luminal narrowing; greater plaque accumulation results in luminal compromise.[24,25] Arterial expansion also applies to the EEL; when comparing the area within the EEL and plaque area of balloon angioplasty arteries by linear regression, an excellent correlation is present ($R^2 = 0.83$, $p < 0.0001$, Fig. 17.2). Further, there is a similar strong correlation between plaque area and EEL in both long-term success and failure ($R^2 = 0.81$ in success and 0.89 in failure). Thus, when one is able definitively to identify the EEL and measure the area within the EEL morphometrically, the EEL *per se* appears to be of less importance in long-term outcome than the creation of a large acute lumen and resultant neointimal growth.

Angiographic studies have demonstrated that the creation of a larger lumen area at the time of angioplasty is associated with an improved long-term success.[26] This finding has been confirmed in a morphologic study showing that a final lumen size at 25% or more of the cross-sectional arterial area (long-term success) had a larger acute lumen (final lumen plus the neointimal area—Table 17.1, Figs 17.1 and 17.3). The amount of neointimal healing correlated with the acute lumen area (Fig. 17.4) and area within the EEL (Fig. 17.5). The correlation of the neointimal

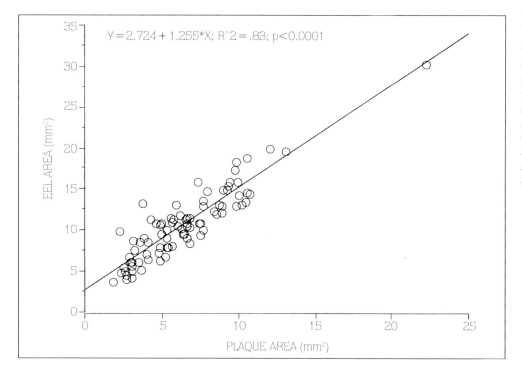

Figure 17.2
Linear regression comparing the area of within the external elastic lamina (EEL) with the plaque area in 85 segments from 28 coronary arteries subjected to PTCA during life and studied at a mean of 71 weeks after angioplasty. The data fit a linear model with a correlation coefficient (R^2) of 0.83.

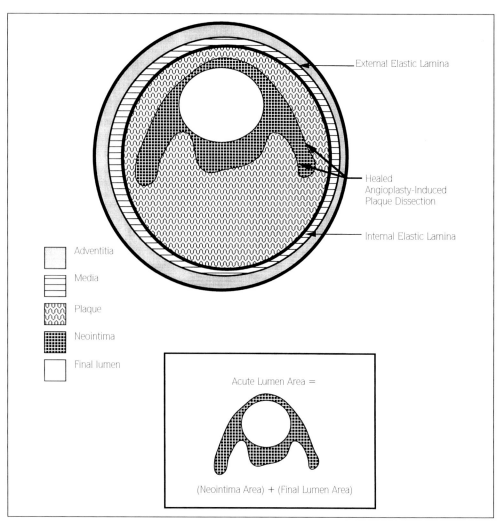

Figure 17.3
Schematic diagram of the method of histologic analysis of each coronary artery segment that demonstrated balloon angioplasty effect. The following measurements were made by computerized planimetry: arterial size (area within the internal elastic lamina), plaque area, neointima area, adventitial area and final lumen area. The acute lumen area is the sum of the final lumen area and neointimal area. (With permission)

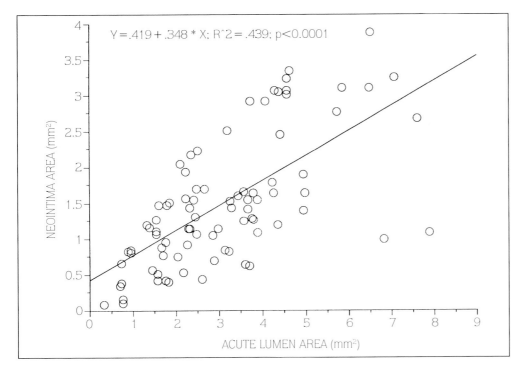

Figure 17.4
Linear regression comparing the area of neointima formation with the acute lumen area in 85 segments from 28 coronary arteries subjected to PTCA during life and studied at a mean of 71 weeks after angioplasty. The data fit a linear model with a correlation coefficient (R^2) of 0.44. (With permission)

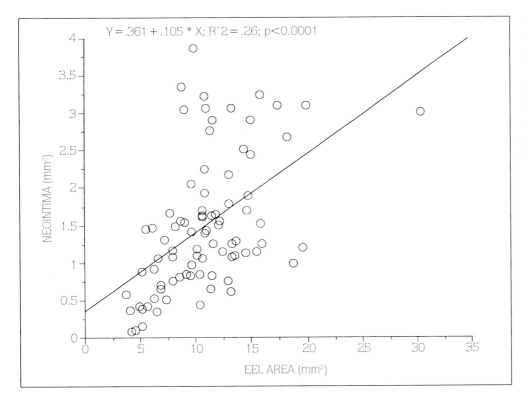

Figure 17.5
Linear regression comparing the area of neointima formation with the EEL area in 85 segments from 28 coronary arteries subjected to PTCA during life and studied at a mean of 71 weeks after angioplasty. The data fit a linear model with a correlation coefficient (R^2) of 0.26.

area with the acute lumen is logical because a small acute lumen can only permit the development of a relatively small neointima before the lumen becomes occluded.[23] The larger acute lumen from balloon injury will invariably result in greater injury stimulating an augmented neointimal response. The extent of injury has also been shown to correlate with the development of greater neointima by Nobuyoshi et al.[22]

In contrast to histologic analysis, angiographic studies are unable to depict adventitial changes after PTCA. IVUS studies can provide serial measurements within the same arterial segment and have suggested that remodeling, defined as decrease in EEL cross-sectional area, is the main determinant of late failure.[17] Mintz et al.[17] showed that restenotic lesions had a greater decrease in EEL cross-sectional area and lumen area from baseline than nonrestenotic lesions (0.8 ± 2.9 and 1.2 ± 2.8 mm^2, respectively, $p < 0.0001$). The change in lumen cross-sectional area correlated more strongly with the late reduction in EEL cross-sectional area than with the increase in plaque plus medial area. In contrast, our data demonstrate a better correlation between EEL and plaque area than with EEL and luminal area ($R^2 = 0.83$, $p < 0.0001$ and $R^2 = 0.20$, $p = 0.001$, respectively). We also observed that long-term successes had a stronger correlation between medial area/EEL and EEL area ($R^2 = -0.325$, $p < 0.0001$) than long-term failures ($R^2 = -0.02$, $p = $ NS) reflecting an association of medial thinning with increased EEL area. In the IVUS study, plaque area was not quantitated and it is possible that plaque area also correlated with the EEL. The EEL area was similar in long-term success (10.0 ± 4.0 mm^2) and failure (11.1 ± 4.4 mm^2, $p = $ NS, Table 17.1) in our morphologic study. Morphologic studies are able to outline clearly the area enclosed by the EEL, and we were unable to show any difference in success and failure, leading to the conclusion that the plaque area and acute lumen area are the main determinants of success and failure. It should be noted, however, that pathologic analyses are limited by an inability to perform serial measurements over time as can be done in IVUS studies.

Role of the adventitia in restenosis after balloon angioplasty

It is essential to know what changes occur in the adventitia during the development of atherosclerosis itself prior to addressing the changes that may occur after angioplasty. We have studied the extent of luminal narrowing as well as the adventitial area in coronary arteries with varying degrees of atherosclerosis. The adventitial area increases with increases in plaque area and percent stenosis (Table 17.2). The mean adventitial area was 2.50 ± 1.05 mm^2 (range 0.74–6.53 mm^2) for arteries with a mean cross-sectional area luminal narrowing of $54 \pm 26\%$. Because the adventitial area is dependent on the vessel size, we normalized the adventitial area to the mean area enclosed by the internal elastic lamina (9.34 ± 4.0 mm^2). There was a significantly greater normalized adventitial area in arteries with a luminal narrowing above 75% (3.61 ± 1.75 mm^2) as compared to arteries with 0–25% narrowing (2.54 ± 1.36 mm^2, $p = 0.02$), and 25–49% luminal narrowing (2.21 ± 1.80 mm^2, $p = 0.005$). The adventitial area was similar in arteries with 25–49% and 50–74% luminal

Table 17.2 Morphometric measurement of area within the external elastic lamina and adventitial area in human autopsy coronary arteries.

% stenosis	EEL area (mm^2)*	Adventitial area (mm^2)†
0–24	10.21 ± 3.15	2.17 ± 0.75
25–49	13.99 ± 4.89	2.49 ± 0.94
50–74	10.25 ± 4.31	2.40 ± 1.09
75–100	9.70 ± 3.48	2.89 ± 1.21
All arteries	**10.79 ± 4.23**	**2.50 ± 1.05**

Notes:
* 0–24% vs. 25–49%, $p = 0.02$.
  25–49% vs. 50–74%, $p = 0.01$.
  25–49% vs. 75–100%, $p = 0.005$.
† 0–24% vs. 75–100%, $p = 0.06$.
Maximal EEL area is present at 25–49% cross-sectional area stenosis by atherosclerotic plaque, which corresponds to the recognized limit of compensatory arterial enlargement. Adventitial area progressively increases as percent luminal stenosis increases.

narrowing (2.21 ± 1.80 mm^2 and 2.66 ± 0.65 mm^2, respectively). However, the EEL area started to decrease in arteries with luminal narrowing above 50% (Table 17.2). Therefore, the relationship between the EEL and adventitial growth appears to be divergent, indicating that arteries do not undergo compensatory enlargement (defined by an enlarged EEL) beyond 30–40% luminal narrowing (Fig. 17.6). The main determinant of adventitial area is plaque area: the greater the plaque area the greater the adventitial area.

We have studied human autopsy coronary arteries >1 month after balloon injury (Table 17.3).[27] The adventitial area in PTCA arteries (2.13 ± 1.01 mm^2) was similar to the proximal non-dilated reference arterial segment (2.16 ± 0.80 mm^2, $p = $ NS). This similarity in adventitial areas was also seen when normalizing adventitial areas for vessel size (calculated from the ratio of the adventitial area to the mean of all EEL area measurements in the study). There was an increase in normalized adventitial area in arteries with medial injury (0.23 ± 0.10 mm^2) versus dilated arteries without medial injury (0.19 ± 0.06 mm^2, $p<0.03$). This observation was further confirmed by measuring the maximal adventitial thickness; when medial injury was present, the adventitial thickness was 0.32 ± 0.19 mm, and when medial injury was absent, the thickness was 0.24 ± 0.16 mm ($p = 0.03$). This increase in adventitial thickness suggests that the arterial wall injury is not limited to the lumen and atherosclerotic plaque, but also extends

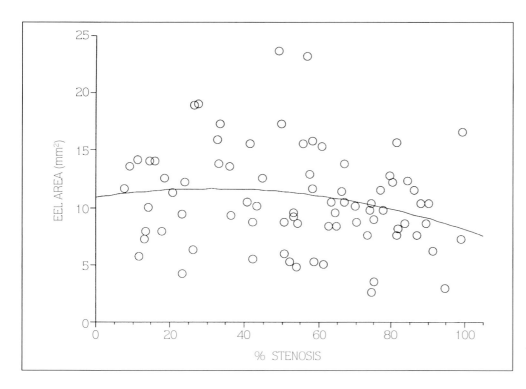

Figure 17.6
Second-order regression comparing the area of within the EEL with percent luminal stenosis. There is an overall reduction in EEL area with increasing severity of arterial stenosis beyond 30–40% cross-sectional luminal narrowing.

into the media and adventitia. There was stronger correlation ($R^2 = 0.2$, $p<0.005$) of neointima area with IEL disruption length, an index of arterial injury severity, than with adventitial thickness at the IEL disruption site ($R^2 = 0.05$, $p = $ NS), suggesting that the effect of balloon injury is greater at the luminal surface than in the adventitia. Not only was there an increase in the adventitial area following medial injury, but the neointimal area was also significantly greater when medial injury was present versus absent (2.06 ± 1.00 vs. 1.63 ± 1.03 mm^2, respectively, $p<0.04$). Indeed, the success of balloon angioplasty is determined by how much the artery can be enlarged, and this involves the deformation of media and adventitia. It is, therefore, not

surprising that proliferating cells are seen in the injured adventitia as has been reported in various animal models (see below).[15,28]

We did not observe any significant differences in the EEL area or intimal area between arteries with long-term histologic success or failure following PTCA. The neointimal area (1.83 ± 1.09 mm^2) correlated with the adventitial area at the PTCA site ($R^2 = 0.23$, $p<0.0002$). This correlation seems logical as the injury is not limited to the plaque surface alone, and injury extends throughout the vessel, including the media and the adventitia. The final lumen at the PTCA site correlated positively with the acute lumen ($R^2 = 0.50$, $p = 0.001$) and weakly with the adventitial

Table 17.3 Morphometric measurements in human coronary arteries subjected to balloon angioplasty at a mean of 55 weeks' ante-mortem. PTCA-induced disruption of the arterial media is associated with a larger and thicker adventitia and a larger neointima.

	Adventitial area (mm^2)	Maximal adventitial thickness (mm^2)	EEL area (mm^2)	Neointima area (mm^2)	Final lumen area (mm^2)
Media disrupted	2.49 ± 1.25	0.32 ± 0.19	11.10 ± 3.44	2.06 ± 1.00	1.21 ± 1.05
Media intact	1.82 ± 0.58	0.24 ± 0.16	10.01 ± 3.52	1.63 ± 1.03	1.08 ± 1.20
p-value	0.0008	<0.03	0.12	<0.04	0.56

area ($R^2 = 0.04$, $p = 0.02$). Furthermore, the contribution to the narrowed final lumen by neointima and plaque was approximately 4 times greater than the increase in adventitial area. It would be of interest to determine if plaques retract after injury, just as scars retract after skin injury, when the collagen polymerizes, and this transformation may be dependent upon plaque composition. At least 50% of the plaque is composed of acellular collagen, 22% is cellular collagen, 10% is heavily calcified tissue, another 10% is necrotic core or gruel and the remainder consists of inflammatory cells.[29] As noted above, the adventitial area is proportional to the plaque area and does not increase in the absence of intimal plaque accumulation.

Animal models of restenosis and the role of adventitia

In normal and atherosclerotic animal models, early studies emphasized the importance of the neointima, and it was almost uniformly thought that smooth muscle cell proliferation within a proteoglycan matrix was the main contributor to restenosis.[22,30] Recent experimental studies have focused attention on the adventitia. Animal models are an invaluable resource in the study of the sequence of events of restenosis. However, we must realize the limitations of the various animal models compared to human atherosclerotic lesions and recognize the differences in architecture among normal animal arteries. The normal dog and domestic pig coronary artery have comparable lumens, and both have an intima composed of a single layer of endothelial cells with an underlying basement membrane in contact with the IEL. The media is composed predominantly of smooth muscle cells with minimal proteoglycans and collagen, and at the sites close to the arterial ostia there may be some interspersed elastic fibers.[11] The adventitia, however, is very different in these two models. In contrast to the single layer EEL in the dog, the pig EEL is several layers thick and is composed of short fibrils with collagen interspersed in between. The collagen is mostly concentrated away from the arterial wall close to the surrounding fat. The area occupied by the adventitia is similar in the two animals (pig 0.68 ± 0.32 mm^2, dog 0.84 ± 0.24 mm^2, $p = $ NS); however, the number of adventitial vessels (vasa vasorum) are significantly greater in the pig than in the dog (12 ± 4/mm^2 vs. 4 ± 2/mm^2, respectively, $p < 0.005$).[11]

Balloon angioplasty of normal pig arteries results in medial disruption (or rupture) and a similar luminal area compared to a normal uninjured artery (1.93 ± 0.94 mm^2 vs. 2.98 ± 0.50 mm^2, respectively).[11] In contrast, coronary angioplasty in the dog leads to medial disruption with a resultant larger lumen than the normal uninjured lumen (4.20 ± 1.90 mm^2 vs. 3.22 ± 0.96 mm^2, respectively).[11] The

EEL area postangioplasty is significantly smaller in the pig than the dog (4.61 ± 1.36 mm^2 vs. 7.16 ± 2.41 mm^2, respectively, $p = 0.05$), but the intimal and the adventitial areas are similar. However, both the lumen area/arterial area (pig 0.22 ± 0.10 mm^2, dog 0.39 ± 0.10 mm^2, $p < 0.05$) and the adventitial area/arterial area (pig 0.48 ± 0.08, dog 0.32 ± 0.06, $p < 0.0005$) are significantly different postangioplasty in the two animals.[11] Further, the number of adventitial vessels/mm^2 is greater in the pig than the dog (23 ± 4 mm^2 vs. 4 ± 2 mm^2, respectively $p < 0.01$).[11] It is therefore possible that species adventitial differences account for the pathologic changes after PTCA.

In normal pig and rabbit arteries, it has been shown that the neointimal hyperplasia and arterial remodeling determine the outcome after arterial injury. Many investigators now believe that the amount of neointima is similar in successful and restenotic arteries, but changes in EEL and adventitia are the final determinants of late failure. Contrasting views on the relative importance of the neointima and adventitia have been expressed in studies utilizing the rabbit atherosclerotic model. Kakuta et al.[31] showed that the intimal area was similar in arteries with long-term successful angioplasty compared with restenotic arteries, and that the only difference was in the IEL and EEL areas. In contrast, Gertz et al.[32] reported that the plaque area was the critical determinant of final success and failure. In the study by Kakuta et al.,[31] the atherosclerotic plaque was not differentiated from the neointimal proliferation, and animals were fed a high-cholesterol diet even after angioplasty, thus making it difficult to determine whether the plaque progression was different in the two groups. Furthermore, serum cholesterol values were not measured, and the rabbit model is prone to highly variable atherosclerotic plaque formation and serum cholesterol values.[33] Therefore, unless the neointima is measured separately from underlying plaque, no definite conclusions can be drawn even when angiographic results at the time of angioplasty were similar. In normal rabbit arteries, Lafont et al.[34] concluded that late residual stenosis (defined as the difference between the reference noninjured lumen and the normalized injured lumen) correlated with chronic constriction (the ratio of EEL area of the lesion to the EEL area of the noninjured artery). This is not unexpected as the lumen is dependent upon the intimal area, and chronic constriction is dependent upon the extent of injury in normal arteries. This is not to suggest that the EEL does not play a role in restenosis, but it must be recognized that adventitial changes are dependent upon the extent of injury induced.

Injured nonatherosclerotic pig arteries behave similarly to the rabbit in that luminal compromise is produced which is dependent upon the extent of arterial injury. There are very few studies in the pig atherosclerotic model, and long-term studies are rare. Post et al.[9] induced atherosclerosis in the porcine internal and external iliac arteries by balloon injury and animals were fed a high-cholesterol diet over 28 weeks followed by balloon dilatation and sacrifice at 4 weeks. There was greater intimal hyperplasia in the atherosclerotic arteries (49%) than in balloon-injured normal arteries (11%). The authors propose that there was pre-existing plaque present when balloon angioplasty was performed as was seen in the noninjured segments. Therefore, the contribution by neointima was only 25% to the final luminal narrowing. Their main findings were that if underlying atherosclerotic plaque were present, it contributes significantly to the final outcome. The arterial injury induced is also greater in the presence of plaque and contributes to ultimate luminal narrowing by both intimal thickening and via injury to the adventitia.

To our knowledge, only one study of balloon angioplasty has been reported in atherosclerotic nonhuman primates.[15] Monkeys with atherosclerotic iliac arteries after 36 months of a high-lipid diet underwent angioplasty and were sacrificed at 4, 7, 14 and 28 days. BrDU was given to label proliferating cells. The arterial lumen transiently increased in size but returned to baseline at 7 days. Proliferating cells were maximal at 4 and 7 days and were more frequently observed in the adventitia (proliferation index 45 ± 6%) compared with the media or the intima (9 ± 3% and 16 ± 6%, respectively). The neointima thickened greatly at 14 and 28 days, but the EEL expansion prevented a further loss of the lumen area. At 28 days, the percent increase in area of each component of the vessel wall at the angioplasty site as compared to the control vessel was 343 ± 89% for the intima, 150 ± 29% for the EEL and 119 ± 21% for the lumen.[15] These results illustrate that the neointima was the major component of the final lumen, and that the adventitia also played a role which is probably dependent upon the extent of injury.

Investigators have questioned the origin of the smooth muscle cells in the neointima, raising the possibility that these cells may arise in the adventitia. In an elegant study of normal pig coronary arteries following balloon injury, Scott et al.[28] identified proliferating cells in various regions of the arterial wall at 1, 3, 7 and 14 days. Proliferation index was highest in the adventitia at 3 days (27%), and was lower at sites of medial disruption (11%) and in media away from the site of disruption (6%). No neointima was identified at 3 days. Increased proliferation was seen in the neointima (proliferation index 19%) compared with the adventitia (10%) at 7 days and remained greater in the intima (7%) than the adventitia (3%) at 14 days. To understand cell proliferation better, the authors administered BrDU on days 2 and 3 after balloon injury and sacrificed the animals at 14 days. They observed the greatest labeling in the adventitia; however, 43% of intimal cells were also positive. From these results, the authors concluded that the proliferating adventitial cells may migrate into the intima from the adventitia. However, it must be noted that the area for potential healing and neointimal growth in between the ruptured media is far smaller than the adventitial area in

this model. The neointima and disrupted media should therefore have a lower proliferation index as compared to the adventitia. Injury, although directed at the intima and media is not limited to these regions in this model; the adventitia is markedly stretched, and will therefore demonstrate thickening secondary to fibroblast proliferation and collagen deposition. It is interesting that we do not observe proteoglycan matrix deposition in the adventitia but only in the intima, probably because the smooth muscle cells proliferate from the medial disruption site. Once a neointima develops, the smooth muscle cells further proliferate within the neointima and lay down proteoglycans, thus giving rise to an expanded neointimal layer.

Summary

Balloon angioplasty results in extensive injury to the vessel wall; this includes plaque fracture, medial stretch, dissection or rupture, and adventitial stretch (with probable focal breaks in the adventitial collagen) followed by repair of the injured arterial wall. Healing occurs not only at the luminal surface (with re-endothelialization and neointimal formation) but also within the plaque and media. The adventitia is also repaired via inflammation, neovascularization, fibroblast proliferation and eventual collagen deposition. The final outcome of balloon injury is healing, but the percent stenosis must be less than 75% narrowed in cross-sectional area for the balloon angioplasty to be successful long term. There is little doubt that neointimal formation contributes to the final loss of the lumen, but current controversy has focused on the other important structural determinants of the success and failure. From human and animal studies, we believe that late effective arterial patency is dependent on the creation of a large acute lumen with requires enlargement of the EEL. Late loss occurs not only secondary to neointimal growth but also due to retraction of the EEL. The amount of neointima and the adventitial growth are determined by the amount of injury. The greater the underlying percent stenosis secondary to the atherosclerotic plaque, the greater is the potential for sufficient lumen loss to cause restenosis.

References

1   Holmes DR, Viestrra RE, Smith HC, et al. Restenosis after percutaneous transluminal coronary angioplasty (PTCA): a report from the PTCA registry of the National Heart, Lung and Blood Institute. Am J Cardiol, 1984; **53**: 77C–81C.

2   Nobuyoshi M, Kimura T, Nosaka H, et al. Restenosis after successful percutaneous transluminal coronary angioplasty:

serial angiographic follow-up of 229 patients. *J Am Coll Cardiol* 1988; **12**: 616–23.

3   Haudenschild CC. Pathologenesis of restenosis. *Z Kardiol*, 1989; **78**: 28–34.

4   Forrester JS, Fishbein M, Helfant R, Fagin J. A paradigm for restenosis based on cell biology: clues for the development of new preventive therapies. *J Am Coll Cardiol* 1991; **17**: 758–69.

5   Sarembock IJ, LaVeau PJ, Sigal SL, *et al.* The influence of inflation pressure and balloon size on the development of intimal hyperplasia following balloon angioplasty: a study in the atherosclerotic rabbit. *Circulation* 1989; **80**: 1029–40.

6   LaVeau PJ, Sarembock IJ, Sigal SL, Yang TL, Ezekowitz MD. Vascular reactivity after balloon angioplasty in an atherosclerotic rabbit. *Circulation* 1990; **82**: 1790–801.

7   Waksman R, Robinson KA, Sigman SR, Cipolla GD, King SB III. Balloon overstretch injury correlates with neointimal formation and not with vascular remodeling in the pig coronary restenosis model. *J Am Coll Cardiol* 1994; **23**: 138A (abstract).

8   Nunes GL, Sgoutas DS, Sigman SR, *et al.* Vitamins C and E improve the response to coronary balloon injury in the pig: effect of vascular remodeling. *Arteroscler Throm Vasc Biol* 1995; **15**: 156–65.

9   Post MJ, Borst C, Kuntz RE. The relative importance of arterial remodeling compared with intimal hyperplasia in lumen renarrowing after balloon angioplasty: a study in the normal rabbit and the hypercholesterolemic Yucatan micropig. *Circulation* 1994; **89**: 2816–21.

10   Currier JW, Faxon DP. Restenosis after percutaneous transluminal coronary angioplasty: have we been aiming at the wrong target? *J Am Coll Cardiol* 1995; **25**: 516–20.

11   Brott BC, Labinaz M, Culp SC, *et al.* Vessel remodeling after angioplasty: comparative anatomic studies. *J Am Coll Cardiol*, 1994; **23**: 138A (abstract).

12   O'Brien ER, Alpers CE, Stewart DK, et al. Proliferation in primary and restenotic coronary atherectomy tissue: implications for antiproliferative therapy. *Circ Res* 1993; **73**: 223–31.

13   Taylor AJ, Farb A, Angello DA, Burwell LR, Virmani R. Proliferative activity in coronary atherectomy tissue. *Chest* 1995; **108**: 815–20.

14   Steele PM, Chesbro JH, Stanson AW, *et al.* Balloon angioplasty; natural history of the pathophysiologic response to injury in a pig model. *Circ Res* 1985; **57**: 105–12.

15   Geary RL, Williams JK, Golden D, *et al.* Time course of cellular proliferation, intimal hyperplasia, and remodeling following angioplasty in monkeys with established atherosclerosis: a nonhuman primate model of restenosis. *Arterioscler Thromb Vasc Biol* 1996; **16**: 34–43.

16   Mintz GS, Pichard AD, Kent KM, *et al.* Intravascular ultrasound comparison of restenotic and *de novo* coronary artery narrowings. *Am J Cardiol* 1994; **74**: 1278–80.

17   Mintz GS, Popma JJ, Pichard AD, *et al.* Arterial remodeling after coronary angioplasty: a serial intravascular ultrasound study. *Circulation* 1996; **94**: 35–43.

18   Essed CE, Van Den Brand M, Becker AE. Transluminal coronary angioplasty and early restenosis: fibrocellular occlusion after wall laceration. *Br Heart J* 1986; **110**: 1186–7.

19   Farb A, Virmani R, Atkinson JB, Kolodgie FD. Plaque morphology and pathologic changes in arteries from patients after coronary balloon angioplasty. *J Am Coll Cardiol* 1990; **16**: 1421–9.

20   Garratt KN, Edwards WD, Vietstra RE, Kaufmann UP, Holmes DR. Coronary morphology after percutaneous directional coronary atherectomy in humans: autopsy analysis of three patients. *J Am Coll Cardiol* 1990; **16**: 1432–6.

21   Ueda M, Becker AE, Fujimoto T. Pathologic changes induced by repeated percutaneous transluminal coronary angioplasty. *Br Heart J* 1987; **58**: 635–43.

22   Nobuyoshi M, Kimura T, Ohishi H, *et al.* Restenosis after percutaneous transluminal coronary angioplasty: pathologic observations in 20 patients. *J Am Coll Cardiol* 1991; **17**: 433–9.

23   Farb A, Virmani R, Atkinson JB, Anderson PE. Long-term histologic patency after percutaneous transluminal coronary angioplasty is predicted by the creation of a greater lumen area. *J Am Coll Cardiol* 1994; **24**: 1229–35.

24   Glagov S, Weisenberg E, Zarins CK, Stankunavicius R, Kolettis GJ. Compensatory enlargement of human atherosclerotic coronary arteries. *N Engl J Med* 1987; **316**: 1371–5.

25   Litovsky SH, Farb A, Burke AP, *et al.* Effect of age, race, body surface area, heart weight and atherosclerosis on coronary artery dimensions in young males. *Atherosclerosis* 1996; **123**: 243–50.

26   Kuntz RE, Safian RD, Levine MJ, *et al.* Novel approach to the analysis of restenosis after the use of three new coronary devices. *J Am Coll Cardiol* 1992; **19**: 1493–9.

27   Sangiorgi G, Farb A, Carter AJ, *et al.* Contribution of neointima and adventitia to final lumen area in human coronary arteries treated by balloon angioplasty: a histopathologic analysis. *J Am Coll Cardiol*, 1997; **29 (Suppl)**: 200.

28   Scott NA, Cipolla GD, Ross CE, *et al.* Identification of a potential role for the adventitia in vascular lesion formation after balloon overstretch injury of porcine coronary arteries. *Circulation* 1996; **93**: 2178–87.

29   Kragel AH, Reddy SG, Wittes JT, Roberts W. Morphometric analysis of the composition of coronary arterial plaques in isolated unstable angina pectoris with pain at rest. *Am J Cardiol* 1990; **66**: 562–7.

30   Liu MW, Roubin GS, King SE III. Restenosis after coronary angioplasty: potential biologic determinants and role of intimal hyperplasia. *Circulation* 1989; **79**: 1374–87.

31   Kakuta T, Currier JW, Haudenschild CC, Ryan TJ, Faxon DP. Differences in compensatory vessel enlargement, not intimal formation, account for restenosis after angioplasty in the hypercholesterolemic rabbit model. *Circulation* 1994; **89**: 2809–15.

32   Gertz SD, Gimple LW, Banai S, *et al.* Geometric remodeling is not the principal pathologenetic process in restenosis after balloon angioplasty. *Circulation* 1994; **90**: 3001–8.

33   Kolodgie FD, Katocs AS, Largis EE, *et al.* Hypercholesterolemia in the rabbit induced by feeding graded amounts of low-level cholesterol: methodological considerations regarding individual variability in response to dietary cholesterol and development of lesion type. *Arterioscler Thromb Vasc Biol* 1996; **16**: 1454–64.

34   Lafont A, Guzman LA, Whitlow PL, *et al.* Restenosis after experimental angioplasty: intimal, medial, and adventitial changes associated with constrictive remodeling. *Circ Res* 1995; **76**: 996–1002.

18

Local drug delivery with stents

Konstantinos G Kostopoulos, Kai Wang and
Ivan De Scheerder

Introduction

Abrupt or threatened vessel closure and restenosis remain the two major limitations of percutaneous transluminal coronary angioplasty (PTCA).[1,2] Indwelling endovascular stents were initially designed to reduce or even eliminate both acute or subacute coronary reclosure and late restenosis after PTCA. Although coronary stents seemed initially promising, several limitations became obvious. Major concerns that need further study are their thrombogenic properties and the induction of local hyperplastic response caused by a foreign body response.[3] Thrombogenic response following stent deployment is a matter of several contributing factors. The atherosclerotic degenerated vessel wall is prone to thrombosis due to endothelial dysfunction. Stent material itself, together with the stent-induced vascular injury, will further increase the risk of thrombotic events. On the other hand, local blood-flow disturbances caused by stent deployment, especially when the stent is not fully aligned to the vessel wall, are another significant contributing factor in the pathogenesis of thrombosis. Cellular recruitment and release of all kind of growth factors in contribution to the local thrombotic processes result in a fibromuscular proliferative response and vessel restenosis. Other factors determining the stent-related neointimal hyperplasia are the healing response induced by balloon dilatation and stent implantation, and the foreign body reaction induced by the stent itself.

Target of reduction of thrombosis and proliferation

Numerous pharmacologic agents have been tested in order to reduce acute thrombosis and hyperproliferative cellular response. The too-low active drug concentrations at the target site achieved with systemic administration are mainly responsible for the failure of therapy in clinical trials. Since endovascular stents are increasingly used it is mandatory to shift and focus our interest on the development of locally delivered inhibitory agents of both thrombotic and neointimal response. The use of stents as potential vehicles for local drug administration is considered a new challenging therapeutic modality in interventional cardiology. Its potential advantage is the fact that these stents supply a relatively large amount of drug under conditions of prolonged tissue contact. Stent-related local drug delivery will have to focus on the two major remaining problems of stenting: acute and subacute thrombosis and stent-induced neointimal hyperplasia.

Acute or subacute stent thrombosis

Stent thrombosis, acute and subacute, represents an essential part of wound healing and is related to four major determinants:

I   The thrombogenic environment caused by the underlying atherosclerotic diseased vessel and injury of the vessel wall during balloon angioplasty and stent implantation.

2 The thrombogenicity of the stent itself.

3 The relationship between the stent and the vessel wall (optimal stent alignment) determining flow characteristics.

4 Blood factors and the coagulation system.

Metallic surface modifications aim against the two inter-related components of clot formation: the increased risk of platelet aggregation and activation, as well as the factor XII activation. Any method with a potentially inhibitory effect on protein adsorption on to metallic surfaces should represent an effective means with respect to either of these two outcomes.

Coating of stents will only affect the surface of the stent and thus decrease the thrombogenicity of the stent itself. Stent-related local antithrombotic drug release can also have a positive effect on the thrombogenicity caused by the underlying atherosclerotic diseased vessel and the thrombogenicity caused by injuring the vessel wall during stent implantation.

Coating of endovascular metallic devices is a concept of preventing thrombosis by creating a relatively inert stent surface. It offers the unique advantage of improving their design by altering surface properties (Fig. 18.1). Stents, after being coated, become less thrombogenic due to a smoother surface and a lower propensity in blood protein adsorption, platelet apposition and aggregation. This way, the metallic surface itself is no longer exposed to blood products and cells. Apart from surface texture, surface electric charge, free surface energy and surface tension can be modified by coatings. Experimental studies have shown a decrease in thrombotic events after coronary stent implantation in a porcine model using polyurethane-coated stents.[4] Coated stents also have the advantage that their coating can be loaded with an antithrombotic drug either to decrease further the thrombogenicity of the stent itself or to create a local antithrombotic drug release system that could also affect the thrombogenic environment.

Heparin, which is an antithrombin III factor, has been one of the most extensively explored substances for attachment on metallic stent surfaces. Its binding on metallic surfaces has been achieved in several ways. A promising and advanced method was the one introduced by Lam *et al.*,[5] who developed the end-point attachment of heparin on artificial surfaces. According to this method, the antithrombin site of heparin molecule is preserved functionally intact and bioactive throughout the coupling reaction. In addition, the above-mentioned linking process makes the heparin molecule more biocompatible with platelets, granulocytes and macrophages than heparin itself.[6,7] Several heparin-coated stents have been tested in *in vitro* and *in vivo* models. Copper stents implanted in porcine

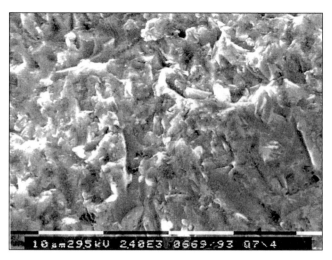

a

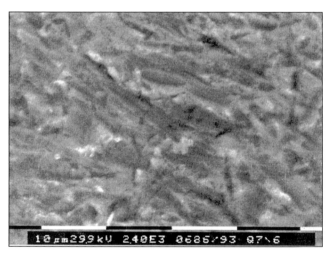

b

Figure 18.1

Coating of bare nitinol coronary stent using a polyurethane coating creating a smooth stent surface (SEM: magnification: ×2500): (a) bare nitinol stent; (b) coated stent.

coronary arteries are well known to be very thrombogenic resulting in thrombotic stent closure within hours after stent implantation. In order to evaluate the efficacy of stent coating in decreasing copper stent thrombosis, heparin and polyurethane-coated copper stents were compared to noncoated stents in pig coronary arteries. Thrombogenic events were significantly decreased in both groups of coated stents, especially in the heparin-coated stents.[8] Heparin-coated stainless-steel stents tested in nonatherosclerotic native animal vessels were also found to be less thrombogenic than the noncoated stents.[9,10] Although thrombus formation was not totally eliminated, heparin-coated stents exhibited a reduction in the rate of thrombosis and absence of angiographically detected thrombus within the first 24 hours after implantation.[11–14] When implanted in a rabbit carotid artery model, heparin-coated nitinol stents experienced less accumulation of thrombotic material than the noncoated stents.[15] Palmaz–Schatz heparin-coated stents with a Carmeda Bioactive Surface (Carmeda AB, Stockholm, Sweden) proved to provide a significant *in vitro* protection against platelet aggregation under conditions of full or incomplete stent expansion. These results suggest an additional protective effect of heparin-coated stents when stents are not fully expanded after implantation.[16] These experimental data indicate that platelet deposition and activation are inhibited in heparin-coated stents. Despite the fact of their less thrombogenic effect, heparin-coated stents tested in different species have shown conflicting results concerning neointimal hyperplastic response and late restenosis rate. In a porcine coronary model, no improvement in late vessel patency and neointimal hyperplasia was reported,[10] while other investigators noted a decrease in restenosis rate in heparin-coated stented baboon carotid arteries.[17]

Clinical data using heparin-coated stents are currently available. In the pilot phase of the BENESTENT II study, which is a multicenter, prospective and nonrandomized study, patients with a single *de novo* coronary lesion in native vessels suffering from stable angina pectoris received an elective implantation of a heparin-coated Palmaz–Schatz stent.[18] Heparin therapy was progressively postponed by 6, 12 and 36 hours following sheath removal, resulting in a 98–100% overall clinical success rate, 0% subacute stent thrombosis rate, a low incidence of vascular complications (5.9–0%) and a reduction of in-hospital stay from 7.4 to 3 days. It is noteworthy to mention that in phase IV, coumadin and heparin were replaced by 100 mg of aspirin and 250 mg ticlopidin. Six-month results were also promising, indicating an overall restenosis rate of 16%.

In our effort to overcome the problem of thrombotic processes and to accelerate wound-healing response and re-endothelization following vascular stenting, fibrin biological active coatings have been applied to stents and are currently under extensive experimental investigation. Although the deposition process of fibrin coating on stents has some inherent drawbacks, like fibrin instability outside the body and the doubtful degree of adherence on metallic surfaces, these problems seem to be under control. *In vitro* and *in vivo* animal studies showed minimal platelet adhesion to fibrin-coated titanium self-expandable and Palmaz–Schatz balloon-expandable stents and found the fibrin coating stable and durable. Eight weeks later no thrombosis or foreign body reaction in the fibrin-coated stents were found.[19,20] Although fibrin does not block the development of neointimal formation, it has been shown that it causes less

hyperplasia in comparison to other tested polymers.[21] Since fibrin is a natural hydrogel, fibrin-coated stents can also be used as molecular vehicles for gene therapy or local delivery of pharmacological agents. Fibrin-coated stents have been used as depots to deliver the RGD synthetic peptide (arginine-glycine-aspartane) in atherosclerotic animal model. Results showed a significantly lower neointimal hyperplasia in RGD-loaded fibrin coating stented arteries than in the uncoated controls.[22] Pathologic data from modified fibrin-coated titanium self-expandable and Palmaz–Schatz balloon-expandable stents, seeded with endothelial cells, have demonstrated increased biocompatibility and reduced thrombogenicity when tested in animal models.[19] When fibrin and basement membrane components were used as Wiktor stent coating implanted in porcine coronary arteries, they also showed excellent results as far as short-term vessel wall patency and neointimal hyperplasia were concerned.[23] To date, no fibrin-coated stents have been used in human beings. Elimination of viral or bacterial contamination during the preparation and development of a human-compatible fibrin-coating in order to avoid the risk of immunological reactions, remain unsolved problems.

The experimental evaluation of a new polylactic acid stent coating impregnated with hirudin and prostacyclin analogs revealed a significant reduction of intimal hyperplasia.[24] The effect on platelet thrombus formation of a potent GPIIB/IIIA inhibitor when locally delivered on composite polymer-metal stents was tested in a canine coronary artery model. When compared to uncovered standard metallic stents, a significant reduction in platelet aggregation and deposition was noted.[25] The same results were noted when the monoclonal antibody AZ1, directed against the platelet GPIIB/IIIA, alone or conjugated with urokinase, was passively immobilized to polymer-coated stents and tested in a rabbit iliac artery model. Neointimal proliferation, however, was found unaltered when compared to control stented arteries.[26,27] In animal experimental models, Palmaz–Schatz stents' thrombogenicity has been successfully modified by coating them with a NO donor, inhibiting platelet activity.[28,29] Other possible antiplatelet or antithrombin drug candidates for local delivery loaded on stents are salicylates, dipyridamole, ticlopidine and additional thrombin or antithrombin III inhibitors such as low molecular weight heparin, R-hirudin, hirulog, argatroban, efegatran, tick anticoagulant peptide and Ppack.

Short-term local arterial delivery of forskolin, a nonpolar adenylate cyclase activator with vasodilator and antiplatelet properties, loaded on polymer-coated removable nitinol stents, was extensively studied.[30] High and active local drug concentrations dependent on the presence of stent-to-tissue gradients were found in forskolin-coated stents. This study also demonstrated that the highest drug activity was present just in the microenvironment of the arterial damage, where the stent was embedded into the injured arterial wall.

Stent-induced neointimal hyperplasia

A great number of different metallic intracoronary stents are now available, mostly useful in cases of abrupt or threatened closure and suboptimal post-PTCA results. Elective stenting in selected patients with *de novo* focal lesions has also been approved for the reduction of restenosis and the need for repeat interventions.[31,32] However, all stents represent permanent foreign devices and coronary stenting is still associated with another foreign body-related complication: increased neointimal hyperplasia. Theoretically, the perfect metallic stent is the one provided with optimal mechanical properties and biocompatibility with living tissues. Biocompatibility refers to the absence of any kind of tissue response triggered by an implant. Following stent deployment, there are two different types of tissues coming in direct contact with metallic surface: blood and vascular wall. Thrombus plays an important role in healing after arterial injury and may affect the development of neointimal hyperplasia.

The process of restenosis begins with injury to the arterial wall, resulting in the release of thrombogenic, chemotactic and growth factors. Aggregated platelets are activated, releasing mitogenic factors. Afterwards, lymphocytes and macrophages are accumulated and release other factors with mitogenic and chemotactic properties. The final result is the formation of thrombus and the initiation of a restenosis process. Intimal hyperplasia represents a hypertrophic response to endothelial injury, which involves migration and proliferation of smooth muscle cells and fibroblasts in the subendothelium and medial layer. Almost one third of all stented coronary arteries exhibit diameter reduction exceeding 50%. Reduction or even elimination of both stent surface thrombogenicity and response to local injury appear to be attractive future approaches. It is noteworthy to mention that although stent thrombosis seems to be dependent on both surface material and the severity of vessel injury, stent materials have not been importantly implicated in intimal growth processes. On the other hand, since optimal stent expansion and aggressive combined per oral antiplatelet treatment did prove to be effective to reduce cardiac events and in particular thrombotic occlusion of stented vessels, it is reasonable to direct our efforts primarily at the restenosis process itself.[33]

Hyperplastic response following balloon angioplasty is the principal drawback limiting the long-term success of intracoronary interventions in a substantial portion of treated patients. Several animal models of arterial injury have been proposed and thoroughly studied to test potential therapies.[34] Swine coronary arteries have shown similar vascular response to human coronary arteries when injured. A more pronounced hyperplastic response due to a substantial neointimal thickening has been documented when severe mechanical injury is caused by an oversized metal stent. The amount of neointimal thickening has proved to be directly proportional to the degree of locally induced trauma that is ordinally proportional to injury depth.[35] A more pronounced smooth muscle cell stimulation occurs when a greater degree of stent radial forces are encountered by excessively oversized devices. Quantitative angiographic studies in humans have shown that the initial optimal results after stenting are partially balanced by a greater degree of late loss.[31,32] Intravascular ultrasound studies have also demonstrated the contribution of intimal hyperplasia in the in-stent restenotic process.[36]

Experimental and clinical efforts in animal models and human beings to decrease the degree of luminal restenosis following intraluminal angioplastic interventions, by systemic medical treatment, have been disappointing. Local delivery of agents with antiproliferative properties seems to be a promising alternative of treating the restenosis process. Stents are potential carriers of such compounds. As mentioned before, no difference has been found in intimal thickness between heparin-coated and noncoated stents implanted in animal arteries.[9,10] This finding may be surprising since earlier experimental studies suggest that platelets, thrombin and mural thrombosis are involved in the restenosis process.[37] These findings open the debate on what is the real importance of platelet adhesion and mural thrombi formation on neointimal hyperplasia after stent implantation. After balloon angioplasty, organization of mural thrombi seems to play a major role in the restenosis process. Studies with heparin-coated stents suggest, however, that this is less the case after stent implantation. Other factors, such as deep injury caused by the deployment of the stent in the diseased artery and the implantation of a foreign body inducing a foreign body response, are potentially more important in the pathogenesis of neointimal hyperplasia after stent implantation. Another point is, of course, the dose of heparin locally available. Intimal hyperplastic response could be theoretically inhibited only when the locally delivered pharmacologic agent is present in adequate doses and when it represents an effective one in decreasing this biologic response to injury. There is recent experimental evidence showing that heparin-coated tantalum stents can reduce neointimal formation when deployed in baboon carotid arteries.[17] It can be speculated that with improved stent-coating techniques, resulting in higher concentrations of locally delivered heparin, a decrease in intimal proliferation over the stent itself may be possible. The combined stent covering with two different pharmacologic agents, one antithrombotic on the luminal surface and another antiproliferative on its surface adjacent to the media, seems to be an attractive alternative modality.

A large number of agents initially used in systemic delivery models, with potent antiplatelet and/or antiproliferative properties, are now tested as a local stent delivery system. Polyorganophosphazene polymer-coated metallic stents loaded with angiopeptin, a somatostatin analog, have been assessed in porcine coronary arteries. Although vessel narrowing was less pronounced in the angiopeptin-coated stents, histiolymphocytic and fibromuscular reactions were found to be the same in both angiopeptin and nonangiopeptin-coated groups.[38] Corticosteroids are also known for their *in vitro* capability to decrease vascular smooth muscle cell proliferation and local inflammatory response. Dexamethasone proved to be useful in the *in vitro* attenuation of early inflammatory response to vascular injury by inhibiting the PDGF-related monocyte migration.[39] When a dexamethasone microlayer was loaded on to the surface of tantalum wire-coil stents and implanted in porcine coronary arteries, tissue response was found to be the same in both dexamethasone coated and nondexamethasone poly-

L-lactic acid-coated stents. It was postulated that the absence of a significant limitation of the neointimal proliferation in this animal model was caused by too low drug concentrations.[40] However, it is well known that poly-L-lactic acid coatings can induce a severe histiolymphocytic reaction which may balance the positive effect of dexamethasone in this study model.[35,41] Local methylprednisolone delivery using a polyorganophosphazene polymer-coated metallic stent has also been studied in swine coronary arteries (Figs 18.2 and 18.3). This corticosteroid compound was found effective in the inhibition of foreign body response induced by polymer-coated stents.[42] Colchicine, a drug with anti-inflammatory, antimytotic and migration inhibitory properties, is also under investigation. Tantalum wire-coil stents coated with this agent in different

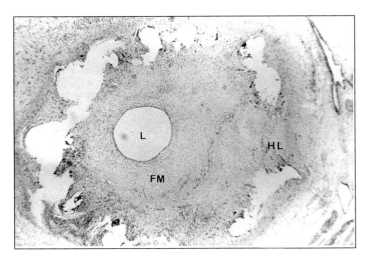

a

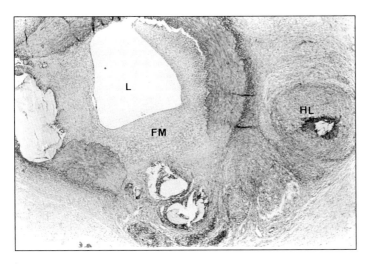

b

Figure 18.2

The effect of methylprednisolone coating of polyorganophosphazene-coated stents. (a) polyorganophosphazene-coated stent showing a severe histiolymphocytic reaction surrounding the stent filaments and the remainings of the polymer, resulting in a severe fibromuscular proliferation and vessel lumen narrowing; (b) methylprednisolone-loaded stent showing a less pronounced histiolymphocytic reaction and a decreased fibromuscular proliferation, resulting in a better lumen area at follow-up. (L: vessel lumen; FM: fibromuscular proliferation; HL: histiolymphocytic reaction.)

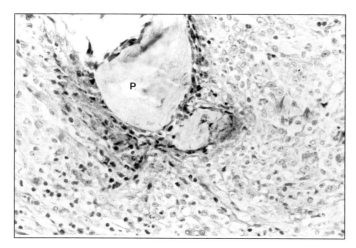

a

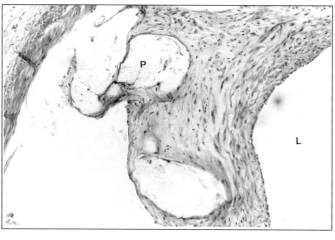

b

Figure 18.3
(a) Higher magnification of a polyphosphazene-coated stent showing a severe histiolymphocytic reaction surrounding the remainings of the polymer; (b) methylprednisolone-loaded stent showing only a minimal histiolymphocytic reaction. (P: polymer remainings; L: vessel lumen.)

quantities and implanted in porcine coronary arteries produced marked hyperproliferative changes with increased cellular infiltration, fibrosis and medial thickening.[43] The effect on neointimal proliferation after stent implantation has also been tested for methotrexate and other cytostatic agents in animal models.[44] Several other possible antiproliferative compounds such as ciprostene and ilprost (prostacyclin analogs), slow calcium channel blockers, estrogens, cyclosporine, cytarabine, fusion proteins binding growth factors, ketanserine and PDGF-inhibitor trapidil are candidates for local release when being absorbed to stents. Recently, the effect of inert coatings such as silicon carbide or diamond-like coating has also been evaluated in decreasing intimal hyperplasia. Silicon carbide-coated stents tested in iliac rabbit arteries have shown normal endothelialization with a very low degree of vascular smooth muscle cell proliferation 6 months after implantation.[45]

While restenosis in previously stented coronary arteries is a process related to the degree of muscle cell-mediated neointimal hyperplasia, any kind of 'active' stent that could inhibit this response should be interesting. Intracoronary local radiation is a relatively simple method to inhibit intimal proliferative response after stent implantation. Radioactive ^{32}P impregnated beta-particle-emitting stents have been developed and are under clinical evaluation. Their efficacy to inhibit neointimal hyperplasia has been demonstrated in several animal models.[46–49]

Drug-loaded biodegradable polymer stents

Limited drug-loading capacity and inadequate sustained local drug release are considerable limitations of coated metallic stents. Together with the relatively short-term concerns of postprocedural problems such as acute closure and restenosis, the permanence of metal stents seems to be unnecessary. Bioabsorbable stents permitting adequate drug delivery and mechanical support for a reasonable time period could be more ideal. A great number of polymers have been developed, but no completely blood-compatible polymers are yet available.

A potential transformation to a more biocompatible polymer stent could be achieved by loading it with antiplatelet or antithrombotic agents. The most promising polymers for future stent use are polyphosphate esters, polyaminocarbonates, polyhydroxybutyrate and hyaluronic acid polymers.

There is strong evidence that biodegradable stents can induce an inflammatory and thrombotic response. The Kyoto University, the Cleveland Clinic-Mayo-Thoraxcenter and the Duke bioabsorbable stents have been studied in animal models.[50–52] A sterilized poly-L-lactide biodegradable, open mesh, self-expanding stent proved to be the most advantageous when soaked with heparin. Heparin-coated bioabsorbable stents have also shown decreased thrombogenic reactions when compared to noncoated.[53] Biodegradable stents consisting of a combination of polylactic acid and polycaprolactone act as devices capable of the delivery of gene transfer vectors to the rabbit arterial wall.[54] However, smooth muscle cell proliferative response could not be prevented in experimental animal models.[55] Biodegradable endoluminal polymer paving layers have also proven to be alternative means of effective local heparin delivery and may yield a flexible future clinical method in providing several pharmacologic agents after interventional intravascular procedures.[56]

Cell seeding

Endothelial cell-coated stents seem to be a promising concept, since acute or subacute thrombosis is an event that occurs before the complete endothelialization of an implanted metallic stent. Preliminary results using Palmaz–Schatz stents seeded by endothelial stents and implanted in rabbit iliac arteries are encouraging. The most important advantage of endothelial cell-seeded stent implantation is the faster re-endothelialization of the arterial segment underlying the stent itself. The ability for stent endothelial coating with autologous endothelial cells obtained from the individual to whom the stent is planned to be deployed seems feasible. However, despite the fact that metallic stents can be coated with functionally active endothelial cells, and are implantable into *in vitro* systems, this process is of limited clinical use at the present time.[57,58] Perhaps the autologous vein graft-coated stent is the most representative and ideally biocompatible, nonthrombogenic stent. Experimental and clinical studies investigate its utility in the reduction of acute and subacute thrombosis and restenosis after coronary angioplasty.[59,60]

Stent-mediated gene therapy

Gene therapy is also currently under study to decrease postangioplasty neointimal hyperplasia. Gene therapy depicts the transportation of a gene modifying the healing response and decreasing the neointimal hyperplasia in the injured arterial wall by seeding cells that have been previously transfected with a desired gene, by transfer of gene vectors or by introducing naked DNA. Such an introduction and endothelial or muscular layer colonization can also be achieved by using DNA-coated stents as gene carriers.[61,62]

Intravascular stents can be successfully implanted, when first loaded with genetically engineered endothelial cells, which are either specifically labelled or directed to secrete a specific therapeutic protein. *In vivo* use of such stents can directly introduce genetically transformed cells into the vascular wall and improve the function of the stents by the local release of anticoagulants, thrombolytics or antiproliferative agents.[61] Genetically modified endothelial cells with increased surface fibrinolytic activity have proved to express a favorable antithrombotic and antiproliferative outcome.[63]

Conclusions

Interest for local drug delivery with stents will remain high in the future, mostly because of the absence of any systemic pharmaceutical active means of reducing the restenosis rate after arterial angioplasty interventions. Material-induced acute and subacute thrombotic events are almost kept under clinical control since the introduction of potent antiplatelet drugs. However, other problems such as material biocompatibility, improvements in techniques of drug loading and release of active antiproliferative agents for a precise modification of the local response to arterial injury and foreign body response need further investigation. While a systemic suppression of locally active potential growth stimuli cannot be accomplished, the reasonably conceptual strategy would be a kind of stent with multidrug and time-controlled delivery properties preventing thrombotic and/or hyperproliferative response.

References

1 Ellis SG, Roubin GS, King SB III, *et al.* Angiographic and clinical predictors of acute closure after native vessel coronary angioplasty. *Circulation* 1988; **77**: 372–9.

2 Lincoff AM, Popma JJ, Ellis SG, Hacker JA, Topol EJ. Abrupt vessel closure complicating coronary angioplasty: clinical, angiographic and therapeutic profile. *J Am Coll Cardiol* 1992; **19**: 926–35.

3 Eeckhout E, Kappenberger L, Goy JJ. Stents for intracoronary placement: current status and future directions. *J Am Coll Cardiol* 1996; **27**: 757–65.

4 De Scheerder IK, Wilczek KL, Verbeken EV, *et al.* Biocompatibility of polymer-coated oversized metallic stents implanted in normal porcine coronary arteries. *Atherosclerosis* 1995; **114**: 105–14.

5 Larm O, Larsson R, Olsson P. A new non-thrombogenic surface prepared by selective covalent binding of heparin via a reducing terminal residue. *Biomat Med Dev Artif Org* 1983; **11**: 161–74.

6 Larm O, Larsson R, Olsson P. Surface-immobilized heparin. In: Lane DA, Lindahl U (eds). *Heparin. Chemical and Biological Properties. Clinical Applications* (London: Edward Arnold, 1989): 597–608.

7 Larsson R, Larm O, Olsson P. The search for thromboresistance using immobilized heparin. *Ann NY Acad Sci* 1987; **516**: 102–15.

8 Wilczek KL, De Scheerder IK, Wang K, *et al.* Implantation of balloon expandable copper stents in porcine coronary arteries. A model for testing the efficacy of stent coating in decreasing stent thrombogenicity. *Eur Heart J* 1996; **17 (Suppl)**: 455 (abstract).

9 Hardhammar PA, van Beusekom HM, Emanuelsson HU, *et al.* Reduction in thrombotic events with heparin-coated Palmaz–Schatz stents in normal porcine coronary arteries. *Circulation* 1996; **93**: 423–30.

10 De Scheerder IK, Wang K, Wilczek KL, Meuleman D, Piessens JH. Heparin coating of metallic coronary stents decrease their thrombogenicity but does not decrease neointima hyperplasia. *Circulation* 1995; **92 (Suppl)**: I-535 (abstract).

11 Bonan R, Bhat K, Lefevre T, *et al.* Coronary artery stenting after angioplasty with self-expanding parallel wire metallic stents. *Am Heart J* 1991; **121**: 1522–30.

12 Rogers C, Karnovsky MJ, Edelman ER. Inhibition of experimental neointimal hyperplasia and thrombosis depends on the type of vascular injury and the site of drug administration. *Circulation* 1993; **88**: 1215–21.

13 Jeong MH, Owen WG, Staab ME, *et al.* Does heparin release coating of the Wallstent limit thrombosis and platelet deposition? Results in a porcine carotid injury model. *Circulation* 1995; **92 (Suppl)**: I-37 (abstract).

14 Bailey SR, Paige S, Lunn A, Palmaz J. Heparin coating of endovascular stents decreases subacute thrombosis in a rabbit model. *Circulation* 1992; **86 (Suppl I)**: I-186 (abstract).

15 Sheth S, Park KD, Dev V, *et al.* Prevention of stent subacute thrombosis by segmented polyurethanurea-polyethylene oxide-heparin coating in rabbit carotid. *J Am Coll Cardiol* 1994; **23 (Suppl)**: 187A (abstract).

16 Kocsis JF, Lunn AC, Mohammad SF. Incomplete expansion of coronary stents: risk of thrombogenesis and protection provided by a heparin coating. *J Am Coll Cardiol* 1996; **27 (Suppl A)**: 84A (abstract).

17 Chronos NAF, Robinson KA, Kelly A, *et al.* Neointima formation in stented baboon carotid arteries is reduced by bonded heparin: correlation with decreased thrombogenicity. *J Am Coll Cardiol* 1996; **27 (Suppl A)**: 85A (abstract).

18 Serruys PW, Emanuelsson H, van der Giessen W, *et al.* Heparin-coated Palmaz–Schatz stents in human coronary arteries. Early outcome of the Benestent-II Pilot Study. *Circulation* 1996; **93**: 412–22.

19 Kipshidze N, Baker JE, Nikolaychik V. Fibrin coated stents as an improved vehicle for endothelial cell seeding. *Circulation* 1994; **90**: I-597.

20 Baker JE, Horn JB, Nikolaychik V, Kipshidze N. Fibrin stent coatings. In: Sigwart U (ed.). *Endoluminal Stenting* (London: WB Saunders, 1996): 84–9.

21 Holmes DR, Camrud AR, Jorgenson MA, Edwards WD, Schwartz RS. Polymeric stenting in the porcine coronary artery model: differential outcome of exogenous fibrin sleeves versus polyurethane-coated stents. *J Am Coll Cardiol* 1994; **24**: 525–31.

22 Baker JE, Nikolaychik V, Zulich A, Komorowski R, Kipshidze N. Fibrin coated stents as a depot to deliver RGD peptide inhibit vascular reaction in atherosclerotic rabbit model. *J Am Coll Cardiol* 1996; **27 (Suppl A)**: 197A (abstract).

23 Van Beusekom HMM, Van Vliet HHDM, Van der Giessen WJ. Fibrin and basement membrane components, as a biocompatible and thromboresistant coating for metal stents. *Eur Heart J* 1994; **15 (Suppl)**: 378 (abstract).

24 Pasquantonio J, Beilharz EJ, Preter D, *et al.* A new hirudin/prostacyclin analog releasing polylactic acid stent coating reduces restenosis in sheep. *Eur Heart J* 1996; **17 (Suppl)**: 177 (abstract).

25 Tanguay JF, Santos RM, Kruse KR, *et al.* Local delivery of a potent GPIIB/IIIA inhibitor using a composite polymeric stent reduces platelet deposition. *Eur Heart J* 1996; **17 (Suppl)**: 454 (abstract).

26 Aggarwal RK, Martin W, Ireland DC, Azrin MA, de Bono DP, Gershlick AH. Effects of polymer-coated stents eluting antibody to platelet GPIIb/IIIa on platelet deposition and neointima formation. *Eur Heart J* 1996; **17 (Suppl)**: 176 (abstract).

27 Aggarwal RK, Ireland DC, Ragheb A, de Bono DP, Gershlick AH. Reduction in thrombogenicity of polymer-coated stents by immobilization of platelet-targeted urokinase. *Eur Heart J* 1996; **17 (Suppl)**: 177 (abstract).

28 Folts JD, Maalej N, Keaney JF, Loscalzo J. Coating Palmaz–Schatz stents with a unique NO donor renders them much less thrombogenic when placed in pig carotid arteries. *Circulation* 1995; **92 (Suppl)**: I-670 (abstract).

29 Makkar RR, Eigler NL, Nakamura M, *et al.* Marked inhibition of acute stent thrombosis by a novel nitric oxide donor. *Circulation* 1995; **92 (Suppl)**: I-688 (abstract).

30 Lambert TL, Dev V, Rechavia E, Forrester JS, Litvack F, Eigler NL. Localized arterial wall drug delivery from a polymer-coated removable metallic stent. Kinetics, distribution and bioactivity of forskolin. *Circulation* 1994; **90**: 1003–11.

31 Fischmann DL, Leon MB, Baim DS, *et al.* A randomized comparison of coronary-stent placement and balloon angioplasty in the treatment of coronary artery disease. *N Engl J Med* 1994; **331**: 496–501.

32 Serruys PW, de Jaegere P, Kiemeneij F, *et al.* A comparison of balloon expandable stent implantation with balloon angioplasty in patients with coronary artery disease. *N Engl J Med* 1994; **331**: 489–95.

33 Schomig A, Neumann FJ, Kastrati A, *et al.* A randomized comparison of antiplatelet and anticoagulant therapy after the placement of coronary artery stents. *N Engl J Med* 1996; **334**: 1084–9.

34 Muller D, Ellis S, Topol E. Experimental models of coronary artery restenosis. *J Am Coll Cardiol* 1992; **19**: 418–32.

35 Schwartz R, Huber K, Murphy J, *et al.* Restenosis and the proportional neointimal response to coronary artery injury: results in a porcine model. *J Am Coll Cardiol* 1992; **19**: 267–74.

36 Dussaillant GR, Mintz GS, Pichard AD, *et al.* Small stent size and intimal hyperplasia contribute to restenosis: a volumetric intravascular ultrasound analysis. *J Am Coll Cardiol* 1995; **26**: 720–4.

37 Haudenschild CC. Restenosis: pathophysiologic considera-

tions. In: Topol E (ed.). *Textbook of Interventional Cardiology* (Philadelphia: WB Saunders, 1994): 382–99.

38 De Scheerder I, Wilczek K, Van Dorpe J, *et al.* Local angiopeptin delivery using coated stents reduces neointimal proliferation in overstretched porcine coronary arteries. *J Inv Cardiol* 1996; **8**: 215–22.

39 Poon M, Hsu WC, Zhang H, Taubman MB. Dexamethasone inhibits vascular smooth muscle cell mediated monocyte migration. *Circulation* 1994; **90**: I-462 (abstract).

40 Lincoff AM, Furst JG, Ellis SG, Topol EJ. Sustained local drug delivery by a novel intravascular eluting stent to prevent restenosis in the porcine coronary artery. *J Am Coll Cardiol* 1994; **23 (Suppl)**: 18A (abstract).

41 Lincoff AM, Schwartz RS, van der Giessen WJ, *et al.* Biodegradable polymers can evoke a unique inflammatory response when implanted in the coronary artery. *Circulation* 1992; **86 (Suppl)**: I-801 (abstract).

42 De Scheerder IK, Wang K, Wilczek K, *et al.* Local methylprednisolone inhibition of foreign body response to coated intracoronary stents. *Cor Art Dis* 1996; **7**: 161–6.

43 Eccleston DS, Lincoff AM, Furst JG. Administration of colchicine using a novel prolonged delivery stent produces a marked local biological effect within the porcine coronary artery. *Circulation* 1995; **92 (Suppl)**: I-85 (abstract).

44 Cox DA, Anderson PG, Roubin GS, Chou CY, Agrawal SK, Carender JB. Effects of local delivery of heparin and methotrexate on neointimal proliferation in stented porcine coronary arteries. *Cor Art Dis* 1992; **3**: 237–48.

45 Unverdorben M, Schywalsky M, Labahn D, *et al.* A new silicon carbide coated stent-experience in the rabbit. *Eur Heart J* 1996; **17 (Suppl)**: 178 (abstract).

46 Hehrlein C, Donges K, Gollan C, Metz J, Fehnsenfeld P. Low-dose radioactive Palmaz–Schatz stents prevent smooth muscle cell proliferation and neointimal hyperplasia in rabbits. *J Am Coll Cardiol* 1995; **25 (Suppl)**: 9A (abstract).

47 Laird JR, Carter AJ, Kufs WM, *et al.* Inhibition of neointimal proliferation with a beta particle emitting stent. *J Am Coll Cardiol* 1995; **25 (Suppl)**: 287A (abstract).

48 Fiscell TA. Radioactive stents for the prevention of neointimal hyperplasia. In: Sigwart U (ed.). *Endoluminal Stenting* (London: WB Saunders, 1996): 134–8.

49 Carter AJ, Laird JR, Hoopes TG. Histology after placement of a β-particle emitting stent: insights into inhibition of neointimal formation. *J Am Coll Cardiol* 1996; **27 (Suppl A)**: 198A (abstract).

50 Susawa T, Shiraki K, Shimizu Y. Biodegradable intracoro-

nary stents in adult dogs. *J Am Coll Cardiol* 1993; **21 (Suppl I)**: 483A (abstract).

51 Lincoff AM, van der Giessen WJ, Schwartz RS, *et al.* Biodegradable and biostable polymers may both cause vigorous inflammatory responses when implanted in the porcine coronary artery. *J Am Coll Cardiol* 1993; **21 (Suppl I)**: 179A (abstract).

52 Stack RS, Califf RM, Phillips HR, *et al.* Interventional cardiac catheterization at Duke Medical Center. *Am J Cardiol* 1988; **62**: 3F–24F.

53 Zidar JP, Mohammad SF, Culp SC, Brott BC, Phillips HR, Stack RS. *In vitro* thrombogenicity analysis of a new bioabsorbable balloon-expandable, endovascular stent. *J Am Coll Cardiol* 1993; **21 (Suppl I)**: 483A (abstract).

54 Landau C, Willard JE, Clagett GP, Eberhart RC, Meidell RS. Biodegradable stents function as vehicles for vascular delivery of recombinant adenovirus vectors. *Circulation* 1995; **92 (Suppl)**: I-670 (abstract).

55 Gao R, Shi R, Qiao S, Song L, Li Y, Tang C. A novel polymeric local heparin delivery stent: initial experimental study. *J Am Coll Cardiol* 1996; **27 (Suppl A)**: 85A (abstract).

56 Slepian MJ, Campbell PK, Berrigan K, *et al.* Biodegradable endoluminal polymer layers provide sustained transmural heparin delivery to the arterial wall *in vitro*. *Circulation* 1994; **90**: I-20 (abstract).

57 Bailey SR. Endothelial seeding. In: Sigwart U (ed.). *Endoluminal Stenting* (London: WB Saunders, 1996): 94–101.

58 Flugelman MY, Virmani R, Leon MB, Bowman RL, Dichek DA. Genetically engineered endothelial cells remain adherent and viable after stent deployment and exposure to flow *in vitro*. *Circ Res* 1992; **70**: 348–54.

59 Toutouzas KP, Stefanadis C, Vlachopoulos C, *et al.* Autologous vein graft-coated stent: a comparative experimental study with conventional stenting. *Eur Heart J* 1996; **17 (Suppl)**: 178 (abstract).

60 Stefanadis C, Tsiamis E, Toutouzas K, *et al.* Autologous vein graft-coated stent in coronary artery disease: the first implantation in *de novo* lesions in human. *Circulation* 1995; **92 (Suppl)**: I-544 (abstract).

61 Dichek DA, Neville RF, Zwiebel JA, Freeman SM, Leon MB, Anderson WF. Seeding of intravascular stents with genetically engineered endothelial cells. *Circulation* 1989; **80**: 1347–53.

62 Plautz G, Nabel E, Nabel GJ. Introduction of vascular smooth muscle cells expressing recombinant genes *in vivo*. *Circulation* 1991; **83**: 578–83.

63 Sawa H, Vinogradsky B, Guala A, Fujii S. Genetically engineered endothelial cells: increased surface fibrinolysis and potential adaptation to endovascular stenting. *Circulation* 1995; **92 (Suppl)**: I-53 (abstract).

IV

Molecular and Vascular Pathophysiology

19

Arterial gene transfer for therapeutic angiogenesis: early clinical results

Jeffrey M Isner, Ann Pieczek, Robert Schainfeld, Richard Blair, Laura Haley and Takayuki Asahara

Introduction

The prognosis for patients with chronic critical leg ischemia, i.e. rest pain and/or established lesions which jeopardize the integrity of the lower limbs, is often poor. Psychological testing of such patients has typically disclosed quality-of-life indices similar to those of patients with cancer in critical or even terminal phases of their illness.[1] It has been estimated that 150 000 in toto[2] require lower-limb amputations for ischemic disease in the USA per year. Their prognosis after amputation is even worse:[3] the perioperative mortality for below-knee amputation in most series is 5–10% and for above-knee amputation 15–20%. Even when they survive, nearly 40% will have died within 2 years of their first major amputation; a major amputation is required in 30% of cases, and full mobility is achieved in only 50% of below-knee and 25% of above-knee amputees.

These grim statistics are compounded by the lack of efficacious drug therapy. As concluded in the Consensus Document of the European Working Group on Critical Leg Ischemia,[3] '... there presently is inadequate evidence from published studies to support the routine use of primary pharmacological treatment in patients with critical leg ischemia ...'. Evidence for the utility of medical therapy in the treatment of claudication is no better.[4,5] Consequently, the need for alternative treatment strategies in such patients is compelling.

The therapeutic implications of angiogenic growth factors were identified by the pioneering work of Folkman and colleagues over two decades ago.[6–8] More recent investigations have established the feasibility of using recombinant formulations of such angiogenic growth fac-

tors to expedite and/or augment collateral artery development in animal models of myocardial and hindlimb ischemia.[9–15] This novel strategy for the treatment of vascular insufficiency has been termed 'therapeutic angiogenesis'.[16]

Among the various growth factors which have been shown to promote angiogenesis,[17,18] vascular endothelial growth factor (VEGF),[19] also known as vascular permeability factor (VPF)[20] and vasculotropin (VAS),[21] is an endothelial cell-specific mitogen. Because endothelial cells represent the critical cell type responsible for new vessel formation,[22–24] and because smooth muscle cells—one of the critical cell types responsible for the development of certain vascular lesions[25–27]—would not be directly activated, cell-type specificity has been considered to represent an important advantage of VEGF for therapeutic angiogenesis.

VEGF is further distinguished from other angiogenic cytokines by the fact that the first exon of the VEGF gene includes a secretory signal sequence which permits the protein to be naturally secreted from intact cells.[28] Previous studies from the authors' laboratory[29,30] have shown that arterial gene transfer of cDNA encoding for a secreted protein could yield a meaningful biological outcome despite a low transfection efficiency. We therefore performed preclinical animal studies to establish the feasibility of site-specific gene transfer of phVEGF$_{165}$, encoding the 165-amino acid isoform of VEGF, applied to the hydrogen polymer coating of an angioplasty balloon,[31] and delivered percutaneously to the iliac artery of rabbits in which the femoral artery had been excised to cause unilateral hindlimb ischemia.[32] Analysis of the transfected internal iliac arteries using reverse transcription–polymerase chain reaction (RT–PCR) confirmed reproducible gene expression at the mRNA level for up to 21 days postgene transfer.[33] Augmented development of collateral vessels was documented by serial angiograms in vivo, and increased capillary density at necropsy.[34] Consequent amelioration of the hemodynamic deficit in the ischemic limb was documented by improvement in the calf blood pressure ratio (ischemic/normal limb), as well as increased resting and maximum vasodilator-induced blood flow[35] in the VEGF-transfected animals versus controls transfected with a reporter gene. These findings formed the basis for the current clinical investigation.

Based on these preclinical studies, the authors developed clinically applicable strategies for therapeutic angiogenesis employing either recombinant human VEGF protein (rhVEGF)[12] or the gene-encoding VEGF (phVEGF).[36] Because the protein is not yet available for human application, in December 1994 the authors initiated clinical trials of human gene therapy involving percutaneous arterial gene transfer of phVEGF for patients with critical limb ischemia. The gene-encoding VEGF is delivered as so-called 'naked DNA', i.e. DNA unassociated with other vectors, including viruses or liposomes. The solution of plasmid DNA is applied to the hydrogel coating of an angioplasty balloon; the polymer acts as a 'sponge' to retain DNA until the balloon is inflated at the site of gene transfer, at which time the DNA is transferred to the arterial wall.

Clinical course

The first 8 patients to receive phVEGF$_{165}$ arterial gene transfer included 5 men and 3 women ranging in age from 54 to 92 years (m + SEM = 71.9 ± 12.6) (Table 19.1).

Four patients presented with ischemic ulcers of the foot and/or toes. In these 4 patients, the size of the ulcers at the time of presentation ranged from 1 cm × 1 cm to 7 cm × 3 cm; the depth ranged from 2 cm (2 patients) to 3 cm (2 patients). During the time required to complete screen tests prescribed by the protocol prior to gene therapy, tissue loss continued to progress in all 4 patients, despite optimized foot care. By the time of gene transfer, the ulcers ranged in size from 1 cm × 1 cm to 5 cm × 8 cm.

In one of the two patients with an ulcer (no. 3, Table 19.1), who received 1000 µg of phVEGF$_{165}$, the size and depth of the ulcer appeared to stabilize for a period of approximately 2 months following arterial gene transfer—the progressive increase in the size of this ulcer pregene therapy vs. the apparent plateau observed for 2 months' postgene therapy. During these 2 months, the patient experienced a reduction in rest pain, sufficient to allow him to proceed with a 2-week trip abroad. Near the end of this trip, which involved extensive walking, the patient experi-

enced an increase in rest pain and the ulceration of the great toe became gangrenous. Subsequently, the patient was referred back to his physician for amputation of his left great toe and distal bypass surgery using a composite graft. Two weeks following surgery, the patient returned for a transmetatarsal amputation. Patient no. 8 had a similar course; despite developing angiographic evidence of new collateral vessels (see below), she ultimately underwent a below-knee amputation.

Three patients presented with claudication and rest pain unassociated with loss of tissue integrity. Rest pain in each of these patients was manifested principally by nocturnal episodes of forefoot pain, waking the patients from sleep; the pain was typically relieved by placing the affected limb in a dependent position. At 3 months' postgene therapy, all 3 patients remain free of rest pain. Prior to gene therapy, all 3 patients also complained of claudication at less than 100 m on a level surface. At 3 months' follow-up, patient no. 5 was walking more than 0.5 miles/day without pain; in patients nos. 6 and 7 the extent of pain-free walking was unchanged.

Ankle-brachial index (ABI)

The ABI measured prior to gene therapy ranged from 0 to 0.47 (0.31 ± 0.15). Compared to the ABI measured prior to gene therapy, the mean value of measurements recorded for each patient at weekly intervals up to 3 months' postgene therapy did not improve by more than 0.1, the increment suggested to represent a significant change following angioplasty or reconstructive surgery.[37]

Magnetic resonance angiography (MRA)

One patient (no. 4) with a permanent cardiac pacemaker was not studied by MRA. In 3 patients (nos. 1–3), no significant change was apparent on serial assessment of MRA scans. In the last 3 patients to receive the 1000 µg dose, however, MRA performed subsequent to gene transfer demonstrated improved perfusion of the infrapopliteal circulation. In no. 5 (Fig. 19.1), optimization of signal intensity was noted by 6 weeks, involving a large corkscrew-appearing collateral and the peroneal artery subserved by this collateral artery. In no. 6 (Fig. 19.2), improvement in flow, inferred from an increase in signal intensity in the posterior tibial and peroneal arteries, was observed by 3 weeks' follow-up. In no. 7 (Fig. 19.3), improved flow involving all three major infrapopliteal arteries, but most prominent in the peroneal and posterior tibial, was optimal by 4 weeks' postgene transfer; geniculate collateral vessels

Table 19.1 Clinical features of patients treated with phVEGF₁₆₅.

Pt	Sex	Age	Cigs	DM	Rutherford Class	ABI	Prev Rx	Rest pain +/0	Dur'n	Meds	Ulcer +/0	Dur'n	Loc'n	Size	Depth‡	Other	Vascular occlusion in affected limb DF	SFA	Pop	AT	PT	Per	BP
1	M	54	+	0	5	0.43	Fem-fem BP; fem-pop BP†; PTA of fem-pop BP*	+	7 mo	Percocet; fentanyl patch	+	7 mo	Foot	8 cm × 5 cm	3	Pitting edema	0	TO	TO	TO	TO	TO	TO
2	M	60	+	+	5	0.00	PF, EA and fem-pop BP; revision of BP; PTA of BP × 2*	+	6 mo	percocet	+	6 mo	Foot	1 cm × 1 cm to 2 cm × 2 cm	3	0	0	TO	TO	TO	TO	TO	TO
3	M	81	0	0	5	0.39	Fem-pop BP; SFA/pop PTA†	+	6 mo	E-S tylenol	+	6 mo	Toe	3 cm × 3 cm	2	0	0	TO	TO	TO	TO	TO	TO
4	M	92	0	0	5	0.28	Recommended for AKA	+	5 mo	Percocet; fentanyl patch; morphine sulfate	+	4 mo	Toes	1 cm × 1 cm	2	Pitting edema	0	TO	TO	TO	TO	TO	na
5	F	72	0	0	4	0.31	Fem-pop BP	+	17 mo	Vicoden	0	na	na	na	na	0	0	TO	TO	0	0	0	TO
6	F	71	+	0	4	0.31	Fem-pop PTA; fem-per BP; PTA of fem-per BP; iliac PTA; repeat PTA of fem-per BP	+	6 mo	Vicoden; percocet; codeine	0	na	na	na	na	0	0	TO	TO	TO	TO	0	TO
7	M	73	+	0	4	0.47	Fem-pop BP; fem-AT BP; CABG; CEA (bilateral)	+	6 mo	Percocet	0	na	na	na	na	0	0	TO	0	TO	TO	TO	TO
8	F	70	+	0	5	0.26	None	+	15 mo	Percocet; fentanyl patch; vicoden	+	7 mo	Toes	3 cm × 3 cm	3	0	0	0	0	0	TO	TO	na

Notes:

‡ Performed following development of ulcer.

* 1 = superficial; 2 = involves subcutaneous tissue; 3 = exposure of tendon or bone; 4 = necrosis of tendon or bone.

Abbreviations: (+) = yes; (0) = no: ABI = ankle-brachial index: AKA = above-knee amputation: AT = anterior tibial: BP = bypass surgery of lower extremity: CABG = coronary artery bypass graft: CEA = carotid endarterectomy: Cigs = cigarette smoker: DF = deep femoral: DM = diabetes mellitus: Dur'n = duration: EA = endarterectomy: F = female: Fem-fem = femoral-femoral: Fem-pop = femoral-popliteal: Loc'n = location: Meds = analgesic medications: mo = months: na = not applicable: PF = profundaplasty: Pop = popliteal: Per = peroneal: Prev Rx = previous angioplasty or surgery in affected limb: Pt = patient: PT = posterior tibial: R = right: SFA = superficial femoral artery: TO = total occlusion.

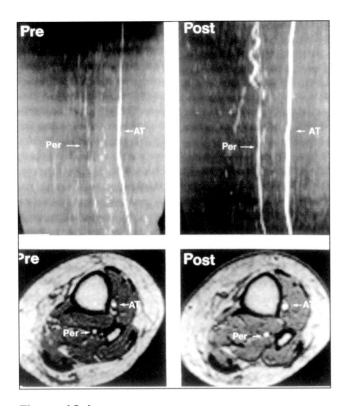

Figure 19.1
Magnetic resonance angiography (MRA, performed without contrast media) pre- and postgene therapy in no. 5. In comparison to the longitudinal reconstruction (top) and tomographic view of the infrapopliteal vessels recorded pregene therapy, the study recorded postgene therapy shows enhanced flow via a tortuous collateral (arrow) to the peroneal (Per) artery distally; flow into the anterior (AT) artery is improved as well.

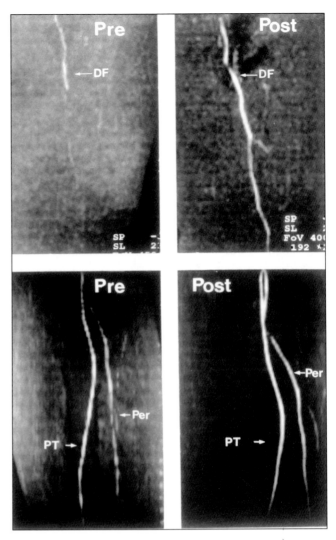

Figure 19.2
MRA pre- and postgene therapy in no. 6: in postgene therapy there is improved flow in the deep femoral (DF) artery, as well as the posterior tibial (PT) and peroneal (Per) arteries.

reconstituting the distal popliteal artery also showed increased flow in comparison to the MRA recorded pregene transfer. In no. 8, improved flow was documented at the ankle level.

Intravascular ultrasound (IVUS)

IVUS examination performed in preparation for gene transfer identified accessible arterial segments for arterial gene transfer that were free of atherosclerotic narrowing in 6/8 patients; the arterial wall at the site of gene transfer in these 6 patients had a clearly recognizable three-layer appearance, indicating minimal to absent intimal thickening.[38] In 2 patients (nos. 2 and 3), no site could be identified in either the superficial femoral artery (SFA) or deep femoral artery that was similarly pristine; the site least

narrowed by atherosclerotic plaque was therefore selected for arterial gene transfer.

IVUS inspection of the site of arterial gene transfer was repeated at 4 weeks (nos. 1, 2 8) or 12 weeks (nos. 3, 5, 6, 7 and 8) postgene transfer. In no. 4, as described above, gene transfer performed immediately proximal to the site of occlusion in the popliteal artery resulted in retrograde propagation of the original occlusion for approximately 2 cm, occluding the gene transfer site. In the remaining 6 patients, arterial gene transfer to a normal (4 patients) or mildly atherosclerotic (2 patients) artery did not compromise vessel patency; specifically, subsequent IVUS examina-

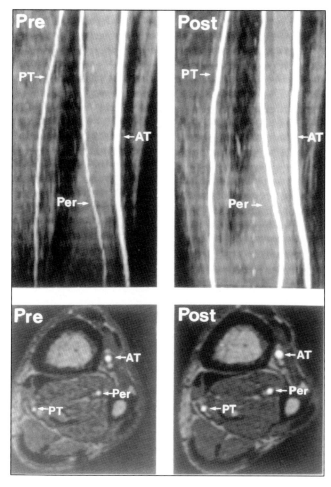

Figure 19.3
MRA pre- and postgene therapy in no. 7: in postgene therapy, markedly improved flow is seen in the posterior tibial (PT) and peroneal (Per) arteries and, to a lesser degree, in the anterior tibial (AT) artery as well.

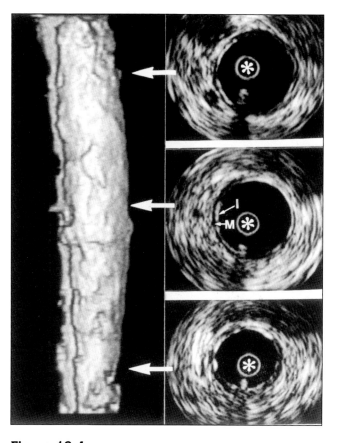

Figure 19.4
3D reconstruction and representative tomographic views of entire length of gene transfer site in no. 5. Uniform luminal caliber is preserved, and tomographic views confirm preserved three-layer appearance of arterial wall with no new intimal thickening at any site.

tions disclosed no new intimal thickening up to 3 months' postgene transfer (Fig. 19.4).

Intravascular Doppler flow analysis

Intra-arterial blood flow was measured in the ischemic limb at the time of 3 months' follow-up angiography in nos. 3, 5, 6, 7 and 8. In comparison to flow measured immediately prior to arterial gene transfer, no improvement in flow was observed in no. 3. In the remaining 4 patients, however, including all 3 patients (nos. 5–7) in whom evidence of clinical improvement was observed, improved flow was

documented at 3 months' postgene transfer (Fig. 19.5). The improvement in flow included both flow measured at rest (132.3–188.5% of baseline), as well as that recorded 30–90 sec following administration of the endothelium-independent vasodilator, nitroglycerin (120.0–158.6% of baseline).

Digital subtraction angiography (DSA)

In the first 7 patients, serial DSA examinations disclosed no gain or loss of collateral vessels. In no. 8, however, the first patient to be treated with the 2000 μg dose, DSA

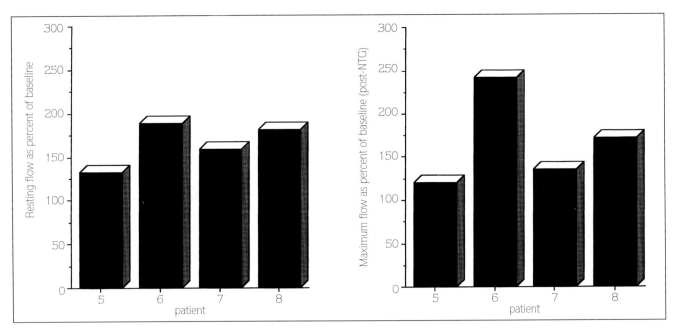

Figure 19.5
Resting and maximum (postnitroglycerin) blood flow in ischemic limb measured by intravascular Doppler flow wire pre- vs. 3 months' postgene therapy in nos. 5–8. In nos. 5–8, resting flow was increased by 32.3, 88.5, 59.0 and 82%; maximum flow was increased by 20.0, 58.6, 35.5 and 72%.

performed 4 weeks' postgene therapy disclosed a marked increase in collateral vessels in the ischemic limb at the knee, mid-tibial and ankle levels (Fig. 19.6). These persisted unchanged at the time of a subsequent angiogram recorded 8 weeks later.

Other findings

In no. 8, evidence of angiogenesis consequent to arterial gene transfer was also apparent on inspection of the integument of the distal portion of the ischemic limb. Three separate telangiectasia developed over the medial ankle (1) and dorsal forefoot (2) approximately 1 week following gene transfer (Fig. 19.7). Excisional biopsy and light microscopic examination (Fig. 19.7) of one of these lesions disclosed markedly positive staining for CD31, identifying endothelial cells comprising vessels within this lesion; the proliferative nature of these endothelial cells was shown by immunostaining of adjacent sections with an antibody to proliferating cell nuclear antigen (PCNA). The two lesions not removed by surgical biopsy underwent spontaneous regression by 8 weeks' postgene transfer.

Ophthalmologic examination was done in all cases. No changes were noted in funduscopic examination performed at 3 months' follow-up in any patient.

Complications

One patient (no. 3) developed a pseudoaneurysm at the site of antegrade cannulation for arterial gene transfer. This was treated successfully by ultrasound-guided compression and resolved without sequelae.

Discussion

Our preliminary experience with arterial gene transfer in the treatment of peripheral vascular disease extends these previous studies performed in live animals to human subjects. No adverse consequences attributable to the recombinant protein encoded by phVEGF$_{165}$ were observed. The absence of these complications is consistent with site-specific activity observed in preclinical animal studies of

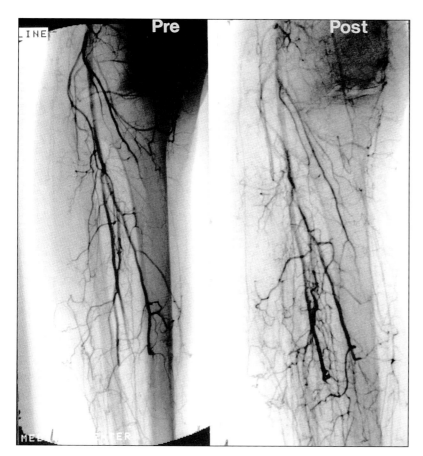

Figure 19.6
Selective digital subtraction angiography performed immediately prior to (left) and 1 month post- (right) gene therapy disclosed plethora of new collateral vessels in ischemic limb. (Reproduced from reference 67 with permission.)

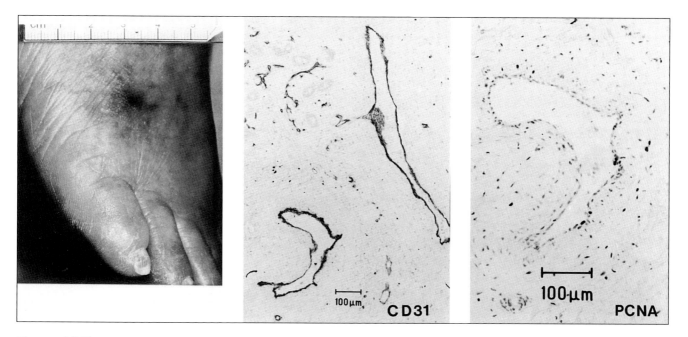

Figure 19.7
One of three spider angiomata which developed approximately one-week postgene therapy in distal portion of ischemic limb. Photomicrographs of tissue sections immunostained with antibody to endothelial antigen CD31 indicate vascularity of lesion, while immunostain of adjacent section for proliferating cell nuclear antigen (PCNA) indicates extent of proliferative activity among endothelial cells in lesion. (Reproduced from reference 67 with permission.)

VEGF, administered either as plasmid DNA[33] or the recombinant protein,[39] such site-specific angiogenesis appears to be mediated by paracrine induction of VEGF receptors in endothelial cells exposed to factors secreted by hypoxic myocytes.[40] IVUS examination disclosed no new intimal thickening up to one-year postgene transfer. It is indeed likely that phVEGF$_{165}$ gene transfer accelerates re-endothelialization and thereby obviates luminal compromise of the transfected segment.[41]

Because the current investigation is a phase I trial, evidence of bioactivity was considered a secondary objective. Furthermore, a dose-escalating strategy was mandated for this trial due to the fact that VEGF, either as a recombinant protein or otherwise, had not been previously administered to human subjects. In contrast to the dose employed in preclinical animal studies (500 µg, or 0.114 mg/kg for 3.5 kg rabbits), the dose of plasmid DNA for the first 2 patients was limited to 100 and 500 µg (0.001 and 0.007 mg/kg), respectively. The subsequent 5 patients were approved for 1000 µg (0.014 mg/kg). At what may still be considered to be a relatively low dose (the dose will ultimately escalate to 4000 µg for the final 7 patients of the total 22 approved for this phase I trial), evidence of bioactivity was nevertheless observed. In 3 of the 4 patients treated with 1000 µg of plasmid DNA in whom the gene transfer site remained patent, evidence of augmented flow to the distal portion of the ischemic limb was documented by three independent modalities. In these 3 patients, intravascular Doppler analysis disclosed an increase in both resting flow (132.3–188.5% of baseline), and maximum flow (120.0–158.6%) provoked by intra-arterial nitroglycerin; these results compare favorably with the mean increase in rest (140%) and maximum (173%) flow documented in the rabbit model of limb ischemia 30 days following administration of VEGF$_{165}$ recombinant protein.[42] Contrast-negative MRA graphically confirmed the increased infrapopliteal blood flow in these 3 patients, and contrast angiography documented accelerated delivery of contrast media from the common femoral artery to the pedal arch vessels in these 3 patients as well. Moreover, these latter 3 patients, each of whom presented with several (6–17) months of ischemic rest pain, remain free of rest pain at 3 months' follow-up. In the fourth patient, in whom rest pain was associated with aggressive growth in the size of an ischemic ulcer during the 3 months prior to gene therapy, further extension of the ulcer was blunted for 2 months' postgene therapy.

Recently reported clinical trials of human gene therapy for cystic fibrosis[43] and Duchenne's muscular dystrophy[44] yielded somewhat disappointing results, perhaps in part related to the challenge of expressing the gene product—which in both of these cases remains intracellular—among a large proportion of airway epithelia or skeletal myocytes respectively. In the current protocol, the requirement for a higher transfection efficiency may be obviated by the fact that VEGF protein includes a leader sequence which permits active secretion from intact cells; thus, even if VEGF gene expression is limited to a small number of cells, the paracrine effects of the secreted gene product may be sufficient to achieve a meaningful biologic effect. The question, however, as to whether naked plasmid[45–50] will suffice, or whether, in spite of the secreted feature of the gene product, the magnitude of gene expression required will demand the use of adjunctive, including viral, vectors[51–60] remains to be addressed. If naked plasmid DNA alone is to be used, then the optimal dose of plasmid DNA remains to be established. Other critical issues which remain to be clarified include the optimal frequency of administration; if the gene product is limited to a 30-day window—as suggested by preclinical studies[33]—then the time interval required for full maturation of a lengthy collateral network might benefit from repeated administration, 3 weeks, for example, after the first dose. The extent to which a favorable response is affected by the proximity of the site of gene transfer to the ischemic focus in the affected limb also remains uncertain.

The more global issue regarding the relative merits of gene therapy vs. administration of the recombinant protein for achieving therapeutic angiogenesis also remains uncertain. The nonavailability of VEGF recombinant protein for human subjects makes this, currently, a moot point. Should the protein be made available for human testing, it will be intriguing to see whether the slow-release depot aspect of gene therapy,[61] administered in a site-specific fashion and targeted to local pathology, will yield outcomes which are superior to that which can be achieved with bolus and/or continuous administration of the protein.

Certain limitations of the current study must be explicitly underscored. With regard to safety, these findings are preliminary and do not establish the long-term safety of VEGF, administered either as a gene or gene product. Likewise, the preliminary nature of the results dictates that evidence of bioactivity, while encouraging, must be viewed cautiously. This is particularly so given that this first phase of clinical investigation was nonrandomized. While consideration was given to the issue of a control group, the HIRB, RAC and FDA concurred that there was limited justification for undertaking catheter manipulation in patients with marginal limb perfusion and extensive atherosclerosis solely for the purpose of performing a sham transfection. For the patient undergoing gene transfer, the procedural risks were offset by the potential for relief from unremitting rest pain or healing of refractory ulcers; for the patient undergoing a sham transfection, the risks would not be offset by any potential benefit. To minimize the likelihood of spontaneous improvement in either rest pain and/or the appearance of an established ulcer, inclusion criteria required, in the case of rest pain alone, a minimum duration of four weeks of rest pain with dependence on narcotics without improvement; in the case of nonhealing ulcerations, a minimum of 4 weeks of conservative therapy without evidence of healing was required. While rest pain and/or ulcerations of this nature may precipitously deteriorate, the potential for spontaneous improvement under these circumstances is remote.[3] The short-term nature of the follow-up obtained to date also leaves undetermined the durability of apparent clinical improvement observed in selected patients.

The precise mechanism responsible for the salutary effects observed in patients who received the 1000 µg dose of DNA remains uncertain. What we have observed, by three independent examinations, is evidence of increased flow to the distal extremities, specifically distal to the pre-existing occluded vessels. This was most graphically illustrated by MRA performed pre- and postgene therapy. In no. 5, for example, striking reconstitution of the distal peroneal artery developed in association with a similarly lengthy occlusion of the SFA/popliteal artery. In no. 6, flow was improved to both the peroneal and posterior tibial. In no. 7, flow appeared substantially increased in the posterior tibial, peroneal and to a lesser degree, in the anterior tibial—all distal to the SFA/popliteal, which was occluded over its entire length. In each of these patients, measurement of increased blood flow using an intravascular Doppler wire, and accelerated transit of angiographic contrast media, supported the results of MRA.

These findings are consistent with the experimental observations described recently by Pearlman et al.,[14] who used magnetic resonance imaging (MRI) to study the time delay in delivery of contrast media to the collateral-dependent myocardium of pigs in which the circumflex coronary artery was occluded by an ameroid constrictor. Following 6 weeks of treatment with VEGF (recombinant protein), contrast arrival time in the myocardium subserved by the occluded circumflex was markedly accelerated. Because survival and function of this ischemic myocardial zone is dependent upon collateral flow, the observed improvement in contrast delivery was inferred to represent augmented neovascularity, although direct demonstration of the same was not shown. Previous DNA labeling studies in this swine model,[62] a similar canine model[63] and the ischemic rabbit hindlimb[64] have established that improvements in flow associated with collateral development are typically associated with proliferation of new vessels smaller than 180 µ in diameter, including a statistically significant increase in capillary density. We presume that among the 3 patients described above, flow from the profunda to the infrapopliteal vessels was improved via an augmented network of collaterals. Direct evidence of new blood vessel formation, however, remains pending, either because the size of the new vascular structures is beyond the resolution of conventional angiography, or because of other, as yet, undisclosed reasons.

We have also considered the alternative possibility that the increase in distal extremity blood flow might be the result of vasodilatation. VEGF has been shown in vivo to produce endothelium-dependent hypotension that can be blocked and/or reversed by administration of N^G-monomethyl-L-arginine (L-NMMA), an inhibitor of nitric oxide synthase.[65] Moreover, in vitro studies have demonstrated VEGF-induced relaxation of canine coronary arteries that was abolished by endothelial denudation or pretreatment with L-NMMA,[66] and recent studies in the authors' laboratory have directly documented VEGF-induced release of nitric oxide from isolated rings of endothelium-intact (but not endothelium-denuded) rabbit aorta (van der Zee R, unpublished data). It is the authors' current feeling, however, that relief of rest pain at 12 weeks accompanied by evidence of augmented flow in the ischemic limb is unlikely to represent a vasodilator effect of VEGF, given that preclinical animal studies have consistently demonstrated expiration of gene expression (and, by inference, synthesis of recombinant VEGF protein) between 21 and 30 days postgene transfer.[33]

Conclusions

These findings have thus established proof of principle for two concepts. The first is the potential for the administration of angiogenic growth factors to promote development of new collateral blood vessels in human patients. While not yet sufficient to prevent distal limb amputation in patients with advanced gangrene, use of higher doses, multiple applications and/or alternative delivery routes, viz., intramuscular injection, of the gene or protein may yield sufficient neovascularity to make this goal a reality.

The second concept is the feasibility of arterial gene transfer of naked DNA. The use of naked DNA is admittedly inefficient, permitting successful transfection of less than 1% of the target smooth muscle cells. In the case of VEGF, there are several aspects of the gene, protein and target tissue which may have contributed to modulation of the host phenotype (increased vascularity and flow) despite a low transfection efficiency. First, VEGF, as noted above, is actively secreted by intact cells; previous studies in the authors' laboratory[30] have documented that genes which encode for secreted proteins—as opposed to proteins which remain intracellular—may yield meaningful biological outcomes due to paracrine effects of the secreted gene product.

Acknowledgments

The authors gratefully acknowledge the contributions of Susan Rossow, BS, Orit Manor, PhD and Ken Walsh, PhD for preparation of the plasmid DNA used in this clinical trial; Jason Lowry, BS for resequencing of the plasmid DNA; Dr Joachim Schorr of Qiagen for assistance in quality control testing of the plasmid; Dr Jeff Griffiths for supervising the microbial testing of the plasmid; Drs Scott Bortman, Dan Jurayj, Kathleen Hogan, Marvin Lopez, David Cave, Alan Roper and the physicians of the New England Eye Center for their generous assistance in screening and management of the patients described herein; Susan Kelly, patient advocate; and Debbie Canatta, Karen Macarone and Mickey Neely for superb administrative assistance.

References

1   Albers M, Fratezi AC, DeLuccia N. Assessment of quality of life of patients with severe ischemia as a result of infrainguinal arterial occlusive disease. *J Vasc Surg* 1992; **16**: 54–9.

2   Dormandy JA, Thomas PRS. What is the natural history of a critically ischemic patient with and without his leg? In: Greenhalgh RM, Jamieson CW, Nicolaides AN (eds). *Limb Salvage and Amputation for Vascular Disease* (Philadelphia, PA: WB Saunders, 1988): 11–26.

3   European Working Group on Critical Leg Ischemia. Second European consensus document on chronic critical leg ischemia. *Circulation* 1991; **84**: IV-1–IV-26.

4   Isner JM, Rosenfield K. Redefining the treatment of peripheral artery disease: role of percutaneous revascularization. *Circulation* 1993; **88**: 1534–57.

5   Pentecost MJ, Criqui MH, Dorros G, et al. Guidelines for peripheral percutaneous transluminal angioplasty of the abdominal aorta and lower extremity vessels: a statement for health professionals from a special writing group of the Councils on Cardiovascular Radiology, Arteriosclerosis, Cardio-Thoracic and Vascular Surgery, Clinical Cardiology, and Epidemiology and Prevention, the American Heart Association. *Circulation* 1994; **89**: 511–31.

6   Folkman J, Merler E, Abernathy C, Williams G. Isolation of a tumor factor responsible for angiogenesis. *J Exp Med* 1971; **133**: 275–88.

7   Folkman J. Tumor angiogenesis: therapeutic implications. *N Engl J Med* 1971; **285**: 1182–6.

8   Folkman J. Anti-angiogenesis: new concept for therapy of solid tumors. *Ann Surg* 1972; **175**: 409–16.

9   Banai S, Jaklitsch MT, Casscells W, et al. Effects of acidic fibroblast growth factor on normal and ischemic myocardium. *Circ Res* 1991; **69**: 76–85.

10   Baffour R, Danylewick R, Burdon T. An angiographic study of ischemia as a determinant of neovascularization in arteriovenous reversal. *Surg Gynecol Obstet* 1988; **166**: 28–32.

11   Yanagisawa-Miwa A, Uchida Y, Nakamura F, et al. Salvage of infarcted myocardium by angiogenic action of basic fibroblast growth factor. *Science* 1992; **257**: 1401–3.

12   Takeshita S, Zheng LP, Brogi E, et al. Therapeutic angiogenesis: a single intra-arterial bolus of vascular endothelial growth factor augments revascularization in a rabbit ischemic hindlimb model. *J Clin Invest* 1994; **93**: 662–70.

13   Banai S, Jaklitsch MT, Shou M, et al. Angiogenic-induced enhancement of collateral blood flow to ischemic myocardium by vascular endothelial growth factor in dogs. *Circulation* 1994; **89**: 2183–9.

14   Pearlman JD, Hibberd MG, Chuang ML, et al. Magnetic resonance mapping demonstrates benefits of VEGF-induced myocardial angiogenesis. *Nature Med* 1995; **1**: 1085–9.

15   Pu LQ, Sniderman AD, Brassard R, et al. Enhanced revascularization of the ischemic limb by means of angiogenic therapy. *Circulation* 1993; **88**: 208–15.

16   Höckel M, Schlenger K, Doctrow S, Kissel T, Vaupel P. Therapeutic angiogenesis. *Arch Surg* 1993; **128**: 423–9.

17   Folkman J, Klagsbrun M. Angiogenic factors. *Science* 1987; **235**: 442–7.

18   Folkman J, Shing Y. Angiogenesis. *J Biol Chem* 1992; **267**: 10931–4.

19   Ferrara N, Henzel WJ. Pituitary follicular cells secrete a novel heparin-binding growth factor specific for vascular endothelial cells. *Biochem Biophys Res Commun* 1989; **161**: 851–5.

20   Keck PJ, Hauser SD, Krivi G, et al. Vascular permeability factor, an endothelial cell mitogen related to PDGF. *Science* 1989; **246**: 1309–12.

21   Plouet J, Schilling J, Gospodarowicz D. Isolation and characterization of a newly identified endothelial cell mitogen produced by AtT-20 cells. *EMBO J* 1989; **8**: 3801–6.

22   D'Amore PA, Thompson RW. Mechanisms of angiogenesis. *Ann Rev Physiol* 1987; **49**: 453–64.

23   Folkman J, Haudenschild C. Angiogenesis *in vitro*. *Nature* 1980; **288**: 551–6.

24   Vernon RB, Sage EH. Between molecules and morphology. Extracellular matrix and creation of vascular form. *Am J Pathol* 1995; **147**: 873–83.

25   Ross R. The pathogenesis of atherosclerosis: a perspective for the 1990s. *Nature* 1993; **362**: 801–5.

26   Clowes AW, Reidy MA, Clowes MM. Kinetics of cellular proliferation after arterial injury. I. Smooth muscle growth in the absence of endothelium. *Lab Invest* 1983; **49**: 327–33.

27 Pickering JG, Weir L, Jekanowski J, Kearney MA, Isner JM. Proliferative activity in peripheral and coronary atherosclerotic plaque among patients undergoing percutaneous revascularization. *J Clin Invest* 1993; **91**: 1469–80.

28 Tischer E, Mitchell R, Hartmann T, *et al*. The human gene for vascular endothelial growth factor: multiple protein forms are encoded through alternative exon splicing. *J Biol Chem* 1991; **266**: 11947–54.

29 Takeshita S, Losordo DW, Kearney M, Isner JM. Time course of recombinant protein secretion following liposome-mediated gene transfer in a rabbit arterial organ culture model. *Lab Invest* 1994; **71**: 387–91.

30 Losordo DW, Pickering JG, Takeshita S, *et al*. Use of the rabbit ear artery to serially assess foreign protein secretion after site specific arterial gene transfer *in vivo*: evidence that anatomic identification of successful gene transfer may underestimate the potential magnitude of transgene expression. *Circulation* 1994; **89**: 785–92.

31 Riessen R, Rahimizadeh H, Blessing E, Takeshita S, Barry JJ, Isner JM. Arterial gene transfer using pure DNA applied directly to a hydrogel-coated angioplasty balloon. *Hum Gene Ther* 1993; **4**: 749–58.

32 Pu LQ, Sniderman AD, Arekat Z, Graham AM, Brassard R, Symes JF. Angiogenic growth factor and revascularization of the ischemic limb: evaluation in a rabbit model, *J Surg Res* 1993; **54**: 575–83.

33 Minutes Recombinant DNA Advisory Committee (RAC) of National Institutes of Health, 13 September 1994. *RAC 9409-088 approved in final form 11/15/94*.

34 Takeshita S, Zheng LP, Asahara T, *et al*. *In vivo* evidence of enhanced angiogenesis following direct arterial gene transfer of the plasmid encoding vascular endothelial growth factor. *Circulation* 1993; **88**: I-476 (abstract).

35 Takeshita S, Bauters C, Asahara T, *et al*. Physiologic assessment of angiogenesis by arterial gene therapy with vascular endothelial growth factor. *Circulation* 1994; **90**: I-90 (abstract).

36 Takeshita S, Tsurumi Y, Couffinhal T, *et al*. Gene transfer of naked DNA encoding for three isoforms of vascular endothelial growth factor stimulates collateral development *in vivo*. *Lab Invest* 1996; **75**: 487–502.

37 Rutherford RB (Chairman), Flanigan DP, Gupta SK, *et al*., prepared by the Ad Hoc Committee on Reporting Standards, Society for Vascular Surgery/North American Chapter, International Society for Cardiovascular Surgery. Suggested standards for reports dealing with lower extremity ischemia. *J Vasc Surg* 1986; **4**: 90–4.

38 Rosenfield K, Isner JM. Intravascular ultrasound in patients undergoing coronary and peripheral arterial revasculariza-

tion. In: Topol E (ed.). *Interventional Cardiology* (2nd edn) (Philadelphia, PA: WB Saunders, 1993): 1153–85.

39 Bauters C, Asahara T, Zheng LP, *et al*. Site-specific therapeutic angiogenesis following systemic administration of vascular endothelial growth factor. *J Vasc Surg* 1995; **21**: 314–25.

40 Brogi E, Schatteman G, Wu T, *et al*. Hypoxia-induced paracrine regulation VEGF receptor expression. *J Clin Invest* 1996; **97**: 469–76.

41 Asahara T, Bauters C, Pastore CJ, *et al*. Local delivery of vascular endothelial growth factor accelerates reendothelialization and attenuates intimal hyperplasia in balloon-injured rat carotid artery. *Circulation* 1995; **91**: 2793–801.

42 Bauters C, Asahara T, Zheng LP, *et al*. Physiologic assessment of angiogenesis induced by vascular endothelial growth factor in a rabbit ischemic hindlimb model. *Am J Physiol* 1994; **36**: H1263–H1271.

43 Knowles MR, Hohneker KW, Shou Z, *et al*. A controlled study of adenoviral-vector-mediated gene transfer in the nasal epithelium of patients with cystic fibrosis. *N Engl J Med* 1995; **333**: 823–31.

44 Meddell JR, Kissel JT, Amato AA, *et al*. Myoblast transfer in the treatment of Duchenne's muscular dystrophy. *N Engl J Med* 1995; **333**: 832–8.

45 Wolff JA, Malone RW, Williams P, *et al*. Direct gene transfer into mouse muscle *in vivo*. *Science* 1990; **247**: 1465–8.

46 Lin H, Parmacek MS, Morle G, Bolling S, Leiden JM. Expression of recombinant genes in myocardium *in vivo* after direct injection of DNA. *Circulation* 1990; **82**: 2217–21.

47 Buttrick PM, Kass A, Kitsis RN, Kaplan ML, Leinwand LA. Behavior of genes directly injected into the rat heart *in vivo*. *Circ Res* 1992; **70**: 193–8.

48 Chapman GD, Lim CS, Gammon RS, *et al*. Gene transfer into coronary arteries of intact animals with a percutaneous balloon catheter. *Circ Res* 1992; **71**: 27–33.

49 Gal D, Weir L, Leclerc G, Pickering JG, Hogan J, Isner JM. Direct myocardial transfection in two animal models: evaluation of parameters affecting gene expression and percutaneous gene delivery. *Lab Invest* 1993; **68**: 18–25.

50 Conry RM, LoBuglio AF, Kantor J, *et al*. Immune response to a carcinoembryonic antigen polynucleotide vaccine. *Cancer Res* 1994; **54**: 1164–8.

51 Ohno T, Gordon D, San H, *et al*. Gene therapy for vascular smooth muscle cell proliferation after arterial injury. *Science* 1994; **265**: 781–4.

52 Schulick AH, Newman KD, Virmani R, Dichek DA. *In vivo*

gene transfer into injured carotid arteries: optimization and evaluation of acute toxicity. *Circulation* 1995; **91**: 2407–14.

53   Chang MW, Barr E, Jonathan S, *et al*. Cytostatic gene therapy for vascular proliferative disorders with a constitutively active form of the retinoblastoma gene product. *Science* 1995; **267**: 518–22.

54   Zwiebel J, Freeman S, Kantoff P, Cornetta K, Ryan U, Anderson W. High-level of recombinant gene expression in rabbit endothelial cells transduced by retroviral vectors. *Science* 1989; **243**: 220–43.

55   Mulligan RC. The basic science of gene therapy. *Science* 1993; **260**: 926–32.

56   von der Leyen HE, Gibbons GH, Morishita R, *et al*. Gene therapy inhibiting neointimal vascular lesion: *in vivo* transfer of endothelial cell nitric oxide synthase gene. *Proc Natl Acad Sci USA* 1995; **92**: 1137–41.

57   Willard JE, Landau C, Glamann B, *et al*. Genetic modification of the vessel wall: comparison of surgical and catheter-based techniques for delivery of recombinant adenovirus. *Circulation* 1994; **89**: 2190–7.

58   Guzman RJ, Hirschowitz EA, Brody SL, Crystal RG, Epstein SE, Finkel T. *In vivo* suppression of injury-induced vascular smooth muscle cell accumulation using adenovirus-mediated transfer of the herpes simplex virus thymidine kinase gene. *Proc Natl Acad Sci USA* 1994; **91**: 10732–6.

59   Grossman M, Raper SE, Kozarsky K, *et al*. Successful *ex vivo* gene therapy directed to liver in a patient with familial hypercholesterolemia. *Nature Genetics* 1994; **6**: 335–41.

60   Lemarchand P, Jones M, Yamada I, Crystal RG. *In vivo* gene transfer and expression in normal uninjured blood vessels using replication-deficient recombinant adenovirus vectors. *Circ Res* 1993; **72**: 1132–8.

61   Riessen R, Isner JM. Prospects for site-specific delivery of pharmacologic and molecular therapies. *J Am Coll Cardiol* 1994; **23**: 1234–44.

62   White FC, Carroll SM, Magnet A, Bloor CM. Coronary collateral development in swine after coronary artery occlusion. *Circ Res* 1992; **71**: 1490–500.

63   Unger EF, Banai S, Shou M, *et al*. Basic fibroblast growth factor enhances myocardial collateral flow in a canine model. *Am J Physiol* 1994; **266**: H1588–H1595.

64   Takeshita S, Rossow ST, Kearney M, *et al*. Time course of increased cellular proliferation in collateral arteries following administration of vascular endothelial growth factor in a rabbit model of lower limb vascular insufficiency. *Am J Pathol* 1995; **147**: 1649–60.

65   Horowitz J, Hariawala M, Sheriff DD, Keyt B, Symes JF. *In vivo* administration of vascular endothelial growth factor is associated with EDRF-dependent systemic hypotension in porcine and rabbit animal models. *Circulation* 1995; **92**: I-630–I-631 (abstract).

66   Ku DD, Zaleski JK, Liu S, Brock TA. Vascular endothelial growth factor induces EDRF-dependent relaxation in coronary arteries. *Am J Physiol* 1993; **265**: H586–H592.

67   Isner JM, Pieczek A, Schainfeld R, *et al*. Early report: clinical evidence of angiogenesis following arterial gene transfer of phVEGF$_{165}$. *Lancet* 1996; **348**: 370–4.

20

Growth factors: a future role in interventional cardiology?

Jonathan Leor, Sharon Aboulafia and Alexander Battler

Introduction

Despite significant progress in preventing and treating atherosclerotic cardiovascular disease, this disorder remains a major therapeutic challenge. Both coronary artery bypass surgery and percutaneous transluminal coronary angioplasty are effective revascularization techniques for treatment of obstructive coronary artery disease. These modalities, however, are palliative and have recognized limitations in cases complicated by distal or diffuse coronary artery disease, small vessel disease and restenosis. Therefore, there is still a need for new therapeutic agents to prevent, arrest or reverse atherosclerosis and coronary artery disease.

Recent insights into the pathogenesis of vascular and myocardial disease have opened up a new horizon of molecular and cellular therapies that target genes, molecules and peptides. Growth factors constitute a potentially novel form of adjuvant therapy to interventional cardiology techniques. Recent studies in animal models suggest that exogenous administration of growth factors before, after or during acute myocardial ischemia or infarction can be used for myocardial protection, collateral development, improved myocardial function and viability. In addition, administration of growth factors can amplify healing, endothelial function and diminish restenosis in animal models of vascular injury.

This chapter provides a few selected topics that highlight recent advances in the current research of growth factors as a therapeutic strategy for ischemic heart disease and heart failure. The biological rationale for these new therapies and the future implications of growth factor therapy in interventional cardiology are discussed. However, the scope of this chapter does not allow for a comprehensive review of the basic biology and the characteristics of various growth factors expressed in the normal and diseased heart. A review of this topic can be found in a number of specialized texts and reviews devoted to molecular and cellular biology of the heart.[1-3]

Growth factors and the heart: biological rationale

Classically, the name growth factors signifies their mitogenic activity. Their role is now understood in much broader terms as external cellular signals that lead to a variety of cellular responses such as differentiation, stimulation of function, shape changes and apoptosis as well as proliferation.

Growth factors are small polypeptides synthesized and secreted by certain cell types, which stimulate responsive target cells. In general, growth factors produce their effects by binding to a membrane receptor which, in turn, activates secondary intracellular secondary messengers, and these activate nucleus transcription factors. These transcription factors regulate gene expression and subsequent protein synthesis. Unlike the normal endocrine response, the growth response to growth factors occurs several hours after the initial stimulation, and is more likely to occur if two or more growth factors have been activated. The pathways of cell proliferation and differentiation as mediated by growth factors are complex. Many factors are expressed after processing by several intermediate cell types. The growth factors are also codependent on each other, one factor being the stimulus or suppressor of several other factors.

The recent isolation and molecular cloning of numerous growth factors, the description of their expression in the heart and the demonstration that cardiac myocytes are a target for growth factors indicate that growth factors are involved initially in cardiogenesis and cardiac growth, and later in congestive heart failure and hypertrophy as well as in development of collateral circulation. The total number of growth factors expressed in the myocardium is unknown. Among those identified in the heart include transforming growth factor-beta (TGF-β), insulin-like growth factor-I (IGF-I), endothelin I, angiotensin II, acidic fibroblast growth factor or basic fibroblast growth factor (aFGF or bFGF also called FGF-1 and FGF-2). Some of these growth factors, such as IGF-I, have been implicated in activating an adaptive hypertrophic response. Cardiac myocytes treated with IGF-I have shown a dramatic increase over controls in the number of sarcomeres.[4] Therefore, growth factors such as growth hormone or IGF-I have been suggested as therapeutic agents for improving contractility of the failing myocardium.[5]

Cardiac myocytes are terminally differentiated and unable to proliferate. Growth or hypertrophy is the major long-term adaptive mechanism of the heart. It has been suggested that early compensatory growth is beneficial while subsequent growth may become pathological and contribute to increased mortality. Modification of this adaptive response is a major objective in the development of a therapeutic approach. The success in discovering and cloning the genes for many growth factors means that recombinant growth factors can be produced in pharmaceutical quantities. The availability of recombinant growth factors would enable us to augment the failing myocardium after injury.[5]

The pathobiology of atherosclerosis in coronary arteries involves a series of events that include endothelial dysfunction, infiltration of inflammatory cells into the vessel wall, alterations of intimal smooth muscle cell phenotype and vascular remodeling. Current therapies are directed either at reducing risk factors which promote atherosclerosis, or enhancing blood flow through interventions such as balloon angioplasty or surgical revascularization.

The extent of myocardial injury resulting from ischemic insult is determined, in part, by the extent of collateral circulation to the region. Coronary collaterals can limit the severity of myocardial ischemia and myocardial necrosis.[6] It has been evident for many years that growth factors play a role in collateral vessel development.[7] It is unclear, however, which of the numerous growth factors is the major one. Furthermore, it is unclear whether this role is defined by a single factor or by a regulated sequence of a cascade of growth factors, and which cell type in the heart is responsible for growth factor production. Collateral growth is thought to be induced by a chemical signal from the ischemic myocardium, which triggers the events leading to DNA synthesis and to mitosis in collateral vessels. Angiogenic growth factors, such as fibroblast growth factors (FGF), a general mitogen and the most potent angiogenic factor, and vascular endothelial growth factor (VEGF), a less potent angiogenic factor but a mitogen specific for endothelial cells, have been isolated from human cardiac tissue[8,9] and were extracted in larger quantities in the presence of myocardial ischemia. The use of angiogenic growth factors to increase blood flow to ischemic myocardium represents a new experimental therapeutic approach which has attracted a lot of attention and optimism for an alternative strategy to current therapies.

Based on current knowledge, it has been hypothesized that the exogenous administration of growth factors can create a novel therapeutic strategy by 1) enhancing angiogenesis and collateral circulation to the ischemic zone; 2) inducing direct myocardial protection against ischemic injury; 3) augmentation of myocardial function; and 4) restoration of endothelial function and prevention of restenosis after vascular injury.

Angiogenesis and collateral blood flow

Collateral development occurs as an intrinsic adaptive response to coronary artery stenosis. Coronary collaterals can ameliorate myocardial ischemia and preserve myocardial function and viability in the presence of impaired perfusion. Furthermore, myocardial viability after myocardial infarction has been correlated with the extent of collateral blood flow.[6] Thus, there has been much interest in finding ways to enhance collateral function in patients with coronary stenosis. Table 20.1 lists some of the recent experimental studies testing the hypothesis that growth factors can enhance collateral development and collateral circulation in the heart.

In a series of pioneering studies, Battler et al.[11] showed that intracoronary injection of bFGF (a mitogen and a potent agiogenic growth factor) at the time of experimental myocardial infarction, enhances angiogenesis in a swine model. Unger et al.[12] demonstrated that intracoronary administration of bFGF increases angiogenesis and collateral flow in a canine model of ameroid-induced progressive left circumflex coronary artery occlusion. In another study, Banai et al.[13] showed that intracoronary injection of VEGF for 23 days can enhance collateral development. Lazarous et al.[14] reported that continuous administration of bFGF systematically enhanced collateral flow; its beneficial effects occurred between day 7 and 14 of therapy and continued

Table 20.1 Growth factor therapy for improving myocardial collateral vessels and flow.

Reference	Growth factor	Model	Ischemia reperfusion	Measurements	Results: growth factors vs. control
Banai et al.[10]	aFGF	In vivo canine	Gradual occlusion of LAD	• Coronary collaterals	• No increase in coronary collaterals • Smooth muscle hyperplasia
Battler et al.[11]	bFGF	In vivo swine	Intracoronary injection of beads	• Angiogenesis after 2 weeks • Myocardial function after 2 weeks	• Increase in angiogenesis • No effect on regional left ventricular wall motion
Banai et al.[13]	VEGF	In vivo canine	Gradual occlusion of LCx	• Collateral blood flow after 7–28 days • Angiogenesis after 7–28 days	• 40% increase in collateral blood flow • Increase in angiogenesis
Unger et al.[12]	bFGF IC	In vivo canine	Gradual occlusion of LCx	• Collateral blood flow after 7–28 days • Angiogenesis after 7–28 days	• Increase in collateral blood flow • Increase in angiogenesis • Coronary vasodilatation
Sellke et al.[24]	bFGF	In vivo swine	Gradual occlusion of LCx	• Endothelial function • Angiogenesis	• Improved endothelial function • Increased angiogenesis
Lazarous et al.[14]	bFGF IV	In vivo canine	Gradual occlusion of LCx	• Collateral development after 38 days • Collateral flow after 38 days	• Acceleration of collateral development • Augmentation of collateral flow
Koh et al.[23]	TGF-β in cardiac grafts	In vivo mice		• Graft survival and gene expression • Angiogenesis	• Grafted cells expressed TGF-β as long as 3 months • Increased angiogenesis at the border of the grafts
Hariawala et al.[25]	rhVEGF	In vivo swine	Gradual occlusion of LCx	• Blood flow in the ischemic zone • Arterial pressure • Peripheral resistance	• Increase in collateral blood flow • Drop in arterial pressure • Drop in peripheral resistance
Lazarous et al.[15]	IV bFGF vs. IV VEGF	In vivo canine	• Gradual occlusion of LCx • Balloon injury to iliofemoral artery	• Collateral flow after 7 days • Neointimal thickening after 7 days	• bFGF enhanced collateral flow • bFGF did not increase neointimal thickening • VEGF did not increase collateral flow • VEGF increased neointimal thickening
Giordano et al.[22]	FGF-5	In vivo swine Intracoronary gene transfer	• Gradual occlusion of LCx	• Regional perfusion • Regional contractility • Angiogenesis • FGF gene expression	• FGF-5 gene transfer improved regional perfusion • FGF-5 gene transfer ameliorated pacing-induced myocardial dysfunction • FGF-5 gene transfer enhanced angiogenesis • Positive FGF gene expression in the heart

Notes:
aFGF = acidic fibroblast growth factor; bFGF = basic fibroblast growth factor; CK = creatine kinase; GH = growth hormone; IC = intracoronary; IGF = insulin-like growth factor; IV = intravenous; LAD = left anterior descending coronary artery; LCx = left circumflex coronary artery; rhVEGF = recombinant human vascular endothelial growth factor; TGF-β = transforming growth factor-β; VEGF = vascular endothelial growth factor.

after cessation of therapy. Using the canine model of progressive coronary artery occlusion, Lazarous et al.[15] compared the effects of bFGF and VEGF on coronary collateral development and on balloon denudation injury of the iliofemoral artery. Seven days of treatment with bFGF enhanced collateral development without increasing neointimal accumulation at the site of vascular injury. Surprisingly, in this model VEGF did not increase collateral development and significantly exacerbated neointimal accumulation. The study gave support to the possibility that the angiogenic effects of bFGF are dissociated from potential deleterious responses to vascular injury.

Recently, a single dose of intra-arterial[16] or intravenous[17] VEGF has been shown to enhance collateral vessel formation in a rabbit ischemic hindlimb model. These data are encouraging for the treatment of ischemic limbs, but need confirmation in the setting of coronary artery disease.

After animal experiments confirmed that gene transfer can be applied successfully to native arteries,[18] naked plasmid DNA encoded for VEGF was applied to a coating of an angioplasty balloon and transfected directly to the internal iliac artery of a rabbit ischemic hindlimb.[18-20] There was significant improvement in collateral vessel development and limb perfusion after VEGF cDNA. After these encouraging animal experiments, a clinical trial was initiated to evaluate whether local delivery of a gene encoding for VEGF can enhance collateral development in patients with ischemic peripheral vessel disease.[19,20] The results of Isner et al.[21] and the advances in gene transfer techniques suggest that this strategy might be applied to myocardial ischemia.

Most recently, Giordano et al.[22] showed that intracoronary injection of a recombinant adenovirus expressing human FGF-5 resulted in mRNA and protein expression of the transferred gene in a swine model of pacing-induced myocardial ischemia. Two weeks after gene transfer, regional abnormalities in pacing-induced function and blood flow were improved, effects that persisted for 12 weeks. These benefits were associated with evidence of angiogenesis. In another exciting study, Koh et al.[23] showed the efficacy of myoblast-based gene therapy to the myocardium. They used intracardiac grafts comprising genetically modified skeletal myoblasts to deliver recombinant TGF-β to the heart. They found viable grafts as long as 3 months after implantation with areas of angiogenesis on the graft border.

The feasibility of using recombinant formulations of angiogenic growth factors to augment collateral development has now been well established. Studies have suggested that two angiogenic factors, bFGF and VEGF, are sufficiently potent to merit further investigation in clinical trials.

Vascular injury and restenosis

Endothelial cells can release substances that inhibit coagulation and thrombosis, and cause vasorelaxation by production of nitric oxide, prostacycline and prostaglandin E_2. Recent advances in the field of gene therapy provide the opportunity to modify cells involved in vascular injury and restenosis genetically.[19] Recent reports on growth factor therapies for vascular injury are very promising and may be applied to the coronary arteries. Asahara et al.[26] tested the hypothesis that smooth muscle cell proliferation might be indirectly inhibited if re-endothelization could be specifically facilitated at sites of balloon-induced arterial injury. They showed that a single local administration of VEGF enhanced re-endothelization and decreased neointimal proliferation in a rat carotid injury model.[26]

Bauters et al.[17] showed that the administration of VEGF, in a rabbit model of hindlimb ischemia, promotes recovery of endothelium-dependent collateral blood flow as tested by administration of serotonin and acetylcholine.

If the results obtained in peripheral vessels in animal models can be repeated in atherosclerotic coronary arteries, it may be the first step in a new strategy to prevent thrombosis or restenosis after percutaneous transluminal coronary angioplasty.

Myocardial protection and limitations of ischemic damage

One of the most exciting discoveries in the research of growth factor therapy for heart disease is the potential for these agents to decrease ischemic myocardial damage. Several studies (Table 20.2) suggest that various growth factors can attenuate myocardial damage following ischemia and reperfusion.

Yanagisawa-Miwa et al.[27] were the first to report that intracoronary administration of bFGF during acute myocardial infarction in a canine model resulted in reduction in the infarct size and increase in the number of capillaries and arterioles in the treated territory. These intriguing results were recently confirmed by Horrigan et al.[28] who reported reduction in myocardial infarct size following intracoronary injection of bFGF in a canine model of ischemia and reperfusion. In this study, the beneficial effect of bFGF was independent of hemodynamic effect or the effect upon angiogenesis. The latter study suggests that bFGF provides direct myocardial protection independently of angiogenesis.

Harada et al.[29] reported that administration of bFGF in a swine model of chronic ischemia improved myocardial function and reduced infarct size. Other growth factors,

Table 20.2 Cardioprotective effect of growth factors during myocardial ischemia.

Reference	Growth factor	Model	Ischemia reperfusion	Measurements	Results: growth factors vs. control
Lefer et al.[33]	TGF-β	• In vivo rat model of myocardial infarction • Langendorff rat heart	30/20	• Myocardial injury • Vasodilator response • Superoxide anion • Effect of exogenous TNF	• Reduced myocardial injury • Preserved endothelial function • Reduced superoxide production • Blocked TNF activity
Yanagisawa-Miwa et al.[27]	bFGF	In vivo canine model	Thrombosis of LAD	• Infarct size after 1 week • Cardiac function • Capillary density	• Reduction in infarct size • Improved myocardial function • Increased capillary density
Lefer et al.[34]	TGF-β	In vivo feline	1.5 hr/4.5 hr	• Myocardial necrosis • Myeloperoxidase activity • Neutrophil adherence to ischemic endothelium	• Reduction in myocardial necrosis • Reduction in neutrophil accumulation • Reduction in neutrophil adherence
Harada et al.[29]	bFGF	In vivo swine	Gradual ischemia of LCx	• Infarct size • Collateral reserve • Recovery after rapid pacing • Left ventricular thickness	• Reduction in infarct size • Better collateral reserve • Improved myocardial function • Increased left ventricular thickness
Padua et al.[32]	bFGF	Isolated rat heart model	60/30 min	• Recovery of developed force • CK	• Improved recovery of myocardial function • Reduction in myocardial injury
Battler et al.[31]	IGF-II	In vivo swine	Coronary injection of beads	• Wall motion score • Angiogenesis • Histology	• Better wall motion after 4 weeks • No effect on angiogenesis • Peri-infarct myocyte hypertrophy
Buerke et al.[30]	IGF-I	In vivo rat model	20 min/24 hr	• CK loss • Myeloperoxidase activity • Apoptosis	• Reduction in myocardial injury • Reduction in neutrophil accumulation • Attenuated apoptosis
Horrigan et al.[28]	bFGF	In vivo canine model	4 hr/7 days	• Infarct size • Ejection fraction • Capillary density after 7 days • Cell proliferation after 7 days • Hemodynamics	• Reduction in infarct size • No effect on ejection fraction • No effect on capillary density • No effect on cell proliferation • No effect on blood pressure

Notes:
aFGF = acidic fibroblast growth factor; bFGF = basic fibroblast growth factor; CK = creatine kinase; GH = growth hormone; IC = intracoronary; IGF = insulin-like growth factor; IV = intravenous; LAD = left anterior descending coronary artery; LCx = left circumflex coronary artery; rhVEGF = recombinant human vascular endothelial growth factor; TNF = tumor necrosis factor; TGF-β = transforming growth factor-β; VEGF = vascular endothelial growth factor.

such as IGF-I and TGF-β, were also implicated in myocardial protection against ischemic injury.[30,33] Buerke et al.[30] showed in a rat model of myocardial ischemia that IGF-I (1–10 μg) administered 1 hour before 20 min of ischemia and 24 hours reperfusion significantly attenuated myocardial injury measured by creatine kinase loss. IGF-I decreased cardiac myeloperoxidase activity, an index of neutrophil accumulation and the incidence of myocyte apoptosis as detected by DNA fragmentation. The authors suggested that IGF-I is an effective protective agent for the ischemic myocardium against 'reperfusion injury' via two mechanisms: inhibition of neutrophil-induced cardiac necrosis, and prevention of reperfusion-induced apoptosis.

Battler et al.[31] investigated the effect of IGF-II on regional myocardial function in a swine model of myocardial infarction. Animals treated with intracoronary IGF-II had a better wall motion score 4 weeks after myocardial infarction. Histologic analysis revealed that animals treated with IGF-II had peri-infarct myocyte hypertrophy with no evidence of angiogenesis.

Padua et al.[32] examined the protective role of bFGF in myocardial injury in an isolated rat heart model of 60 min of ischemia and 30 min of reperfusion. bFGF improved recovery of mechanical function as compared with controls. Myocardial injury, assessed by determination of phosphocreatine kinase in the effluent, was reduced following bFGF treatment.

The mechanism of growth factor protective action in acute myocardial infarction is unclear and necessarily involves mechanisms other than angiogenesis. The mechanisms suggested to account for myocardial salvage after administration of growth factors would include the following: 1) augmentation of collateral flow to the infarct zone by growth of new vessels; 2) an increase in collateral flow by dilatation of pre-existing collateral channels; 3) a direct protective effect on ischemic myocytes; and 4) suppression of cardiac myocyte apoptosis.

The direct protective effects of growth factors against ischemic myocardial injury as demonstrated in animal models can be useful in the settings of coronary revascularization and open-heart surgery. These therapeutic effects, however, need further confirmation in animal models of PTCA and bypass surgery.

Enhancing cardiac performance

Evidence is accumulating that growth hormone function regulates myocardial growth and maintains muscle mass and strength.[36] Most of the biological effects of growth hormone on the heart are mediated by local production of IGF-I, which in turn regulates tissue growth by paracrine and autocrine mechanisms. Exogenous administration of IGF-I and growth hormone in the normal rat evokes a direct hypertrophic response with enhanced systolic function.[37] Studies of various models of heart failure in laboratory animals suggest that the growth hormones IGF-I and IGF-II contribute to improved cardiac performance, induction of myocyte hypertrophy and alterations of the distribution of myosin isoforms which improve the efficiency of energy metabolism in the heart (Table 20.3).

Recent observations suggest that growth hormone and IGF-I are essential to the cardiovascular system, and exogenous administration can enhance cardiac function and induce hypertrophy. Yang et al.[38] found that administration of growth hormone improved myocardial function in a rat model of congestive heart failure after myocardial infarction. Battler et al.[31] recently demonstrated that administration of IGF-II into myocardial infarction can improve left ventricular function independent of angiogenesis.

Cardiac growth and function are impaired in patients with growth hormone congenital deficiency. Administration of growth hormone to such patients increases wall thickness and normalizes cardiac performance.[36] On the other hand, a long-term excess of growth hormone causes cardiac hypertrophy and hyperkinetic syndrome, with increased cardiac output and reduced vascular resistance. In an experimental model of congestive heart failure, IGF-I induced additional myocyte growth, which was associated with significant improvement of cardiac function.[39]

Recently, in a small uncontrolled clinical trial, Fazio et al.[40] reported the effects of growth hormone as therapy for left ventricular dysfunction in patients with dilated cardiomyopathy. The authors reported exciting preliminary results of improvement in left ventricular ejection fraction, isovolumic relaxation time and increase in left ventricular mass during a 3-month treatment with growth hormone. Hemodynamic measurements, myocardial oxygen consumption, the efficiency of myocardial energy use and functional capacity of the patients were all improved during treatment with growth hormone.

However, the above promising results should be interpreted with caution.[41] It was a short-term (3 months) and uncontrolled study. The beneficial effects tended to diminish 3 months after growth hormone was discontinued. The safety of such long-term treatment is questioned. The clinical data derived from patients with acromegaly and excessive myocardial hypertrophy and diastolic dysfunction have demonstrated that myocyte hypertrophy, patchy fibrosis and myofibril degeneration are present.

The mechanisms behind the beneficial effects of growth hormone remain speculative. However, the study of Fazio et al.[40] suggests a new strategy to treat this common health problem, particularly in patients who are unsuitable for current therapy.

Table 20.3 Growth factor therapy to enhance myocardial function.

Reference	Growth factor	Model	Ischemia reperfusion	Measurements	Results: growth factors vs. control
Battler et al.[31]	IGF-II	In vivo swine	Coronary injection of beads	• Wall motion score • Angiogenesis • Histology	• Better wall motion after 4 weeks • No effect on angiogenesis • Peri-infarct myocyte hypertrophy
Yang et al.[38]	GH	Rat model of heart failure 1 month after myocardial infarction	Permanent coronary artery occlusion	• Cardiac index • Stroke volume index • dP/dT • Vascular resistance	• Increased cardiac index • Increased stroke volume index • Increased dP/dT • Decreased vascular resistance
Duerr et al.[39]	IGF-I GH	Rat model of heart failure 1 month after myocardial infarction	Permanent coronary artery occlusion	• Cardiac output • Cardiac index • Vascular resistance	• Increased cardiac output • Increased cardiac index • Decreased vascular resistance
Giordano et al.[22]	FGF-5	In vivo swine Intracoronary gene transfer	Gradual occlusion of LCx	• Regional perfusion • Regional contractility • Angiogenesis • FGF gene expression	• FGF-5 gene transfer improved regional perfusion • FGF-5 gene transfer ameliorated pacing-induced myocardial dysfunction • FGF-5 gene transfer enhanced angiogenesis • Positive FGF gene expression in the heart
Cittadini et al.[37]	• GH • IGF-I	• In vivo rat • Langendorff perfusion model		• Echocardiography • Hemodynamics • Morphometric histology	• Left ventricular hypertrophic response • Increased cardiac index • Decreased vascular resistance
Fazio et al.[40]	GH for 3 months	Clinical trial in patients with dilated cardiomyopathy		• Left ventricular wall thickness • Chamber size • Heart catheterization • Exercise capacity • Symptoms	• Increased left ventricular wall thickness • Reduced chamber size • Reduced end systolic wall stress • Improved cardiac output • Increased exercise capacity • Improved symptoms

Notes:
aFGF = acidic fibroblast growth factor; bFGF = basic fibroblast growth factor; CK = creatine kinase; GH = growth hormone; IC = intracoronary; IGF = insulin-like growth factor; IV = intravenous; LAD = left anterior descending coronary artery; LCx = left circumflex coronary artery; rhVEGF = recombinant human vascular endothelial growth factor; TGF-β = transforming growth factor-β; VEGF = vascular endothelial growth factor.

Questions and controversies

Several issues remain to be questioned and debated. Which is the best growth factor for therapeutic angiogenesis and enhancement of collateral circulation? bFGF or VEGF? VEGF is an endothelial specific mitogen which includes a signal sequence permitting active secretion. Theoretically, bFGF action remains intracellular. However, Lazarous et al.[15] recently suggested that bFGF is superior to VEGF for therapeutic angiogenesis in a canine model of myocardial ischemia. Asahara et al.[43] demonstrated that combined administration of VEGF and bFGF stimulates significantly greater and more rapid augmentation of collateral circulation, resulting in superior hemodynamic improvement compared with either VEGF or bFGF alone.

Which is the preferred agent to enhance cardiac performance? IGF-I, IGF-II or growth hormone? Current data do not enable us to identify a significant advantage of any of these agents.

The issue of safety in human trials if of great concern. Scientists are worried about possible adverse reactions related to the transfer of viruses and recombinant DNA molecules into humans. In addition, growth factors may accelerate atherosclerosis, fibrosis and cancer. Administration of angiogenic peptides could have a dual effect in patients with coronary artery disease, promoting collateral formation, but simultaneously inducing neointimal smooth muscle cell accumulation, ultimately exacerbating the atherogenic process. Excess amounts of growth hormone were associated with increased morbidity and mortality from cardiovascular disease and cancer.[42]

Recombinant protein or gene? Which is the best therapeutic method? In terms of safety and bioactivity, gene transfer may be superior to one or multiple large doses of recombinant protein. The advantage of protein therapy is better control of the amount of therapeutic growth factor.

These questions and many others must be answered before growth factors should be used in clinical practice.

Summary and future implications

Recent interest in growth factors as an alternative therapeutic strategy to alter the contractile properties of cardiomyocytes and to improve myocardial function and viability opens new frontiers in cardiovascular therapy. In the setting of interventional cardiology, growth factors can provide adjuvant therapy with direct myocardial protection and increase the viability and function of the ischemic myocardium.

The ability to introduce growth factor genes into vessel walls may be a useful strategy for therapeutic angiogenesis and prevention of restenosis, as well as to enhance healing and viability after vascular injury. In this situation, even a few transfected cells may be enough to produce recombinant growth factors in concentrations that are physiologically effective. Such an approach will be efficacious even with the transient expression of the gene product, since the beneficial effects of angiogenic growth factors persist long after administration is discontinued. Although growth factors have not yet become part of clinical practice, they have attracted a great deal of interest and are involved in several preliminary clinical trials.

Most recently, cellular grafting has emerged as an accepted approach for delivery of therapeutic peptides. The use of genetically modified cells for the delivery of recombinant molecules has potential as a powerful approach for ex vivo gene therapy. Recently, Leor et al.[44] demonstrated the feasibility of fetal cardiomyocyte transplantation into myocardial infarction. If the fetal graft could be engineered ex vivo to produce growth factor, the ability to introduce growth factor gene into myocardial infarction may be a useful strategy for therapeutic angiogenesis to enhance myocardial healing and viability.

In summary, exogenous administration of growth factors provides a new therapeutic strategy for cellular cardiomyoplasty and myocardial repair after myocardial injury. Recent experiments also suggest potential adjuvant treatment to current interventional cardiology techniques and offer hope that gene therapy can be used to enhance collateral circulation, to improve myocardial viability and to prevent future ischemic episodes.

References

1   Chien RK, Grace AA. Principles of cardiovascular molecular and cellular biology. In Braunwald E (ed.). Heart Disease: Textbook of Cardiovascular Medicine (5th edn) (Philadelphia, PA: WB Saunders, 1997): 1626–49.

2   Schott RJ, Morrow LA. Growth factors and angiogenesis. Cardiovasc Res 1993; **27**: 1155–61.

3   Lembo G, Hunter JJ, Chien KR. Signalling pathways for cardiac growth and hypertrophy. Recent advances and prospects for growth factor therapy. Ann NY Acad Sci 1995; **752**: 115–27.

4   Donath MY, Zapf J, Eppenberger-Eberhardt M, Froesch ER, Eppenberger HM. Insulin-like growth factor I stimulates myofibril development and decreases smooth muscle alpha-actin of adult cardiomyocytes. Proc Natl Acad Sci USA 1994; **91**: 1686–90.

5   Sacca L, Fazio S. Cardiac performance: growth hormone enters the race. Nat Med 1996; **2**: 29–30.

6   Sabia PJ, Powers ER, Ragosta M, Sarembock IJ, Burwell LR, Kaul S. An association between collateral blood flow and myocardial viability in patients with recent myocardial infarction. *N Engl J Med* 1992; **327**: 1825–31.

7   Schaper W, Gorge G, Winkler B, Schaper J. The collateral circulation of the heart. *Prog Cardiovasc Dis* 1988; **31**: 57–77.

8   Casscells W, Speir E, Sasse J, *et al*. Isolation, characterization, and location of heparin-binding growth factors in the heart. *J Clin Invest* 1990; **85**: 433–41.

9   Fujita M, Ikemoto M, Kishishita M, *et al*. Elevated basic fibroblast growth factor in pericardial fluid of patients with unstable angina. *Circulation* 1996; **94**: 610–13.

10 Banai S, Jaklitsch MT, Casscells W, *et al*. Effects of acidic fibroblast growth factor on normal and ischemic myocardium. *Circ Res* 1991; **69**: 76–85.

11 Battler A, Scheinowitz M, Bor A, *et al*. Intracoronary injection of basic fibroblast growth factor enhances angiogenesis in infarcted swine myocardium. *J Am Coll Cardiol* 1993; **22**: 2001–6.

12 Unger EF, Banai S, Shou M, *et al*. Basic fibroblast growth factor enhances myocardial collateral flow in a canine model. *Am J Physiol* 1994; **266**: H1588–95.

13 Banai S, Jaklitsch MT, Shou M, *et al*. Angiogenic-induced enhancement of collateral blood flow to ischemic myocardium by vascular endothelial growth factor in dogs. *Circulation* 1994; **89**: 2183–9.

14 Lazarous DF, Scheinowitz M, Shou M, *et al*. Effects of chronic systemic administration of basic fibroblast growth factor on collateral development in the canine heart. *Circulation* 1995; **91**: 145–53.

15 Lazarous DF, Shou M, Scheinowitz M, *et al*. Comparative effects of basic fibroblast growth factor and vascular endothelial growth factor on coronary collateral development and the arterial response to injury. *Circulation* 1966; **94**: 1074–82.

16 Takeshita S, Zheng LP, Brogi E, *et al*. Therapeutic angiogenesis. A single intraarterial bolus of vascular endothelial growth factor augments revascularization in a rabbit ischemic hind limb model. *J Clin Invest* 1994; **93**: 662–70.

17 Bauters C, Asahara T, Zheng LP, *et al*. Recovery of disturbed endothelium-dependent flow in the collateral-perfused rabbit ischemic hindlimb after administration of vascular endothelial growth factor. *Circulation* 1995; **91**: 2802–9.

18 Isner JM, Feldman LJ. Gene therapy for arterial disease. *Lancet* 1994; **344**: 1653–4.

19 Isner JM, Walsh K, Symes J, *et al*. Arterial gene transfer for therapeutic angiogenesis in patients with peripheral artery disease. *Hum Gene Ther* 1996; **7**: 959–88.

20 Isner JM, Walsh K, Symes J, *et al*. Arterial gene therapy for therapeutic angiogenesis in patients with peripheral artery disease. *Circulation* 1995; **91**: 2687–92.

21 Isner JM, Pieczek A, Schainfeld R, *et al*. Clinical evidence of angiogenesis after arterial gene transfer of phVEGF165 in patient with ischaemic limb. *Lancet* 1996; **348**: 370–4.

22 Giordano F, Ping P, McKiirnan S, *et al*. Intracoronary transfer of fibroblast growth factor-5 increases blood flow and contractile function in an ischemic region of the heart. *Nature Med* 1996; **2**: 534–9.

23 Koh GY, Kim SJ, Klug MG, Park K, Soonpaa MH, Field LJ. Targeted expression of transforming growth factor-β1 in intracardiac grafts promotes vascular endothelial DNA synthesis. *J Clin Invest* 1995; **95**: 114–21.

24 Sellke FW, Wang SY, Friedman M, *et al*. Basic FGF enhances endothelium-dependent relaxation of the collateral-perfused coronary microcirculation. *Am J Physiol* 1994; **267**: H1303–11.

25 Hariawala MD, Horowitz JJ, Esakof D, *et al*. VEGF improves myocardial blood flow but produces EDRF-mediated hypotension in porcine hearts. *J Surg Res* 1996; **63**: 77–82.

26 Asahara T, Bauters C, Pastore C, *et al*. Local delivery of vascular endothelial growth factor accelerates reendothelialization and attenuates intimal hyperplasia in balloon-injured rat carotid artery. *Circulation* 1995; **91**: 2793–801.

27 Yanagisawa-Miwa A, Uchida Y, Nakamura F, *et al*. Salvage of infarct myocardium by angiogenic action of basic fibroblast growth factor. *Science* 1992; **257**: 1401–3.

28 Horrigan MCG, MacIsaac AI, Nicolini FA, *et al*. Reduction in myocardial infarct size by basic fibroblast growth factor after temporary coronary occlusion in a canine model. *Circulation* 1996; **94**: 1927–33.

29 Harada K, Grossman W, Friedman M, *et al*. Basic fibroblast growth factor improves myocardial function in chronically ischemic porcine hearts. *J Clin Invest* 1994; **94**: 623–30.

30 Buerke M, Murohara T, Skurk C, Nuss C, Tomaselli K, Lefer AM. Cardioprotective effect of insulin-like growth factor in myocardial ischemia followed by reperfusion. *Proc Natl Acad Sci USA* 1995; **92**: 8031–5.

31 Battler A, Hasdai D, Goldberg I, *et al*. Exogenous insulin-like growth factor II enhances post-infarction regional myocardial function and myocyte growth in the swine. *Eur Heart J* 1995; **16**: 1851–9.

32   Padua RR, Sehi R, Dhalla NS, Kardami E. Basic fibroblast growth factor is cardioprotective in ischemia-reperfusion injury. *Mol Cell Biochem* 1995; **143**: 129–35.

33   Lefer AM, Tsao P, Nobuo A, Palladino MA. Mediation of cardioprotection by transforming growth factor-β. *Science* 1990; **249**: 61–4.

34   Lefer AM, Ma XL, Weyrich AS, Scalia R. Mechanism of the cardioprotective effect of transforming growth factor beta 1 in feline myocardial ischemia and reperfusion. *Proc Natl Acad Sci USA* 1993; **90**: 1018–22.

35   Buerke M, Murohara T, Skurk C, Nuss C, Tomaselli K, Lefer AM. Cardioprotective effect of insulin-like growth factor I in myocardial ischemia followed by reperfusion. *Proc Natl Acad Sci USA* 1995; **92**: 8031–5.

36   Sacca L, Cittadini A, Fazio S. Growth hormone and the heart. *Endocr Rev* 1994; **15**: 555–73.

37   Cittadini A, Stromer H, Katz ES, *et al.* Differential cardiac effects of growth hormone and insulin-like growth factor-I in the rat. A combined *in vivo* and *in vitro* evaluation. *Circulation* 1996; **93**: 800–9.

38   Yang R, Bunting S, Gillet N, Clark R, Hongkui J. Growth hormone improves cardiac performance in experimental heart failure. *Circulation* 1995; **92**: 262–7.

39   Duerr RL, McKirnan D, Gim RD, Ross CG, Chien KR, Ross J. Cardiovascular effects of insulin-like growth factor-I and growth hormone in chronic left ventricular failure in the rat. *Circulation* 1996; **93**: 2188–96.

40   Fazio S, Sabatini D, Capaldo B, *et al.* A preliminary study of growth hormone in the treatment of dilated cardiomyopathy. *N Engl J Med* 1996; **334**: 809–14.

41   Loh E, Swain JL. Growth hormone for heart failure—cause for cautious optimism. *N Engl J Med* 1996; **334**: 856–7.

42   Wright AD, Hill DM, Lowy C, Fraser TR. Mortality in acromegaly. *Q J Med* 1970; **39**: 1–16.

43   Asahara T, Bauters C, Zheng LP, *et al.* Synergistic effect of vascular endothelial growth factor and basic fibroblast growth factor on angiogenesis *in vivo*. *Circulation* 1995; **92**: II365–71.

44   Leor J, Patterson M, Quinones M, Kedes L, Kloner RA. Transplantation of fetal myocardial tissue into the infarcted myocardium of rat: a potential method for repair of infarcted myocardium. *Circulation* 1996; **94 (Suppl II)**: II-332–II-336.

21

Genetic engineering of stents

Moshe Y Flugelman, Anat Weisz, Iris Keren-Tal, David A Halon and Basil S Lewis

Introduction

The use of endoluminal stents has made a major impact on the practice of interventional cardiology in recent years.[1,2] Stent materials and design have improved to provide stents which are flexible, maneuverable and relatively easy to implant. Improvement in techniques of stent deployment (high-pressure balloons, intravascular ultrasound) and the routine use of the antiplatelet drugs ticlopidine and aspirin, rather than full prolonged anticoagulation with heparin and warfarin, has resulted in a reduced incidence of early stent thrombosis and a low incidence of puncture site-related complications.[1–3]

Complications following successful stent deployment are related to 1) acute and subacute stent thrombosis and 2) smooth muscle cell proliferation and late coronary restenosis. Several strategies have been developed to reduce local stent thrombosis.[4,5] Heparin-coated stents appear to reduce the restenosis rate in patients,[6] and polymer-coated stents eluting platelet glycoprotein IIb/IIIa receptor antibody reduce platelet deposition and improve the patency rate[7] in an animal model.

A different strategy for improving stent surfaces by seeding stents with endothelial cells was described by van der Gissen et al.[8] and later by Dichek et al.[9] Seeding intravascular prostheses with endothelial cells is a time-honored method in vascular surgery,[10,11] since endothelial cells naturally provide the best interface between blood and tissue. Rapid endothelialization after balloon angioplasty and stent deployment will probably reduce the risk of thrombosis and decrease the incidence of restenosis.[12–14] An even better endothelial surface may be achieved if the endothelial cells secrete selective protein substances locally.[14,15] Secretion of these therapeutic proteins can be achieved by gene transfer to the endothelial cells with overexpression of the transgene by the cells.[9,16]

In this chapter the authors describe their experience in seeding stents with genetically modified endothelial cells and discuss the issues that need to be addressed in the field. Genetic engineering of stents is a new approach which aims to improve the results of angioplasty, and is a technique at the junction of interventional cardiology and molecular and cellular biology.

Seeding stents with genetically modified endothelial cells

The application of techniques of gene transfer to vascular biology provides a tantalizing potential method for modulating tissue growth following acute vascular injury. Experimental methods of gene transfer were applied to vascular tissue but are yet to be improved. Direct in vivo gene transfer to vascular cells can be achieved with retroviral vectors but gene transfer efficiency is very low,[17] while gene transfer with adenoviral vectors is selective to endothelial cells due to anatomical barriers.[18] The concept of seeding stents with genetically modified cells may provide a somewhat complex but feasible method for gene transfer to the vessel wall. In this model, the modified cells, delivered on a stent and targeted to the vascular segment of interest, secrete both locally and intraluminally the therapeutic proteins that will either penetrate the full thickness of the arterial wall or be secreted into the blood and exert their effects distal to the region of stent deployment. The method aims, then, to limit gene transfer to the cells seeded on the stent, a simpler technique than to alter gene expression in the vessel wall. Protein secretion from the seeded stents would continue for a given period of time, which may be sufficient to alter vascular growth during the critical phase in the days and weeks following angioplasty.

Cell harvesting

Endothelial cell harvesting is the first step for genetically engineering stents. The cells of the patients must be used to prevent rejection and resulting local inflammation. Thus autologous endothelial cells can be harvested from veins, arteries or adipose tissue.[10,11,19] Although the lag period from cell harvesting to the time point with sufficient cells for seeding is relatively long with venous and arterial sources, cells isolated from these vessels are definitely endothelial cells. With experience, human endothelial cell harvesting from saphenous veins is predictable and reproducible. Experience with adipose cell harvesting is yet to be gained in the authors' laboratory.

Choice of vector

In vitro gene transfer to the isolated cells can be achieved by several methods. Viral vectors are far more efficient for gene transfer to cells when compared to naked DNA or liposome-DNA complex gene transfer. We have used retroviral vectors to transfer marker, selection and therapeutic genes to endothelial cells *in vitro*.[19-21] The use of a selection gene allows the growth of a homogeneous population of endothelial cells, all expressing the gene of interest and the transgenes integrate into the genomic DNA with retroviral gene transfer. Cells dividing from the transduced cell express the transgene and thus a prolonged period of transgene expression can be expected with retroviral vector gene transfer. Adenoviral vectors for gene transfer are more efficient *in vitro* and *in vivo* and their use shortens the period for achieving a cellular population that expresses the therapeutic gene. As the transgene is not integrated into the genomic DNA, cells that divide from the modified cells will not express the transgene. The use of a viral vector can be tailored to therapeutic needs. For short-term local expression of therapeutic proteins after angioplasty, adenoviral gene transfer may be appropriate, while retroviral gene transfer can be employed when prolonged, continuous expression of the therapeutic gene is needed.

Genes to be considered

The selection of the transgene is of major importance. In animal experiments of autologous, genetically modified, endothelial cell stent seeding, the t-PA gene was used.[19-21] The authors were able to detect the presence of the modified cells in the arterial segment of stent deployment in two thirds of the experiments, 10 days after stent deployment. In further studies of seeding vascular grafts with endothelial cells expressing t-PA, it was shown that overexpression of t-PA may be deleterious to cell adherence to the grafts and cell retention was reduced.[16] Proteolytic properties of t-PA render the molecule unsuitable for genetic modification of seeded cells. Other thrombolytic proteins that prevent local thrombosis but do not affect cell adherence are needed. Such a protein may be the factor Xa inhibitor.

The authors are currently examining the use of vascular endothelial growth factor (VEGF) in our stent seeding experiments.[22] The theoretical basis for our choice is that endothelial cells produce the finest interface between blood and the arterial wall and rapid endothelialization may well prevent postangioplasty complications. Local overexpression of VEGF may also prove to be important in the process of angiogenesis.[23] The effect of VEGF gene transfer to human saphenous vein endothelial cells is shown in Fig. 21.1. The apparent increase in cell number was

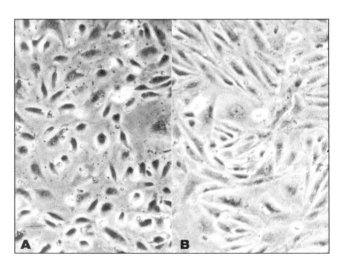

Figure 21.1

Human endothelial cells in tissue culture, after harvesting from 5 cm long saphenous vein segments stripped during coronary bypass surgery. (a) Control cells. (b) Cells exposed to adenoviral vector expressing vascular endothelial growth factor (VEGF). Cells exposed to the vector exhibit morphologic changes, with elongation and clustering, and an increased proliferation rate.

associated with morphological changes. The duration of VEGF secretion and cell retention on the stents are presently undergoing *in vitro* testing and need to be tested *in vivo*.

Other approaches to genetic engineering of stents

There are several other possible ways to modify stents genetically. It should be noted that all methods are theoretical and there are scant data to support their feasibility. Incorporation of nucleic acids (either DNA or RNA) into polymers that cover stents may have a potential for genetic modification of stents. Slow-release DNA encoding therapeutic genes may have a significant physiologic effect as shown with hydrogel-coated balloon catheters in which plasmid DNA was incorporated.[24] A short RNA sequence complementary to certain regions of the RNA molecule (antisense) may be used to inhibit local proliferation of smooth muscle cells and therefore restenosis.[25] This method, proven to be effective *in vitro*, may have a potential use *in vivo*.

Unresolved issues

Several issues must be addressed before seeded stents are deployed in patients. These issues include methods for detection of *in vivo* cell retention on stents,[16,19,26] assessment of physiologic effects of the secreted proteins, technical aspects of seeded stent deployment[27] and, very importantly, the safety of the procedure. The authors are currently engaged in *in vitro* and *in vivo* animal experiments which will make implantation of genetically modified stents safe and feasible.

Acknowledgment

This work was supported by a grant of the Israel Ministry of Health no. 2731.

References

1   Serruys PW, de Jaegere P, Kiemeneij, *et al*. A comparison of balloon expandable-stent implantation with balloon angioplasty in patients with coronary artery disease. *N Engl J Med* 1994; **331**: 489–95.

2   Fischman DL, Leon MB, Baim DS, *et al*. A randomized comparison of coronary-stent placement and balloon angioplasty in the treatment of coronary artery disease. *N Engl J Med* 1994; **331**: 496–501.

3   Schomig A, Newman FJ, Kastrati A, *et al*. A randomized comparison of antiplatelet and anticoagulant therapy after the placement of coronary artery stents. *New Engl J Med* 1996; **334**: 1126–8.

4   Wilcox JN. Thrombin and other potential mechanisms underlying restenosis. *Circulation* 1991; **84**: 432–5.

5   Flugelman MY. Inhibition of intravascular thrombosis and vascular smooth muscle cell proliferation by gene therapy. *Thromb Haemo* 1995; **74**: 406–10.

6   Serruys PW, Emanuelsson H, van der Giessen W, *et al*. Heparin coated Palmaz–Schatz stents in human coronary arteries. Early outcome of the Benestent II pilot study. *Circulation* 1996; **93**: 412–22.

7   Aggarwal RK, Ireland DC, Azrin MA, Ezekowitz MD, de Bono DP, Gershlick AH. Antithrombotic potential of polymer coated stents eluting platelet glycoprotein IIb/IIIa receptor antibody. *Circulation* 1996; **94**: 3311–17.

8   Van der Gissen WJ, Serruys PW, Visser WJ, Verdouw PD, van Schalkwijk WP, Jongkind JF. Endothelialization of endovascular stents. *J Interven Cardiol* 1988; **1**: 109–20.

9   Dichek DA, Neville RF, Zwiebel JA, Freeman SM, Leon MB, Anderson WF. Seeding of intravascular stents with genetically engineered endothelial cells. *Circulation* 1989; **80**: 1347–53.

10   Zilla P, Deutsch M, Meinhart J, *et al*. Clinical *in vitro* endothelialization of femoropopliteal bypass grafts: an actuarial follow-up over three years. *J Vasc Surg* 1994; **19**: 540–8.

11   Pasic M, Muller-Glauser W, Odermatt B, Lachat M, Seifert B, Turina M. Seeding with omental cells prevents late neointimal hyperplasia in small-diameter dacron grafts. *Circulation* 1995; **82**: 2605–16.

12   Ueda Y, Nanto S, Komamura K, Kodama K. Neointimal coverage of stents in human coronary arteries observed by angioscopy. *J Am Coll Cardiol* 1994; **23**: 341–6.

13   Fischlein T, Zill P, Meinhart J, *et al*. *In vitro* endothelialization of a mesosystemic shunt: a clinical case report. *J Vasc Surg* 1994; **19**: 549–54.

14   Clowes AW. Improving the interface between biomaterials and the blood; the gene therapy approach. *Circulation* 1996; **93**: 1319–20.

15   Dichek DA. Therapeutic potential of genetic engineering: enhancement of endothelial cell fibrinolysis. In: Zilla P, Fasol R, Callow A (eds). *Applied Cardiovascular Biology 1990–91* (Basel: Karger, 1992): Vol. 2, 197–204.

16   Dunn PF, Newman KD, Jones M, *et al.* Seeding of vascular grafts with genetically modified endothelial cells. *Circulation* 1996; **93**: 1439–46.

17   Flugelman MY, Jaklitsch MT, Newman KD, Casscells SW, Bratthuaer GL, Dichek DA. Low levels *in vivo* gene transfer into the arterial wall through a perforated balloon catheter. *Circulation* 1992; **85**: 1110–17.

18   Rome JJ, Shayani V, Flugelman MY, *et al.* Anatomic barriers determine the distribution of *in vivo* gene transfer into the arterial wall: modeling with microscopic tracer particles and verification with a recombinant adenoviral vector. *Athero Thromb* 1994; **14**: 148–61.

19   Flugelman MY, Virmani R, Leon MB, Bowman RL, Dichek DA. Genetically engineered endothelial cells remain adherent and viable after stent deployment and exposure to pulsatile flow. *Circ Res* 1992; **70**: 348–54.

20   Flugelman MY, Rome JJ, Virmani R, Newman KD, Dichek DA. Detection of genetically engineered endothelial cells seeded on endovascular prosthesis ten days after *in vivo* deployment. *J Mol Cell Cardiol* 1993; **25 (Suppl I)**: S-38.

21   Flugelman MY, Rome JJ, Virmani R, *et al.* In vivo deployment of balloon expandable stents seeded with genetically modified autologous endothelial cells – animal experi-ments, and initial human *in vitro* studies. (Submitted for publication 1997.)

22   Ferrara N, Houck K, Jakeman L, Leung DW. Molecular and biological properties of the vascular endothelial growth factor family. *Endocr Rev* 1992; **13**: 18–32.

23   Majesky M. A little VEGF goes a long way. *Circulation* 1996; **94**: 3062–4.

24   Asahara T, Chen D, Tsurumi Y, *et al.* Accelerated restitution of endothelial integrity and endothelial dependent function after phVEGF$_{165}$ gene transfer. *Circulation* 1996; **94**: 3291–302.

25   Speir E, Epstein SE. Inhibition of smooth muscle cell proliferation by an antisense oligodeoxynucleotide targeting the messenger RNA encoding proliferating cell nuclear antigen. *Circulation* 1992; **86**: 538–47.

26   Sharefkin JB, Lather C, Smith M, Rich NM. Endothelial cell labeling with indium-111-oxine as a marker of cell attachment to bioprosthetic surfaces. *J Biomed Mat Res* 1983; **17**: 345–57.

27   Scott NA, Candal FJ, Robinson KA, Ades EW. Seeding of intracoronary stents with immortalized human microvascular endothelial cells. *Am Heart J* 1995; **129**: 860–6.

22

The role of inflammation in atherosclerosis

Arnon Blum and Hylton I Miller

The cellular level

'Atherosclerosis, the principal cause of heart attack, stroke, and gangrene of the extremities, is responsible for 50% of all mortality in the USA, Europe, and Japan. The lesions result from an excessive inflammatory-fibroproliferative response to various forms of insult to the endothelium and smooth muscle of the artery wall. A large number of growth factors, cytokines, and vasoregulatory molecules participate in this process. Our ability to control the expression of genes encoding these molecules and to target specific cell types provides opportunities to develop new diagnostic and therapeutic agents to induce the regression of the lesions and possibly to prevent their formation' (Russell Ross).[1]

In the nineteenth century there were two major hypotheses to explain the pathogenesis of atherosclerosis: the 'incrustation' hypothesis and the 'lipid' hypothesis. The incrustation hypothesis of von Rokitansky,[2] proposed in 1852 and modified by Duguid,[3] suggested that intimal thickening resulted from fibrin deposition, with subsequent organization by fibroblasts and secondary lipid accumulation. The lipid hypothesis proposed by Virchow[4] in 1856 suggested that lipid in the arterial wall represented a transduction of blood lipid, which subsequently formed complexes with acid mucopolysacharides; lipid accumulated in arterial walls because mechanisms of lipid deposition predominated over those of removal. The two hypotheses are now integrated into a more complex 'response to injury' hypothesis, developed by Ross,[1] which represents the prevalent view of the initiation of atherosclerosis.[5]

Basically, the atherosclerotic process is, at the outset, a protective response to insults to the endothelium and smooth muscle cells of the arterial wall. The response consists of the formation of fibrofatty and fibrous lesions, preceded and accompanied by inflammation. The advanced pathologic atherosclerotic plaques result from an excessive inflammatory-fibroproliferative response to numerous diverse insults.[1] Studies of animals with artificially induced hypercholesterolemia[6–8] have confirmed that three processes are involved in the formation of atherosclerotic lesions: 1) the proliferation of smooth muscle cells, macrophages and possibly lymphocytes; 2) the formation by smooth muscle cells of a connective tissue matrix comprising elastic fiber proteins, collagen and proteoglycans; and 3) the accumulation of lipids, mostly free and esterified cholesterol, in the surrounding matrix and the associated cells.

The cellular events that occur during progression of lesions in hypercholesterolemic animals are almost exactly mirrored by those observed in human atherosclerotic coronary arteries in hearts removed during transplant surgery.[9] Shortly after the induction of hypercholesterolemia, monocytes and lymphocytes adhere in clusters to the endothelium, migrate over its surface and reach the subendothelial intima by penetrating at endothelial cell junctions; there, the monocytes are converted to macrophages, 'ingest' lipids and their appearance changes to foam cells. Progression of atherosclerotic lesions is thus marked by the accumulation of alternating layers of smooth muscle cells and lipid-laden macrophages. The arteries contain sites with retracted endothelial cells, which expose underlying lipid-filled macrophages and provide sites for platelet interactions leading to the formation of mural thrombi.

The formation of fibrous lesions in response to injury is not in itself remarkable; wound healing follows such a course. The response to arterial injury differs from the injury of most other tissues and organs in two respects: 1) the principal source of connective tissue in the arterial wall is the smooth muscle cell; and 2) the sources of arterial injury (hypertension, hypercholesterolemia, cigarette smoking, diabetes and obesity) are likely to be chronic. Thus the progression from a fatty streak to a fibrous plaque is unlikely to be interrupted.[1]

Growth factors and cytokines

The growth-regulatory molecules can induce multiple and, in some instances, divergent effects. They can stimulate or inhibit cell proliferation, and many of the proliferative agents act as chemoattractants. The molecules that are potentially important in cell proliferation include platelet-derived growth factor (PDGF),[10,11] basic fibroblast growth factor (bFGF),[12,13] heparin-binding epidermal growth factor (HB-EGF),[14] insulin-like growth factor-1 (IGF-1), interleukin-1 (IL-1),[15] tumor necrosis factor alfa TNFalfa)[16] and transforming growth factor beta (TGFbeta).[17] All of them may induce smooth muscle cell proliferation and are generally not expressed in the normal artery, whereas they are upregulated in lesions of atherosclerosis.

Several of these growth factors are also chemoattractants. Chemotaxis is a critical event in the development of the lesions of atherosclerosis and in the restenosis that often occurs after surgical intervention and angioplasty. Thus, chemotaxis is necessary to bring leukocytes into the artery wall and, at some sites, smooth muscle cells from the media into the intima of the artery. Colony stimulating factors (CSFs), monocyte chemotactic protein-1 (MCP-1),[18] oxidized low-density lipoprotein (oxLDL)[19] and TGFbeta can each induce monocyte chemotaxis and endothelial transmigration, whereas PDGF and IGF-1 can induce smooth muscle cell chemotaxis.[20] Basic FGF, which has no signal sequence and is present in the cytosol of most cells, is also found in basement membranes and could be released as a result of cell injury. It is a potent mitogen and chemoattractant for monocytes and a mitogen for smooth muscle cells.

IL-1, TNFalfa, interferon gamma (INFgamma) and IL-2 are well recognized cytokines that, together with the CSFs, are modulators of the inflammatory response that occurs once the endothelium has been exposed to injurious agents. The assumption is that none of these factors work alone, and that there is a network of cellular interactions. The release of one molecule can lead to the expression of a second molecule in a target cell that can then either stimulate its neighbors in a paracrine way, or itself in an autocrine way. An example would be the release of IL-1 or TNF, by activated lesion macrophages exposed to agonists such as oxLDL.[21]

In cultures, either of these macrophage products (and also TGFbeta) will induce PDGF-A gene expression in smooth muscle cells.[22] Similarly, when endothelial cells in culture are exposed to agonists, including IL-1, TNFalfa or TNFbeta,[22] they express the gene for, and secrete, PDGF-BB. Thus, if these cytokines were released in vivo by activated underlying macrophages. PDGF-BB secretion by the adjacent endothelium could in turn stimulate underlying smooth muscle cells to migrate or replicate.

Support for the relevance of these observations in cell culture has come from data demonstrating that PDGF gene expression is increased in smooth muscle cells and in adjacent macrophages in human atherosclerotic lesions.[23] Specimens obtained by endarterectomy of the carotid artery contain increased messenger RNA for PDGF-BB chain and for C-fms, the proto-oncogene that encodes the M-CSF receptor, prominent on macrophages and recently observed on smooth muscle cells.[24]

T-lymphocytes

Immunohistochemical analysis using monoclonal antibodies for specific cell types has shown that the lipid-rich core region of advanced human atherosclerotic plaques is dominated by macrophages.[25] The fibrous cap that surrounds the lipid core is dominated by vascular smooth muscle cells, but it also contains substantial numbers of T-lymphocytes and macrophages.[26] Monocyte-derived macrophages and T-lymphocytes are already present at a very early stage of atherosclerosis and are detectable in the fatty streak.[27] Among the lymphocytes, both CD4 and CD8 T cells can be detected, but there are very few, if any, B cells or plasma cells within the plaque.

The presence of activated T-lymphocytes in the atherosclerotic plaque suggests a local immune response. It has been postulated that such a response may be directed against local antigens in the plaque. Molecular genetic studies have demonstrated that these T cells were heterogeneous in terms of their immunological specificities.[28] It is therefore possible that only a small proportion of plaque T cells respond to local antigens: these cells probably elicit a process that brings in other T cells by immunologically nonspecific mechanisms. Very few B lymphocytes are present in the plaque.[29] However, there is an intense adventitial B cell infiltration in the inflammatory periaortitis or periarteritis that may develop around advanced atherosclerotic plaques.[30] The periaortic lesion is an adventitial inflammatory infiltrate that contains large amounts of B-lymphocytes, plasma cells and immunologloglobulins together with oxidized lipids. It has been proposed that it represents an autoimmune response to the oxidized lipids that are generated during the atherosclerotic process.[30]

Hansson et al.[31] showed in 1984 that a substantial proportion of the T cells in the atherosclerotic plaque are in an activated state. The activation pattern, with a high frequency of HLA-DR and VLA-1 expression and a much lower frequency of interleukin-2 receptor expression, is similar to that reported to occur in chronic inflammatory conditions. T cells may be activated locally, presumably by antigens presented in the context of class II MHC expressing smooth muscle cells and/or macrophages in the atherosclerotic lesion.

It has been observed that activated lymphocytes lose the sIL-2R after a few days but retain other signs of a continuing activation process,[32] such as the expression of HLA-DR and virus-like agent-1 on the surface of activated T cells that were isolated from plaques.[33] Activated T-lymphocytes secrete growth factors and cytokines that may affect other cell types and the process of atherosclerosis. It was demonstrated that smooth muscle cells are sensitive to interferon gamma (secreted by T cells) and respond by inhibition of proliferation and by expression of class II HLA antigens.[34,35]

Plaque 'at risk' and unstable angina pectoris

Most coronary thrombi are associated with tears of the intima, and an entrance of a large pool of extracellular lipids.[36] The risk of plaque rupture appears to be related to the composition of the atherosclerotic plaque. However, the precise mechanisms causing plaque rupture are not fully understood.[37]

Van der Wal et al.[38] investigated the cellular components of recently ruptured atherosclerotic plaques with cell-specific monoclonal antibodies in an attempt to evaluate further the potential role of an inflammatory process in the pathogenesis of intimal tearing. Their study confirmed that the fibrous cap overlying the lipid core appeared to be highly variable in both thickness and cellular constituents. At the site of erosion, the superficial parts of the cap were dominated by macrophages and T-lymphocytes. At sites of deep plaque rupture, the fibrous cap showed a localized accumulation of macrophages and T cells, with loss of smooth muscle cells. It therefore appears that the site of plaque rupture is associated with the occurrence of large numbers of macrophages and T cells and lack of smooth muscle cells.

Both T cells and macrophages expressed class II major histocompatibility complex antigens abundantly, and the site of the intimal tear always could be distinguished from the surrounding plaque tissue by an increase in the number of HLA-DR+ cells. The HLA-DR expression indicates activation of these cells. The activated T cells may trigger neighboring macrophages to synthesize and secrete tissue-degrading enzymes, such as metalloproteinases. This study showed that plaque rupture causing thrombosis, whether as a superficial erosion or as a deep fissure, is associated with a localized inflammatory process.[38]

It has been demonstrated that the C-reactive protein (CRP) level is increased in 'active' unstable coronary artery disease[39] and could be used as a prognostic factor in patients with unstable angina pectoris—the higher the CRP level the worse the prognosis.[40] Further studies have shown that serum amyloid type A (SAA) could also be used as a quantitative marker for instability of angina pectoris,[41] and that the inflammatory process is prolonged, lasting months, even after clinical 'stabilization' of the angina pectoris.[42]

Therapeutic implications

Aspirin

It is well established that aspirin effectively reduces short-term and long-term risks of myocardial infarction after an episode of unstable coronary artery disease.[43–46] Aspirin is an anti-inflammatory drug that acts through blockade of the arachidonic acid cascade, and by suppression of antibody production, interference with antigen-antibody aggregation, inhibition in vitro of antigen-induced release of histamine and nonspecific stabilization of changes in capillary permeability in the presence of immunological insults.[47]

Heparin

In the acute phase, intravenous heparin infusion for 5–7 days is at least as effective as aspirin,[47,48] but the benefits are short lived because of reactivation of the disease soon after the infusion is stopped.[49] Other studies have shown that a combination of heparin and aspirin is more effective than aspirin alone;[45,46,48,50] however, these benefits also seem to pass after termination of the infusion.

Low molecular weight heparin

In the FRISC study,[51] low molecular heparin was given to unstable angina patients, and was found to be safe and protective against new cardiac events in patients with unstable coronary artery disease. Heparin and low molecular weight heparin act mainly by antithrombin III mediated inhibition of factor Xa; also through thrombin inhibition[52] and the release of tissue factor inhibitor, which might contribute to the antithrombotic effect.[53] Heparin also has antiatherogenic and antiproliferative properties, depresses cell-mediated immunity and suppresses graft-versus-host reactions.[47]

The molecular level

The role of cell adhesion molecules (CAM) in atherosclerosis is critical. Adhesion molecules are a group of proteins located in the outer surface of cell membranes, as soluble proteins in the serum, and also can be found in the cytoplasm. They are considered one of the keystones of cellular communication, cell recruitment, chemotaxis, the production and secretion of cytokines, as well as gene regulation involved with cellular proliferation, inhibition and apoptosis.

The adhesion proteins expressed on the vascular endothelial cell surface fall into two classes: the selectins (E-selectin, P-selectin, L-selectin) and the immunoglobulin family (vascular cell adhesion molecule = VCAM-1; intercellular adhesion molecule = ICAM-1).[54]

A breakthrough came with the description of the 'three-step model' of the development of the inflammatory response by Butcher[55] and Springer.[56] This model placed the adhesive events in a logical order, related them to physiologically relevant conditions of flow and ascribed particular molecules to distinct cellular events. The three steps enunciated were 1) capture of leukocytes from the axial stream to roll along the endothelium; 2) the firm adhesion of these leukocytes to endothelial cells; and 3) their subsequent transmigration into tissues.

Rolling was shown to be mediated by E and P selectin on endothelial cells. These adhesion proteins were thought to have special structural (long stems) and ligand-recognition features (lectin-carbohydrate stems), making them uniquely suitable for the rapid on/off adhesion that is an essential feature of rolling. Firm adhesion was mediated by intercellular adhesion molecule-1 and VCAM-1 interacting with the leukocyte integrins. Finally, transmigration was thought to be due to chemokines, such as interleukin-8, MCP-1 or Eotaxin, which also served locally to activate the integrins to mediate firm adhesion.[57]

In human atheroma, VCAM-1 is expressed not only on endothelial cells but also on macrophages and smooth muscle cells.[58] It has been demonstrated that smooth muscle cells of the blood vessel express various beta-integrins that appear to mediate cell interactions with the extracellular matrix.[59] Cytokines like IL-1 and TNFalfa are secreted as a response to adhesive molecules' expression in monocytes, and activate monocytes and macrophages[60] that can modify low-density lipoprotein (LDL) by peroxidation.[61] Oxidized LDL has cytotoxic effects on endothelial and mesenchymal cells and is responsible for the central necrosis that frequently exists in advanced atherosclerotic plaques. Oxidized LDL also amplifies the release of local cytokines elaborated by endothelial cells.

IL-1 and TNFalfa cause a rapid induction of the adhesive molecules E-selectin, VCAM-1 and ECAM-1, whereas interferon gamma up-regulates ICAM-1 over a longer period of time (10–24 hours).[62,63] Expression of VCAM-1 and the presence of T cells in the atherosclerotic plaque suggest that immunologic events mediated by cell adhesion molecules may play a role in the progression of atherosclerosis. As a result of increased cell adhesion molecules on the activated endothelium, binding of leukocytes and monocytes is potentiated, and these cells start to excrete cytokines, some of which may act as chemoattractants and allow monocytes to enter the intima by squeezing between endothelial cells.[64] The macrophages in the subendothelial layer have been shown to produce several growth factors, such as platelet-derived growth factor (PDGF),[65] and transforming growth factor (TGF).[66]

Monocyte-derived TGFbeta stimulates matrix production by smooth muscle cells.[67] The extracellular matrix is composed of fibronectin, laminin and collagen types 1 and 4; all of these components promote cell adhesion and migration,[68] and also influence the phenotypic transformation of smooth muscle cells by means of the beta-integrin subfamily.[69] Fibronectin (which is increased in atherosclerosis) promotes modulation of smooth muscle cells from a contractile to a synthetic phenotype, whereas laminin has the opposite effect.[70] Viral infections of endothelial cells have been shown to increase their adhesiveness to monocytes through P-selectin expression;[71] there might be a role for viral infection in the pathogenesis of atherosclerosis.[72,73]

Platelets and CAM

Under normal circumstances, the intact endothelium sequesters the adhesive glycoprotein ligands (von Willebrand factor, fibronectin and collagen) from the platelet in the subendothelium, thus preventing platelet adhesion in the absence of vascular damage. GPIb/Ix mediates the initial binding of platelets at rest to von Willebrand factor. This interaction induces the transition of GPIIb/IIIa from an inactive to an active state, which leads to platelet aggregation. On platelet stimulation with numerous agonists, GPIIb/IIIa becomes activated such that it can bind fibrinogen and several other ligands, including fibronectin, vitronectin, von Willebrand factor and thrombospondin.

Recently, blockade of GPIIb/IIIa has been intensively studied as an approach to antiplatelet therapy. The murine monoclonal antibody 7E3[74] blocks the GPIIb/IIIa receptor. The evaluation of 7E3 in the prevention of ischemic complication (EPIC) trial,[75] a double-blind, placebo-controlled trial in 2099 patients undergoing high-risk coronary angioplasty treated with c7E3 (chimeric Fab), demonstrated a 35% reduction of major ischemic events (death, myocardial infarction, urgent revascularization) at 1 month for the

71   Etingen OR, Silverstein RL, Hajjar DP. Identification of monocyte receptor on herpes virus infected endothelial cells. *Proc Natl Acad Sci USA* 1991; **88**: 7200–3.

72   Benditt EP, Barrett T, McDougall JK. Viruses in the etiology of atherosclerosis. *Proc Natl Acad Sci USA* 1983; **80**: 6386–9.

73   Hajjar DP. Viral pathogenesis of atherosclerosis: impact of molecular mimicry and viral genes. *Am J Pathol* 1991; **139**: 1195–211.

74   Coller BS. A new murine monoclonal antibody receptors an activation dependent change in the confirmation and/or microenvironment of the platelet glycoprotein IIb/IIIa complex. *J Clin Invest* 1985; **76**: 101–8.

75   EPIC Investigators. Use of a monoclonal antibody directed against the platelet glycoprotein IIb/IIIa receptor in high-risk coronary angioplasty. *N Engl J Med* 1994; **330**: 956–61.

76   Fan ST, Edington TS. Coupling of the adhesive receptor CD11b/CD18 to functional enhancement of effector macrophage tissue factor response. *J Clin Invest* 1991; **87**: 50–7.

77   Altieri DC, Edington TS. The saturable high affinity association of factor X to ADP-stimulated monocytes defines a novel function of the Mac-1 receptor. *J Biol Chem* 1988; **263**: 7007–15.

78   Shuman MA. Thrombin-cellular interactions. *Ann NY Acad Sci* 1986; **485**: 228–39.

79   McNamara CA, Sarembock IJ, Gimple LW, et al. Thrombin stimulates proliferation of cultured rat aortic smooth muscle cells by a proteolitically activated receptor. *J Clin Invest* 1993; **91**: 94–8.

80   Clowes AW, Clowes MM, Fingerle J, Reidy MA. Regulation of smooth muscle cell growth in injured artery. *J Cardiovasc Pharmacol* 1989; **14 (Suppl 6)**: S12–S15.

81   Heino J, MaQsaque J. Transforming growth factor-beta switches the pattern of integrins expressed in MG63 human osteosarcoma cells and causes a selective loss of cell adhesion to laminin. *J Biol Chem* 1989; **264**: 21800–11.

82   Holmes DRJ, Vliestra RE, Smith HC, et al. Restenosis after percutaneous transluminal coronary angioplasty (PTCA): a report from the PTCA registry of the National Heart, Lung, and Blood Institute. *Am J Cardiol* 1984; **53**: 77C–81C.

83   Fabricant CG, Fabricant J, Litrenta MM, Minick CR. Virus induced atherosclerosis. *J Exp Med* 1978; **148**: 335–40.

84   Melnick JL, Petrie BL, Dressman GR, et al. Cytomegalovirus antigen within human arterial smooth muscle cells. *Lancet* 1983; **2**: 2644–7.

85   Hendrix MGR, Salimans MM, van Boven CPA, Bruggeman CA. High prevalence of latently present cytomegalovirus in arterial walls of patients suffering from grade III atherosclerosis. *Am J Pathol* 1990; **136**: 23–8.

86   Adam E, Melnick JL, Probtsfield JL, et al. High level of cytomegalovirus antibody in patients requiring vascular surgery for atherosclerosis. *Lancet* 1987; **2**: 291–3.

87   Speir E, Modall R, Huang ES, et al. Potential role of human cytomegalovirus and p53 interaction in coronary restenosis. *Science* 1994; **265**: 391–4.

88   Zhou YF, Leon MB, Waclawin MA, et al. Association between prior cytomegalovirus infection and the risk of restenosis after coronary atherectomy. *N Engl J Med* 1996; **335**: 624–30.

89   Nieto FJ, Adam E, Sorlie P, et al. Cohort study of cytomegalovirus infection as a risk factor for carotid intimal-medial thickening, a measure of subclinical atherosclerosis. *Circulation* 1996; **94**: 922–7.

90   Geist LJ, Monick MM, Stinski MF, Hunninghake GW. The immediate early genes of human cytomegalovirus upregulate expression of the interleukin-2 and interleukin-2 receptor genes. *Am J Cell Biol* 1991; **5**: 292–6.

91   Gouczol E, Plotkin SA. Cells infected with human cytomegalovirus release a factor that stimulates cell DNA synthesis. *J Gen Virol* 1984; **65**: 1833–7.

92   Alcami J, Barzu T, Michelson S. Induction of an endothelial cell growth factor by human cytomegalovirus infection of fibroblasts. *J Gen Virol* 1991; **72**: 2765–70.

93   Kowalik TF, Wing B, Haskill JS, et al. Multiple mechanisms are implicated in the regulation of NF-kappa B activity during human cytomegalovirus infection. *Immunology* 1993; **78**: 405–12.

94   O'Brien KD, Allen MD, McDonald TO. Vascular cell adhesion molecule-1 is expressed in human coronary atherosclerotic plaques: implicated for the mode of progression of advanced coronary atherosclerosis. *J Clin Invest* 1993; **92**: 945–51.

95   Span AH, van Dam-Mieras MC, Mullers W, Endert J, Muller AD, Bruggeman CA. The effect of virus infection on the adherence of leukocytes or platelets to endothelial cells. *Eur J Clin Invest* 1991; **21**: 331–8.

96   Etingin OR, Silverstein RL, Hajjar DP. Von Willebrand factor mediated platelet adhesion to virally infected endothelial cells. *Proc Natl Acad Sci USA* 1993; **90**: 5133–6.

97   van Dam-Mieras MCE, Muller AD, van Hinsbergh VWM, Muller WJ, Bomans PH, Bruggeman CA. The procoagulant response of cytomegalovirus infected endothelial cells. *Throm Haemost* 1992; **68**: 364–70.

98   Zhou YF, Guetta E, Yu ZX, Finkel T, Epstein SE. Human cytomegalovirus, through its immediate early gene product IE 72, directly activates transcription of the scavenger receptor gene in human aortic smooth muscle cells. *Circulation* 1995; **92 (Suppl I)**: I-162.

99   Yamashiroya HM, Ghosh L, Yang R, Robertson AL. Herpes viridae in the coronary arteries and aorta of young trauma victims. *Am J Pathol* 1988; **130**: 71–9.

100   Tumilowicz JJ, Gawlil ME, Powell BB, Trentin JJ. Replication of cytomegalovirus in human arterial smooth muscle cells. *J Virol* 1985; **56**: 839–45.

101   Benditt EP, Benditt JM. Evidence of a monoclonal origin of human atherosclerotic plaques. *Proc Natl Acad Sci USA* 1973; **70**: 1753–6.

102   Fujinami RS, Nelson JA, Walker L, Oldstone MB. Sequence homology and immunologic cross-reactivity of human cytomegalovirus with HLA-DR beta chain: a means for graft rejection and immunosuppression. *J Virol* 1988; **62**: 100–5

23

Analysis of pathogenesis of atherosclerosis by intravascular ultrasound

Raimund Erbel, Junbo Ge, Günther Görge, Michael Haude, Fengqi Liu, Dietrich Baumgart, Stephen Sack and Allan Jeremias

Introduction

Coronary angiography is regarded as the gold standard for the diagnosis of coronary artery disease. Based on the clinical symptoms the indication for medical, interventional or surgical therapy is based on coronary angiography. Except for coronary calcification, no information about the morphology of the arterial wall is received. Coronary angiography is a contour method and gives the information about the coronary lumen, but not about the arterial wall. Early discrepancies between pathologic–anatomic studies and coronary angiography have already been published.[1,2] Differences between coronary angiography and morphology are also known by cardiac surgeons.

Intravascular ultrasound (IVUS) is a new method which visualizes the coronary lumen as well as the coronary arterial wall in cross-sections. This means that changes of the coronary arterial intima, the sign of coronary atherosclerosis, are detected. IVUS and its value for analysing the pathogenesis of coronary artery disease are described herein.

Intravascular ultrasound

Interventional cardiology has supported the development of IVUS. Three different methods are available for IVUS imaging (Fig. 23.1):

- rotation of a mirror (Ultracross, Boston Scientific, Sunnyvale CA, USA), which reflects the ultrasound beam;

- rotation of a single element ultrasound transducer (Sonicath, Boston Scientific, Watertown MA, USA);

- multielement electronic systems, with multiple circular ultrasound crystals embedded at the catheter tip (Endosonics, Rancho Cordova CA, USA).

The ultrasound frequency which is used is 30 MHz. The resolution in the axial direction is between 150 and 170 μm, in the lateral direction in the range of 200 μm and in the longitudinal direction in the range of 250 μm.[4-7] The catheter size ranges from 2.9 to 6.0F, so that vessels with a diameter of more than 1.5 mm can be examined. The catheter is guided using a monorail technique, but over-the-wire catheters are also available. The ultrasound console allows on-line assessment of vessel diameters and vessel areas as well as calculation of area and diameter stenosis.

Archiving is done using S-VHS video systems, and hard copy printouts. The new digital storage capability of one system of up to 40 images/sec is very promising (Endosonics, USA). The integration of the ultrasound image with the angiographic image is, at the moment, the best solution by transformation of the video signal to the X-ray signal (Echo Map, Siemens, Erlangen, Germany). Full-screen ultrasound images are available without fluoroscopy. When combined with fluoroscopy, the ultrasound image is placed in one of the four corners. These images can be stored with the coronary angiogram using a freeze IVUS frame or a real-time IVUS sequence. The great advantage is that one medium is utilized for imaging, storage and archiving, with high-resolution angiographic and ultrasound resolution on CD-ROM. The combined picture-in-picture allows for exact positioning of the ultrasound transducer. Thus, an

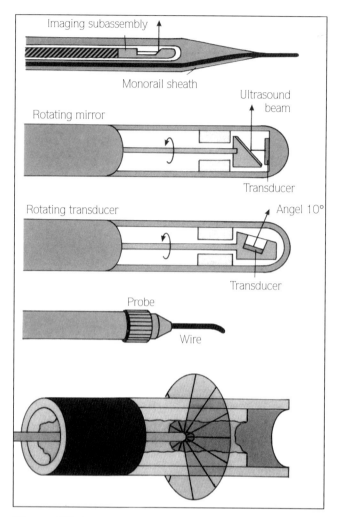

Figure 23.1

Different possibilities for IVUS showing rotating mirrors, rotating transducers and multielement electronic sectors scanners with schematic drawing of vessel imaging. Modified according to Bom et al.[1]

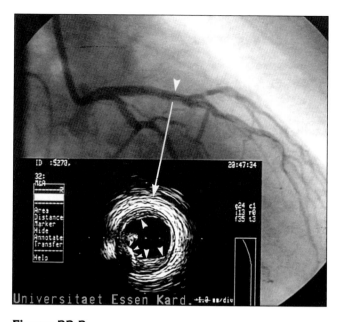

Figure 23.2

Visualization of a nearly normal coronary angiogram and visualization of calcified and noncalcified plaque formation of the left anterior descending coronary artery. The arrows show the transducer position in the Echo Map system (Siemens, Erlangen, Germany) with the picture-in-picture IVUS image technique (calibration 1 mm, 30 MHz transducer).

improvement in reproducibility can be expected. This is particularly important for follow-up studies, particularly after interventions, but also for regression and progression studies of coronary atherosclerosis (Fig. 23.2).

Using IVUS, cross-sectional images of the coronary arteries are provided. However, longitudinal images, which are obtained by coronary angiography, are not available. Three dimensional (3D) systems have been developed.[8,9] During a slow pull-back with 0.25–1 mm/sec images are stored with or without ECG triggering and specially developed 3D algorithms can be used to provide longitudinal and cross-sectional images. Thus, not only area but also volume of atherosclerotic plaque can be calculated and related to the vessel size and vessel lumen.[8,9]

Accuracy of intravascular ultrasound

The cross-sectional luminal area and vessel area can be analyzed using IVUS. In comparison to histology, a high accuracy and reproducibility could be assessed for peripheral and coronary arteries.[4,5,10] For normal arteries, or arteries with minimal abnormalities, a high correlation coefficiency between 0.77 and 0.92 could be assessed in comparison to coronary angiography.[4,5,7,11] The correlations were between 0.90 and 0.96 for coronary bypass visualization.[12,13] After percutaneous transluminal coronary angioplasty (PTCA), poor correlation coefficiencies, between

0.18 and 0.63, were reported due to dissections which reduced the accuracy of angiography.[7,14,15] The determined thickness correlated only for the sum of the intima and media and not for the media and intima separately.

Determination of the accuracy of IVUS with more sophisticated *in vitro* methods demonstrated that up to 25% errors can occur due to an underestimation of the true vessel size. This was explained by software and algorithm mistakes and *in vitro* experimental studies which used room temperature instead of body temperature.[16,17] In an editorial to this study, *in vitro* testings of IVUS catheters were considered to be important because, in interventional cardiology, decisions concerning interventional devices or stent size are based on IVUS.[17] Even perforations, which were reported with higher pressures and larger balloons when used for better stent implantation, may be related to the underestimation of the vessel diameter with subsequent oversizing of devices.[18]

Tissue characterization by IVUS is possible. For detection of calcium a high sensitivity and specificity of 97% and 99% was reported.[4] A clinically useful sensitivity of 89% for detection of lipid pools and 67% for fibrotic tissue was also reported. Similar results have been reported by others.[19]

Development of atherosclerosis

Intimal thickening is already detected at a young age.[20–22] After many years of describing the plaque morphology (Fig. 23.3) by pathology,[23–26] the American Heart Association published guidelines for classification of coronary atherosclerosis. The guidelines particularly emphasize that the recommendation should be using coronary artery imaging techniques.[27]

Type I lesion

These lesions are characterized microscopically by small deposits of macrophages with intracellular lipid at typical sites of the coronary artery tree.[22] Foam cells are seen. The lesions are eccentric and detected in up to 30% of the children. Similar lesions can be produced experimentally with a high cholesterol diet in rabbits. Adhesion of monocytes to the endothelium are seen. Activated monocytes are captured and infiltrate the intima—a selectine-dependent process. The adhesion and infiltration of monocytes need several weeks. An endothelium dysfunction which is produced by hypercholesterolemia is, however, detected within minutes of hypercholesterolemia.[28] The production of oxidized LDL (low density lipoprotein) enhances endothelial dysfunction due to reduced vasodilatation.[28]

Type II lesions (fatty streaks)

In comparison to type I lesions, fatty streaks are visible without microscopy, due to the yellow streaks at the luminal surface of arteries in type II lesions. They are already detected in older children at an age of 9–15 (Fig. 23.3). These plaques are particularly prominent in the proximal part of the left coronary artery opposite to the origin of the circumflex coronary artery.[21,26,29] The changes occur in the left coronary artery earlier than in the right coronary artery.[29] Via histology, foam cells and macrophages are found as well as smooth muscle cells loaded with lipids. In addition, T-lymphocytes as well as some mast cells are found. For the first time extracellular lipids and lipoproteins are detected. The lipids are mainly cholesterol esters (77%).[30] The prevalence of type I and II lesions reaches more than 50% in 12–14-year-old children, and 8% already show changes corresponding to more advanced lesions.[20] Similar lesions and cholesterol-loaded lesions are detected experimentally in rabbits fed with hypercholesterolemic diet.

By IVUS, eccentric lesions producing a three-layer appearance can be detected when intimal thickening exceeds the limit of resolution (150–200 μm). Typically, focal eccentric lesion are seen in the proximal part of the coronary arteries with 200–350 μm thickness (Fig. 23.4).

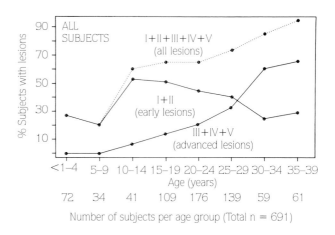

Figure 23.3
Development of plaque formation (Stary I–V) of the coronary artery in victims of accidents assessed by pathology (Stary[20]).

Type III lesions (preatheroma)

These lesions are found in young adults. An increase of lipid deposits covered by macrophages and foam cells is found. In addition to cholesterol and fatty acid lysolecithine, sphingomyeline and fatty acids are found.[20–22] Type III lesions are detected in the proximal part of coronary arteries by IVUS. The early stage of the disease is characterized by a dense reflecting zone, compromising the lumen, but with no hemodynamic consequences as a large lumen is still present (Fig. 23.4). A differentiation to type II lesions is difficult, and related to plaque thickness in type III lesions greater than 350 µm.

Type IV lesions (atheroma)

The ongoing process of coronary atherosclerosis is characterized by increased lipid deposits usually found in a core located adjacent to the media. Cholesterol crystals are found and cell necrosis is part of this process.[20,23] Usually a thick fibrous cap is present. A typical lesion is shown in Fig. 23.5. Characteristic of type IV lesion imaged by IVUS is a central and deeply located echolucent zone with a fibrous cap of more than 500 µm. Usually the echolucent zone cannot be separated from the media. It is most often found in eccentric and rarely in concentric lesions. In addition, these lesions have been found more often in the proximal than in the distal part of the coronary artery tree (Fig. 23.4).

Type V lesions

The type V lesions are subdivided into three classes.

Type Va lesion (fibroatheroma, fibrolipoid plaque, unstable plaque, plaque at risk)

Typically an ongoing increase of the lipid content of the plaque is found. The size of the central core increases and the fibrous cap decreases.[23,31,32] The fibroatheroma is known as unstable plaque at risk. With the increase of the lipid content the danger of rupture increases. It has been reported that in ruptured plaques the lipid pool is more than 40% of the total plaque area.[31,32] In addition, with an increase of the number of foam cells the smooth muscle cell content decreases and the content of macrophages increases, suggesting an inflammatory process.

Characteristically, IVUS detects the lipid core (Fig. 23.4) with an echolucent zone covered by a small fibrous cap.

Even multiple plaques at risk can be visualized (Fig. 23.5). These lesions are found especially in patients with unstable angina.[33] As the fibrotic tissue increases the arterial distensibility decreases due to the increase in collagen content, a feature which can be used in the future to differentiate between type IV and type V lesions, by analyzing the vessel compliance.

Type Vb (calcified plaque)

Calcification can be sometimes found in type III lesions extra- and intracellularly by microscopy but is more prominent in type IV, and even more so in type V lesions.[22] Calcification is due to a degenerative process and is, most often, a sign of cell necrosis. This type of lesion is characterized by a high calcium content with superficial or deep localization in the plaques and classified in 4 degrees dependent on the arc of calcification (Fig. 23.2). Due to shadowing, calcification can be detected with high accuracy (Fig. 23.5).

Type Vc (fibrotic plaque)

This type of plaque is found particularly in the peripheral arteries, but can be seen also in the coronary arteries and is characterized by a focal dense eccentric or concentric plaque formation, but without shadowing or only minor shadowing, due to microcalcification (Fig. 23.5). Usually the luminal area is reduced and significant stenosis develops.

Detections of coronary artery disease by IVUS

Early signs of atherosclerosis

IVUS can detect focal plaque morphology when the intimal thickness exceeds the 50–200 µm resolution of IVUS. The studies of Velican and Velican[34] showed that this limit is reached by the age of 20–30 years. That means that in the early stage the normal coronary artery is characterized by a circular lumen, which has a smooth luminal border and only one visible layer (Fig. 23.2). The three-layer appearance, which is due to an intimal thickening of more than 200-µm, is typical for the more advanced stage of the physiological aging process.[7,35,36] The media is significantly less reflectant than the intima and adventitia. The three-layer appearance is, by itself not a pathologic finding at older ages. The sum of the media and intima reflects the autopsy finding of media and intimal thickness. The adventi-

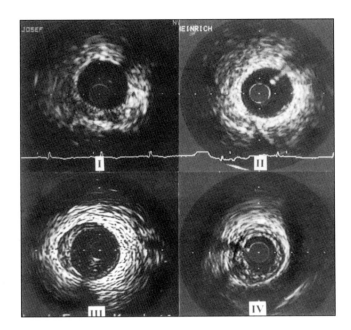

Figure 23.4
IVUS visualization of coronary lesions according to the AHA recommendations (type I, II, III, IV lesions;[19] calibration 1 mm, 30 MHz transducer).

tia can usually not be separated from the surrounding tissue. The best possibility to estimate the true wall thickness is at the crossing point of the coronary artery with the vein.

Remodeling

With the development of atherosclerosis, vessel size usually increases, and the possible luminal narrowing is compensated by an increase in vessel size. Glagov et al.[37] termed this phenomenon remodeling. He found that remodeling is exhausted when the increase in vessel size exceeds 40%. Further analysis showed that remodeling is exhausted when the circumference of the vessel exceeds 83%.[38] Epicardial imaging and have IVUS imaging demonstrated that the above autopsy observations can be recognized in vivo, as well.[3,39] IVUS was used to analyze the vessel size in patients with normal coronary angiograms, and plaque formation was also analyzed proximal and distal to the plaque-containing segments. It could be demonstrated that the compensatory process is exhausted when the plaque area exceeds 45%. The beginning of vessel luminal narrowing is seen when the plaque area is plotted versus the vessel area. When the plaque area reaches 8–10 mm^2 no further increase of vessel size occurs.[40] In rare situations, luminal widening is not present, rather a shrinkage is first observed, indicating that luminal narrowing is combined with a reduction of the total vessel size.[41] Remodeling explains why coronary angiography is not able to detect

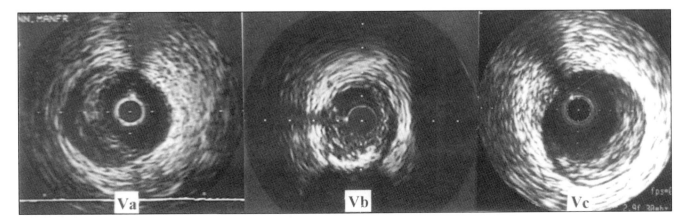

Figure 23.5
IVUS of coronary atherosclerosis type Va, Vb and Vc according to the AHA recommendations.[19] (Calibration 1 mm, 30 MHz transducer.)

early signs of atherosclerosis, and explains the reported discrepancies between angiography and autopsy.[2,24]

Angiographically normal coronary arteries

In 10–15% of the patients undergoing coronary angiography due to suspected coronary artery disease, normal coronary angiograms are found.[42] When signs of ischemia are present with a normal coronary angiogram, syndrome X is diagnosed.[42] Others define angina chest pain, normal angiography and ST-segment depression on exercise testing or atrial pacing as syndrome X.[43,44] Using IVUS with intracoronary Doppler, the differentiation of patients who otherwise would have been regarded as normal can be performed. In a study group of 44 patients, only 30% of patients with syndrome X had no plaque formation and a normal coronary flow reserve.[45] Similar discrepancies were described by others.[46–49] Intracoronary Doppler was able to clarify the disease in patients with angiographically normal coronary arteries with plaque formation, as in 36% of our patients coronary flow reserve was reduced, suggesting additional microvascular abnormalities. This reduction could not be explained by the extent of the disease because, in the vessels studied by IVUS, luminal narrowing was not more than 50%, the cut-off point of coronary flow reduction.[51] Interestingly, a correlation trend was noticed between the extent of plaque formation and coronary flow reserve. Thus, there may be a weak relation between the extent of coronary artery disease in epicardial coronary arteries and microvascular involvement.

Patients included in previous studies might not have been carefully characterized, and syndrome X is likely to be very heterogeneous.[44,50,52] Discrepancies might be related to the differences in patient groups, as suggested by Maseri et al.[53] Our study demonstrated that 36% of the patients with angiographically normal coronary arteries had reduced coronary flow reserve fulfilling the criteria established by others.[42,53,54] Yet, IVUS showed that 48% of these patients had coronary plaque formation. Only 16% of the total population studied could have been included in the syndrome X category according to the criteria proposed by Kaski et al.[52] Both groups represent different populations. The disease in patients with plaque formation was even more pronounced than in those with plaque formation but normal coronary flow reserve. Future studies to elucidate syndrome X may first have to rule out atherosclerosis by employing IVUS. This may in turn lead to a better selection of patients and possibly elimination of striking discrepancies in the results of clinical, hemodynamic, metabolic and prognostic studies.

Signs of early arteriosclerosis were observed in 48% of the patients, and these were not detected by coronary angiography, as previously reported.[36,55] The present study demonstrated that most (86%) of the lesions were focal and eccentric, indicating that early stages of coronary arteriosclerosis were present. This is an agreement with pathological observations that arteriosclerosis first develops as a focal lesion with lipid deposits and foam cells formed by macrophages.[22] Within the studied part of the left coronary artery, focal lesions were found mainly in the proximal segment of the artery, which is known to be predominantly involved in the early stages of the disease.[21,26,29] The number of lesions and the percentage of calcified lesions (13%) also support the hypothesis that an early stage of the disease was present. Furthermore calcium deposits were more frequent (44%) in patients with plaque formation and reduced coronary flow reserve than without flow reduction.[45]

Complicated lesions and plaque rupture

Plaque formation is approaching an unstable situation at Stary Va level. These lesions are known to rupture (plaques at risk, vulnerable plaques) when additional risk factors are present, such as inflammation, exercise and changes of the blood components. This has been known for many years,[23,32,45] and the American Heart Association has classified the development of complicated lesions into 3 subclasses: types VIa, VIb, VIc.

Type VIa

Type VIa lesions represent plaque which ruptures exposing the lipid pool to the blood, leading to plaque ulcer with or without thrombus formation. A typical image is demonstrated in Figure 23.6. Such a plaque rupture was first described by IVUS by Zamorano et al.[56] The plaque rupture, by angiography appeared as a contrast deposit outside the coronary lumen, usually described as an aneurysm, but in reality representing a plaque ulcer filled with contrast.[56,57] This morphology of coronary plaque (Fig. 23.6) is found in patients with unstable angina, myocardial infarction and sudden death.[58–63] Thus, it is not surprising that in patients with sudden death, disseminated emboli consisting of atherosclerotic plaque material and thrombi are found.

Type VIb lesion

Type VIb lesions represent an intramural hematoma, a sign also found in patients with developing aortic dissection.[64] Detection by IVUS is very difficult. To date there is no reported case where histological material received by atherectomy confirmed the intravascular image. We

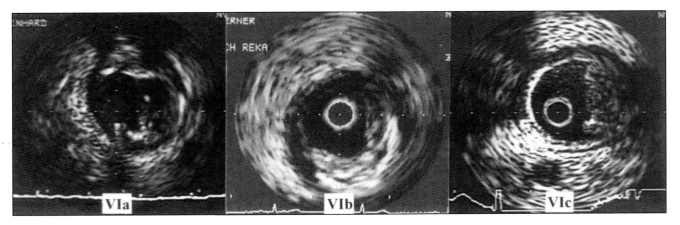

Figure 23.6
Complicated coronary lesions type VIa–c according to the AHA recommendations.[19] (Calibration 1 mm, 30 MHz transducer.)

observed this IVUS appearance in two patients. It was characterized by multiple echolucent zones which were close together and well distributed inside the total plaque. Angiography is normal in these cases, or characterized by luminal narrowing which is produced by the intramural hematoma (Fig. 23.6). The intramural hematoma has to be separated from extramural hematoma, which can occur after interventions leading to compression of the lumen.[65]

Type VIc lesion

Type VIc lesions are most frequently found in patients with unstable angina, acute myocardial infarction and sudden death. Angioscopy showed mural white or red thrombus formation.[66,67] IVUS reveals mural thrombi that form a typical stratified pattern first described by Kearney et al.[68] This stratified pattern can be multiple and is found in more than 80% of the patients with unstable angina. This corresponds to the incidence of thrombus formation which was observed by angioscopy in patients with unstable angina. Myocardial infarction occurs when the vessel is totally occluded. As described by Bocksch et al. for the first time[2] the intravascular ultrasound catheter will produce footprints within the vessel.

Typical for thrombus formation is 1) the stratified pattern; 2) the rough vessel wall surface; 3) fine oscillating structures as well as 4) catheter footprints. Echolucent zones and calcium are found nearby (Fig. 23.6). Plaque usually ruptures at the point of increased wall tension in the adjacent part between the normal and diseased vessel,

often containing calcifications. Other authors have also described similar results.[69–72]

Nomenclature

The American Heart Association has suggested indexing the lesion underlying the plaque rupture in its first appearance with the type of complicated lesion classified by a second index. Thus, lesion type Va which is rupturing, producing a plaque ulcer, could be described as lesion type Va/VIa. Studying patients with unstable angina demonstrated that plaque rupture can also occur with a normal coronary angiogram. Oscillating plaque structures have been seen in these patients (Fig. 23.7).[73] This lesion is described as II/VIa.

Healing of ruptured plaque

Follow-up studies of complicated lesions (ruptured plaques) have led to a better understanding of the healing process. The first case report was presented by Ge et al.[74] The authors could demonstrate that a free-floating ruptured intimal flap in the right coronary artery was found in a controlled study adjacent to the arterial wall, resulting in an increase of the plaque echodensity and thickness. Another healing process was described by Baumgart et al.[73] who observed after 2 months in a patient with a plaque rupture II/VIa that an attachment of the free oscillating intimal parts to the wall in a patient with a normal coronary

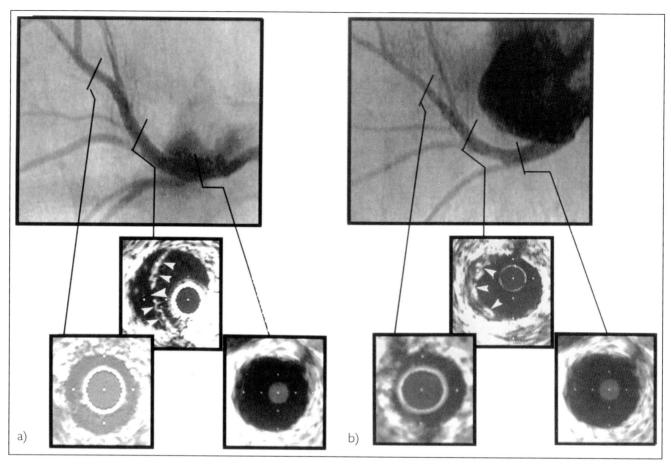

Figure 23.7
Unstable angina with a normal coronary angiogram. Demonstration of plaque rupture type II/VIa with fibrous cap (arrow), tear (large arrow) and emptied lipid pool (plaque ulcer) (a) and spontaneous healing 2 months later demonstrating intimal thickening (arrows) leading to plaque type Vc according to Stary (b). Calibration 1 mm. 30 MHz. (Baumgart *et al.*[73])

angiogram resulted in an increase in wall thickness. This was accompanied by normalization of the ECG and ventricular wall motion (Fig. 23.7).

Jeremias *et al.*[75] were able to demonstrate an intermittent stage of ruptured plaque healing by visualizing a thrombus formation within the ruptured plaque which may lead to an increase of the thrombus within the emptied plaque ulcer and result in organization of the plaque thrombus, as described by pathology.[75]

Conclusion

IVUS has given new insights into the pathogenesis of arteriosclerosis that was never before possible by other imaging modalities. The high accuracy of IVUS allows the visualization of type II and III lesions, following the recommendations of the American Heart Association.[27] Differentiation of tissue can be given for calcified lesions, fibrotic lesions, lipid core, plaque rupture, thrombus formation and detection of advanced lesions, i.e., detection of plaques at risk, and plaques ruptured with and without thrombus formation also seems to be possible. IVUS in combination with intracoronary Doppler allows a better differentiation and classification of patients with normal coronary angiograms, particularly when signs of ischemia in stress tests are present. New insight into the relation between risk factors and coronary arteriosclerosis can be expected. The analysis of progression or regression of coronary atherosclerosis will, in the future, be based on IVUS. In particular, the demonstration of plaque rupture in patients with normal coronary arteries and unstable angina is of high diagnostic value. IVUS has become the new gold standard for coronary artery disease and has replaced coronary angiography in this aspect. In addition to ultrafast CT (electron beam tomography), new imaging modalities of coronary atherosclerosis are not only providing better images but also allow detection of the disease process at an earlier stage.

References

1 Bom N, ten Hoff H, Lancee CT, Gussenhoven WJ, Bosch JG. Early and recent intraluminal ultrasound devices. *Int J Card Imag* 1989; **4**: 79–88.

2 Freundenberg H, Lichtlen PR. The normal wall segment in coronary stenoses. A postmortal study. *Z Kardiol* 1981; **70**: 863–9.

3 Gerber TC, Erbel R, Görge G, Ge J, Rupprecht HJ, Meyer J. Extent of atherosclerosis and remodeling of the left main coronary artery determined by intravascular ultrasound. *Am J Cardiol* 1994; **73**: 666–71.

4 Di Mario C, The SHK, Madretsma S. Detection and characterization of vascular lesions by intravascular ultrasound. An *in vitro* study correlated with histology. *J Am Soc Echocardiol* 1992; **5**: 135–46.

5 Ge J, Erbel R, Seidel I, *et al.* Experimentelle Überprüfung der Genauigkeit und Sicherheit des intraluminalen Ultraschalls. *Z Kardiol* 1991; **80**: 595–601.

6 Lookwood G, Ryan L, Gotlieb A, *et al.* In vitro high resolution intravascular imaging in muscular and elastic arteries. *J Am Coll Cardiol* 1992; **20**: 153–60.

7 Tobis JM, Mallery J, Mahon D. Intravascular ultrasound imaging of human coronary arteries *in vivo*. *Circulation* 1991; **83**: 913–26.

8 Koch L, Erbel R, Ge J, Zamorano J, Roth T, Meyer J. Anwendung der dreidimensionalen Rekonstruktion von Koronararterien aus IVUS-Bildern. *Z Kardiol* 1993; **82**: 35.

9 Birgelen C v, Erbel R, Di Mario C, *et al.* Three-dimensional reconstruction of coronary arteries with intravascular ultrasound. *Herz* 1995; **20**: 277–89.

10 Mallary JA, Tobis JM, Griffith J. Assessment of normal and atherosclerotic arterial wall thickness with an intravascular ultrasound imaging catheter. *Am Heart J* 1990; **119**: 1392–400.

11 Escaned J, Baptista J, Di Mario C, *et al.* Detection of coronary atheroma by quantitative angiography. Insights gained from intracoronary ultrasound imaging. *J Am Coll Cardiol* 1994; **23**: 174 (abstract).

12 Hase-Hueppmeier S, Uebis R, Doerr R, Hanrath P. Intravascular ultrasound to assess aortocoronary venous bypass grafts *in vivo*. *Am J Cardiol* 1992; **70**: 455–8.

13 Jain SP, Roubin GS, Nanda NC. Intravascular ultrasound imaging of saphenous vein graft stenosis. *Am J Cardiol* 1992; **69**: 133–6.

14 Hodgson JM, Reddy KG, Suneja R, Nair RN, Lesnefsky EJ, Sheehan HM. Intracoronary ultrasound imaging. Correlation of plaque morphology with angiography, clinical syndrome and procedural results in patients undergoing coronary angioplasty. *J Am Coll Cardiol* 1993; **21**: 35–44.

15 Gerber T, Erbel R, Görge G, Ge J, Rupprecht HJ, Meyer J. Classification of morphologic effects of percutaneous transluminal coronary angioplasty assessed by intravascular ultrasound. *Am J Cardiol* 1992; **70**: 1546–54.

16 Stähr P, Rupprecht HJ, Voigtländer T, *et al.* Importance of calibration for diameter and area determination by intravascular ultrasound. *Intern J Card Imag* 1996; **12**: 221–9.

17 Bhargava V, Penny WF, Arbab-Zadeh A. Editorial comment: in response to the article by P Stähr *et al.* Importance of calibration for diameter and area determination by intravascular ultrasound. *Intern J Card Imag* 1996; **12**: 231–2.

18 Colombo A, Hall P, Nakamura S, *et al.* Intravascular stenting without anticoagulation accomplished with intravascular ultrasound guidance. *Circulation* 1995; **91**: 1676–88.

19 Stary HC, Chandler AB, Dinsmore RE, *et al.* A definition of advanced types of atherosclerotic lesions and a histological classification of atherosclerosis. *Circulation* 1995; **92**: 1355–74.

20 Stary HC. The sequence of cell matrix changes in atherosclerotic lesions of coronary arteries in the first forty years of life. *Eur Heart J* 1990; **11 (Suppl)**: 3–19.

21 Stary HC. Changes in components and structure of atherosclerotic lesions developing from childhood to middle age in coronary arteries. In: Just H, Hort W, Zeiher AM (eds). *Arteriosclerosis. New Insight into Pathogenetic Mechanisms and Prevention. Basic Res Cardiol* 1994; **89 (Suppl 1)**: 17–31.

22 Stary HC, Blankenhorn DH, Chandler AB, *et al.* A definition of the intima of human arteries and of its atherosclerosis-prone regions. *Circulation* 1992; **85**: 391–405.

23 Hempel H. *Lehrbuch der allgemeinen Pathologie und der pathologischen Anatomie* (Berlin: Springer-Verlag, 1968).

24 Godin CM, Dyrda I, Pasternac A, Campeau L, Bourassa MG. Discrepancies between cineangiographic and postmortem finding in patients with coronary artery disease and recent myocardial revascularization. *Circulation* 1974; **49**: 703–56.

25   Vladaver Z, Edwards JE. Pathology of coronary atherosclerosis. *Progr Cardiovasc Dis* 1971; **14**: 256–74.

26   Wolkoff K. Über die Atherosklerose der Coronararterien des Herzens. *Beitr Path Anat* 1929; **82**: 555–96.

27   Erbel R, Ge J, Jollet N, Görge G, Haude M. Intravascular ultrasound based Stary classification of coronary plaque formation. *J Am Coll Cardiol* 1996; **27**: 702–1 (abstract).

28   Cook JP, Tsoo PS. Is NO an endogenous antiatherogenic module? *Arterioskler Thrombos* 1994; **14**: 653–5.

29   Montenegro MR, Eggen DA. Topography of atherosclerosis in the coronary arteries. *Lab Invest* 1968; **18**: 586–93.

30   Katz SS, Shipley GG, Small DN. Physical chemistry of the lipids of human atherosclerotic lesions. Demonstration of a lesion intermediate between fatty streaks of advanced plaques. *J Clin Invest* 1976; **58**: 200–1.

31   Davies MJ, Bland MJ, Hangartner WR, Angelini A, Thomas AC. Factors influencing the presence or absence of acute coronary thrombi in sudden ischemic death. *Eur Heart J* 1989; **10**: 203–8.

32   Richardson PD, Davies MJ, Born GVR. Influence of plaque configuration and stress distribution on fissuring of coronary atherosclerotic plaques. *Lancet* 1989; **II**: 941–4.

33   Falk E, Shah PK, Fuster V. Pathogenesis of plaque disruption. In: Fuster V, Ross R, Topol EJ (eds). *Atherosclerosis and Coronary Artery Disease* (Philadelphia, PA: Lippincott-Raven, 1996): 491–501.

34   Velican D, Velican C. Comparative study on age-related changes and atherosclerotic involvement of the coronary arteries of male and female subjects up to 40 years of age. *Atherosclerosis* 1981; **38**: 39–50.

35   Ge J, Erbel R, Görge G, et al. Intravascular ultrasound imaging of arterial wall architecture. *Echocardiography* 1992; **9**: 475–83.

36   Ge J, Erbel R, Gerber T, et al. Intravascular ultrasound imaging of angiographically normal coronary arteries. A prospective study *in vivo. Br Heart J* 1994; **71**: 572–8.

37   Glagov S, Weisenberg E, Zanrins CK, Stakunavicius R, Kolettis GJ. Compensatory enlargement of human atherosclerotic coronary arteries. *New Engl J Med* 1987; **316**: 1371–5.

38   Zarins CK, Weisenberg E, Kolettis G, Stankunavicius R, Glagov S. Differential enlargement of artery segments in response to enlarging atherosclerotic plaques. *J Vasc Surg* 1988; **7**: 386–94.

39   McPherson DD, Serna AJ, Hiratzka LF, et al. Coronary arterial remodeling studied by high-frequency epicardial echocardiography: an early compensatory mechanism in patients with obstructive coronary atherosclerosis. *J Am Coll Cardiol* 1991; **17**: 79–86.

40   Ge J, Erbel R, Zamorano J, et al. Coronary artery remodeling in atherosclerotic disease. An intravascular ultrasonic study *in vivo. Coron Art Dis* 1993; **4**: 981–6.

41   Erbel R, Ge J, Görge G, et al. Intravaskuläre Sonographie bei koronarer Herzkrankheit. *Dtsch Med Wschr* 1995; **120**: 845–54.

42   Kern MJ. Syndrome X: understanding and evaluating the patient with chest pain and normal coronary arteriograms. *Heart Dis Stroke* 1992; **1**: 299–302.

43   Kemp GH jr, Vokonas PS, Cohn PF, Gorlin R. The anginal syndrome associated with normal coronary angiograms: report of six year experience. *Am J Med* 1973; **54**: 735–42.

44   Kemp HG, Kronomal RA, Vlietstra RE, Frey RL. Coronary artery surgery study (CASS) participants: seven year survival of patients—with normal or near normal coronary arteriograms: A CASS Registry study. *J Am Coll Cardiol* 1986; **7**: 479–83.

45   Erbel R, Ge J, Bockisch A, et al. Value of intracoronary ultrasound and Doppler in the differentiation of angiographically normal coronary arteries: a prospective study in patients with angina pectoris. *Eur Heart J* 1996; **17**: 880–9.

46   Nissen SE, Gurley JC, Grines CL, et al. Intravascular ultrasound assessment of lumen size and wall morphology in normal subjects and patients with coronary artery disease. *Circulation* 1991; **84**: 1087–99.

47   Fitzgerald PJ, St Goar FG, Connolly AJ, et al. Intravascular ultrasound imaging of coronary arteries: is three layers the norm? *Circulation* 1992; **86**: 154–8.

48   Tobis JM, Mallery J, Mahon D, et al. Intravascular ultrasound imaging of human coronary arteries *in vivo. Circulation* 1991; **83**: 913–26.

49   Wenguang L, Gussenhoven EJ, Zhong Y. Validation of quantitative analysis of intravascular ultrasound images. *Int J Card Imag* 1991; **6**: 247–53.

50   Sax FL, Cannon RO, Hanson C, Epstein SE. Impaired forearm vasodilator reserve in patients with microvascular angina: evidence of a generalized disorder of vascular function? *N Engl J Med* 1987; **317**: 1366–70.

51   Gould KL, Kirkeeide RL, Buchi M. Coronary flow reserve as a physiologic measure of stenosis severity. Part I. - Relative and absolute coronary flow reserve during changing aortic pressure and cardiac work load. Part II. Determination from arteriographic stenosis dimensions under standardized conditions. *J Am Coll Cardiol* 1990; **15**: 459–74.

52 Kaski JC, Tousoulis D, Galassi AR, et al. Epicardial coronary artery tone and reactivity in patients with normal coronary arteriograms and reduced coronary flow reserve (syndrome X). J Am Coll Cardiol 1991; **18**: 50–4.

53 Maseri A, Crea F, Kaski JC, Crake T. Mechanism of angina pectoris in syndrome X. J Am Coll Cardiol 1991; **17**: 499–506.

54 Opherk D, Zebe H, Weihe E, et al. Reduced coronary dilatory capacity and ultrastructural changes of the myocardium in patients with angina pectoris but normal coronary angiograms. Circulation 1981; **63**: 817–25.

55 Davidson CJ, Sheikh KH, Harrison JK, et al. Intravascular ultrasonography versus digital subtraction angiography. J Am Coll Cardiol 1990; **16**: 633–66.

56 Zamorano J, Erbel R, Ge J, et al. Spontaneous plaque rupture visualized by intravascular ultrasound. Eur Heart J 1994; **15**: 131–3.

57 Ge J, Haude M, Görge G, Liu F, Erbel R. Silent healing of spontaneous plaque disruption demonstrated by intracoronary ultrasound. Eur Heart J 1995; **16**: 1149–51.

58 Ambrose JA, Winters SL, Stern A, et al. Angiographic morphology and the pathogenesis of unstable angina pectoris. J Am Coll Cardiol 1985; **5**: 609–16.

59 Kragel AH, Gertz SD, Roberts WC. Morphologic comparison of frequency and types of acute lesions in the major epicardial coronary arteries in unstable angina pectoris, sudden coronary death and acute myocardial infarction. J Am Coll Cardiol 1991; **18**: 801–8.

60 Nobuyoshi M, Tanaka M, Nosaka H, et al. Progression of coronary atherosclerosis. Is coronary spasm related to progression? J Am Coll Cardiol 1991; **18**: 904–10.

61 Shub C, Vlietstra RE, Smith HC, Fulton RE, Eleveback LR. The unpredictable progression of symptomatic coronary artery disease. Mayo Clin Proc 1981; **56**: 155–60.

62 Sinapius D. Beziehung zwischen Koronarthrombosen und Myokardinfarkten. Dtsch Med Schr 1972; **97**: 443–8.

63 Wilson RF, Holida MD, White CW. Quantitative angiographic morphology of coronary stenoses leading to myocardial infarction or unstable angina. Pathophysiol Nat Hist 1986; **73**: 286–93.

64 Erbel R, Mohr-Kahaly S, Oelert H, et al. Diagnostic strategies in suspected aortic dissection: comparison of computed tomography, aortography and transesophageal echocardiography. Am J Cardiac Imag 1990; **4**: 157–72.

65 Werner GS, Figulla HR, Grosse W, Kreuzer H. Extensive intramural hematoma as the cause of failed coronary angioplasty: diagnosis by intravascular ultrasound and treatment by stent implantation. Cath Card Diagn 1995; **36**: 173–8.

66 Siegel RJ, Chae JS, Forrester JM, Ruiz CE. Angiography, angioscopy, and ultrasound imaging before and after percutaneous balloon angioplasty. Am Heart J 1990; **120**: 1086–90.

67 Mizuno K, Satomura K, Miyamoto A, et al. Angioscopic evaluation of coronary-artery thrombi in acute coronary syndromes. New Engl J Med 1992; **326**: 287–91.

68 Kearney P, Erbel R, Rupprecht HJ, et al. PTCA mechanism in stable and unstable angina analyzed with intracoronary ultrasound before and after intervention. Eur Heart J 1996; **17**: 721–30.

69 Mintz GS, Potkin BN, Cooke RH. Intravascular ultrasound imaging in a patient with unstable angina. Am Heart J 1992; **123**: 1692–4.

70 Hodgeson J, Reddy D, Suney R, Nair R, Lesnefsky E, Sheehan H. Intracoronary ultrasound imaging. J Am Coll Cardiol 1993; **21**: 35–44.

71 Bocksch W, Beckmann S, Greysse S, Paeprer H, Scharl M. Morphological changes after PTCA in patients with chronic stable angina versus acute myocardial infarction. Intravascular Ultrasound Study. Eur Heart J 1993; **14**: 109–15.

72 Gerber ThC, Erbel R, Görge G, Ge J, Rupprecht H jr, Meyer J. Classification of morphologic effects of percutaneous transluminal coronary angioplasty assessed by intravascular ultrasound. Am J Cardiol 1992; **70**: 1546–54.

73 Baumgart D, Liu F, Haude M, Görge G, Ge J, Erbel R. Acute plaque rupture and myocardial stunning in patients with normal coronary arteriography. Lancet 1995; **346**: 143–4.

74 Ge J, Haude M, Görge G, Liu F, Erbel R. Silent healing of spontaneous plaque disruption demonstrated by intracoronary ultrasound. Eur Heart J 1995; **16**: 1149–51.

75 Jeremias A, Ge J, Erbel R. New insight into plaque healing after plaque rupture with subsequent thrombus formation by intravascular ultrasound. Heart 1997 (in press).

76 Kramer JR, Kitazume H, Proudfit WL, Matsuda Y, Williams GW, Sones FM jr. Progression and regression of coronary atherosclerosis. Relation to risk factors. Am Heart J 1983; **105**: 134–44.

77 Hubert HB, Feinleib M, McNamara PM, Castelli WP. Obesity as an independent risk factor for cardiovascular disease. A 26-year follow-up of participants in the Framingham heart study. Circulation 1983; **67**: 968–77.

scopically visible thrombi had a red thrombus protruding into the vessel lumen. Angiography revealed an intraluminal filling defect in one, a stenosis with hazy arterial borders in one, and stenoses with overhanging edges in three.

Thrombi were less often seen in patients with unstable angina. In 18 consecutive patients with unstable angina, a red globular intraluminal thrombus was seen in three (17%) patients; four (22%) patients had thrombi that were flat or slightly raised and adherent to the stenosis; thrombi were not detected in the remaining 11 (61%) patients.

A somewhat unexpected finding was the not infrequent detection of thrombi in patients with stable angina, or in the nonculprit vessels of those with unstable angina or with recent myocardial infarction. Of 16 'stable' coronary lesions examined, thrombi that were invariably small and adherent to the wall were seen in 5 (31%) lesions.

Coronary dissections

Experimental studies in animals and anecdotal postmortem observations in man suggest that dissection to a greater or lesser extent almost invariably occurs during balloon angioplasty. Angiographically, dissections are seen with moderate frequency after angioplasty; although the presence of visible dissection after angioplasty is not associated with a greater long-term risk of restenosis, it has been associated with an increased risk of acute closure. Angioscopically, dissections may present as thin white wisps of tissue that appear to float in the vessel lumen. Alternatively, there may be longitudinal fissures in the vessel wall with varying degrees of haemorrhage. On occasion, dissections may present as yellow irregular masses apparently floating in the lumen.

In one patient studied after angioplasty, we found a mobile intraluminal mass that corresponded to the typical angiographic description of thrombus. Angioscopy revealed no evidence of thrombus, but rather a yellow mobile flap of tissue floating in the lumen. This led to the decision to perform atherectomy rather than conventional balloon angioplasty. In another patient studied one week after a thrombolyzed myocardial infarction, an eccentric stenosis with overhanging edges was seen on angiography in the proximal part of a large right coronary artery. Angioscopy revealed a yellow ulcerated plaque protruding into the vessel lumen, with only a small amount of adherent thrombus. Because of the angioscopic findings, we elected to implant an intracoronary stent, which produced a satisfactory acute angiographic result.

Restenosis

Appearance of the restenotic plaque

At the Lille Heart Institute, we recommend 6-month follow-up angiography to all patients after successful coronary angioplasty. Twenty-three such patients underwent angioscopy of the dilated lesion. The appearance of the stenosis in these patients was remarkably uniform: 15 lesions were white or greyish-white in appearance and either completely smooth or only slightly irregular. These appearances, which are similar to those described by White et al.[21] presumably are the visual correlate of the fibrous plaque that has been documented histologically in such lesions. Of the remaining eight lesions, four were yellow, and four were reddish-pink.

Angioscopic predictors of restenosis

Angiographic classification has not proved useful to identify lesions at high risk of restenosis. Discordant results have been reported regarding, for example, the risk of restenosis at angiographically-defined complex lesions. Thus, in 1995, we investigated whether the morphological characteristics of the plaque assessed by angioscopy at the time of angioplasty were predictive of angiographic restenosis at 6-month follow-up.[22] One hundred and seventeen patients who underwent a successful single lesion angioplasty and an adequate angioscopy procedure were restudied with quantitative coronary angiography at 6 months follow-up. Plaque shape and color or dissection were not predictive of restenosis. However, a protruding thrombus at the PTCA site was associated with an excessive risk of restenosis. The late loss was significantly higher ($p < 0.05$) when a protruding thrombus was observed, than in the case of lining thrombus (late loss = 0.59) or no thrombus (late loss = 0.47).

Potential clinical applications of angioscopy

Only in recent years has the technique of coronary angioscopy developed to the extent that it can be performed in the clinical setting (Table 24.3). Even now, technical considerations preclude its use as a routine adjunct to coronary angiography. Studies with intraoperative angioscopy, which has been performed now for more than

Table 24.3 Potential indications for coronary angioscopy

Diagnosis of thrombus
Unstable angina
Equivocal angiographic findings
- intraluminal filling defect
- 'hazy' angiographic appearances
Evaluation of angioplasty results
- differentiation of dissection/thrombus
- need for adjunctive therapy
- evaluation of new interventional devices

Table 24.4 Limitations of angioscopy.

Limitation	Cause
Extremely proximal segments	Inadequate space for occlusive cuff
Severe angulation	Limited flexibility of optic bundle
Field of view	Tip of optic bundle non-steerable
Viewing time	Ischemia related to coronary occlusion
Collateral circulation	Saline flush may be insufficient for adequate viewing
No quantification	Lack of calibration device

a decade, have suggested a potential role in verifying the integrity of anastomotic sites during coronary bypass surgery, and in inspecting venous grafts for possible damage, and for the presence of incompletely ligated side-branches, before implantation. Grundfest et al.[23] reported that in three cases, angioscopic findings led to a revision of the anastamosis. Last year, White et al.[24] collecting data at six medical centers showed the value of angioscopy before angioplasty. They studied 122 patients, mainly patients with unstable angina (78%), but 22% with stable angina, and performed a univariate and multivariate analysis. They demonstrated that angioscopic thrombus was associated with a increased incidence of adverse outcome after angioplasty. These conclusions are important and clinically relevant since the identification of these high risk patients could lead to pre-procedure treatment with antithrombotic or antiplatelet drugs.

It is too soon to predict whether coronary angioscopy will have a role in future clinical practice (Table 24.4). However, the additional information provided by angioscopy is clearly of benefit, in specific situations, in deciding the optimal therapeutic approach, as has been shown in anecdotal reports.

The advent of intracoronary stenting has introduced yet another iatrogenic problem for the interventional cardiologist, namely that of early stent occlusion. It is conventionally held that early coronary stent occlusion is exclusively due to the development of stent thrombosis. A recent report described a series of patients in whom early stent occlusion

was not due to thrombosis, but was a consequence of obstructive intimal dissection.[25] A dissection was not observed in any of the cases on the immediate post-stenting angiogram.

The major advantage of angioscopy is the ability to detect the presence of intracoronary thrombus. Angioscopy has been clearly shown to be superior to angiography in this respect.[11,12,18–20] The availability of newer technologies such as transluminal extraction atherectomy, that appear to be associated with a lower acute complication rate than traditional balloon angioplasty, for the treatment of lesions that have a large burden of thrombus, suggest a potential role for angioscopy in pre-angioplasty assessment, when the angiographic appearances are suspicious. A particular niche for angioscopy may lie in the assessment of patients with recent myocardial infarction. Residual stenosis on angiography in such patients may be due to the presence of a significant underlying atherosclerotic stenosis, but may equally be due to the presence of residual thrombus superimposed on an insignificant lesion. Angioscopic assessment may aid in this distinction and may be useful in deciding the optimal therapeutic approach.

Finally, there are numerous potential research applications for percutaneous angioscopy. The assessment of the results of thrombolytic therapy in unstable angina, the assessment of the post-cardiac transplantation patient, and the assessment of the immediate results of angioplasty and of newer non-balloon technologies represent only a few of the potential applications.[26]

References

1   Maseri A, L'Abbate A, Pesola A, *et al.* Coronary vasospasm in angina pectoris. *Lancet* 1977; **i**: 713–17.

2   De Wood MA, Spores J, Notske R, *et al.* Prevalence of total coronary occlusion during the early hours of transmural myocardial infarction. *N Engl J Med* 1980; **303**: 897–902.

3   Dietz WA, Tobis JM, Isner J. Failure of angiography to accurately depict the extent of coronary artery narrowing in three fatal cases of percutaneous transluminal coronary angioplasty. *J Am Coll Cardiol* 1992; **19**: 1261–70.

4   Glagov S, Weisenberg E, Zarins CK, Stankunavicius R, Kolettis GJ. Compensatory enlargement of human atherosclerotic coronary arteries. *N Engl J Med* 1987; **316**: 1371–5.

5   Beatt KJ, Serruys PW, Luijten HE, *et al.* Restenosis after coronary angioplasty: the paradox of increased lumen diameter and restenosis. *J Am Coll Cardiol* 1992; **19**: 1382–90.

6   Little WC, Constantinescu M, Applegate R, *et al.* Can coronary angiography predict the site of a subsequent myocardial infarction in patients with mild-to-moderate coronary artery disease? *Circulation* 1988; **78**: 1157–66.

7   Allen D, Graham E. Intracardiac surgery – a new method. *J Am Med Assoc* 1922; **79**: 1028–30.

8   Carlens E, Silander T. Method for direct inspection of the right atrium: experimental observations in the dog. *Surgery* 1961; **49**: 622–4.

9   Hombach V, Höher M, Hannekum A, *et al.* Erste klinische Erfahrungen mit der Koronarendoskopie. *Deutsche Medizinische Wochenschrift* 1986; **111**: 1135–40.

10 Uchida Y, Tomaru T, Nakamura F, Furuse A, Fujimori Y. Percutaneous coronary angioscopy in patients with ischemic heart disease. *Am Heart J* 1987; **114**: 1216–22.

11 Sherman CT, Litvack F, Grundfest W, *et al.* Coronary angioscopy in patients with unstable angina pectoris. *N Engl J Med* 1986; **315**: 913–19.

12 Mizuno K, Satomura K, Miyamoto A, *et al.* Angioscopic evaluation of coronary–artery thrombi in acute coronary syndromes. *N Engl J Med* 1992; **326**: 287–91.

13 White CJ, Ramee SR, Collins TJ, Mesa JE, Jain A, Ventura HO. Percutaneous coronary angioscopy: applications in interventional cardiology. *J Interven Cardiol* 1993; **6**: 61–7.

14 Uchida Y, Hasegawa K, Kawamura K, Shibuya I. Angioscopic observation of the coronary luminal changes induced by percutaneous transluminal coronary angioplasty. *Am Heart J* 1989; **117**: 769–76.

15 Nakamura F, Kvasnicka J, Uchida Y, Geschwind HJ. Percutaneous angioscopic evaluation of luminal changes induced by excimer laser angioplasty. *Am Heart J* 1992; **124**: 1467–72.

16 Hamon M, Lablanche JM, Bauters C, McFadden EP, Quandalle P, Bertrand ME. Effect of balloon inflation in angiographically normal segments during coronary angioscopy; a quantitative angiographic study. *Cathet Cardiovascular Diagn* 1994; **31**: 116–21.

17 Lee G, Garcia HJ, Corso P, *et al.* Correlation of coronary angioscopic to angiographic findings in coronary artery disease. *Am J Cardiol* 1986; **58**: 238–41.

18 White CJ, Ramee SR, Collins TJ, Mesa JE, Jain A. Percutaneous angioscopy of saphenous vein coronary bypass grafts. *J Am Coll Cardiol* 1993; **21**: 1881–5.

19 Lablanche JM, Hamon M, McFadden EP, Bauters C, Quandalle P, Bertrand ME. Persisting intracoronary thrombus is frequently detected by angioscopy three weeks after thrombolysis for acute myocardial infarction. *Eur Heart J* 1993; **14 (Suppl)**: 404A.

20 Lablanche JM, Hamon M, McFadden EP, Bauters C, Quandalle P, Bertrand ME. Angiographically silent thrombus frequently persists after thrombolytic therapy for acute myocardial infarction: a prospective angioscopic study. *Circulation* 1993; **88 (Suppl I)**: I-595.

21 White CJ, Ramee SR, Mesa JE, Collins TJ. Percutaneous coronary angioscopy in patients with restenosis after coronary angioplasty. *J Am Coll Cardiol* 1991; **17**: 46B–49B.

22 Bauters C, Lablanche JM, McFadden E, Hamon M, Bertrand ME. Relation of coronary angioscopic findings at coronary angioplasty to angiographic restenosis. *Circulation* 1995; **92**: 2473–9.

23 Grundfest W, Litvack F, Sherman T, *et al.* Delineation of peripheral and coronary detail by intraoperative angioscopy. *Ann Surg* 1985; **202**: 394–400.

24 White C, Ramee S, Collins T, *et al.* Coronary thrombi increase PTCA risk angioscopy as a clinical tool. *Circulation* 1996; **93**: 253–8.

25 Den Heijer P, Van Dijk RB, Twisk PM, Lie KI. Early stent occlusion is not always caused by thrombosis. *Cathet Cardiovasc Diagn* 1993; **29**: 136–40.

26 Ventura HO, White CJ, Jain SP, *et al.* Assessment of intracoronary morphology in cardiac transplant recipients by angioscopy and intravascular ultrasound. *Am J Cardiol* 1993; **72**: 805–9.

25

Intravascular ultrasound imaging: an update

Gad Keren

Introduction

Whether intravascular ultrasound (IVUS) imaging is only a research technique or a clinical tool is a question raised by most interventional cardiologists since the introduction of this technology. During the pursuit of clinical relevance this imaging modality was used in a multitude of basic and clinical research programs whereby interesting observations were made. The image correlation to histology with accurate dimensions and use in vascular physiology were confirmed. Most importantly, the role in interventional cardiology and radiology was clarified. The practicality of using IVUS in coronary artery disease, acute coronary syndromes and the ability to obtain high-resolution images of vessel walls and to differentiate atheroma components and plaques subtypes has improved remarkably our understanding of the mechanisms of various interventional modalities. It has had a marked impact on the current performance of interventional procedures as well as future developments in the field.

From technology to histology

Catheter-based IVUS has proved to be a safe procedure whether performed with a mechanical or an integrated multiple element system. The European Safety Registry[1] described an acceptable 1.1% rate of complications including vessel spasm, dissection and wire entrapment. The progress of the technology and image quality overcame many of the limitations previously raised. The size of the

catheters, now mostly smaller than 3 F, allow clinical introduction to stenotic sites even prior to intervention.

Optimal resolution and penetration of ultrasound were defined for ultrasound frequencies in the range of 20–40 MHz.[2] Higher frequencies may improve resolution but result in lower penetration, increased attenuation and backscatter from small particles such as rough surfaces or even cellular elements in the vessel. With most current systems, and for practical purposes, axial resolution is in the range of 0.05 and 0.1 mm and lateral resolution 0.2–0.3 mm. These technological limitations have to be taken into account when interpreting coronary images, since the thickness of the healthy intima is about 0.1 mm, the media 0.2 mm and adventitia more than 0.3 mm. Thus, healthy intima may not be clearly visualized during real-time IVUS imaging (Fig. 25.1).

The issue of standardized gain setting is currently not resolved—a problem comparable to all ultrasound-based imaging techniques. Increased gain may result in bright echogenic areas, mistakenly interpreted to be fibrous or calcified atheromas. Low gain may have an opposite effect and cause echo drop-outs mistakenly thought to be lipid accumulations or dissections after intervention.

Thus, thorough training in image acquisition and interpretation is mandatory for all personnel who use this modality. With the advent of computer technology, the ability to obtain three-dimensional (3D) images of the heart and vessels was applied to IVUS.[3] Three-dimensional reconstruction of IVUS images is feasible but is dependent on the quality of the two-dimensional (2D) images and is marred in a significant manner by vessel motion, expansion between systole and diastole, vessel torsion and catheter

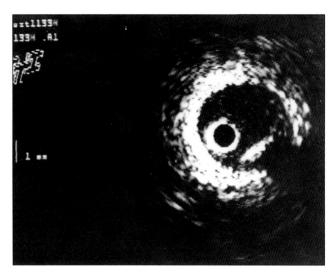

Figure 25.1
Vessel wall during real-time imaging where the normal three-layer appearance cannot be seen from 6 to 3 o'clock. There is a small calcified lesion between 3 and 6 o'clock.

eccentricity. Computerized 3D reconstruction allows display of the tomographic images in their longitudinal relation and provides a spatial image and a potential way for quantification.[3,4]

Pathologic studies and examinations with IVUS have shown standard angiography does not provide reliable quantitative assessment of coronary atherosclerosis and is grossly inadequate for evaluation of vessel wall architecture. These studies have demonstrated that coronary angiography consistently underestimates the severity of coronary atherosclerosis.[5-7]

In daily practice we are already aware of the fact that IVUS may show diffuse disease in the major coronary arteries of patients whose angiograms show focal disease only in portions of the vessel. Moreover, the amount of plaque present at angiographically stenotic sites is larger than perceived from angiography. These angiographic inaccuracies result from interpretation of stenosis in relation to 'reference' segments that look angiographically normal but are actually diseased.[8-10]

Compensatory enlargement of coronary vessels

Coronary atherosclerosis is associated with vessel remodeling and dilatation. Thus, the angiographic appearance of the

vessel may be normal despite marked accumulation of plaque. Quantitative analysis of arterial morphometry documents that as the cross-sectional area of the plaque increases within a diseased vessel segment, the outer wall of the artery expands in an attempt to compensate for the accumulation of plaque. This focal compensatory enlargement maintains cross-sectional area at stenotic sites of arteries. Indeed, focal compensatory enlargement has been described as a mechanism to maintain luminal cross-sectional area in human femoral, carotid and coronary arteries. A significant correlation was found between vessel area and plaque area in the original presentation of this concept by Glagov and coworkers.[11] The idea was later corroborated by IVUS and epicardial echocardiography for coronary arteries,[12-14] for femoral arteries,[15] carotid arteries and, more recently, for saphenous veins used as arterial conduits in bypass operation.[16] According to these authors, clinically and angiographically significant coronary artery disease develops when a focal failure of compensatory dilatation occurs in response to atherosclerotic plaque deposition. Compensatory enlargement may develop as a response to increased shear stress caused by atherosclerotic plaque in conjunction with endothelial-dependent factors or, alternatively, to medial attenuation with loss of underlying structural support.

Losordo et al.[15] used IVUS on 62 paired adjacent normal and diseased sites in the superficial femoral arteries of 20 patients undergoing peripheral vascular interventions. They have shown a decrease in lumen cross-sectional area from 21 mm^2 at angiographically normal sites to 16 mm^2 at adjacent diseased sites. This decrease in lumen area was associated with an increase in plaque area and vessel area from 32 mm^2 to 37 mm^2. Regression analysis disclosed a significant correlation between cross-sectional area of the plaque and total arterial area at the lesion site, without affecting adjacent normal segments of the vessel. Wong et al.[12] performed a segment-by-segment analysis of IVUS images in 15 patients. They showed that maximal plaque area was not significantly different between those having more than 50% narrowing by quantitative angiography and those who did not show any significant disease, indicating compensatory enlargement of the vessel due to plaque accumulation in some of the patients.

Nishioka et al.[14] studied the mechanism of compensatory enlargement in human coronary arteries using IVUS in 30 patients with coronary artery disease. They have defined compensatory enlargement to be present when the lesion site total vessel cross-sectional area was larger than the proximal normal segment, inadequate compensatory enlargement when the lesion vessel cross-sectional area was smaller than the distal reference site, and intermediate remodeling when the vessel cross-sectional area at the lesion site was intermediate between the two reference sites. Compensatory enlargement was observed in 19 (54%) of 35 lesions, inadequate enlargement in 26% and intermediate remodeling in 20% of lesions. In the compensatory enlargement group the vessel wall area increased markedly (182%), exceeded the lumen area reduction and was partially compensated (82%) by the vessel cross-sectional area increase. In the inadequate compensatory enlargement group, the cross-sectional area reduction contributed to 39% of the lumen area reduction at the lesion site, whereas wall area increase explained 61% of the lumen area reduction at the lesion site. The inadequate compensatory enlargement resulting in relative vessel constriction at the lesion site appears to be an important contributing factor, along with plaque proliferation to vascular stenosis.

Mendelsohn and coworkers[16] evaluated the response of saphenous vein bypass grafts to progressive atherosclerosis. They suggested that in veins, the reaction to flow and shear forces may be similar to arteries but veins may lack the endothelial-mediated function required for remodeling. Twenty-four discrete lesions and reference sites in 21 saphenous vein grafts were studied. Lesion vessel area was larger than the reference area in 23 of 24 vessels and there was a significant correlation between plaque and vessel area. In this study, similar to reports for native coronary arteries, the ability to increase plaque burden is also impeded for vein grafts when more than 30–40% of the vessel area is occupied by plaque. The authors concluded that saphenous veins used as coronary arterial conduits undergo compensatory enlargement in a manner similar to muscular arteries.

The vessel wall in stable and unstable coronary syndromes

Early *in vitro* studies comparing IVUS images and histology have demonstrated the three-layer appearance of the vessel wall.[17–22] The intima and internal elastic membrane are echogenic; the media, which is mostly muscular, is hypoechoic and the adventitia highly echogenic, due to reflectivity of the external elastic membrane and collagen fibers in the adventitia. Potkin *et al.*[17] have shown that coronary arteries are mostly muscular and have a three-layered appearance, whereas Lockwood *et al.*[18] confirmed these results but showed that elastic nonmuscular arteries have a homogeneous highly echogenic appearance as suggested also by Nishimura *et al.*[22] The same investigators and others have made significant progress in understanding IVUS images of atheromatous vessels.

Kragel *et al.*[23] identified the following components in the atheroma of patients with chronic and acute ischemic syndromes:

- Dense fibrous collagenous tissue.

- Loose fibrous tissue with more delicate arrangement of collagen.
- Cellular fibrous tissue and collagen and elastin fibers.
- Heavily calcified tissue.
- Pultaceous debris that is reach in extracellular lipid.
- Foam cells without lymphocytes.
- Inflammatory infiltrates.

The underlying pathology in unstable coronary syndromes such as unstable angina, acute myocardial infarction (MI) or sudden coronary death is plaque rupture and thrombus formation that may be either occlusive or nonocclusive. Plaques prone to rupture are considered unstable and have abundant lipid accumulation.[24,25] Calcified fibrotic plaques are considered as more stable and less prone to rupture. Since IVUS enabled to differentiate between various atheroma subtypes, it was hoped that the unstable plaques could be identified, fissures and plaque ruptures detected and thrombi localized. However, in spite of marked improvement in image quality, the ability to differentiate with confidence various atheroma subtypes remains relatively limited. The extent of vessel wall disease can be assessed reliably and gross distinction between 'soft' and 'hard' atheroma can be made. Hard atheromata laden with fibrous tissue are highly echogenic and, when calcified, they cast shadows. 'Soft' atheroma are abundant with pultaceous lipid debris and cellular elements. Loose and cellular fibrous tissue cause medium or low echo reflectance in the atheroma. Lipids have usually even lower levels of echo-reflectance and may be echolucent (Fig. 25.2).[17–22,26] This level of interpretation is insufficient. Areas behind calcific accumulations or metal struts of stents may not be well visualized and sometimes completely shadowed.[27–29]

In a recent study, Hiro *et al.*[30] examined the accuracy of IVUS in assessing the biophysical properties of atherosclerotic plaques. They showed that IVUS reliably distinguishes tissue characteristics of fibrosis and calcification but not of 'soft' atheroma which may be as firm as a more intense fibrous tissue. This problem was further substantiated by Giro and coworkers[31] who studied 106 coronary segments by ultrasound compared to histology. They have shown that cholesterol crystals and calcospherites are echogenic and are quite abundant in atheromatous lipid pools. The echogenecity of lipid pools is dependent on the amount of these materials, which may add to the difficulty in their identification.

Ultrasound images of intravascular thrombi were originally described as having a speckled echo signal softer than a dense atheroma. This ultrasound characteristic is difficult to differentiate from echogenicity originating in plaques composed mainly of loose connective tissue or fibromuscular tissue. Furthermore, our experience in patients with unstable coronary syndrome and acute MI led us to believe that thrombi are not easily detected by IVUS imaging.[32]

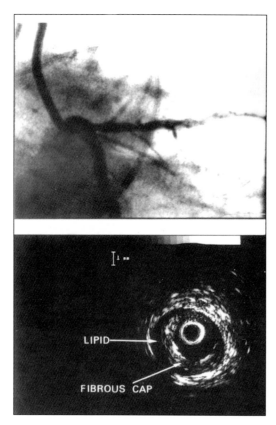

Figure 25.2
An atheroma in the proximal LAD. The atheroma has a
hypoechoic core with a fibrous cap. The hypoechoic core is most
probably lipid accumulation.

ing thrombi was further investigated by Chemarin-Aliballi et al.[35] who studied patients after thrombolysis and compared the IVUS findings to histology specimens obtained from atherectomy in these patients. The sensitivity of IVUS to detect thrombus was 80% and the specificity 50%, with a positive predictive value of 77%. Since the IVUS studies were performed at least one day after the acute event it is conceivable that most of the thrombi detected were from aggregated red blood cells and not from a platelet-rich composition. Another negative study with regard to the ability of IVUS to detect unstable plaques and thrombus formation was performed by de Feyter and coworkers[36] who compared angiography, angioscopy and IVUS in their ability to diagnose these lesions. There was no significant correlation among lesion characteristics obtained with angiography, angioscopy and ultrasound. Only angioscopy differentiated between lesion characteristics of patients with stable and unstable angina. IVUS does not discriminate in a reliable manner lesions from patients with stable and unstable angina.

As discussed earlier, plaque rupture and fissuring is the underlying mechanism for most acute coronary events. Fenggi et al.[37] studied 121 patients with unstable angina or acute MI, and performed IVUS prior to intervention. Contrast injection during IVUS was used to improve rupture delineation. Plaque rupture was observed in 29 lesions and was characterized by a narrow tear and deep ulceration. The authors thus concluded that ulceration and residual plaque rupture can be visualized within unstable plaques. These conclusions are different from Lugt et al.[38] who, in 40 human specimens of coronary arteries, showed that the sensitivity of detecting dissection was 79% and plaque rupture 37% by IVUS. Thus, only large tissue detachment can reliably be detected by IVUS. These conclusions seem logical when considering the limitations of axial and lateral resolution of IVUS when 20–30 MHz transducers are used.

This impression was substantiated by data from Siegel et al.[33] who compared angioscopy, IVUS and histology in 70 arterial specimens. The sensitivity of IVUS in detecting thrombi was only 57% compared to 100% by angioscopy. They concluded that IVUS and angioscopy are relatively accurate in identifying atheroma subtypes; however, the sensitivity of IVUS in identifying thrombi is low due to a false negative interpretation of laminar clots, and the inability to distinguish disrupted and stable atheroma from thrombus.

In an in vitro model using videodensitometry, Frimerman et al.[34] showed that thrombi of varying compositions have different echogenecity. Platelet-rich thrombi are hypoechoic and may not be visualized by ultrasound. Echogenic reflectance of thrombi was enhanced with an increasing amount of red blood cells and whole blood clots had a typical speckled appearance. The value of IVUS in identify-

Intravascular ultrasound in transplant recipients

Coronary artery disease develops in patients who undergo cardiac transplantation. This process may be due to the rejection process, medical therapy or progression of native vessel disease. Atherosclerotic changes were detected in more than 80% of 132 post-transplant patients.[39] In 64% of patients the changes were in the proximal segments of the vessels, in 43% in the middle and in 26% in the distal segments. In two thirds of patients this process is concentric, in 48% it was diffuse and in 52% it was focal.

Rickenbacher and coworkers[40] performed IVUS in 174 heart transplant recipients at baseline and up to 15 years after transplantation. They have shown that transplant coronary artery disease appeared to progress with time.

Most of the progression occurred within the first years whereas calcification was detected only at a later stage. Serial IVUS imaging studies at the time of post-transplant angiography and one year later demonstrated progression of intimal thickening at specific sites in only some cardiac transplant patients. Progression of intimal proliferation can occur in individuals in the presence or absence of initially increased intimal thickening or angiographic disease at the time of initial studies.[41]

IVUS in interventional procedures

Since the emergence of percutaneous transluminal coronary angioplasty (PTCA), a large variety of interventional procedures were developed to treat invasively atherosclerotic flow-limiting lesions. Angiography is a luminogram and, although providing important anatomic information, is unable to assess accurately changes in wall structure and geometry and to provide a clear *in vivo* understanding of the mechanisms of success and failure, of these procedures. IVUS, within a few years, proved to be a most valuable tool with qualitative and quantitative measures that have improved our evaluation of how these interventions work, the choice of the right instrument and the long-term results.

Percutaneous transluminal coronary angioplasty (PTCA)

PTCA causes enlargement of the vessel lumen by the following mechanisms: 1) plaque fracture and fissuring with intimal flaps and localized medial dissection; 2) eccentric stretching of plaque-free wall segments; and 3) generalized stretching of the vessel wall with plaque compression.

In vitro PTCA studies

IVUS provides insight into the mechanism of coronary angioplasty. An extensive *in vitro* study by Tobis et al.[42] in 17 human atherosclerotic artery segments, before and after balloon dilatation angioplasty, showed clear demarcation between the lumen and the endothelium, the atheroma plaque, the muscular media and the adventitia. Dissected and disrupted plaques were clearly visible as well as flaps in the lumen. Similar findings were observed by Pandian et al.[43] and Gussenhoven et al.[44] In an *in vitro* study, Lugt et al.[38] compared the incidence of vascular damage diagnosed by IVUS in 40 postballoon dilatation arterial segments com-

pared to histology; 81% of the increase in lumen area was accounted for by the increase in medial-bound area, and 19% by plaque area decrease. Sensitivity of detecting dissection was 79% and plaque rupture 37%. Thus, only large tissue detachment could reliably be detected by IVUS.

In vivo PTCA studies

In native coronary arteries, Potkin et al.[45] have observed that atheroma composition may be an important determinant of balloon angioplasty results in patients with significant coronary artery disease. Plaque type was assessed by echoreflectivity where highly echogenic areas are considered fibrous or calcified and low echogenicity as mixed cellular or lipid-laden plaque. Fissures were considered as focal superficial breaks in the plaque, and dissection as a deep break extending in a radial, longitudinal or circumferential direction. In highly echogenic hard atheroma (fibrous or calcific), successful angioplasty was associated with discrete dissection. Fissures were observed in 70% of lesions, and dissections in 83% of lesions. Their conclusion was that successful PTCA in hard plaque occurs mainly by dissection, and soft plaque by expansion.

The variability of plaque composition between patients with stable and unstable angina was stressed by Hodgson et al.[46] who showed that in 75% of patients with unstable angina undergoing PTCA, plaques were of soft echogenic material, and only 25% were hard. In patients with stable angina 41% of plaques were soft and 59% were hard. Losordo and coworkers[47] have indeed corroborated that dissection was the main mechanism of successful angioplasty; however, in all their patients plaque compression was found with only minimal arterial stretch.

In a later study, Mario et al.[48] tried to establish, using IVUS, mechanisms of acute lumen gain and late loss in 18 patients treated with PTCA. They have confirmed that hard plaque undergoes dissection, whereas acute lumen gain in soft plaque is mostly by plaque compression. In their study, PTCA acute results were associated with plaque reduction in 52% of cases and vessel expansion in 48% of cases.

The role of calcium in determining the response to PTCA was studied by Fitzgerald and coworkers[49] who showed that 74% of dissections during PTCA were associated with marked calcification (a calcium arc of more than 86°). They suggested that localized calcium has a direct role in promoting dissection, probably due to local high shear forces at the calcium deposition site (Fig. 25.3).[49]

The long-term results of PTCA are under extensive study since this revascularization procedure was introduced. IVUS is an accurate technique to calculate changes that occur in vessel diameter and area and the mechanism of increase or decrease in vessel size following interventions. Gil et al.[50] have shown that lesion composition (soft, calcific or mixed atheroma) does not influence the acute

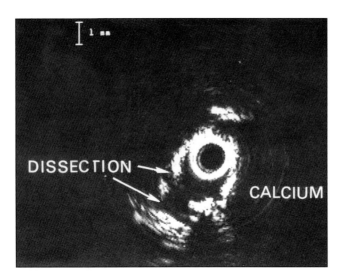

Figure 25.3
Failed PTCA in a severely calcified atheroma with dissection planes noted at the edge of the calcified segment.

stretch results or extent of immediate recoil and the relative lumen gain by PTCA.

All the above-mentioned studies have looked at planar changes at the lesion site, and at a proximal or distal reference site. Mintz et al.[51] in a genuine research project, tried to determine whether plaque compression occurs in vivo during PTCA, and attempted to explain previously published reports showing a decrease in plaque cross-sectional area at the lesion site after PTCA. The authors evaluated the changes at the lesion site in the classic planar methodology, as well as using a volumetric method extending 8 mm axially in each direction from the peak of stenosis. They have shown that when the planar methods were used, external elastic membrane cross-sectional area increased by 12%, lumen by 203% and plaque plus media cross-sectional area by 10%. Using the volumetric technique they have shown that external elastic membrane volume increased by 11% and lumen volume by 33%; there was no change in plaque plus media volume following PTCA. The authors concluded that during PTCA there is an axial redistribution of the atherosclerotic plaque away from the center of the lesion to the proximal and distal ends of the lesion.

Integrated ultrasound angioplasty devices have been developed and proved reliable in assessing changes in wall morphology during the procedure.[52-54] These combined technologies will improve our ability to assess the effect of PTCA while performing the procedure and will provide guidance for reliable decision-making in interventional cardiology.

Directional coronary atherectomy

Excision of atherosclerotic plaques from native coronaries with directional atherectomy was found effective in treating flow-limiting lesions (Fig. 25.4). IVUS may help in guiding this procedure by providing a clear distinction between normal tissue and plaque, and by assessing the distribution and depth of the plaque and plaque composition. Sequential 2D and 3D reconstruction prior to and following atherectomy may help in assessing the extent of disease and plaque removal.

Braden et al.[55] studied 39 lesions of 37 patients with IVUS prior to and immediately after directional coronary atherectomy (DCA). They identified plaque reduction as the main mechanism of DCA, resulting in 22 lesions, vessel stretching in 5 and combined effects in 12 lesions. Their main conclusion was that plaque reduction accounted for 81% of lumen gain during DCA whereas vessel expansion has a limited role in improvement of lumen area during atherectomy. Weissman and coworkers[56] studied pre- and post-DCA IVUS images and calculated volume changes of the artery, plaque and lumen at the lesion site and reference segments. They found no significant change in the volume of the artery, lumen or plaque burden at the reference segment. However, a significant increase in lumen volume, due mainly to plaque removal, was found at the treated lesion site. On average 40% of the target plaque volume was removed but a significant amount of remaining atheroma was noted. This is consistent with other studies which documented a significant amount of remaining atheroma after directional atherectomy. The increase in lumen area was not associated with a significant change in artery area.

Matar et al.[57] performed an extensive study in 170 patients to identify IVUS predictors of DCA results. They evaluated clinical, procedural, angiographic and ultrasound variables in a multivariate linear regression model. Atherectomy was effective in removal of plaque burden resulting in significant increase in lumen cross-sectional area from 1.7 to 6.6 mm^2, mainly due to a decrease in plaque plus media area (from 18 to 14 mm^2). Atherectomy device size and increased balloon pressure were associated with increased plaque removal whereas larger arc of calcification, longer lesions and larger preatherectomy plaque plus media area resulted in higher postatherectomy percent cross-sectional narrowing. This study confirmed that plaque composition and extent may help in assessing the suitability of lesions for DCA.

In a combined IVUS and quantitative angiography study, Popma et al.[57a] have confirmed that DCA is associated with

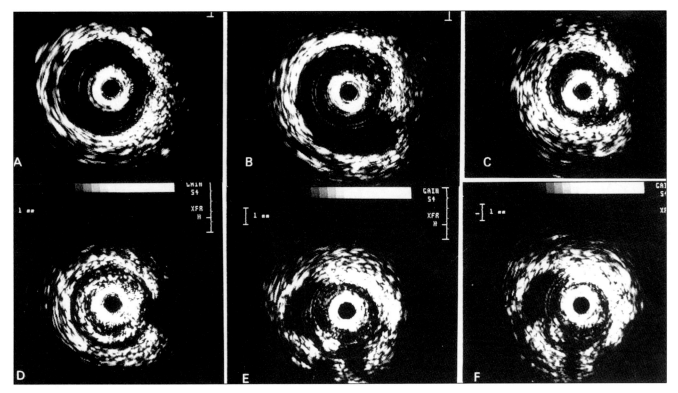

Figure 25.4
Sequential images from the left main (panel A), through the bifurcation (panel B) into the diseased LAD (panels C to F). The atherectomy cuts are noted in panels E and F.

a high success rate and infrequent complications in selected lesion subsets, although the degree of plaque resection may be limited if extensive calcification is present. Late clinical events occur more frequently in patients with diabetes mellitus, unstable angina or a history of restenosis.

De Lezo[58] studied 52 patients who underwent coronary atherectomy for flow-limiting lesions with guidance of IVUS. Resected material was weighed and underwent histologic analysis. Similar to previous *in vitro* studies, echogenic plaques had a higher collagen and calcium content whereas echolucent plaques were softer in content and had an increased level of fibrin, cellular elements and lipids. Ultrasound plaque reduction by atherectomy was greater for echolucent than for highly echogenic plaques. However, the incidence of restenosis at late follow-up was higher for echolucent than for echogenic primary lesion atherectomy.

Marsico et al.[59] performed IVUS in 32 patients undergoing balloon angioplasty and 29 patients undergoing DCA. They showed that stretching of the vessel wall and an increase in vessel area accounted for 68% of the luminal

gain in patients undergoing balloon angioplasty, while plaque reduction accounted for the remaining 32%. Plaque dissections were noted in 32% and fissures in 60% of treated lesions. Directional atherectomy caused a significant improvement in lumen area. Stretching of the vessel with increase in total vessel area accounted for 49% of improvement and plaque reduction for the remaining 51%. Interestingly, in calcific plaques, stretching of the vessel wall accounted for only 9% of luminal gain compared to 56% in noncalcific plaques. Dissections and fissuring occurred only rarely during DCA.

These results are different from those reported by Tenaglia et al.[60] who suggested that vessel expansion does not occur during atherectomy. In a similar study, Mario et al.[48] tried to establish mechanisms of acute lumen gain and late loss that occur over time following PTCA or DCA. They have studied 18 patients treated with PTCA and 16 with DCA for angina pectoris. Coronary angiography and IVUS were performed at baseline and 6–8 months after the procedure. The authors found that reduction in plaque area explained 66% of lumen gain by DCA and 52%

by PTCA. Expansion of total vessel area explained 34% of the increase in lumen gain by DCA and 48% by PTCA. During PTCA concentric soft plaques were more frequently compressed compared to eccentric and hard calcific plaques and plaque fracture and dissections accounted for acute improvement in mixed-calcific plaques. The long-term follow-up studies by Mario and coworkers have shown that 92% of late lumen loss in the DCA group was accounted for by plaque increase whereas, in the PTCA group, 67% of late lumen loss was accounted for by the reduction of total vessel area (recoil) and 32% by plaque increase.

The Optimal Atherectomy Restenosis trial (OARS) is a 200 patient multicenter study designed to assess 'optimal' IVUS-guided DCA on acute and late clinical outcomes. The authors preliminary conclusions were that optimal IVUS-guided DCA can be performed with a high success rate, larger lumen gain and improved late clinical and angiographic results.[61] Combined atherectomy and IVUS catheters are currently in development and may prove a helpful guide in performing this procedure.

Rotational atherectomy (Rotablator)

The rotational atherectomy device has a diamond-coated elliptical tip that, during high-speed rotation, abrades occlusive athereosclerotic lesions and restores patency of stenotic coronary vessels. In a comprehensive study Mintz and coworkers[62] analyzed IVUS images obtained in 28 patients after rotational atherectomy. Most lesions were significantly calcified with a mean arc of calcium of 160 ± 126°. After atherectomy, the intima-lumen interface was distinct and circular with smooth borders and a sharp clear interface of lumen and plaque. The lumen was larger than the burr tip even when adjunct balloon dilatation was not performed. Dissections were observed in 29% of lesions and fissures in 32% but there was no evidence of extensive tissue disruption. Total cross-sectional area of the vessel did not increase, supporting the view that improvement in lumen size is mainly due to atheroma ablation without significant vessel expansion. These findings are consistent with in vitro experimental studies which showed that after rotational atherectomy the residual lumen is smooth and shiny, with a denuded endothelium and ablated parts of the atheroma; damage to the media is minor with minimal fissuring and no dissections. The authors concluded that the Rotablator (Heart Technology, Inc) causes effective ablation of calcified plaque and creates a cylindrical uniform lumen larger than the burr. Arterial expansion occurs only rarely.

In a sequential IVUS study before and after rotational

atherectomy, and following balloon angioplasty, Kovach et al.[63] characterized the mechanisms of lumen enlargement after each phase of intervention. Rotational atherectomy in 48 lesions resulted in an increased lumen area from 1.8 to 3.9 mm² with a decrease in plaque plus media area from 15.7 to 13 mm² without a significant change in total vessel area. The target arc of calcium was reduced by 26% following atherectomy; thrombus could not be delineated during IVUS in any of the patients. Balloon dilatation was associated with a marked increase in total vessel size and arterial expansion was documented in 80% of the patients. The amount of atheroma (plaque plus media) did not change and lumen area increased from 3.9 to 5.2 mm². Dissections occurred in 40% of lesions after atherectomy within the calcified area and in 77% of lesions after balloon dilatation, usually at the sites adjacent to the calcium deposits. The authors concluded that rotational atherectomy causes lumen enlargement by selective ablation of hard, especially calcified atherosclerotic plaque, with little tissue disruption and rare arterial expansion. Adjacent balloon angioplasty further increased lumen area by a combination of arterial dissection and arterial expansion specially of compliant noncalcified plaque elements.

Laser angioplasty

The use of transcatheter laser angioplasty for treating flow-limiting coronary lesions has been in practice for many years. It was proposed that laser energy will result in localized photoablation without extensive thermal injury. IVUS renders a practical tool to assess in vivo the results of coronary laser angioplasty.

In an in vitro model, Schmid and coworkers[64] used excimer laser coronary angioplasty in 41 coronary segments and evaluated the results with IVUS imaging. IVUS enabled accurate identification of the ablation sites, though precise quantification of the amount of ablation was impossible when IVUS images were compared to histology, mainly due to limitation of axial and lateral resolution.

Mintz et al.[65] performed IVUS imaging in 202 lesions undergoing Excimer laser angioplasty and in 49 lesions. The studies were performed before and after intervention. The lumen improvement after laser angioplasty from an average of 1.4–2.7 mm² was the result of both tissue ablation and vessel expansion. There was no change in the arc of calcium and there was no evidence of calcium removal. In some lesions, lumen improvement was due entirely to plaque ablation and in others it was due entirely to vessel expansion. The amount of tissue ablation was small and averaged 40% of the cross-sectional area of the laser catheter. Dissections were noted in superficial fibrocalcific plaques that developed a characteristic fragmented appearance. The authors concluded that photoablation and forced vessel expansion mediated by either acoustic shock waves or vapor bubbles are the mechanisms of lumen enlargement and plaque dissection after Excimer laser angioplasty in human coronary vessels.

Coronary stents

Coronary stenting was initially used as a safe and effective bail-out procedure to prevent impending vessel closure after balloon dilatation and in patients with recurrent restenosis. However, deployment of these metallic devices has recently been shown to reduce the frequency of restenosis in *de novo* lesions in selected groups of patients compared to balloon angioplasty. Until the introduction of effective antithrombotic therapy, stent placement was associated with 1–3% thrombotic complications.

IVUS seemed a perfect imaging modality to assess stent deployment characteristics and long-term results since metal, similar to calcium, is highly echogenic. Indeed, stent struts or coils are well visualized by IVUS and in most stents imaging by IVUS is significantly improved compared to fluoroscopy and angiography. Recently, radio-opaque tantalum stents have been introduced and provide a better fluoroscopic delineation of the stent struts compared to stents made of stainless steel or Nitinol.[66] The IVUS measurements of the stent and reference lumen dimensions and cross-sectional area were found highly reproducible with low inter- and intraobserver variability.[67] This imaging modality has been used extensively over the last few years in an effort to improve our understanding of stent deployment characteristics and define IVUS guidelines for implantation. Full stent expansion to the appropriate size complete apposition and symmetry, both axially and longitudinally, were found to be important criteria that may help to avoid events of acute and subacute stent thrombosis. Moreover, arterial remodeling is reduced by stent deployment, though tissue growth is augmented.

The initial IVUS stent studies were performed after Palmaz–Schatz stent implantation. Acutely, stents were usually concentric with an inner layer of highly reflective struts that obscure a middle hypoechoic layer composed of media and compressed atheroma and an outer echogenic adventitia (Fig. 25.5). The lumen of the stented vessels was usually clear of flaps or thrombi. The stent struts were sometimes expanded in an asymmetric fashion. Chronic changes included a thin layer of neointimal hyperplasia in a significant number of patients. These initial observations were later expanded with careful comprehensive and longitudinal studies performed to assess the determinants of acute success and late restenosis after stent implantation.

Nakamura *et al.*[68] compared IVUS imaging with coronary angiography in 63 patients who underwent Palmaz–Schatz stent insertion for native coronary artery

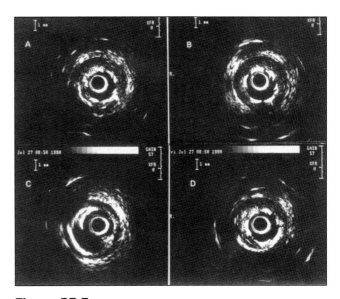

Figure 25.5
Palmaz–Schatz stents as visualized from the proximal (panel A) to the distal part (panel D) immediately after stent implantation.

stenosis. The angiographic and IVUS data were used to decide whether stent placement results were satisfactory and whenever necessary further balloon dilatation was performed. After the first balloon dilatation the tightest lumen cross-sectional area was 6.9 mm^2 and this increased after further dilatation to 9 mm^2, with an initial symmetry index (ratio of smallest compared to largest diameter) of 0.83 that later improved to 0.86. Eighty percent of the stents received further dilatations based on IVUS imaging data. Angiographic percent diameter stenosis was improved from baseline average of 72 to 9% after deployment and −4% after further dilatation. There was no case of subacute thrombosis in this group. In two patients, small dissections were created after high-pressure balloon inflations with larger balloons, necessitating implantation of short stents. The authors concluded that IVUS evaluation after stent insertion demonstrates a significant degree of underestimation compared with coronary angiography. Using IVUS, more than 80% of patients underwent further dilatation despite the initial appearance of an optimal angiographic result. The results of the study supported the view that IVUS-guided careful stent deployment with adherence to criteria of size, symmetry and apposition may reduce the need for anticoagulation.

In a later study from the same center, Goldberg and coworkers[69] guided stent deployment with the use of angiography and IVUS to obtain optimal results in 40 patients. The angiographic percent diameter stenosis was 74% at baseline and increased to an average of 8% after apparent successful angiographic results, and to −6% negative residual stenosis after IVUS-guided correction. These changes were associated with a marked increase in lumen cross-sectional area obtained by IVUS and improvement in eccentricity index from 0.84 to 0.89 at the final post-IVUS dilatation. The study further demonstrated that stents do not uniformly expand along the long axis, and that IVUS-guided higher pressure and larger balloon inflation result in an intrastent cross-sectional area that translates to a significant increase in flow through the vessel. This may, in the long run, result in a lower incidence of thrombotic events and restenosis.

To facilitate and optimize stent delivery two improvements were proposed. First, an effort was made to introduce a sheath-covered stent delivery system that will increase the safety of implantation.[70] The system includes a compliant balloon. To improve stent expansion and geometry, further dilatation with a low compliant high-pressure oversized balloon is advocated. Secondly, Mudra et al.[54] suggested an integrated balloon with an IVUS catheter system that will enable immediate ultrasound imaging to assess stent deployment characteristics. This combined therapeutic and imaging capability is time consuming, and may prevent possible harm to the newly deployed stent by introducing catheters multiple times. Deployment was successful in 18 of 20 patients eligible for the study. IVUS showed a smaller minimal luminal diameter compared to angiography. IVUS criteria considered as optimal for stent deployment were good apposition of the stent struts with a ratio of 0.9 between minimal stent cross-sectional area and average lumen area of the normal or almost normal proximal and distal vessel. Whenever optimal criteria were not achieved, further dilatation with high-pressure or higher-volume balloons were performed, resulting in increased luminal area and an improved correlation of stent intraluminal dimensions between IVUS and angiography. The conclusion of this preliminary study was that combined imaging and balloon angioplasty is feasible, with an acceptable success rate. IVUS on-line imaging may reveal lumen size underestimation that will allow better stent dilatation and long-term results.

Recent studies suggest that arterial remodeling after balloon angioplasty may have a more significant role compared to neointimal proliferation in causing restenosis. The process of remodeling involves changes that occur in the adventitia and media and may be halted by the deployment of stents. Two factors may contribute to stent restenosis. First, stents trigger the development of neointima and, second, is the possible chronic recoil and reduction in stent size. Hoffman et al.[71] performed serial IVUS studies in 142 stents to determine the relative contribution of both these factors in causing restenosis. The acute angiographic and ultrasound results were excellent and the Palmaz–Schatz

stents were quite uniform in size longitudinally, except for the narrowest portion at the articulation site where most of the prolapsed tissue was detected. On later follow-up studies, lumen size decreased markedly, with only a minor change in stent size. In-stent intimal proliferation was significant throughout the stent lumen and accumulated more at the central articulation site. Late lumen loss correlated strongly with tissue growth and weakly with stent recoil and remodeling. The authors concluded that stents prevent the remodeling process and restenosis of stents is the result of relatively uniform neointimal tissue proliferation throughout the stent. In a second study, the same authors showed[72] that endovascular stents induce tissue proliferation both within the endoluminal stent surface and in the tissue layers surrounding the metallic Palmaz–Schatz stent struts. Similar to previous findings, tissue proliferation was greater in restenotic than in nonrestenotic stents. Tissue proliferation surrounding the stent was accompanied by adaptive remodeling and increase in external elastic membrane cross-sectional area.[72]

In summary, ultrasound guidance for stent placement has shown the following:

- Lumen gain and vessel expansion during stent implantation are usually larger than in PTCA. IVUS guidance results in low final percent stenosis.

- Lesion composition has an effect on stent expansion characteristics, mainly when calcified.

- High-pressure dilatation can safely be used for stent deployment and may improve angiographic results.

- IVUS guidance may help to avoid anticoagulation using criteria for stenosis, apposition and symmetry.

- Arterial remodeling is reduced compared to PTCA but tissue growth is augmented.

- Prevention of restenosis with stents compared to other devices is mainly by effect on remodeling.

Choice of interventional modality

With the development of smaller IVUS catheters, preintervention studies can be relatively safely performed and the information obtained used to change treatment strategies. Nishioka et al.[73] suggested that whereas 48% of the treatment decisions were influenced by IVUS data in 1993, 84% were influenced in 1994. They confirmed that in their center, IVUS was increasingly performed for ambiguous lesions, ostial lesions and stent placement. Similar findings were summarized from the Guide I trial[74] where IVUS added important data in 68% of cases, resulting in a change of treatment decisions in 48% of the patients. The changes included prolonged perfusion when dissections were detected, balloon upsizing when lumen dilatation was not satisfactory, performance of PTCA instead of DCA when lesions were calcified and DCA when lesions turned out to be eccentric. Mintz et al.[75] studied the impact of preintervention IVUS imaging on revascularization treatment strategy in 329 patients in 341 lesions. In the study, 'intended' strategy based on angiographic data was compared to the actual procedure performed; use of IVUS caused a change in therapy in 124 lesions (121 patients). Revascularization was performed, when not planned, in 20 lesions (6%), and was avoided when planned in 21 lesions (7%). Revascularization strategy was altered in 20 lesions (6%) and a final option of revascularization strategy was selected based on IVUS data in 63 lesions (20%). For example, in nine cases, coronary artery bypass graft (CABG) surgery was elected instead of catheter intervention. The clinical decisions taken were performance of rotational atherectomy, laser angioplasty or coronary artery bypass graft surgery when lesions were calcified, and DCA when lesions were eccentric and mildly calcified. Intracoronary stents were placed when dissections, aneurysms or fibrotic lesions were encountered during IVUS imaging. Thrombi in saphenous vein grafts were treated by pharmacologic thrombolysis or with extraction atherectomy.[75]

Also of importance is the decision when to abort any intervention. Indeed over a 3-year period at the Washington Hospital Center, out of 1660 cases, IVUS imaging helped to differentiate insignificant from significant disease, and in 10% of cases a decision was made to abort any intervention.[76]

Restenosis and late outcome after interventions

Whether IVUS is a research technique or a clinical tool is still debatable mainly at a time of cost containment and in view of the risks involved in performing an invasive procedure for diagnostic purposes. The main thrust of research was directed to translate the information obtained from imaging for guidance during procedures, to help in choosing the appropriate interventional modality and predicting acute and long-term outcome following interventions.

Restenosis remains the major limitation of transcatheter coronary revascularization. Many clinical, angiographic and more recently IVUS variables were evaluated as possible predictors for restenosis. Review of the subject demonstrates that conclusions drawn from the various studies differ. In an early study of 100 patients undergoing PTCA, Honye et al.[77] suggested that restenosis occurs more frequently in lesions with relatively soft atheroma and insufficient plaque fracture. Only significant fracture of the plaque is associated with prevention of restenosis.

Tenaglia and coworkers[78] performed PTCA, DCA or laser therapy in 68 patients, assisted by an initial IVUS imaging. Six months' angiographic follow-up and 1-year clinical follow up showed that dissections detected in 42% of patients were associated with adverse clinical outcome including cardiac death, MI coronary bypass surgery and, mainly, restenosis. Feld et al.[79] determined the value of IVUS compared to angioscopy in predicting outcome of interventional procedures such as PTCA, DCA, laser angioplasty and stent implantation. They performed interventional procedures in 60 patients followed by either IVUS, angioscopy or both. Follow-up at 1 year was clinical and wherever needed coronary angiography was undertaken. Predictive of adverse outcome were clinical presentation, thrombolytic therapy, angioscopic plaque rupture prior to procedure and the detection of thrombus pre- and post-procedure. The conclusion of the research was that angioscopy but not IVUS or angiography was predictive of adverse outcome in patients with complex lesions after interventions.

In the PICTURE trial,[80] 200 patients were enrolled to try to evaluate whether post-PTCA IVUS imaging can predict 6 months' restenosis. Variables studied were the appearance of dissection, tears, plaque types, plaque area, total vessel area, lumen area and other ratios. Interestingly, not one of the post-PTCA IVUS variables was predictive of angiographic restenosis at 6 months. Jain et al.[81] investigated IVUS-derived parameters that can predict restenosis in 33 patients and lesions, after balloon angioplasty ($n = 25$), and DCA ($n = 8$). Six months' follow-up was performed in 30 patients. They found major dissections in 78% of patients with angiographic restenosis compared to 10% of patients without restenosis, whereas plaque fracture was more abundant in patients without restenosis. Plaque burden, calculated as plaque area/EEL area (external elastic lamina area) was significantly more severe in patients with angiographic restenosis compared with patients without restenosis. The authors concluded that the absence of plaque fracture, existence of a major dissection and greater plaque burden identify patients in whom restenosis is more likely to occur after catheter-based interventions. The rate of arterial recoil was similar in both groups.

In an effort to elucidate the mechanism of restenosis following coronary interventions, Mintz et al.[82] performed IVUS imaging in 212 lesions treated with PTCA, DCA, rotational atherectomy and laser angioplasty. They have found that in patients who developed restenosis, the reduction in lumen size was attributed to a reduction in total vessel area (EEM area). This phenomenon was not encountered in the nonrestenotic lesions. The authors concluded that restenosis is determined after interventions, mainly by the extent and direction of remodeling of the vessel.

The changing concept of the underlying pathophysiology of restenosis called for a change in treatment strategy with significantly more emphasis given to prevention of remodeling mainly with the use of stents. Mintz et al.[83] performed IVUS imaging in 360 nonstented native coronary artery lesions for whom angiographic follow-up was obtained within a few months. The angiographic predictors of restenosis were the use of rotational atherectomy, lesions longer than 10 mm, vessel tortuosity, total occlusion lesions and preintervention TIMI flow less than 3. Lumen cross-sectional area, minimal lumen diameter and eccentricity index obtained from IVUS imaging prior to intervention correlated with the occurrence of restenosis. The highest correlation was found for percent cross-sectional narrowing calculated as plaque plus media cross-sectional area divided by external elastic membrane cross-sectional area. Similarly, these variables obtained in the postintervention IVUS imaging phase correlated significantly with restenosis.

Pitfalls in IVUS imaging

Even though IVUS is a magnificent technological advance in tissue imaging, there are significant limitations and pitfalls that should be well known to the user.

These pitfalls can be divided into three categories:

- Ultrasound related.
- Catheter position related.
- Image interpretation related.

The ultrasound-related pitfalls involve the technical problems of resolution, penetration and backscatter. Penetration and resolution are frequency dependent. A higher-frequency transducer may have better resolution but reduced penetration. The optimal relationship is evidently dependent on the size of the vessel visualized. For coronary vessels 30 MHz seems the optimal relationship, mainly since at higher frequencies the backscatter from intravascular cells is significant and impairs vessel wall visualization. Since the vessel is a round structure within which the imaging catheter rotates, axial and lateral resolution may be reduced. For practical purposes the axial resolution of current devices is about 100 μ and lateral resolution about 300 μ. These limitations have to be taken into consideration in view of the fact that in normal coronary vessels the thickness of the intima is about 100 μ, of the media about 200 μ and of the adventitia 300 μ. These limitations of resolution are important in the era of interventional cardiology where plaque disruptions, fissuring and dissections are looked for by angiography and more recently by IVUS. This issue of axial and lateral resolution becomes even more important when the imaging catheter is not in the mid-position and the imaging head is tilted off-center.

Distortion of the images may occur due to disorientation of the catheter imaging assembly. A round structure may seem ellipsoid as shown in a few in vitro studies. These image distortions have a significant impact on the 3D image structure obtained from IVUS.[22,84,85]

The accuracy of IVUS-derived measurements was tested compared to histology and angiography. The results varied from highly significant correlation between measurements derived by various technics to no correlation as shown in a recent report where Haase et al.[86] compared IVUS measurements to angiographic measurements; the calculated correlation was poor. Other groups have shown that postintervention calculation of vessel dimensions do not correlate with other modalities whereas preintervention measurements show a significant correlation between angiography and ultrasound.

Catheters tend to adhere to vessel walls and near-field reflections are of higher intensity compared to distant reflections. This phenomenon has to be taken into account when considering fibrous plaques.

The ability of ultrasound to identify cellular elements is limited to differentiation of soft versus hard atheroma. The highest specificity was found for identification of calcified deposits. However, calcified deposits cause shadowing of vessel walls and do not allow comprehensive imaging of the entire vessel. Ultrasound imaging is relatively inaccurate in differentiation of thrombus from soft atheromata. Echo-free spaces are difficult to diagnose and are differentiated mainly from calcified plaques or after interventions where the reliable diagnosis of plaque disruption is very important.

Conclusions and future directions

IVUS is being used in many interventional laboratories to optimize therapeutic procedures. The technology has turned from an investigational tool to a clinical tool and provides important information on vessel wall morphology and on changes that take place acutely after a coronary procedure, and long term when restenosis or post-transplant vasculopathy develop. Though it may seem that catheter design has reached a plateau, new technological developments are being introduced to improve the diagnostic accuracy of IVUS. Catheters are smaller and may be miniaturized to a guidewire thickness, similar to the Doppler wire concept. At the final stage of development we may have in use a wire that will support interventional procedures and enable imaging, Doppler flow and even pressure recording. Imaging is currently circumferential, without any ability for forward viewing. However, the technological capacity to develop such an image orientation has recently been demonstrated and may have an important role in visualization of total occlusions.[87]

The 3D orientation of the ultrasound image around the longitudinal axis is an issue under study and is of critical importance in reliable and reproducible 3D reconstruction of the vessels. Over the last few years multiple studies have emphasized the future role of 3D reconstruction in assessing vessel wall pathology and postintervention changes.[3,4]

Significant effort is being made to improve image quality and apply new signal analysis modes such as Doppler tissue imaging, ultrasound backscatter analysis and lumen enhancement with modern contrast agent injection. These and other techniques may augment our ability to differentiate between various components of the atheroma and improve identification of intracoronary thrombi. IVUS imaging catheters have been incorporated with interventional systems such as balloons and atherectomy devices. The combination is feasible, though the long-term results are not yet clear, as is the application with local delivery systems.

IVUS is now an established, feasible and safe method and a new 'gold standard' for imaging the vascular system. It is both a research and a clinical tool, and has become an integral part of the daily activities in the catheterization laboratory.

References

1 Batkoff BW, Linker DT. The safety of intracoronary ultrasound: data from a multicenter European registry. *J Am Coll Cardiol* 1995; **143A**: 734–3 (abstract).

2 Bom N, Lancee CT, Gussenhoven EJ, Li W, Hoff HT. Basic principles of intravascular ultrasound imaging. In: Tobis JM, Yock PG (eds). *Intravascular Ultrasound Imaging* (New York: Churchill Livingstone, 1992): 7–15.

3 Roelandt JRTC, Di Mario C, Pandian NG, Wenguag L, Keane D, Slager CJ. Three-dimensional reconstruction of intracoronary ultrasound images: rationale approaches, problems, and directions. *Circulation* 1994; **90**: 1044–55.

4 Gil R, Birgelen CV, Prati F, Di Mario C, Ligthart J, Serruys PW. Usefulness of three-dimensional reconstruction for interpretation and quantitative analysis of intracoronary ultrasound during stent deployment. *Am J Cardiol* 1996; **77**: 761–4.

5 McPherson DD, Hirazka LF, Lamberth WC, et al. Delineation of the extent of coronary atherosclerosis by high frequency epicardial echocardiography. *N Engl J Med* 1987; **316**: 304–9.

6 Arnett EN, Isner JM, Redwood DR, et al. Coronary artery narrowing in coronary heart disease: comparison of cineangiography in and necropsy findings. *Ann Int Med* 1979; **91**: 350–6.

7 Sahn DJ, Copeland JG, Temkin LP, et al. Anatomic ultrasound correlations for the intraoperative open chest imaging of coronary artery atherosclerotic lesions in human beings. *J Am Coll Cardiol* 1984; **3**: 1169–77.

8 Alfonso F, Macaya C, Goiclea J, et al. Intravascular ultrasound imaging of angiographically normal coronary segments in patients with coronary artery disease. *Am Heart J* 1994; **127**: 536–44.

9 Topol EJ, Nissen SE. Our preoccupation with coronary luminology: the dissociation between clinical and angiographic findings in ischemic heart disease. *Circulation* 1995; **92**: 2333–42.

10 Hausmann D, Johnson JA, Sudhir K, Mullen WL, Friedrich G, Fitzgerald PJ. Angiographically silent atherosclerosis detected by intravascular ultrasound in patients with familial hypercholesterolemia and familial combined hyperlipidemia: correlation with high density lipoproteins. *J Am Coll Cardiol* 1996; **27**: 1562–70.

11 Glagov S, Weisenberg E, Zairns CK, Stankunavicius R, Colletis GJ. Compensatory enlargement of human atherosclerotic coronary arteries. *N Engl J Med* 1987; **316**: 1371–5.

12 Wong CB, Porter TR, Xie F, Deligonul U. Segmental analysis of coronary arteries with equivalent plaque burden by intravascular ultrasound in patients with and without angiographically significant coronary artery disease. *Am J Cardiol* 1995; **76**: 598–601.

13 Weissman NJ, Mendelsohn FO, Palacios IF, Weyman AE. Development of coronary compensatory enlargement *in vivo*: sequential assessments with intravascular ultrasound. *Am Heart J* 1995; **130**: 1283–5.

14 Nishioka T, Luo N, Eigler HL, Berglund H, Kim C-J, Siegel RJ. Contribution of inadequate compensatory enlargement to development of human coronary artery stenosis: An *in vivo* intravascular ultrasound study. *J Am Coll Cardiol* 1996; **27**: 1571–6.

15 Losordo DW, Rosenfield K, Kaufman J, Pieczsk A, Isner JM. Focal compensatory enlargement of human arteries in response to progressive atherosclerosis *in vivo* documentation using intravascular ultrasound. *Circulation* 1994; **89**: 2570–7.

16 Mendelsohn FO, Foster GP, Palacios IF, Weyman AE, Weissman NJ. *In vivo* assessment by intravascular ultrasound of enlargement in saphenous vein bypass grafts. *Am J Cardiology* 1995; **76**: 1066–9.

17 Potkin BN, Bartorelli AL, Gessert JM, et al. Coronary artery imaging with intravascular high frequency ultrasound. *Circulation* 1990; **81**: 1575–85.

18 Lockwood GR, Ryan LK, Gotlieb AI, et al. In vitro high resolution intravascular ultrasound imaging in muscular and elastic arteries. *J Am Coll Cardiol* 1992; **20**: 153–60.

19   Gussenhaven EJ, Essed CE, Lancee CT, *et al.* Arterial wall characteristics determined by intravascular ultrasound imaging: an *in vitro* study. *J Am Coll Cardiol* 1989; **14**: 947–52.

20   Mallery JG, Tobis JM, Griffith J, *et al.* Assessment of normal and atherosclerotic arterial wall characteristics with an intravascular ultrasound imaging catheter. *Am Heart J* 1990; **119**: 1392–400.

21   Fitzgerald PJ, Goar FG, Connolly AJ, *et al.* Intravascular ultrasound imaging of coronary arteries. Is three layers the norm? *Circulation* 1992; **86**: 154–8.

22   Nishimura RA, Edwards WD, Warnes CA, *et al.* Intravascular ultrasound imaging: *in vitro* validation and pathologic correlation. *J Am Coll Cardiol* 1990; **16**: 145–54.

23   Kragel AH, Reddy SG, Wittes JT, *et al.* Morphometric analysis of the composition of atherosclerotic plaques in the four epicardial coronary arteries in acute myocardial infarction and in sudden cardiac death. *Circulation* 1989; **80**: 1747–56.

24   Libby P. Atheroma, much more than mush. *Lancet* 1996; **348 (Suppl 1)**: S4–S7.

25   Fuster V. Coronary thrombosis. *Lancet* 1996: **348 (Suppl 1)**: S7–S10.

26   Keren G, Leon MB. Intravascular ultrasound of atherosclerotic vessels: changes observed during interventional procedures. *Am J Cardiac Imag* 1994; **8**: 129–39.

27   Tobis JM, Mallery J, Mahon D, *et al.* Intravascular ultrasound imaging of human coronary arteries *in vivo*. *Circulation* 1991; **83**: 913–26.

28   Nissen SE, Gurley JC, Grines CL, *et al.* Intravascular ultrasound assessment of lumen size and wall morphology in normal subjects and patients with coronary artery disease. *Circulation* 1991; **84**: 1087–99.

29   Mintz GS, Popma JF, Pichard AD, *et al.* Patterns of calcification in coronary artery disease. *Circulation* 1995; **91**: 1959–65.

30   Hiro T, Leung CY, Guzman SD, *et al.* Are 'soft echoes' really soft? Ultrasound assessment of mechanical properties in human atherosclerotic tissue. *Circulation* 1995; **92**: I-649.

31   Giro EK, Cuenoud HF. Intravascular ultrasound detection of lipid pools in human coronary arteries. *Circulation* 1995; **92**: I-649.

32   Keren G, Leon MB. Characterization of atherosclerotic lesions by intravascular ultrasound: possible role in unstable coronary syndromes and in interventional therapeutic procedures. *Am J Cardiol* 1991; **68**: 85B–91B.

33   Siegel RJ, Ariani M, Fishbein MC, *et al.* Histopathologic validation of angioscopy and intravascular ultrasound. *Circulation* 1991; **84**: 109–17.

34   Frimerman A, Miler HI, Hallman M, Laniado S, Keren G. Intravascular ultrasound characterization of thrombi of different composition. *Am J Cardiol* 1994; **73**: 1053–7.

35   Chemarin-Alibelli MJ, Pieraggi MT, Elbaz M, Carrie D, Puel J, Tobis JM. Identification of coronary thrombus after myocardial infarction by intracoronary ultrasound compared with histology of tissues sampled by atherectomy. *Am J Cardiol* 1997; **77**: 344–9.

36   de Feyter PJ, Ozaki Y, Baptista J, Escaned J, Di Mario C, de Jaegere PPT. Ischemia-related lesion characteristics in patients with stable or unstable angina: a study with intracoronary angioscopy and ultrasound. *Circulation* 1995; **29**: 1408–13.

37   Fenggi JG, Gorge G, Haude M, Baumgart D, Sack S, Erbel R. Visualization of unstable plaque rupture by intracoronary ultrasound. *Circulation* 95; **92**: I-400.

38   Van der Lugt A, Gussenhoven EJ, Stijnen T, *et al.* Comparison of intravascular ultrasound findings after coronary balloon angioplasty evaluated *in vitro* with histology. *Am J Cardiol* 1995; **76**: 661–6.

39   Tuzcu EM, De Franco A, Goormastic M, *et al.* Dichotomous pattern of coronary atherosclerosis 1 to 9 years after transplantation: insights from systematic intravascular ultrasound imaging. *J Am Coll Cardiol* 1996; **27**: 839–46.

40   Rickenbacher PR, Pinto FJ, Chenzbraun A, *et al.* Incidence and severity of transplant coronary artery disease early and up to 15 years after transplantation as detected by intravascular ultrasound. *J Am Coll Cardiol* 1995; **25**: 171–7.

41   Pinto FJ, Chenzbraun A, Botas J, *et al.* Feasibility of serial intracoronary ultrasound imaging for assessment of progression of intimal proliferation in cardiac transplant recipients. *Circulation* 1994; **90**: 2348–55.

42   Tobis JM, Mallery JA, Gessert PhD, *et al.* Intravascular ultrasound cross-sectional arterial imaging before and after balloon angioplasty *in vitro*. *Circulation* 1989; **89**: 873–82.

43   Pandian NG, Kreis A, Weintraub A, *et al.* Intravascular ultrasound assessment of arterial dissection, intimal flaps and arterial thrombi. *Am J Cardiac Imag* 1991; **5**: 72–7.

44   Gussenhoven EJ, Stijnen T, Strijen M, Driel E, Egmond FC. Comparison of intravascular ultrasonic findings after coronary balloon angioplasty evaluated *in vitro* with histology. *Am J Cardiol* 1995; **76**: 661–6.

45   Potkin BN, Keren G, Mintz GS, *et al.* Arterial responses to balloon coronary angioplasty: an intravascular ultrasound study. *J Am Coll Cardiol* 1992; **20**: 942–51.

46   Hodgson JM, Reddy KG, Suneja R, Nair RN, Lesnefsky EJ, Sheehan HM. Intracoronary ultrasound imaging: correlation of plaque morphology with angiography, clinical syndrome and procedural results in patients undergoing coronary angioplasty. *J Am Coll Cardiol* 1993; **21**: 35–44.

47   Losordo DW, Rosenfield K, Pieczek A, Baker K, Harding M, Isner JM. How does angioplasty work? Serial analysis of human iliac arteries using intravascular ultrasound. *Circulation* 1992; **86**: 1845–58.

48   Di Mario C, Gil R, Camenzid E, *et al.* Quantitative assessment with intracoronary ultrasound of the mechanisms of restenosis after percutaneous transluminal coronary angioplasty and directional coronary atherectomy. *Am J Cardiol* 1995; **75**: 772–7.

49   Fitzgerald PJ, Ports TA, Yock PG. Contribution of localized calcium deposits to dissection after angioplasty. *Circulation* 1992; **86**: 64–70.

50   Gil R, Prati F, von Birgelen C, van Swindregt EM, de Feyter P. Ultrasonic plaque characteristics do not determine stretch and recoil after coronary balloon angioplasty. *Circulation* 1995; **92**: I-400.

51   Mintz GS, Pichard AD, Kent KM, Satler LF, Popma JJ, Leon MB. Axial plaque redistribution as a mechanism of percutaneous transluminal coronary angioplasty. *Am J Cardiol* 1996; **77**: 427–30.

52   Isner JM, Rosenfield K, Losordo DW, *et al.* Combination balloon ultrasound imaging catheter for percutaneous transluminal angioplasty. *Circulation* 1991; **84**: 739–54.

53   Wolfe CL, Klette MA, Trask RV, *et al.* Assessment of the results of percutaneous transluminal coronary angioplasty using an integrated ultrasound imaging angioplasty catheter. *Cathet Cardiovas Diag* 1994; **32**: 108–12.

54   Mudra H, Klauss V, Blasini R, *et al.* Ultrasound guidance of Palmaz–Schatz intracoronary stenting with a combined intravascular ultrasound balloon catheter. *Circulation* 1994; **90**: 1252–61.

55   Braden GA, Kutcher MA, Downes TR, Kerensky RA, Herrington DM. Mechanisms of luminal enlargement from directional coronary atherectomy: vessel stretching or plaque removal? *J Am Coll Cardiol* 1993; **21**: 32A.

56   Weissman NJ, Palacios IF, Nidorf SM, Dinsmore RE, Weyman AE. Three dimensional intravascular ultrasound assessment of plaque volume after successful atherectomy. *Am Heart J* 1995; **130**: 413–19.

57   Matar FA, Mintz GS, Pinnow E, Javier SP, *et al.* Multivariate predictors of intravascular ultrasound end points after directional coronary atherectomy. *J Am Coll Cardiol* 1995; **25**: 318–24.

57a Popma J, Mintz G, Satler L, *et al.* Clinical and angiographic outcome after directional coronary atherectomy: a qualitative and quantitative analysis using coronary angiography and intravascular ultrasound. *Am J Cardiol* 1993; **72**: 55E–64E.

58   De Lezo JS, Romero M, Medina M, *et al.* Intracoronary ultrasound assessment of directional atherectomy: immediate and follow up findings. *J Am Coll Cardiol* 1993; **21**: 298–307.

59   Marsico F, Kubica J, De Servi S, *et al.* Influence of plaque morphology on the mechanism of luminal enlargement after directional coronary atherectomy and balloon angioplasty. *Br Heart J* 1995; **74**: 134–9.

60   Tenaglia AN, Buller CE, Kisslo KB, Stack RS, Davidson CJ. Mechanisms of balloon angioplasty and directional coronary atherectomy as assessed by intracoronary ultrasound. *J Am Coll Cardiol* 1992; **20**: 685–91.

61   Simonton CA, Leon MB, Kuntz RE, *et al.* Acute and late clinical and angiographic results of directional atherectomy restenosis study (OARS). *Circulation* 95; **92**: I-545.

62   Mintz GS, Potkin BN, Keren G, *et al.* Intravascular ultrasound evaluation of the effect of rotational atherectomy in obstructive atherectomy coronary artery disease. *Circulation* 1992; **86**: 1383–93.

63   Kovach JA, Mintz GS, Pichard AD, *et al.* Sequential intravascular ultrasound characterization of the mechanisms of rotational atherectomy and adjunct balloon angioplasty. *J Am Coll Cardiol* 1993; **22**: 1024–32.

64   Schmid KM, Voelker W, Wehrman OM, Baumbach A, Haase KK, Karsch KR. Intracoronary ultrasound following excimer laser angioplasty: an *in vitro* in human coronary arteries. *Eur Heart J* 1995; **16**: 188–93.

65   Mintz GS, Kovach JA, Javier SP, *et al.* Mechanisms of lumen enlargement after laser coronary angioplasty: an intravascular ultrasound study. *Circulation* 1995; **92**: 3408–14.

66   Ozaki Y, Keane D, Nobuyoshi M, Hamasaki N, Popma JJ, Serruys PW. Coronary lumen at six month follow up of a new radioopaque Cordis tantalum stent using quantitative angiography and intracoronary ultrasound. *Am J Cardiol* 1995; **76**: 1135–43.

67   Mintz GS, Griffin J, Chuang YC, *et al.* Reproducibility of the intravascular ultrasound assessment of stent implantation in saphenous vein grafts. *Am J Cardiol* 1995; **75**: 1267–70.

68   Nakamura S, Colombo A, Gaglione A, *et al.* Intracoronary ultrasound observations during stent implantation. *Circulation* 1994; **89**: 2026–34.

69   Goldberg SL, Colombo A, Nakamura S, Almagor Y, Maiello L, Tobis JM. Benefit of intracoronary ultrasound in

the deployment of Palmaz–Schatz stents. *J Am Coll Cardiol* 1994; **24**: 996–1003.

70 Kienmeneij G, Laarman G, Slagboom T. Mode of deployment of coronary Palmaz–Schatz stent delivery system: an intravascular ultrasound study. *Am Heart J* 1995; **129**: 638–44.

71 Hoffman R, Mintz GS, Dussaillant GR, *et al.* Patterns and mechanisms of in-stent restenosis: a serial intravascular ultrasound study. *Circulation* 1996; **94**: 1247–54.

72 Hoffman R, Mintz GS, Popma JF, *et al.* Chronic arterial responses to stent implantation: a serial intravascular ultrasound analysis of Palmaz–Schatz stents in native coronary arteries. *J Am Coll Cardiol* 1996; **28**: 1134–9.

73 Nishioka T, Luo H, Tabak S, *et al.* The evolving utility of intracoronary ultrasound. *Am J Cardiol* 1995; **75**: 539–41.

74 The Guide Trial Investigators. Impact of ultrasound on device selection and end point assessment of interventions. Phase I of the guide trial. *J Am Coll Cardiol* 1993; **21**: 134A.

75 Mintz GS, Pichard AD, Kovach JA, *et al.* Impact of preintervention intravascular ultrasound imaging on transcatheter treatment strategies in coronary artery disease. *Am J Cardiol* 1994; **73**: 423–30.

76 Mintz GS, Bucher TA, Kent KM, *et al.* Clinical outcomes of patients not undergoing coronary artery revascularization as a result of intravascular ultrasound imaging. *J Am Coll Cardiol* 1995; **25**: 61A.

77 Honye J, Mahon DJ, Jain A, *et al.* Morphological effects of coronary balloon angioplasty *in vivo* assessed by intravascular ultrasound imaging. *Circulation* 1992; **85**: 1012–25.

78 Tenaglia AN, Buller CE, Kisslo KB, Phillips HR, Stack RS. Intracoronary ultrasound predictors of adverse outcomes after coronary artery interventions. *J Am Coll Cardiol* 1992; **20**: 1385–90.

79 Feld S, Ganim M, Carell ES, *et al.* Comparison of angioscopy, intravascular ultrasound imaging and quantitative coronary angiography in predicting clinical outcome after coronary intervention in high risk patients. *J Am Coll Cardiol* 1996; **28**: 97–105.

80 Peters RJ and the PICTURE Study Group. Prediction of the risk of angiographic restenosis by intracoronary ultrasound imaging after coronary balloon angioplasty. *J Am Coll Cardiol* 1995; **25**: 35A.

81 Jain SP, Jain A, Collins TJ, Ramee SR, White CJ. Predictors of restenosis; a morphometric quantitative evaluation by intravascular ultrasound. *Am Heart J* 1994; **128**: 664–73.

82 Mintz GS, Popma JJ, Pichard AD, *et al.* Arterial remodeling after coronary angioplasty: a serial intravascular ultrasound study. *Circulation* 1996; **94**: 35–43.

83 Mintz GS, Popma JJ, Pichard AD, *et al.* Intravascular ultrasound predictors of restenosis after transcatheter coronary revascularization. *J Am Coll Cardiol* 1996; **27**: 1678–87.

84 Finet G, Narincomme E, Tabib A, *et al.* Artifacts in intravascular ultrasound imaging: analyses and implications. *Ultrasound in Med and Biol* 1993; **19**: 533–47.

85 Chae JS, Brisken AF, Maurer G, Siegel RJ. Geometric accuracy of intravascular ultrasound imaging. *J Am Soc Echo* 1992; **5**: 577–87.

86 Haase J, Ozaki Y, Di Mario J, *et al.* Can intracoronary ultrasound correctly assess the luminal dimensions of coronary artery lesions? A comparison with quantitative angiography. *Eur Heart J* 1995; **16**: 112–19.

87 Evans JL, Ng KH, Vonesh MJ, *et al.* Arterial imaging with a new forward viewing intravascular ultrasound catheter. *Circulation* 1994; **89**: 712–17.

26

Three-dimensional intravascular ultrasound in interventional cardiology

Clemens von Birgelen and Patrick W Serruys

Introduction

The use of intravascular ultrasound (IVUS) allows a unique insight into the extent and distribution of atherosclerotic plaque and permits the assessment of the results of catheter-based coronary interventions.[1-8] Nevertheless, in conventional IVUS there is a lack of an 'angiography-like' longitudinal visualization of the examined coronary segment. This can only be provided by a three-dimensional (3D) IVUS approach.[9-16] The ability to visualize the entire coronary segment 1) avoids the difficult mental conceptualization process, required when using two dimensional (2D) IVUS; 2) provides a more detailed insight into the complex plaque architecture; and 3) facilitates serial IVUS studies.[14,17-20]

In parallel with the progress in quantitative angiography techniques which started with manual caliper assessment and finally reached computer-assisted methods,[21,22] automated methods of quantitative 3D IVUS analysis have been developed[14,15,19,23-27] to reduce the analysis time and the subjectivity of manual tracing.[28] These techniques allow careful evaluation of coronary segments of interest before and after catheter-based coronary interventions,[10-13,16,29-31] and permit on-line measurement of the target lesions and reference segments.[16,25,26] These features facilitate the selection of the optimal type and size of interventional device, and the evaluation of potential complications.

Before any of these 3D features can be used in clinical practice, data acquisition and processing have to be performed, following similar basic steps for all 3D systems currently available. Nevertheless, there are significant differences in the manner of image acquisition, the method of image segmentation and the features provided for 3D visualization and measurement.

Device-controlled image acquisition

After the IVUS machine settings have been optimized, image acquisition is started distal to the stenosis while a motorized pullback device withdraws the imaging catheter through the coronary segment to be reconstructed. Sheath-based IVUS catheters are frequently used, as they are designed for repeated pullbacks and have the advantage that the imaging core has no direct contact with the vessel wall. Such catheters are equipped with a long transparent distal sheath that houses the transducer and reduces the risks of nonuniformity of speed in continuous pullbacks. Nevertheless, during the first few seconds (7–10) of a continuous pullback the imaging core may straighten out inside the catheter before a constant withdrawal speed is achieved. Passing stenoses or stents with anything other than the sheath-based IVUS catheters and motorized pullback devices requires continuous fluoroscopic control (at least at the most crucial sites). IVUS catheters with a floppy distal tip are not suitable for 3D IVUS applications.

Different pullback methods can be applied. A continuous pullback, resulting in an equidistant spacing of adjacent images,[32] is still the most common approach. Side-branches or spots of calcium are used as topographic landmarks to ensure a reliable comparison of the same arterial segment in serial studies. Systolic-diastolic artifacts can hamper the visualization and quantitative analysis of 3D IVUS images, acquired during such pullbacks. Combined use of an ECG-gated image acquisition station (Echoscan, TomTec, Munich, Germany) and a dedicated pullback device (stepping motor) is the most sophisticated and accurate way to overcome this problem of cyclic motion artifacts. Using this ECG-gated system, initially designed for 3D reconstruction of echocardiographic images, the arterial segment can be displayed in 3D and vascular dimensions may be measured at any time of the cardiac cycle. Before image acquisition starts the upper and lower limits of the R-R interval are defined.

Up to 25 IVUS images per cardiac cycle can be sampled (if the length of the R-R interval meets the preset range). This option permits dynamic visualization of coronary segments during an entire cardiac cycle ('4D IVUS').[33,34]

Boundary detection and display options

The segmentation of the digitized IVUS images is the processing step which identifies structures of interest. It can be achieved by the application of dedicated algorithms which discriminate between the blood-pool inside the lumen and structures of the vessel wall.[35] The quality of the reconstruction and the accuracy of the quantitative analysis are highly influenced by the characteristics of the segmentation algorithm used.

The applicability of the threshold-based method, which is based on the definition of a threshold value in the gray-scale,[9] depends significantly upon the basic IVUS image quality. Segmentation can also be achieved by the application of more sophisticated algorithms such as acoustic quantification[24,25] or contour detection algorithms.[14,15,36] The acoustic quantification method (Fig. 26.1) distinguishes between the blood-pool and the vessel wall by use of an algorithm for statistical pattern recognition[16,24–26] (EchoQuant, INDEC, Capitola, CA, USA). Contour detection based on the application of a minimum cost algorithm allows to detect not only the intimal leading edge but also the external vascular boundary (Fig. 26.2) which corresponds to the external elastic lamina.[14,15,19,27,36–38]

Specific shading and rendering techniques can be used to give the 3D reconstructed views a spatial aspect. Different display formats can be used to present the 3D datasets, but a longitudinal format is most commonly generated. General programs for 3D presentation display the reconstructed vascular segment in various views including oblique and tangential sections, comparable to display options available in magnetic resonance imaging systems. Dynamic visualization after ECG-gated image acquisition is also possible.[33]

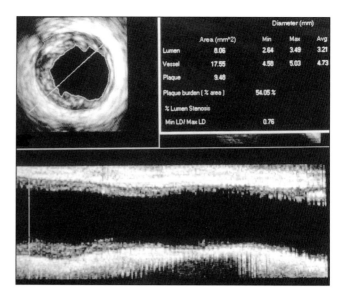

Figure 26.1
Coronary segment after directional atherectomy. The acoustic quantification system (EchoQuant) provides a boundary detection of the lumen (3 cm long segment). Plaque and vessel dimensions of a selected transverse IVUS image can be obtained by tracing the external vessel boundary manually.

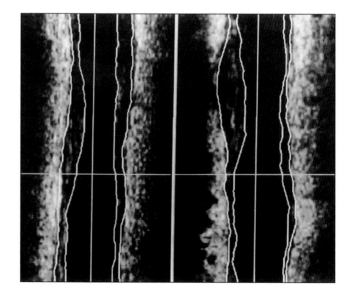

Figure 26.2
Two longitudinal sections of a proximal left anterior descending coronary artery at follow-up after directional coronary atherectomy (Thoraxcenter contour detection system). (Reprinted with permission of reference 14.)

3D systems (Thoraxcenter experience)

Different 3D IVUS systems are available, based on different technical approaches. These systems have specific advantages and disadvantages in applicability, imaging and quantification. Comprehensive and decent validation has been published only for a few 3D IVUS systems, such as, for instance, 1) the binary threshold-based system validated by Matar et al.;[23] 2) the acoustic quantification system;[24,25] and 3) the contour detection approaches of Sonka et al.,[27,37,38] Dhawale et al.[18] and the Thoraxcenter Rotterdam.[14,15,36] At the Thoraxcenter the most experience was gained with both the acoustic quantification system and the Thoraxcenter contour detection system (Table 26.1). The latter system was used on-line in combination with an ECG-gated IVUS image acquisition station.

The acoustic quantification system (EchoQuant) samples images with a digitization frame rate of 8.5 frames per sec (8 cm at a pullback speed of 1.0 mm/sec); segmentation and reconstruction of a vascular segment (max. length 3 cm) can be performed within 3 min. A pattern recognition algorithm detects the blood-pool inside the lumen and requires no geometric assumption of the lumen shape (Fig. 26.1).[24] It may therefore provide accurate detection of an irregularly shaped lumen. However, application of the algorithm may be hampered by the quality of the basic IVUS images.[24,25] It is not capable of detecting the external vascular boundary, but as the reconstruction is performed within a few minutes, online use in the catheterization laboratory is feasible.[25]

The Thoraxcenter contour detection system allows for the analysis of a 3D set of IVUS images, digitized off-line from videotape or online by an ECG-gated image acquisition station. A maximum of 200 IVUS images can be examined, permitting the reliable analysis of approximately 25 mm long (uniform pullback) or 40 mm long (ECG-gated pullback) segments. The method depends less on the image quality than the acoustic quantification. Reliable segmentation and 3D reconstruction remain possible even when the image quality is not optimal and a certain interaction is required. The contour detection procedure[14,15,36] comprises an automated detection of the longitudinal contours of the luminal and external vascular boundaries (external elastic lamina) on two perpendicular longitudinal sections of the vascular segment (Fig. 26.2), based on the application of a minimum cost algorithm.[39] These longitudinal contours define in each individual cross-sectional image regions of interest which guide the final automated contour detection of both lumen and plaque in the transverse IVUS images.[14,15,19,36]

Automated measurement of vascular dimensions

The 3D systems extend the measurement features of 2D IVUS by longitudinal and volumetric measurements, and provide an automated quantification of the plaque and/or the lumen (Fig. 26.3).[19,40] These measurements are used to plan intervention strategies, appropriately size devices and guide the procedures. Therefore it is very important to determine the reliability of these automated measurements.

Table 26.1 Selected characteristics of two 3D IVUS systems.

	Acoustic quantification	Thoraxcenter contour detection
Applicability	Little user interaction required Depends much on image quality	User interaction required Depends less on image quality
Online Use	Online use feasible	Online use feasible with ECG-gated image acquisition
Boundary detection	Detection of lumen only (blood-pool)	Detection of both lumen and external vessel boundary

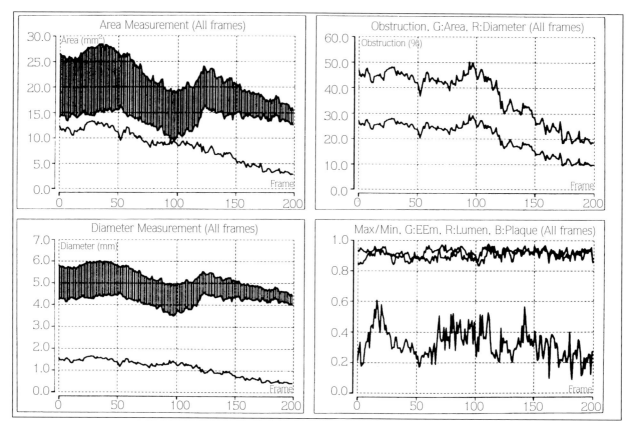

Figure 26.3

Result display of 3D IVUS measurement (Thoraxcenter contour detection method) corresponding to the coronary segment displayed in Fig. 26.2. Left panels show area and mean diameter measurements of lumen, total vessel and plaque. The gray areas represent coronary plaque; upper and lower boundaries of these gray zones correspond with the dimensions of coronary lumen and total vessel. Absolute plaque measurements are shown as a single-line function for both area and diameter measurements (left panels). Functions of the diameter stenosis (%) and area obstruction (%) are displayed in the right upper panel. The right lower panel shows the symmetry of lumen and total vessel and the eccentricity of the plaque. (Reprinted with permission of reference 14.)

The acoustic quantification system

The pattern recognition algorithm of the acoustic quantification system, which is able to distinguish between the blood-pool inside the lumen and the vessel wall, has been validated by Hausmann et al.[24] in 29 aortal segments of New Zealand rabbits. Lumen area measurements by repeated automated analyses, and automated and manual analyses, showed a high correlation ($r = 0.97$ for both) and differences of $1 \pm 10\%$ and $-2 \pm 10\%$, respectively. The correlation between quantitative angiographic measurements and automated 3D IVUS measurements was also high ($r = 0.93$). The between-measurement difference was $7 \pm 14\%$.[24]

The acoustic quantification 3D IVUS system permits online quantification of the coronary lumen, and has fre-

quently been used at the Thoraxcenter Rotterdam during stent procedures (Fig. 26.4). To evaluate the reliability of the automated measurement of the minimal luminal cross-sectional area, we performed a clinical validation by comparing the 3D IVUS measurements in 38 coronary stents with results obtained by conventional 2D IVUS, and both geometric and videodensitometric quantitative coronary angiography.[25] The results by 3D IVUS were slightly smaller than the results by 2D IVUS (8.1 ± 2.7 mm^2 vs. 8.3 ± 2.5 mm^2, NS); the correlation between the measurements by 3D and 2D IVUS was high ($r = 0.81$). Measurements by 3D IVUS showed a higher correlation with videodensitometry ($r = 0.70$) than with geometric quantitative coronary angiography ($r = 0.58$),[25] most likely because measurement of the luminal area is the basic quantification approach of both IVUS and videodensitometry

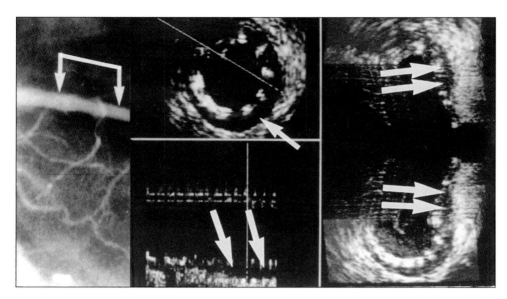

Figure 26.4
Coronary artery with Wallstent implanted (arrows in the angiogram indicate length of the reconstructed segment). IVUS demonstrated an incomplete stent deployment, shown as a zone of low echogenicity between the bright stent struts and the vessel wall (arrowheads). The black area is displayed in cross-sectional (mid up), longitudinal (mid low) and spatial cylindrical views (right-hand side), suggesting additional balloon dilatations at this site.

whereas the geometric angiographic approach depends on the angiographic projection used.

The Thoraxcenter 3D IVUS analysis system

The Thoraxcenter 3D IVUS analysis system has been validated both *in vitro* and *in vivo*. We used the 3D IVUS approach in a tubular phantom, consisting of four segments with luminal diameters between 2 and 5 mm, and found excellent correlation ($r = 0.99$) between the 3D lumen area and volume measurements and the true values.[14] Deviation between the 3D measurements and the true values was small ($-0.7–3.9\%$, areas; $0.3–1.7\%$, volumes).[14] A histomorphometric validation study was performed *in vitro* in 13 atherosclerotic human coronary segments with area stenoses of at least 40%, demonstrating the reliability of the contour detection system.[15] Measurements of lumen, total vessel and plaque, obtained by the 3D contour detection system, showed a good correlation with morphometric measurements on histologic sections ($r = 0.80–0.94$, areas; $0.83–0.98$, volumes). A good agreement (mean difference $\leq 3.7\%$ with SD $\leq 6.2\%$) and high correlation ($r = 0.97–0.99$) were found between area measurements provided by this 3D analysis system and manual tracing on single IVUS images.[15]

The intraobserver and interobserver measurements by the Thoraxcenter 3D analysis system, performed in atherosclerotic coronary arteries of 20 patients *in vivo*, showed high correlations ($r = 0.95–0.98$, areas; 0.99, volumes) and small between-measurement differences ($-0.87–1.1\%$).[14]

The standard deviations of the between-measurement differences of the lumen, total vessel and plaque measurements did not exceed 2.7, 0.7 and 2.8% for the volume, and 7.3, 4.4 and 10.8% for the area measurements.[14] By use of ECG-gated 3D IVUS[33] the variability of the cross-sectional area measurements can be further reduced to standard deviations of the between-measurement differences, not exceeding 5.2, 2.7 and 7.2% respectively (own data, 1996).

3D IVUS in balloon angioplasty and atherectomy

Three-dimensional IVUS prior to coronary interventions facilitates the perception of plaque distribution, and provides valuable information about target lesion, reference and potential 'tapering' of the vessel segment which may influence the intervention strategy. The benefit of 3D IVUS is most significant in long, complex or unclear lesions. In our experience, on-line 3D reconstruction prior to atherectomy is feasible for the examination of plaque eccentricity along the entire coronary segment.

We recently reported a case of deferred angioplasty, based on information obtained from 3D IVUS and intracoronary Doppler in an intermediate LAD lesion.[41] In this patient, referred for balloon angioplasty, no compensatory enlargement of the coronary arterial wall, but a 'reverse Glagovian modeling' was found, recently described in peripheral vessels.[42] Based on the information provided by 3D IVUS imaging and the normal coronary flow reserve, as demonstrated by intracoronary Doppler, no coronary intervention was performed; the absence of inducible ischemia in the myocardial territory subtended by the left anterior descending artery (LAD) was confirmed by dobutamine stress-echocardiography.

The guidance of atherectomy (Fig. 26.1) can be facilitated by 3D reconstruction of IVUS images, as the spatial relation between side-branches and the orientation of the plaque may help to direct the cutter correctly, reduce the frequency of deep cuts and minimize the procedure-related damage to the nondiseased vessel wall. Volumetric IVUS evaluation before and after atherectomy allows the reliable quantification of both plaque ablation and luminal enlargement. To date only volumetric approaches based on 2D analysis of images acquired at 1 mm increments have been reported to evaluate this issue.[43,44]

After balloon angioplasty the most significant benefit can be expected in the evaluation of procedural complications such as severe dissections, which may require the implantation of coronary stents.[45] A comprehensive *in vitro* validation of both the sensitivity of 3D IVUS in the detection of dissections (≥92% in noncalcified arteries) and in the accuracy of length and depth measurements of dissections in 3D (kappa ≥0.72 in noncalcified arteries) has recently been reported by Coy *et al.*, who studied 41 peripheral arterial specimens with a 3D IVUS system (threshold-based segmentation).[10] The clinical feasibility of 3D IVUS (threshold-based approach) for the assessment of dissections after interventions and plaque fractures has been evaluated by Rosenfield *et al.* in 12 coronary arteries as well as 40 peripheral and renal arteries *in vivo*.[9]

Guidance and optimization of coronary stenting

Preintervention 3D IVUS examination of the coronary segment to be treated provides insight into the relation between lesion and side-branches, permits appropriate sizing of the stent (diameter and length) and may help to reduce the frequency of procedural complications of high-pressure stenting.[46] Changes of the cross-sectional lumen area in stents as seen during uniform-speed pullbacks of the IVUS transducer are often smooth and gradual and may therefore be more difficult to recognize by the visual assessment of consecutive 2D IVUS images on-line or from a videotape,[26] explaining the overestimation of the minimum in-stent lumen area by 2D IVUS compared to 3D IVUS.[16,25,26] By use of 3D IVUS the spatial geometry of coronary stents can be reconstructed accurately,[13] and automated measurement of lumen area by 3D IVUS facilitates the detection of stent underexpansion.

The advantages and feasibility of online 3D IVUS (acoustic quantification) for guidance of stenting have been demonstrated recently. In a series of 49 stents we could show that 3D

IVUS is more sensitive than 2D IVUS in assessing optimal stent expansion (Fig. 26.5) and requires less time for analysis (2.6 ± 0.4 min (3D) vs. 4.4 ± 1.5 min (2D); $p < 0.05$).[26]

We then performed 2D and 3D IVUS (acoustic quantification) examinations in 20 Wallstents (Fig. 26.6) and 20 Palmaz–Schatz stents to study the approach of optimized angiography-guided stenting.[16] The background of the rationale for performing this study was that the strategy of optimized stent expansion by high-pressure inflation of oversized balloons had been derived from experience obtained with the Palmaz–Schatz stent, while there was little experience with such a strategy in longer stents such as the Wallstent. Ultrasound criteria of adequate stent expansion were defined as a complete apposition of the stent to the vessel wall, a stent symmetry index (= minimum/maximum lumen diameter) ≥0.7 and a stent-reference lumen area ratio (= minimum in-stent lumen area/average of proximal and distal reference lumen area) ≥0.8. In all cases a smooth angiographic lumen and a negative angiographic diameter stenosis, based on a distal reference, were achieved. Most failures in meeting these IVUS criteria resulted from a low stent-reference lumen area ratio. The Wallstents met the IVUS criteria less often (3D IVUS: 15% vs. 45%, $p < 0.05$), were significantly longer and demonstrated a trend towards a larger vessel tapering, measured as proximal minus distal IVUS reference lumen area (1.33 ± 2.91 mm² vs. 0.44 ± 1.97 mm², NS); Wallstents meeting the IVUS criteria, however, showed less vessel tapering (0.18 ± 1.64 mm²). Thus, although angiographic results and visual assessment of the IVUS examination suggested a good outcome for both the Palmaz–Schatz and Wallstent, few Wallstents met the IVUS criteria in contrast to the Palmaz–Schatz stents. This is most likely caused by vessel tapering (Fig. 26.7), which suggests that the stent-reference lumen area ratio may be unsuitable for the assessment of the adequacy of relatively long stents, such as the Wallstent.[16]

The ECG-gated IVUS acquisition (max. 200 images) and automated online 3D analysis by the Thoraxcenter contour detection program are a feasible approach to evaluate the procedural results after stent deployment. It provides reliable and reproducible measurements of the lumen dimensions along the entire stented segment, and facilitates the detection of the minimum in-stent lumen.[21] A user-friendly display of the lumen symmetry measurements (Fig. 26.3) allows a rapid check of this parameter along the entire coronary segment analyzed. Analyses are currently performed within less than 8 min, which may be acceptable when considering the advantages of this system (Fig. 26.8).

Moreover, the algorithm of the Thoraxcenter contour detection system[14,15] allows the computerized assessment of in-stent neointima at follow-up. This permits measurement of in-stent neointima volume, which is evaluated in both the ERASER trial (effect of ReoPro [Eli Lilly, Indianapolis IN, USA] in Palmaz–Schatz stents) and the TRAPIST trial (effect of Trapidil [UCB, Brussels, Belgium] in Wallstents).

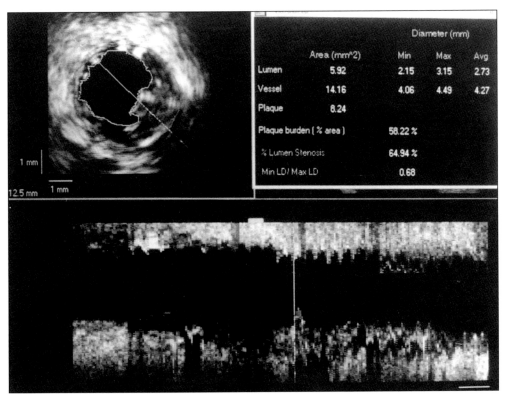

Figure 26.5
Three-dimensional reconstruction of a coronary segment after implantation of 3 AVE microstents (Applied Vascular Engineering, Edmonton, Canada). Asymmetric stent expansion and protrusion of stent struts of the mid-stent into the vessel lumen (at the site of the cursor in the lower panel) are shown. The longitudinal view (lower panel) reveals an adequate deployment of the rest of the stent. The table (right upper panel) provides measurements of the transverse IVUS image displayed (left upper panel). (Avg, Max and Min = average, maximum and minimum, respectively; Min LD/Max LD: ratio of minimal to maximal lumen diameters.) (Reprinted with permission of reference 26.)

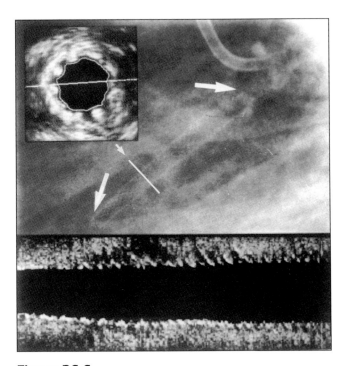

Figure 26.6
Long Wallstent implanted in a left anterior descending coronary artery. Arrowheads indicate the proximal and distal ends of the stent on the radiographic image (upper panel); location of the transverse IVUS image (insert) is indicated by small arrowhead. A longitudinal view (lower panel) is reconstructed, showing a smooth tapering of the luminal dimensions from proximal (right) to distal (left). (Reprinted with permission of reference 16.)

Technical challenges

Several factors, including general problems related to IVUS[47,48] as well as specific limitations of the 3D reconstruction,[49] influence the quality of the reconstruction and measurement. The measurement of both lumen and plaque volumes shows minimal short-term biologic variability upon repeated pullbacks of the same coronary artery segment.[50] The quality of the basic IVUS images is crucial, as poor or incomplete visualization of the lumen–plaque and plaque–adventitia boundaries in the presence of calcification is a problem which hampers both reconstruction and quantification. Currently available transducers have limited lateral resolution,[51] and image distortion by nonuniform rotation of mechanical IVUS catheters or a noncoaxial position of the transducer in the lumen may create complex artifacts in 3D reconstructions.[49] ECG-gated image acquisition and pullback have the potential to minimize the typical cyclic saw tooth-shaped artifacts (Fig. 26.9).[49,52,53] However compared with continuous pullback, image acquisition by the ECG-gated approach requires a longer acquisition time which may cause problems in patients with very severe coronary stenoses before interventions. Vessel curvatures with a radius of less than 5 cm cause a significant

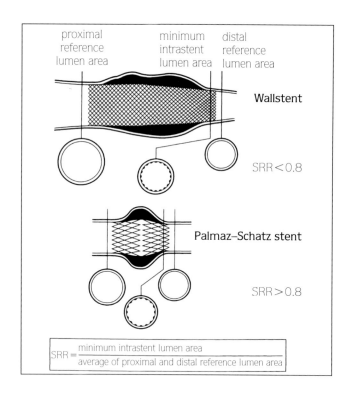

Figure 26.7

Explanation for difficulty in achieving a stent-reference lumen area ratio (SRR) ≥0.8 following Wallstent implantation. In this scheme the Wallstent clearly tapers and does not fulfil the SRR criterion, as the minimal lumen area is located near the distal reference site, with lumen dimensions significantly smaller than the proximal reference. The example of the Palmaz–Schatz stent, however, shows little vessel tapering and is much more likely to fulfil the SRR criterion. (Reprinted with permission of reference 16.)

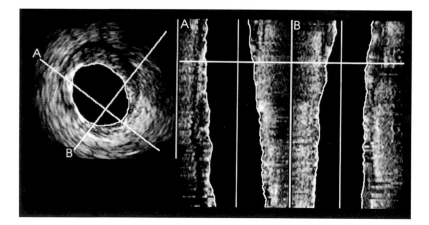

Figure 26.8

Good result after coronary stenting demonstrated by the Thoraxcenter 3D contour detection approach. Contour detection of the lumen in two perpendicular sections (A and B) provides 'regions of interest' which guide the final automated detection in the transverse images.

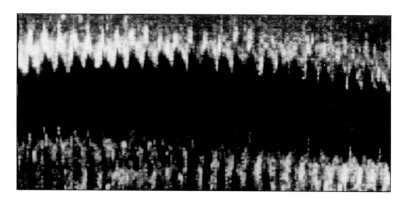

Figure 26.9

Cyclic artifacts in a longitudinally reconstructed image of stented bypass graft. The enormous saw-shaped artifact results from cyclic vessel pulsation and movement of the IVUS catheter inside (= 'catheter fluttering').

distortion of the 3D reconstructed image.[54] Overestimation and underestimation of certain portions of the plaque may be caused by vessel curvatures and bending of the IVUS imaging catheter.[49,55] Furthermore, current 3D systems do not show the real curvatures and spatial orientation of the reconstructed vessel.

Future directions

The combined use of data obtained from biplane angiography and IVUS permit true spatial reconstructions.[56,57] This was demonstrated by the ANGUS technique[57] which was shown to be highly accurate in both vessel phantoms and first human applications. These findings have been confirmed by another group, using a similar technical approach.[58]

In the future most current limitations may be overcome by the use of such combined techniques, advanced segmentation algorithms (e.g. segmentation based on radiofrequency data)[59] and forward-looking transducers.[60] Miniaturization of the imaging catheters and further improvement of the computer technology will help to increase the use of 3D IVUS.

Thus, 3D IVUS is not restricted to research applications, but is a valuable clinical approach. It will gain further importance and become a routine technique, if the interest of the clinicians and the effort of both engineers and clinical research groups is sustained.

References

1 Fitzgerald PJ, St Goar FG, Connolly AJ, et al. Intravascular ultrasound imaging of coronary arteries: is three layers the norm? *Circulation* 1992; **86**: 154–8.

2 Mintz GS, Popma JJ, Pichard AD, et al. Arterial remodeling after coronary angioplasty: a serial intravascular ultrasound study. *Circulation* 1996; **94**: 35–43.

3 Yock PJ, Linker DT. Intravascular ultrasound: looking below the surface of vascular disease. *Circulation* 1990; **81**: 1715–18.

4 Erbel R, Ge J, Bockisch A, et al. Value of intracoronary ultrasound and Doppler in the differentiation of angiographically normal coronary arteries: a prospective study in patients with angina pectoris. *Eur Heart J* 1996; **17**: 880–9.

5 Hodgson J McB, Reddy KG, Suneja R, Nair RN, Lesnefsky EJ, Sheehan HM. Intracoronary ultrasound imaging: correlation of plaque morphology with angiography, clinical syndrome and procedural results in patients undergoing coronary angioplasty. *J Am Coll Cardiol* 1993; **21**: 35–44.

6 Ge J, Erbel R, Rupprecht H-J, et al. Comparison of intravascular ultrasound and angiography in the assessment of myocardial bridging. *Circulation* 1994; **89**: 1725–32.

7 Colombo A, Hall P, Nakamura S, et al. Intravascular stenting without anticoagulation accomplished with intravascular ultrasound guidance. *Circulation* 1995; **91**: 1676–88.

8 Görge G, Haude M, Ge J, et al. Intravascular ultrasound after low and high inflation pressure coronary artery stent implantation. *J Am Coll Cardiol* 1995; **26**: 725–30.

9 Rosenfield K, Losordo DW, Ramaswamy K, Isner JM. Three-dimensional reconstruction of human coronary and peripheral arteries from images recorded during two-dimensional intravascular ultrasound examination. *Circulation* 1991; **84**: 1938–56.

10 Coy KM, Park JC, Fishbein MC, et al. In vitro validation of three-dimensional intravascular ultrasound for the evaluation of arterial injury after balloon angioplasty. *J Am Coll Cardiol* 1992; **20**: 692–700.

11 Rosenfield K, Kaufman J, Pieczek AM, et al. Human coronary and peripheral arteries: on-line three-dimensional reconstruction from two-dimensional intravascular US scans. *Radiology* 1992; **184**: 823–32.

12 Schryver TE, Popma JJ, Kent KM, Leon MB, Eldredge S, Mintz GS. Use of intracoronary ultrasound to identify the true coronary lumen in chronic coronary dissection treated with intracoronary stenting. *Am J Cardiol* 1992; **69**: 1107–8.

13 Mintz GS, Pichard AD, Satler LF, Popma JJ, Kent KM, Leon MB. Three-dimensional intravascular ultrasonography: reconstruction of endovascular stents in vitro and in vivo. *J Clin Ultrasound* 1993; **21**: 609–15.

14 von Birgelen C, Di Mario C, Li W, et al. Morphometric analysis in three-dimensional intracoronary ultrasound: an in-vitro and in-vivo study using a novel system for the contour detection of lumen and plaque. *Am Heart J* 1996; **132**: 516–27.

15 von Birgelen C, van der Lugt A, Nicosia A, et al. Computerized assessment of coronary lumen and atherosclerotic plaque dimensions in three-dimensional intravascular ultrasound correlated with histomorphometry. *Am J Cardiol* 1996; **78**: 1202–9.

16 von Birgelen C, Gil R, Ruygrok P, et al. Optimized expansion of the Wallstent compared with the Palmaz–Schatz stent: online observations with two- and three-dimensional intracoronary ultrasound after angiographic guidance. *Am Heart J* 1996; **131**: 1067–75.

17 Losordo DW, Rosenfield K, Pieczek A, Baker K, Harding M, Isner JM. How does angioplasty work? Serial analysis of human iliac arteries using intravascular ultrasound. *Circulation* 1992; **86**: 1845–58.

18   Dhawale PJ, Rasheed Q, Mecca W, Nair R, Hodgson J McB. Analysis of plaque volume during DCA using a volumetrically accurate three dimensional ultrasound technique. *Circulation* 1993; **88**: I-550 (abstract).

19   von Birgelen C, Slager CJ, Di Mario C, de Feyter PJ, Serruys PW. Volumetric intracoronary ultrasound: a new maximum confidence approach for the quantitative assessment of progression/regression of atherosclerosis? *Atherosclerosis* 1995; **118 (Suppl)**: S103–S113.

20   Galli FC, Sudhir K, Kao AK, Fitzgerald PJ, Yock PG. Direct measurement of plaque volume by three-dimensional ultrasound: potentials and pitfalls. *J Am Coll Cardiol* 1992; **19**: 115A (abstract).

21   von Birgelen C, Umans V, Di Mario C, *et al.* Mechanism of high-speed rotational atherectomy and adjunctive balloon angioplasty revisited by quantitative coronary angiography: edge detection versus videodensitometry. *Am Heart J* 1995; **130**: 405–12.

22   Keane D, Serruys PW. Quantitative coronary angiography: an integral component of interventional cardiology. In: Topol EJ, Serruys PW (eds), *Current Review of Interventional Cardiology* (2nd edn) (Philadelphia, PA: Current Medicine, 1995): 205–33.

23   Matar FA, Mintz GS, Douek P, *et al.* Coronary artery lumen volume measurement using three-dimensional intravascular ultrasound: validation of a new technique. *Cathet Cardiovasc Diagn* 1994; **33**: 214–20.

24   Hausmann D, Friedrich G, Sudhir K, *et al.* 3D intravascular ultrasound imaging with automated border detection using 2.9 F catheters. *J Am Coll Cardiol* 1994; **23**: 174A (abstract).

25   von Birgelen C, Kutryk MJB, Gil R, *et al.* Quantification of the minimal luminal cross-sectional area after coronary stenting: two- and three-dimensional intravascular ultrasound versus edge detection and videodensitometry. *Am J Cardiol* 1996; **78**: 520–5.

26   Gil R, von Birgelen C, Prati F, Di Mario C, Ligthart J, Serruys PW. Usefulness of three-dimensional reconstruction for interpretation and quantitative analysis of intracoronary ultrasound during stent deployment. *Am J Cardiol* 1996; **77**: 761–4.

27   Sonka M, Liang W, Zhang X, De Jong S, Collins SM, McKay CR. Three-dimensional automated segmentation of coronary wall and plaque from intravascular ultrasound pullback sequences. In: *Computers in Cardiology 1995* (Los Alamitos, CA: IEEE Computer Society Press, 1995): 637–40.

28   Hausmann D, Lundkvist AJS, Friedrich GJ, Mullen WL, Fitzgerald PJ, Yock PG. Intracoronary ultrasound imaging: intraobserver and interobserver variability of morphometric measurements. *Am Heart J* 1994; **128**: 674–80.

29   Rosenfield K, Kaufman J, Pieczek A, Langevin RE, Razvi S, Ilsner JM. Real-time three-dimensional reconstruction of intravascular ultrasound images of iliac arteries. *Am J Cardiol* 1992; **70**: 412–15.

30   Mintz GS, Leon MB, Satler LF, *et al.* Clinical experience using a new three-dimensional intravascular ultrasound system before and after transcatheter coronary therapies. *J Am Coll Cardiol* 1992; **19**: 292A (abstract).

31   von Birgelen C, Di Mario C, Reimers B, *et al.* Three-dimensional intracoronary ultrasound imaging: methodology and clinical relevance for the assessment of coronary arteries and bypass grafts. *J Cardiovasc Surg* 1996; **37**: 129–39.

32   Mintz GS, Keller MB, Fay FG. Motorized ICUS transducer pull-back permits accurate quantitative axial measurements. *Circulation* 1992; **86**: I-323 (abstract).

33   Bruining N, von Birgelen C, Di Mario C, *et al.* Dynamic three-dimensional reconstruction of ICUS images based on an ECG gated pull-back device. In: *Computers in Cardiology 1995* (Los Alamitos, CA: IEEE Computer Society Press, 1995): 633–6.

34   Fehske W, Pizzulli L, Hagendorff A, Lüderitz B. Real-time three-dimensional intracoronary ultrasonography: high resolution dynamic images of coronary artery lesions. *J Am Coll Cardiol* 1995; **25**: 180A (abstract).

35   Chandrasekaran K, D'Adamo AJ, Sehgal CM. Three-dimensional reconstruction of intravascular ultrasound images. In: Yock PG, Tobis JM (eds). *Intravascular Ultrasound Imaging* (New York: Churchill-Livingston, 1992): 141–7.

36   Li W, von Birgelen C, Di Mario C, *et al.* Semi-automatic contour detection for volumetric quantification of intracoronary ultrasound. In: *Computers in Cardiology 1994* (Los Alamitos, CA: IEEE Computer Society Press, 1994): 277–80.

37   Sonka M, Zhang X, Siebes M, DeJong S, McKay CR, Collins SM. Automated segmentation of coronary wall and plaque from intravascular ultrasound image sequences. In: *Computers in Cardiology 1994* (Los Alamitos, CA: IEEE Computer Society Press, 1994): 281–4.

38   Sonka M, Zhang X, DeJong SC, Collins SM, McKay CR. Automated detection of coronary wall and plaque borders in ECG-gated intravascular ultrasound pull-back sequences. *Circulation* 1996; **94**: I-653 (abstract).

39   Li W, Bosch JG, Zhong Y, *et al.* Image segmentation and 3D reconstruction of intravascular ultrasound images. In: Wei Y, Gu B (eds), *Acoustical Imaging, Vol. 20* (New York: Plenium Press, 1993): 489–96.

40   von Birgelen C, Mintz GS, de Feyter PJ, *et al.* Reconstruction and quantification with three-dimensional intracoronary ultrasound: an update on techniques, challenges, and future directions. *Eur Heart J* 1997; in press.

41   von Birgelen C, Di Mario C, Serruys PW. Structural and functional characterization of an intermediate stenosis with intracoronary ultrasound and Doppler: a case of 'reverse Glagovian modeling'. *Am Heart J* 1996; **132**: 694–6.

42   Pasterkamp G, Wensing PJW, Post MJ, Hillen B, Mali WPTM, Borst C. Paradoxical arterial wall shrinkage may contribute to luminal narrowing of human atherosclerotic femoral arteries. *Circulation* 1995; **91**: 1444–9.

43   Matar FA, Mintz GS, Farb A, *et al*. The contribution of tissue removal to lumen improvement after directional coronary atherectomy. *Am J Cardiol* 1994; **74**: 647–50.

44   Weissman NJ, Palacios IF, Nidorf SM, Dinsmore RE, Weyman AE. Three-dimensional intravascular ultrasound assessment of plaque volume after successful atherectomy. *Am Heart J* 1995; **130**: 413–19.

45   Cavaye DM, White RA, Lerman RD, *et al*. Usefulness of intravascular ultrasound imaging for detecting experimentally induced aortic dissection in dogs and for determining the effectiveness of endoluminal stenting. *Am J Cardiol* 1992; **69**: 705–7.

46   Reimers B, von Birgelen C, van der Giessen WJ, Serruys PW. A word of caution on optimizing stent deployment in calcified lesions: a case of acute coronary rupture with cardiac tamponade. *Am Heart J* 1996; **131**: 192–4.

47   ten Hoff H, Gussenhoven EJ, Korbijn A, Mastik F, Lancee CT, Bom N. Mechanical scanning in intravascular ultrasound imaging: artifacts and driving mechanisms. *Eur J Ultrasound* 1995; **2**: 227–37.

48   Di Mario C, Madretsma S, Linker D, *et al*. The angle of incidence of the ultrasonic beam: a critical factor for the image quality in intravascular ultrasonography. *Am Heart J* 1993; **125**: 442–8.

49   Roelandt JRTC, Di Mario C, Pandian NG, *et al*. Three-dimensional reconstruction of intracoronary ultrasound images: rationale, approaches, problems and directions. *Circulation* 1994; **90**: 1044–55.

50   Dhawale P, Rasheed Q, Berry J, Hodgson J McB. Quantification of lumen and plaque volume with ultrasound: accuracy and short term variability in patients. *Circulation* 1994; **90**: I-164 (abstract).

51   Benkeser PJ, Churchwell AL, Lee C, Abouelnasr DM. Resolution limitations in intravascular ultrasound imaging. *J Am Soc Echocardiogr* 1993; **6**: 158–65.

52   Di Mario C, von Birgelen C, Prati F, *et al*. Three-dimensional reconstruction of two-dimensional intracoronary ultrasound: clinical or research tool? *Br Heart J* 1995; **73 (Suppl 2)**: 26–32.

53   Dhawale PJ, Wilson DL, Hodgson J McB. Optimal data acquisition for volumetric intracoronary ultrasound. *Cathet Cardiovasc Diagn* 1994; **32**: 288–99.

54   Waligora MJ, Vonesh MJ, Wiet SP, McPherson DD. Effect of vascular curvature on three-dimensional reconstruction of intravascular ultrasound images. *Circulation* 1994; **90**: I-227 (abstract).

55   Klein HM, Günther RW, Verlande M, *et al*. 3D-surface reconstruction of intravascular ultrasound images using personal computer hardware and a motorized catheter control. *Cardiovasc Interven Radiol* 1992; **15**: 97–101.

56   Koch L, Kearney P, Erbel R, *et al*. Three dimensional reconstruction of intracoronary ultrasound images: roadmapping with simultaneously digitized coronary angiograms. In: *Computers in Cardiology 1993* (Los Alamitos, CA: IEEE Computer Society Press, 1993): 89–91.

57   Slager CJ, Laban M, von Birgelen C, *et al*. ANGUS: a new approach to three-dimensional reconstruction of geometry and orientation of coronary lumen and plaque by combined use of coronary angiography and ICUS. *J Am Coll Cardiol* 1995; **25**: 144A (abstract).

58   Evans JL, Ng KH, Wiet SG, *et al*. Accurate three-dimensional reconstruction of intravascular ultrasound data: spatially correct three-dimensional reconstructions. *Circulation* 1996; **93**: 567–76.

59   Bom N, Li W, van der Steen AFW, *et al*. Intravascular ultrasound: possibilities of image enhancement by signal processing. In: van der Wall E, Marwick TH, Reiber JHC (eds), *Advances in Imaging Techniques in Ischemic Heart Disease* (Dordrecht: Kluwer Academic, 1995): 113–25.

60   Ng K-H, Evans JL, Vonesh MJ, *et al*. Arterial imaging with a new forward-viewing intravascular ultrasound catheter. II. Three-dimensional reconstruction and display of data. *Circulation* 1994; **89**: 718–23.

27

A practical approach to quantitative coronary angiography

Jorge F Saucedo, Alexandra J Lansky, Shigenori Ito and Jeffrey J Popma

Introduction

Without question, our understanding of mechanisms and factors responsible for clinical and angiographic recurrence after coronary intervention has expanded dramatically over the past several years. Angiographic restenosis, once viewed as an 'all or none' occurrence,[1] is now characterized as a complex, continuous process involving varying degrees of arterial remodeling, tissue growth, and platelet thrombus formation.[2] While it is well-recognized that restenosis occurs to a greater or lesser degree in most patients, it is also clear that the late angiographic and clinical outcomes after coronary intervention are largely dependent upon the acute procedural result.[3,4] With the use of sophisticated statistical methods, clinical and angiographic predictive models of angiographic restenosis have been developed, yielding insights into the precise factors relating to recurrence after coronary intervention.[5–7] It seems likely that these models will allow physicians to select patients who may benefit most from coronary intervention (versus medical therapy or coronary bypass surgery), to identify which new coronary devices, if any, are appropriate in specific patient and lesion subsets, to target the best residual lumen diameter that will optimize the patient's late outcome, and to aid in the development in new therapies that will further lower recurrence rates after coronary intervention.

The expanded use of quantitative angiography in clinical trials has contributed substantially to our understanding of outcomes after coronary intervention. Clinicians have become more sophisticated in assessing their angiographic results after coronary intervention, often using 'on-line'

quantitative angiography in an attempt to achieve a 'stent-like' result (without the use of a stent). Clinicians have also become more quantitative in their discussions of minimal lumen diameters and residual stenoses, often confirming (or refuting!) their angiographic impressions with use of intravascular ultrasound (IVUS) or Doppler flow measurements. Clinicians can also now appreciate that differences in follow-up lumen diameter as small as 0.2 mm translate into absolute reductions of restenosis rates of 10–20%.[8,9] Given the interdependence of early and late angiographic outcomes, it certainly seems justifiable to be a 'coronary cosmetologist'[10] as long as the approach is a quantitative one!

A basic understanding of the quantitative angiographic methods currently used to evaluate outcomes after coronary intervention seems imperative. Accordingly, the purposes of this chapter are

- to review the methods available for quantitative angiographic analysis after coronary intervention,

- to discuss the clinical uses of quantitative angiography in ongoing clinical trials.

Visual or 'eyeball' assessment of lesion severity

Most clinicians rely upon visual estimates of lesion severity and reference artery size to guide them within the catheterization laboratory. In the National, Heart, Lung, and Blood Institute PTCA Registry, visual estimations of residual lumen diameter were more predictive of 1-year outcome than blinded quantitative angiographic readings.[11] Experienced operators have little difficulty selecting appropriate balloon sizes for coronary intervention, despite the fact that a visual estimate of reference diameter alone is used. The major limitation of the use of visual estimates of stenosis severity as a quantitative clinical or research tool is the substantial inter- and intra-observer variability shown in multiple series.[12–20] Compared to digital caliper or edge-detection methods, visual readings overestimate pre-procedural, and underestimate post-procedural percent diameter stenoses.[12,21,22] It is not surprising that the clinical site angiographic success rates (using the definition of <50% diameter stenosis) are substantially higher than the corresponding Core Laboratory angiographic success rates; such clinical site–Core Laboratory disparity may account for up to a 10% difference in overall procedural success rates.[23,24] The commonly reported visual estimate of '95%' pre-procedural diameter stenosis would represent a minimal lumen diameter less than 0.2 mm in a 3.0 mm vessel, which would require such high coronary perfusion pressures that thrombosis would likely occur.[25,26]

It is possible that the clinician's eye can be 'retrained', providing a more accurate and reproducible estimate of stenosis severity with continued exposure and feedback of quantitative angiographic readings.[27] For clinical studies, panel or consensus readings may also enhance the reproducibility of visual readings.[21] Despite these potential areas for improvement, even 'trained' visual estimates of stenosis severity should be considered suboptimal for research purposes, and other more quantitative methods should be employed.

Caliper methods

The use of digital hand-held calipers is perhaps the simplest and most inexpensive method to quantitate lesion severity before and after coronary intervention.[28–30] Using the injection catheter as the calibration standard, normal and minimum lumen diameters are estimated by adjusting the calipers to encompass the visually-determined arterial borders. It is recommended that the cineangiogram be magnified and projected upon a flat surface prior to performing quantitative analysis, although the arterial edges may often become indistinct at high magnification. Properly performed, the digital caliper method appears moderately correlated with percent diameter stenosis measurements obtained using automated-edge detection methods ($r = 0.89$).[29,30] This method has been used in large scale interventional trials, such as the Bypass Angioplasty Revascularization Investigation (BARI) trial[31] and the Hirulog Angioplasty Study.[32]

Despite the clinical ease of digital caliper use, there are several important limitations of this technique. Caliper measurements obtained from nonmagnified images may result in less favorable correlations with automated edge-detection algorithms ($r = 0.72$); this is possibly due to increased interobserver variability ($r = 0.63$ versus $r = 0.95$ for quantitative angiography).[33] Absolute vessel diameters may also be systematically overestimated using digital calipers.[30,34] In one series, digital calipers overestimated edge-detection readings of vessel diameter by 0.44 ± 0.24 mm in those vessels larger than 2.5 mm;[30] this systematic overestimation by the digital caliper method has also been shown using radiographic phantoms.[35] The most important limitation of digital caliper measurements is the variability in estimates of percent diameter stenosis that have ranged from 7.4%–12.4% in validated angiographic core laboratories.[29,30] These variabilities are substantially higher than those demonstrated using automated edge detection methods,[29,30,33] and investigations using digital calipers must increase the study sample size to balance the measurement error introduced into the study.[30]

Quantitative angiographic methods

Several computer-assisted methods have been developed to provide a more accurate and unbiased assessment of absolute and relative coronary artery dimensions, minimize the degree of observer interaction, reduce operator variability, and shorten the time required for quantitative image processing and analysis.[36–40] Institutional and commercially marketed quantitative angiographic systems include the Cardiovascular Angiographic Analysis System (CAAS-II),[38,40] Cardiovascular Measurement System (CMS),[41] ARTREK,[36] and the Duke University Quantitative/Qualitative Evaluation System,[37] among others.[42]

Quantitative arterial analysis may be divided into several separate processes including:

* film digitization,
* image calibration,
* arterial contour detection,
* observer editing,
* acceptance of the final angiographic reading.

Each one of these steps may contribute substantially to measurement error and every effort should be made to minimize the variability at each stage of the analytic process. Although some quantitative angiographic systems have been developed for 'on-line' digital use,[43,44] the vast majority of experience has been obtained using 'off-line' 35-mm cinefilm analysis.

For most systems, a cinevideo converter optically

magnifies (2 : 1–8 : 1) the selected cineframe and converts it to an analog signal; the analog signal is then digitized using a high quality frame grabber interfaced to the analysis system hardware; images with a 512 × 512 (or 480) pixel matrix and 8 bit gray scale are generally used for analysis.[35,38,45,46] It should be noted that the random noise resulting from a poor quality cinevideo converter or digitizing card may have substantial effects on image reproducibility, and every attempt should be made to maximize the image quality at each step of the imaging processing sequence.[47]

Image calibration is performed using the injection catheter or other external source as the reference standard. Differences in catheter composition, radiographic density, and size may affect the accuracy and reproducibility of image calibration.[48,49] Catheters with a mean difference between the true and measured diameter of less than 3.5% are generally acceptable for clinical use.[48] Catheters between 6–8F are suitable as calibration sources.[41,50,51] Five French catheters should not be used for image calibration,[52–54] and the use of larger (>9F) guiding catheters have not been validated. Although contrast-empty nylon catheters have previously been shown to increase observer variability because of lower catheter image gradients,[55] recent data has suggested that some 6F and 7F nylon catheters are of sufficient radiographic quality to allow accurate image calibration.[41] After the edge-detection algorithm has identified the catheter contour, a scaling factor is entered to obtain the calibration factor. This scaling factor may be obtained from micrometer-determined measurements of the external catheter diameter, the outer or inner catheter diameter provided by the manufacturer, or by determining the radiographic catheter diameter.[56] Micrometry of the true outer diameter of the catheter obviates any potential variability associated with using the French size for a given catheter, particularly with tapering catheters. Optical magnification sufficient to produce calibration factors ranging from 0.04 mm/pixel to 0.09 mm/pixel are generally recommended.

It is important to note that catheter calibration has been performed either without[57] or with[58] contrast within the injection catheter in various clinical studies, and the selection of a contrast-filled or contrast empty catheter for image calibration will often depend on the choice of quantitative angiographic packages. It is critically important that the method of calibration (contrast filled versus contrast empty) be kept constant throughout the study.

After image calibration has been completed, the arterial region of interest is selected and a centerline is drawn along the long-axis of the artery; alternatively, two points, one at the proximal and distal boundaries of the arterial segment can also be selected.[59] Most computer-assisted edge detection algorithms use either the first derivative extremum or a weighted threshold of the first and second derivative extrema obtained from the digitized pixel density profile curves to identify the arterial edge. Each angio-

graphic system varies subtly with respect to the exact location of the arterial edge, construction of the arterial contours, identification of the reference segment, and method of reporting the quantitative results. In general, observer editing should be kept to a minimum during the arterial analysis phase, although the exact amount of editing may vary with the angiographic system used.

Cardiovascular Angiographic Analysis System (CAAS)

The CAAS-I 'off-line' analysis system has been validated using phantom and in vivo models[60,61] and has been used for the past 10 years at the Rotterdam Thoraxcenter.[38,62] Unique features of this PDP 11/44-based system include automated correction for pincushion distortion, an arterial edge detection algorithm that uses a 50% weighted threshold between the first and second derivative extrema of the pixel density profile curve, arterial contour detection using a minimal cost matrix algorithm, and the need for minimal observer editing. The 'interpolated' reference vessel is reconstructed in the segment of interest using a second-degree polynomial function, which provides a reference arterial diameter in the region of the obstruction diameter.[62] While this method is highly reproducible, it may be difficult to apply in ostial stenoses, selected bifurcation lesions, and diffusely diseased segments.[63] Using currently applied methods, post-procedural negative stenosis (i.e. ectasia), which may occur with the use of intracoronary stents, cannot be accurately measured.[63] Physiologic parameters, including transstenotic pressure gradients, calculated coronary flow reserve, quantitative indices of symmetry, curvature and plaque area, are also provided.[63,64] There are few limitations of the CAAS-I system, aside from the abrupt changes in stenosis severity which may be underestimated[37] and the time required for image analysis. Repeated analyses of reference and minimal lumen diameters using the CAAS-I system have demonstrated reproducibilities of ±0.06–0.13 mm and ±0.09–0.14 mm, respectively.[45,65] Reproducibilities of percent diameter stenoses range from 3.5–5.3%.[65]

A second generation Macintosh-based CAAS-II system has recently been introduced, designed for both 'on-line' and 'off-line' quantitative analysis, as well as acquisition and analysis of digitally stored images.[66] The main advantage over the CAAS-I system is the rapidity and the reduced user interaction of the system, making each analysis more objective. Vessels and minimal lumen diameters smaller than 1 mm may still be overestimated.[67] The CAAS-II inter and intra-observer variabilities for 'off-line' minimal lumen diameter measurements are 0.96 mm and 0.108 mm respectively; variabilities for reference diameter are

0.099 mm and 0.096 mm, respectively, and variabilities for percent diameter stenosis are 4.67% and 5.37%, respectively.[68] Further improvements of the contour detection algorithm for small vessel sizes and complex stenoses are underway.

Cardiovascular Measurement System (CMS)

The Cardiovascular Measurement System (CMS, MEDIS, The Netherlands) is a PC-base quantitative angiographic system developed for 'on-line' and 'off-line' quantitative analysis.[41,43,59] The CMS system includes:

- a two-point user-defined pathline (centerline) identification,[59]
- an arterial edge detection using a 50% weighted threshold of the first and second derivative extrema of the pixel density profile curve,
- arterial contour detection using a minimal cost matrix algorithm,
- an 'interpolated' reference vessel diameter.

There is no correction for pincushion distortion with this system. Repeated analyses of reference and minimal lumen diameters using the CMS system have demonstrated variables of 0.12–0.18 mm and 0.09–0.16 mm, respectively, and reproducibilities of 3.7–5.8% for percent diameter stenoses.[65]

The gradient field transform (GFT) is a novel algorithm developed for contour detection with the third generation CMS system, specifically designed for the analysis of complex lesions.[39] Using the traditional arterial edge detection method, a minimal cost algorithm identifies the arterial contour from gradients that are identified in a single perpendicular plane to the pathline. In contrast, the GFT uses multiple scanlines that radiate out from the pathline, thereby identifying the single point with the highest gradient. These points are then linked to form the arterial contour, based on an algorithm that combines the gradient strength and the direction of the edge. Based on phantom studies, accuracy and precision of the CMS–GFT algorithm were excellent (−0.004 mm and ±0.114 mm, respectively); short and severe lesions were reliably measured compared to the systematic underestimation obtained using the conventional minimal cost algorithm. Intraobserver variability for measuring the minimal luminal diameter was better for the GFT than the conventional method (±0.14 mm and ±0.20 mm, respectively).[39]

ARTREK

The ARTREK 'off-line' 35-mm cineangiographic analysis system (Quinton Imaging, Ann Arbor MI) was derived from an 'on-line' quantitative angiographic package developed at the University of Michigan.[44] Although no correction for pincushion distortion is performed with this system, pincushion distortion accounts for an error less than 5–8%, particularly when image acquisition is obtained using 4–7-inch magnifications.[69,70] Arterial edges are identified using a 75% weighted threshold of the first and second derivative extrema (weighted toward the first derivative extremum)[44] and arterial edge contours are constructed using locally adaptive threshold methods applied to adjacent points.[44] Observer editing is performed only to discard spatial outliers, and arterial edges are reconstructed using linear interpolation. The reference diameter is identified using an operator-defined 5–10 mm arterial segment proximal and distal to the lesion. The average of these two segments is used to calculate the reference diameter in the region of the stenosis. This method has been validated using repeated intraobserver measurements (variable frame selection) with a reported variability = 0.15 mm.[34] In vivo phantom validation studies have demonstrated standard errors of 0.23 mm and 0.21 mm for repeated measurements of minimal lumen diameter.[36] Clinical validation studies have demonstrated observer variability of 0.16 mm before angioplasty and 0.23 mm after angioplasty;[44,71] the interobserver variability for measuring percent diameter stenosis was 8.1–8.5%.[71,72]

Other automated systems

Other commercially available and proprietary quantitative angiographic systems have also been validated and used for quantitative analysis.[35,37,42,70,73–78] In general, automated edge-detection algorithms have used either a weighted (e.g. 66%) threshold of the first and second derivative extrema (weighted toward the first derivative extremum) or the first derivative extremum itself as the threshold for arterial edge identification. User-defined or hand drawn arterial contours obtained from magnified images (with or without edge enhancement) have also been used. Clinical experience with these systems is less extensive by our group, but each system has been validated with phantom or in vivo models.

Intersystem comparisons

It has become apparent from a number of clinical studies that there are important differences in the various quantitative angiographic systems with respect to the preferred method of calibration, location of the arterial border and construction of its contour, use of 'smoothing' algorithms, and selection of normal 'reference' segments. These systematic differences affect the accuracy and precision of the absolute and relative angiographic measurements.[47] One *in vitro* and *in vivo* phantom validation study using vessel stenoses between 0.5 and 1.9 mm, performed at 10 different Angiographic Core Laboratories in the United States and Europe, showed substantial system-to-system variability.[47,79] The accuracy of different systems ranged from 0.07 mm to 0.31 mm, and the precision ranged from 0.14 mm to 0.24 mm.[80] These intersystem differences may have profound implications for sample size calculations in clinical trials[30] and may in part have contributed to the clinical and angiographic endpoint discordance noted in some studies.[24,81]

At least some of these inter-system differences may be explained by the specific edge-detection algorithm designed and validated for each analytical system. Edge-detection algorithms that identify the arterial edge using a 50%-weighted threshold of the first and second derivative extrema may have systematically larger reference and obstruction diameters than those using a 75%-weight (weighted toward the first derivative extremum) or the first derivative extremum. Differences in quantitative angiographic algorithms may also affect angiographic restenosis rates reported after balloon angioplasty; binary (>50% follow-up diameter stenosis) restenosis rates have ranged from 33% to 57% in randomized new device trials using different angiographic systems, despite similar angiographic inclusion criteria (i.e. *de novo* lesions in native coronary arteries).[8,9,24,82] Most importantly for randomized clinical trials, quantitative angiographic systems with substantial variability may fail to detect a treatment effect when one truly exists.[47] In aggregate, these inconsistencies in quantitative angiographic results after coronary intervention have led to suspicion and confusion relating to interpretation of late angiographic outcomes after new device intervention trials.[10]

To determine the system-to-system variability between two quantitative angiographic algorithms, we compared the angiographic results obtained in 662 patients using the CMS (non GFT) and the ARTREK systems (Table 27.1).[83] Differences between the pre-procedural minimal lumen diameter obtained with CMS and ARTREK systems was greater for lesions with substantial irregularity. Although CMS and ARTREK were highly correlated for reference diameter, final minimal lumen diameter, and final percent diameter stenosis ($r > 0.90$) the correlation was lower for pre-procedural minimal lumen diameter ($r = 0.80$) and percent diameter stenosis ($r = 0.79$). The differences identified in pre-procedural lesion severity are likely related to system differences in edge contour detection, with underestimation using the CMS minimal cost algorithm, particularly in irregular lesions. Given these findings, it would seem that the CMS–GFT system should be the preferred method of analysis for complex stenoses.

Table 27.1 Comparison of CMS and ARTREK systems in 662 patients.

| | Mean Δ CMS-ARTREK | ±SD | intercept | CMS (y axis) vs. Art (x axis) | | |
				slope	Pearson R	p value
Reference, Pre	0.18 mm	0.19 mm	0.090	1.030	0.913	<0.0001
Reference, Post	0.20 mm	0.19 mm	0.211	0.996	0.899	<0.0001
MLD, Pre	0.15 mm	0.21 mm	0.263	0.879	0.799	<0.0001
MLD, Post	0.13 mm	0.23 mm	0.151	0.994	0.915	<0.0001
% Stenosis, Pre	−3.1%	6.5%	0.115	0.790	0.769	<0.0001
% Stenosis, Post	0.00%	6.5%	0.014	0.956	0.914	<0.0001

MLD = minimal lumen diameter.

Other sources of error in the quantitative angiographic method

Other factors may also contribute to measurement error associated with quantitative angiography. It is clear that the total variance ([standard deviation]^2) of minimal lumen and reference diameters within a particular population is a combination of all the sources of variability contributing to differences in arterial dimensions.[42] These sources of variability include the biologic differences among lumen dimensions, inconsistencies in radiographic image acquisition parameters, and angiographic measurement variability. While some of these parameters cannot be controlled, meticulous attention to factors affecting acquisition and measurement variability will substantially improve the overall accuracy and precision of the quantitative angiographic results.

The average diameter of reference vessels treated in balloon and new device angiography trials varies from 2.56 ± 0.52 mm to 3.23 ± 0.56 mm.[82,84] Some new angioplasty devices, such as intracoronary stents or directional atherectomy, have been targeted for larger (≥3.0 mm) vessels, while others, such as rotational atherectomy and excimer laser angioplasty have been used in smaller (<3.00 mm) ones.[85] Studies that include a wide range of vessel sizes will have more biologic variability in lumen diameters than those that are more restrictive in vessel size selection. It should also be noted that most currently available quantitative angiographic systems have difficulty accurately assessing lumen dimensions below 1 mm,[44,69,74,86] owing to radiographic imaging limitations of small objects (e.g. veiling glare and point spread function).[87,88] A second factor affecting biologic variance in lumen diameter is vasomotor tone. Humoral mediators contribute to cyclic alterations in vasomotor tone during coronary intervention,[89–92] and distal vasoconstriction and vasospasm frequently occur as a result of altered autoregulation.[93] As pre-treatment with oral calcium channel antagonists does not prevent post-angioplasty coronary vasoconstriction,[89] the use of sublingual, intravenous, or intracoronary calcium channel antagonists may be needed to prevent distal epicardial and arteriolar vasoconstriction. Transient maximum coronary vasodilation may also be achieved with intracoronary (50–200 μg),[94,95] intravenous (≥10 μg per minute),[89] or sublingual (5–10 mg) nitroglycerin,[96] or intracoronary (3 mg)[97,98] isosorbide dinitrate. It is essential that intracoronary nitroglycerin be given to standardize vasomotor tone during sequential angiographic studies.

There is little question that accurate and reproducible angiographic analyses are dependent upon meticulous attention to high-quality cineangiogram acquisition.[58] Limiting technical factors include:

- motion artifact (cardiac and respiratory),
- vessel foreshortening,
- inadequate filling of the coronary artery ('streaming') or overfilling of the aortic cusp (precluding analysis of proximal vessels) with contrast,
- failure to separate overlapping branch vessels from the stenosis,
- vessel foreshortening.[58]

Out-of-plane magnification and pincushion distortion may also contribute to small errors in angiographic imaging.[69] Analysis of two 'orthogonal' projections has been recommended, particularly in lesions with significant eccentricity.[25,99] Although this approach is clearly preferable for angiographic restenosis, regression, and physiologic studies,[64] a second, technically suitable projection may not be available in many (14–53%) cases, owing to vessel foreshortening, overlap and poor image quality.[70,100–102] If orthogonal projections are not available, analyses of the 'worst-view' projection may provide sufficiently accurate information.[101] For sequential studies, using the identical angiographic imaging laboratory ensures consistency of the X-ray generator, tube, and image intensifier parameters. Using identical gantry height, angle and skew for sequential imaging studies can be assured by using an on-line notation or a technician worksheet to record these parameters.[58]

Repeated analyses of the same frame demonstrate variabilities ranging from 0.07–0.10 mm for minimal lumen diameter and 2.7–5.1% for percent diameter stenosis even when using precise angiographic systems.[42,45,58,65,86,103] Variability is minimal when neighboring end-diastolic frames are selected,[104] slightly higher when no attempt is made to match cineframes during repeated analyses,[65] and highest when repeated analyses are performed on cineangiograms acquired on different days.[45,58,65] Frame-to-frame differences may result from out-of-plane magnification during the cardiac cycle, inadequate admixture of contrast, and lesion eccentricity.[46] Day-to-day variabilities may result from incomplete control of vasomotor tone, calibration errors, or alterations in the previously described radiographic imaging parameters.[42,45,58,105]

To assess the relative contributions of same-frame, frame-to-frame, and day-to-day angiographic measurement error, 20 cineangiograms obtained from patients undergoing diagnostic catheterization and coronary angioplasty 2.9 days later, were reviewed.[42] Coefficients of variation for repeated analyses were highest for the percent diameter stenosis (14.0%) and lowest for the mean arterial diameter (8.1%). The acquisition and quantitative analysis processes of selected cineframes (noise in the cinevideo optical pathway, edge detection algorithm) accounted for 57% of the total variability, the day-to-day variations in the patient, procedure, and equipment accounted for 30% of total variability, with the frame selection accounting for the remaining 13% of total variability.[42] When direct digital angiography is performed (eliminating random errors associated with noise in the cine-video pathway), frame selection may be a much more important contributor to overall measurement variability.[106] Reproducibility studies performed after coronary angioplasty have shown that barotrauma-induced haziness and arterial wall disruption increase the variability in measured lumen dimensions.[71] No difference in variability has been demonstrated after balloon compared to new device angioplasty.[34,107]

The cineless cardiac catheterization laboratory

It is estimated that 10–15% of new cardiac catheterization laboratories will be using digital acquisition without cinefilm ('cineless' laboratories). The overwhelming impetus for this change has been the significant reduction in radiation exposure and costs required for image acquisition and storage. A number of archiving formats have been used for the digitally acquired angiograms, including Super VHS and D2 tapes, magnetic disks or digital optical disks. All current storage systems have the potential of losing some degree of resolution during the digital to digital or digital to analog compression phase,[108,109] although it has been suggested that data compression factors or three or four may be acceptable for quantitative angiographic purposes.[110] The lack of a single standard and the loss of spacial resolution compared with cinefilm, however, has limited the ability of these 'cineless' centers to participate in investigational trials that rely on quantitative angiographic endpoints. It is clear that super VHS tapes are unsuitable transfer media for quantitative angiographic analysis.

To reach agreement on a single high resolution digital transfer format standard, the American College of Cardiology (ACC), the American College of Radiology (ACR), and the National Electrical Manufacturers Association (NEMA) Ad Hoc Group has established the Digital Imaging and Communications in Medicine (DICOM) standard; the recordable compact disc (CD-R) has been chosen exchange standard[111,112] using a JPEG 2 : 1 lossless compression format. Simultaneously, a European Task Force is also seeking to establish such a standard.[113] Most quantitative angiographic algorithms have the ability to analyze CD-Rs using the DICOM3 digital format. Validation studies comparing cinefilm and CD-R are underway.

Immediate angiographic results

The net balance of lesion stretch[63,114–118] and elastic recoil[116,117,119–122] determines the post-procedural percent

diameter stenosis and residual minimal lumen diameter. Quantitative angiographic analysis of lumen dimensions after conventional balloon angioplasty have shown that angiographic success rates (<50% residual diameter stenosis) range from 70–80%.[23,24,123] Given that the immediate changes in lumen diameters achieved with balloon angioplasty have been modest (0.75–1.16 mm),[5,82,124] alternative devices have been designed to further improve the final lumen dimensions and acute procedural success rates and a number of randomized studies of balloon angioplasty versus intracoronary stents or directional atherectomy have shown that larger acute lumen dimensions translate into higher angiographic success rates using these new devices.[8,24,125,126]

Whether early and late procedural success is best measured using percent diameter stenosis[58,127,128] or minimal lumen diameter[4,7,62] is unsettled. Many have selected the minimal lumen diameter as a primary endpoint because it is well recognized that coronary atherosclerosis is a diffuse process, thereby severely underestimating the extent of atherosclerotic involvement when percent diameter stenoses are used.[129,130] A minor problem with the use of minimal lumen diameter is that it does not account for the large variability in vessel size.[58] The physiological implications of a change in minimum lumen diameter of 1.5 mm as a result of coronary angioplasty will be markedly different, depending upon whether the vessel was 2.0 mm in reference diameter or 4.0 mm in reference diameter. Accordingly, measures of angiographic success after coronary angioplasty should account for both the relative (i.e. percent diameter stenosis) and absolute (i.e. minimal lumen diameter) changes in vessel dimensions and the reference vessel size. Both post-procedural percent diameter stenosis and post-procedural lumen diameter have been correlated with late clinical outcome after new device angioplasty.[3,131]

Lumen re-narrowing after coronary angioplasty

Sequential angiographic studies form the cornerstone of our understanding of the time-dependent pathophysiologic responses after balloon angioplasty.[7,132,133] The vast majority of lesions develop some degree of lumen re-narrowing within 3–6 months after coronary intervention.[132,133] While clinical events related to treatment site re-narrowing generally occur within eight months of the procedure,[134] further progression of lesion severity after 12 months is unusual.[134,135] Progression of atherosclerotic disease at other sites more commonly occurs late (>12 months) after coronary angioplasty, and is generally unrelated to treatment site lumen re-narrowing.[134,136–138]

A number of definitions have been used to calculate

binary restenosis rates after coronary angioplasty, resulting in angiographic recurrence rates ranging from 18–57%.[23,24,139–142] The Emory definition of binary restenosis (≥50% follow-up diameter stenosis) has been used most often in clinical restenosis trials, and is based upon the physiologic reduction of coronary flow reserve in animal models with >50% luminal narrowing.[143] However, the positive and negative predictive value for recurrence of angina with this restenosis definition is moderate (63.3% and 77.8%),[142] and the use of a binary 'cutoff' criteria for restenosis may be problematic, since the restenosis 'process' is continuous and occurs to some extent in virtually all patients.[3,124,132,133]

The absolute reduction in lumen diameter, or late lumen loss, follows a near gaussian distribution after balloon angioplasty, averaging 0.27–0.50 mm.[24,124,140,144] The magnitude of late lumen loss after coronary angioplasty relates to:

- clinical factors (e.g. recent onset angina, diabetes mellitus, serum cholesterol, male gender, prior restenosis),[145–148]
- lesion location and length (e.g. left anterior descending artery, saphenous vein grafts),[146,148–151]
- pre-procedural lesion severity,[149]
- post-procedural results (e.g. initial gain, post-treatment lumen diameter).[4,149]

Of these factors, the post-procedural lumen diameter appears to be the most important.[4] The understanding of the relative trade-off of acute gain and late loss has led to philosophic differences in the definitions of restenosis after coronary intervention.[7,62] In fact, the 'process' of restenosis (late lumen loss) may be greater after new device angioplasty than after balloon angioplasty, which is associated with smaller gain and smaller losses.[129] To further characterize the balance of initial gain and late loss, the loss index (the regression coefficient of the linear relationship between late loss (y axis) and acute gain (x axis) has been used.[5] The loss index remains relatively constant after balloon and new device angioplasty, suggesting that late angiographic outcome relates to the initial angiographic result rather than to the device used for revascularization,[5] although this concept has been challenged.[152,153]

In 30% of lesions, an angiographic improvement in minimum lumen diameter has been observed during the follow-up period.[124] Factors contributing to this improvement include resolution of intraluminal thrombus, remodeling of intimal flaps, and correction of peri-procedural vasospasm. Intravascular ultrasound studies have noted that minimum lumen diameters and reference vessel size (external elastic lamina) also increase in 20% of patients after coronary angioplasty.[154] Other continuous indices for restenosis have been proposed[7,62] which include:

- the follow-up minimal lumen diameter,
- follow-up percent diameter stenosis,
- restenosis index (ratio between the decrease in lumen during follow-up and the initial gain [in mms] after the procedure)
- the utility index (ratio between the final net gain at follow-up and the reference vessel diameter).

Implications for clinical trials

Quantitative angiographic and statistical methods developed over the past several years have allowed more rigorous comparisons of new devices in randomized[24,82,125,126] and nonrandomized[3,4,155] clinical studies. Future studies evaluating the benefit of alternative pharmacological and mechanical methods will focus on the integration of two critical issues:

- the limitations of angiography in assessing late outcome after coronary angioplasty;
- the clinical indices that may be used to identify treatment site failures versus progression of coronary atherosclerosis at other coronary sites.

It is clear that in order for potential new therapies to be clinically meaningful, the biologic reduction in lumen re-narrowing seen by angiography should correlate with some clinical reduction in late cardiac events (e.g. a reduction in repeat revascularization). In the absence of this correlation, the benefit of reduced angiographic restenosis may be simply 'cosmetic' and of questionable clinical importance.[10] At least one new device randomized trial has demonstrated that reduced angiographic restenosis was not associated with a similar reduction in composite late clinical endpoint occurrence[156] and others have suggested that asymptomatic restenosis (≥50% diameter stenosis at the treatment site) may occur in 10–25% of patients after coronary angioplasty.[141,157–159] The reasons for the apparent 'discordance' between angiographic and clinical findings are multifactorial, relating, in part, to the inappropriate linking of major cardiac events with treatment site renarrowing.

Major cardiac events (death, myocardial infarction, coronary bypass operation or repeat coronary angioplasty) occur in approximately 25% of patients within 6–12 months after coronary angioplasty.[84,144] The majority (>85%) of these events occur as a result of repeat revascularization (coronary bypass operation or repeat coronary angioplasty) owing to treatment site re-narrowing; the greatest hazard rate for treatment-site revascularization is seen between 80–240 days,[134,160] closely correlated with known behavior of coronary re-narrowing seen in serial angiographic studies.[132,133] Death and myocardial infarction occur much less often following coronary angioplasty (1%

and 2% per year, respectively), showing an ongoing accumulation of these events with time, unrelated to treatment site re-narrowing (kappa = 0).[136,160,161] It is apparent from these important observations that the best clinical index of treatment-site re-narrowing (the biologic response) after coronary angioplasty may be treatment site revascularization.

Summary

In this chapter, we have reviewed the quantitative angiographic methods available for assessing outcomes after coronary intervention. While important differences in the methodologies may exist between differing angiographic systems and core laboratories, standardization of the image acquisition and analytic methods will substantially reduce observer variability, and reduce the sample sizes required to detect differences between two treatment populations. Quantitative angiographic analyses have also yielded important insights into the mechanism of benefit of balloon and new device angioplasty, demonstrating that alterations in plaque compliance and recoil may be mechanistically responsible for the lower residual diameter stenoses shown with new angioplasty devices, particularly intracoronary stents. The use of target-site revascularization as the optimal surrogate for identifying treatment site renarrowing will undoubtedly gain widespread acceptance in clinical trials, and provide a much closer association between angiographic and clinical events.

References

1 King SB III, Weintraub WS, Tao X, Hearn J, Douglas JS Jr. Bimodal distribution of diameter stenosis 4 to 12 months after angioplasty: implications for definitions and interpretations of restenosis. *J Am Coll Cardiol* 1991; **17**: 345A (abstract).

2 Mintz GS, Popma JJ, Hong MK, *et al*. Intravascular ultrasound to discern device-specific effects and mechanisms of restenosis. *Am J Cardiol* 1996; **78**: 18–22.

3 Kuntz RE, Safian RD, Levine MJ, Reis GJ, Diver DJ, Baim DS. Novel approach to the analysis of restenosis after the use of three new coronary devices. *J Am Coll Cardiol* 1992; **19**: 1493–9.

4 Kuntz RE, Gibson CM, Nobuyoshi M, Baim DS. Generalized model of restenosis after conventional balloon angioplasty and new devices. *J Am Coll Cardiol* 1993; **21**: 15–25.

5 Kuntz RE, Foley DP, Keeler GP, *et al*. Relationship of acute luminal gain to late loss following directional atherectomy or balloon angioplasty in CAVEAT. *Circulation* 1993; **88**: 1-495 (abstract).

6 Kuntz RE, Keaney KM, Senerchia C, Baim DS. Estimating late results of coronary intervention from incomplete angiographic follow-up. *Circulation* 1993; **87**: 815–30.

7 Kuntz RE, Baims DS. Defining coronary restenosis. Newer clinical and angiographic paradigms. *Circulation* 1993; **88**: 1310–23.

8 Fischman DL, Leon MB, Baim DS, *et al*. A randomized comparison of coronary stent placement and balloon angioplasty in the treatment of coronary artery disease. *N Engl J Med* 1994; **331**: 496–501.

9 Serruys PW, de Jaegere P, Kiemeneij F, *et al*. A comparison of balloon-expandable-stent implantation with balloon angioplasty in patients with coronary artery disease. Benestent Study Group [see comments]. *N Engl J Med* 1994; **331**: 489–95.

10 Topol EJ, Nissen S. Our preoccupation with coronary luminology. The dissociation between clinical and angiographic findings in ischemic heart disease. *Circulation* 1995; **92**: 2333–43.

11 Faxon DP, Vogel R, Yeh W, Holmes DR jr, Detre K. Value of visual versus central quantitative measurements of angiographic success after percutaneous transluminal coronary angioplasty. NHLBI PTCA Registry Investigators. *Am J Cardiol* 1996; **77**: 1067–72.

12 Fleming RM, Kirkeeide RL, Smalling RW, Gould KL. Patterns in visual interpretation of coronary arteriography as detected by quantitative angioplasty. *J Am Coll Cardiol* 1991; **18**: 945–51.

13 Zir LM, Miller SW, Dinsmore RE, Gilbert JP, Harthorne JW. Interobserver variability in coronary angiography. *Circulation* 1976; **53**: 627–32.

14 DeRouen TA, Murray JA, Owen W. Variability in the analysis of coronary arteriograms. *Circulation* 1977; **55**: 324–8.

15 Fisher LD, Judkins MP, Lesperance J, *et al*. Reproducibility of coronary arteriographic reading in the coronary artery surgery study (CASS). *Cathet Cardiovasc Diagn* 1982; **8**: 565–75.

16 Detre KM, Wright E, Murphy ML, Takaro T. Observer agreement in evaluating coronary angiograms. *Circulation* 1975; **52**: 979–86.

17 Goldberg RK, Kleiman NS, Minor ST, Abukahil J, Raizner AE. Comparison to quantitative angiography to visual estimates of lesion severity pre and post PTCA. *Am Heart J* 1990; **119**: 178–84.

18 Schweiger MJ, Stanek E, Iwakoshi K, et al. Comparison of visual estimate with digital caliper measurement of coronary artery stenosis. *Cathet Cardiovasc Diagn* 1987; **13**: 239–44.

19 Bairati I, Roy L, Meyer F. Measurement errors in standard visual analysis of coronary angiograms: consequences on clinical trials. *Can J Cardiol* 1993; **9**: 225–30.

20 Beauman GJ, Reiber JH, Koning G, Vogel RA. Comparisons of angiographic core laboratory analyses of phantom and clinical images: interlaboratory variability. *Cathet Cardiovasc Diagn* 1996; **37**: 24–31.

21 Beauman GJ, Vogel RA. Accuracy of individual and panel visual interpretations of coronary arteriograms: implications for clinical decisions. *J Am Coll Cardiol* 1990; **16**: 108–13.

22 Bertrand ME, Lablanche JM, Bauters C, Leroy F, MacFadden E. Discordant results of visual and quantitative estimates of stenosis severity before and after coronary angioplasty. *Cathet Cardiovasc Diagn* 1993; **28**: 1–6.

23 Bairati I, Roy L, Meyer F. Double-blind, randomized, controlled trial of fish oil supplements in prevention of recurrence of stenosis after coronary angioplasty. *Circulation* 1992; **85**: 950–6.

24 Topol EJ, Leya F, Pinkerton CA, et al. A comparison of directional atherectomy with coronary angioplasty in patients with coronary artery disease. *N Engl J Med* 1993; **329**: 221–7.

25 Kirkeeide RL, Gould KL, Parsel L. Assessment of coronary stenoses by myocardial perfusion imaging during pharmacologic coronary vasodilation – VII. Validation of coronary flow reserve as a single integrated functional measure of stenosis severity reflecting all its geometric dimensions. *J Am Coll Cardiol* 1986; **1986**: 103–13.

26 Gould KL. Quantitative analysis of coronary artery restenosis after coronary angioplasty – Has the rose lost its bloom? *J Am Coll Cardiol* 1992; **19**: 946–7.

27 Martinelli MJ, Deutsch E, Ferraro A, Bove AA, Group M Heart. Comparison of angiographic center and local site analysis of PTCA results in a multicenter angioplasty–restenosis trial. *Cathet Cardiovasc Diagn* 1992; **27**: 8–13.

28 Gensini GG, Kelly AE, DaCosta BCB, Huntington PP. Quantitative angiography: The measurement of coronary vasomobility in the intact animal and man. *Chest* 1971; **60**: 522–30.

29 Scoblionko DP, Brown BG, Mitten S, et al. A new digital electronic caliper for measurement of coronary arterial stenosis: comparison with visual estimates and computer-assisted measurements. *Am J Cardiol* 1984; **53**: 689–93.

30 Uehata A, Matsuguchi T, Bittl JA, et al. Accuracy of electronic digital calipers compared with quantitative angiography in measuring coronary arterial diameter. *Circulation* 1993; **88**: 1724–9.

31 Alderman EL, Stadius M. The angiographic definitions of the Bypass Angioplasty Revascularization Investigation. *Coronary Artery Disease* 1992; **3**: 1189–207.

32 Bittl JA, Strony J, Brinker JA, et al. Treatment with bivalirudin (Hirulog) as compared with heparin during coronary angioplasty for unstable or post-infarction angina. Hirulog Angioplasty Study Investigators. *N Engl J Med* 1995; **333**: 764–9.

33 Kalbfleisch SJ, McGillem MJ, Pinto IMF, Kavanaugh KM, DeBoe SF, Mancini GBJ. Comparison of automated quantitative coronary angiography with caliper measurements of percent diameter stenosis. *Am J Cardiol* 1990; **65**: 1181–4.

34 Popma JJ, Leon MB, Keller MB, et al. Reliability of the quantitative angiographic measurements in the New Approaches to Coronary Intervention (NACI) Registry: a comparison of clinical site and angiographic core laboratory readings. *Am J Cardiol* 1997 (in press).

35 Uehata A, Davis S, Orav J, Yeung A. Validation of the accuracy of electronic digital calipers and quantitative angiography using calibrated phantoms. *Circulation* 1993; **88**: I-652 (abstract).

36 Mancini GBJ, Simon SB, McGillem MJ, LeFree MT, Friedman HZ, Vogel RA. Automated quantitative coronary angiography: morphologic and physiologic validation of a rapid digital angiographic method. *Circulation* 1987; **1987**: 452–60.

37 Hermiller JB, Cusma JT, Spero LA, Fortin DF, Harding MB, Bashore TM. Quantitative and qualitative coronary angiographic analysis: review of methods, utility, and limitations. *Cathet Cardiovasc Diagn* 1992; **25**: 110–31.

38 Reiber JHC, Kooijman CJ, Slager CJ, et al. Coronary artery dimensions from cineangiograms—Methodology and validation of a computer-assisted analysis procedure. *IEEE Trans Med Imag* 1984; **M12**: 131–41.

39 van der Zwet PMJ, Reiber JHC. A new approach for the quantification of complex lesion morphology: The Gradient Field Transform; Basic principles and validation results. *J Am Coll Cardiol* 1994; **24**: 216–24.

40 Foley DP, Escaned J, Strauss BH, et al. Quantitative coronary angiography (QCA) in interventional cardiology: clinical application of QCA measurements. *Prog Cardiovasc Dis* 1994; **36**: 363–84.

41 Koning G, van der Zwet PMJ, von Land CD, Reiber JHC. Angiographic assessment of 6 F and 7 F Mallinckrodt Softtouh coronary contrast catheters from digital and cine arteriograms. *Int J Cardiac Imaging* 1992; **8**: 153–61.

42   Herrington DM, Siebes M, Sokol DK, Siu CO, Walford GD. Variability in measures of coronary lumen dimensions using quantitative coronary angiography. *J Am Coll Cardiol* 1993; **22**: 1068–74.

43   Reiber JHC, van der Zwet PMJ, von Land CD, *et al.* On-line quantification of coronary angiograms with the DCI system. *Medicamundi* 1989; **34**: 89–98.

44   Mancini GBJ. Quantitative coronary arteriography: Development of methods, limitations, and clinical applications. *Am J Cardiac Imaging* 1988; **2**: 98–109.

44   Reiber JHC, Serruys PW, Kooijman CJ, *et al.* Assessment of short-, medium-, and long-term variations in arterial dimensions from computer-assisted quantitation of coronary cineangiograms. *Circulation* 1985; **71**: 280–8.

46   Reiber JHC, van Eldik-Helleman P, Visser-Akkerman N, Kooijman CJ, Serruys PW. Variabilities in measurement of coronary arterial dimensions resulting from variations in cineframe selection. *Cathet Cardiovasc Diagn* 1988; **14**: 221–8.

47   Keane D, Haase J, Slager CJ, *et al.* Comparative validation of quantitative coronary angiography systems. Results and implications from a multicenter study using a standardized approach. *Circulation* 1995; **91**: 2174–83.

48   Reiber JHC, den Boer A, Serruys PW. Quality control in performing quantitative coronary arteriography. *Am J Cardiac Imag* 1989; **3**: 172–9.

49   Herrman JR, Keane D, Ozaki Y, den Boer A, Serruys PW. Radiological quality of coronary guiding catheters: a quantitative analysis. *Cathet Cardiovasc Diagn* 1994; **33**: 55–60.

50   Ellis SG, Pinto IMF, McGillem MJ, DeBoe SF, LeFree MT, Mancini GBJ. Accuracy and reproducibility or quantitative coronary arteriography using 6 and 8 French catheters with cine angiographic acquisition. *Cathet Cardiovasc Diagn* 1991; **22**: 52–5.

51   Legrand V, Raskinet B, Martinez C, Kulbertus H. Variability in estimation of coronary dimensions from 6 F and 8 F catheters. *Cathet Cardiovasc Diagn* 1996; **37**: 39–45; (Discussion 46).

52   Brown RIG, MacDonald AC. Use of 5 French catheters for cardiac catheterization and coronary angiography: a critical review. *Cathet Cardiovasc Diagn* 1987; **13**: 214–17.

53   Molajo AO, Ward C, Bray CL, Dobson D. Comparison of the performance of superflow (5 F) and conventional 8 F catheter for cardiac catheterization by the femoral route. *Cathet Cardiovasc Diagn* 1987; **13**: 275–6.

54   Ellis SG, DeBoe SF, Sanz ML, Mancini GBM. Accuracy (A) and reproducibility (R) of 5 Fr catheter systems for out-patient use compared with 8 Fr systems. *Circulation* 1987; **76**: IV-369 (abstract).

55   Reiber JHC, Kooijman CJ, den Boer A, Serruys PW. Assessment of dimensions and image quality of coronary contrast catheters from cineangiograms. *Cathet Cardiovasc Diagn* 1985; **11**: 521–31.

56   Fortin DF, Spero LA, Cusma JT, Santoro L, Burgess R, Bashore TM. Pitfalls in the determination of absolute dimensions using angiographic catheters as calibration devices in quantitative angiography. *Am J Cardiol* 1991; **68**: 1176–82.

57   di Mario C, Hermans WRM, Rensing BJ, Serruys PW. Calibration using angiographic catheters as scaling devices – importance of filming the catheters not filled with contrast medium. *Am J Cardiol* 1992; **69**: 1377 (letter).

58   Lesperance J, Bourassa MG, Schwartz L, *et al.* Definition and measurement of restenosis after successful coronary angioplasty: Implications for clinical trials. *Am Heart J* 1993; **125**: 1394–408.

59   van der Zwet PMJ, Pinto IMF, Serruys PW, Reiber JHC. A new approach for the automated definition of pathlines in digitized coronary angiograms. *Int J Cardiac Imag* 1990; **5**: 75–83.

60   Haase J, di Mario C, Slager CJ, *et al.* In-vivo validation of on-line and off-line geometric coronary measurements using insertion of stenosis phantoms in porcine coronary arteries. *Cathet Cardiovasc Diagn* 1992; **27**: 16–27.

61   di Mario C, Haase J, den Boer A, Reiber JHC, Serruys PW. Edge detection versus videodensitometry in the quantitative assessment of stenosis phantoms: an *in-vivo* comparison in porcine coronary arteries. *Am Heart J* 1992; **124**: 1181–9.

62   Serruys PW, Foley DP, Kirkeeide RL, King SB. Restenosis revisited: insights provided by quantitative coronary angiography. *Am Heart J* 1993; **126**: 1243–67.

63   Strauss BH, Morel M-AM, van Swijndregt EJM, *et al.* Methodologic aspects of quantitative coronary angiography (QCA) in interventional cardiology. In: Serruys PW, Strauss BH, King SB III (eds). *Restenosis After Intervention with New Mechanical Devices* (Amsterdam: Kluwer, 1992): 11–50.

64   de Feyter PJ, Serruys PW, Davies MJ, Richardson P, Lubsen J, Oliver MF. Quantitative coronary angiography to measure progression and regression of coronary atherosclerosis. Value, limitations, and implications for clinical trials. *Circulation* 1991; **84**: 412–23.

65   Lesperance J, Waters D. Measuring progression and regression of coronary atherosclerosis in clinical trials: problems and progress. *Int J Card Imaging* 1992; **8**: 165–73.

66 Escaned J, Baptista J, Di Mario C, et al. Significance of automated stenosis detection during quantitative angiography. Insights gained from intracoronary ultrasound imaging. Circulation 1996; **94**: 966–72.

67 Haase J, Esccaned J, Montoban van Swijndregt E, et al. Experimental validation of geometric and densitometric coronary measurements on the new generation cardiovascular angiography analysis system (CAAS II). Cathet Cardiovasc Diagn 1993; **11**: 104–14.

68 Gronenschild E, Janssen J, Tijdens F. CAAS II: a second generation system for off-line and on-line quantitative coronary angiography. Cathet Cardiovasc Diagn 1994; **33**: 61–75.

69 Popma JJ, Eichhorn EJ, Dehmer GJ. In vivo assessment of a digital angiographic method to measure absolute coronary artery diameters. Am J Cardiol 1989; **64**: 131–8.

70 Brown BG, Bolson E, Frimer M, Dodge HT. Quantitative coronary arteriography. Estimation of dimensions, hemodynamic resistance, and atheroma mass of coronary artery lesions using the arteriogram and digital computation. Circulation 1977; **55**: 329–37.

71 Sanz ML, Mancini GBJ, LeFree MT, et al. Variability of quantitative digital subtraction coronary angiography before and after percutaneous transluminal coronary angioplasty. Am J Cardiol 1987: 55–60.

72 deCesare NB, Williamson PR, Moore NB, DeBoe SF, Mancini GBJ. Establishing comprehensive, quantitative criteria for detection of restenosis and remodeling after percutaneous transluminal coronary angioplasty. Am J Cardiol 1992; **69**: 77–83.

73 Klein JL, Gatlin S, Manoukian SV, King SB. Quantitative coronary angiography: an inexpensive and user friendly system. J Am Coll Cardiol 1993; **21**: 7A (abstract).

74 Spears JR, Sandor T, Als AV, et al. Computerized image analysis for quantitative measurement of vessel diameter from cineangiograms. Circulation 1983; **68**: 453–61.

75 Reiber JH, van der Zwet PM, Koning G, et al. Accuracy and precision of quantitative digital coronary arteriography: observer-, short-, and medium-term variabilities. Cathet Cardiovasc Diagn 1993; **28**: 187–98.

76 Koning G, Reiber JH, von Land CD, Loois G, van Meurs B. Advantages and limitations of two software calipers in quantitative coronary arteriography. Int J Card Imaging 1991; **7**: 15–30.

77 Desmet W, Willems JL, Vrolix M, van Lierde J, Byttebier G, Piessens J. Intra- and interobserver variability of a fast on-line quantitative coronary angiographic system. Int J Card Imaging 1993; **9**: 249–56.

78 Alvarez LG, Jackson SA, Berry JA, Eichhorn EJ. Evaluation of a personal computer-based quantitative coronary analysis system for rapid assessment of coronary stenoses. Am Heart J 1992; **123**: 1500–10.

79 Desmet W, De Scheerder I, Beatt K, Huehns T, Piessens J. In vivo comparison of different quantitative edge detection systems used for measuring coronary arterial diameters. Cathet Cardiovasc Diagn 1995; **34**: 72–80.

80 Keane D, Haase J, Slager C, et al. Comparative validation of quantitative coronary angiographic systems: results and implications from a multicenter study using a standardized approach. Circulation 1995; **91**: 2174–83.

81 Emanuelsson H, Beatt KJ, Bagger JP, et al. Long-term effects of angiopeptin treatment in coronary angioplasty. Reduction of clinical events but not angiographic restenosis. European Angiopeptin Study Group. Circulation 1995; **91**: 1689–96.

82 Adelman AG, Cohen EA, Kimball BP, et al. A comparison of directional atherectomy with balloon angioplasty for lesions of the left anterior descending coronary artery. N Engl J Med 1993; **329**: 228–33.

83 Lansky AJ, Conway TY, Zhang Y, et al. Are quantitative angiographic results after coronary intervention affected by the specific analysis algorithm? Circulation 1996; **94**: 1-437 (abstract).

84 Kent KM, Williams DO, Cassagneua B, et al. Double blind, controlled trial of the effect of angiopeptin on coronary restenosis following balloon angioplasty. Circulation 1993; **88**: 1-506 (abstract).

85 Popma JJ, Leon MB. A lesion-specific approach to new device angioplasty. In: Topol E (ed.) Interventional Cardiology (Philadelphia: WB Saunders, 1993): 973–85; vol 2.

86 Brown BG, Bolson EL, Dodge HT. Quantitative computer techniques for analyzing coronary arteriograms. Prog Cardiovasc Dis 1986; **28**: 403–18.

87 Seibert JA, Nalcioglu O, Roeck WW. Characterization of the veiling glare in x-ray image intensified fluoroscopy. Med Phys 1984; **11**: 172–9.

88 Milne ENC. The role and performance of minute focal spots in roentgenology with special reference to magnification. CRC Crit Rev Radiol Sci 1971; **2**: 269–310.

89 Fischell TA, Derby G, Tse TM, Stadius ML. Coronary artery vasoconstriction routinely occurs after percutaneous transluminal coronary angioplasty. A quantitative arteriographic analysis. Circulation 1988; **78**: 1323–34.

90 Fischell TA, Bausback KN. Effects of luminal eccentricity on spontaneous coronary vasoconstriction after successful percutaneous transluminal coronary angioplasty. Am J Cardiol 1991; **68**: 530–4.

91   Eichhorn EJ, Grayburn PA, Willard JE, *et al.* Spontaneous alterations in coronary blood flow velocity before and after coronary angioplasty in patients with severe angina. *J Am Coll Cardiol* 1991; **17**: 43–52.

92   El-Tamimi H, Davies GJ, Hackett D, *et al.* Abnormal vasomotor changes early after coronary angioplasty: A quantitative arteriographic study of their time course. *Circulation* 1991; **84**: 1198–202.

93   Fischell TA, Bausback KN, McDonald TV. Evidence of altered epicardial coronary artery autoregulation as a cause of distal coronary vasoconstriction after successful percutaneous transluminal coronary angioplasty. *J Clin Invest* 1990; **86**: 575–84.

94   Feldman RL, Marx JD, Pepine CJ, Conti CR. Analysis of coronary responses to various doses of intracoronary nitroglycerin. *Circulation* 1982; **66**: 321–7.

95   Jost S, Rafflenbeul W, Reil GH, *et al.* Elimination of variable vasomotor tone in studies with repeated quantitative coronary angiography. *Int J Card Imaging* 1990; **5**: 125–34.

96   Badger RS, Brown BG, Gallery CA, Bolson EL, Dodge HT. Coronary artery dilatation and hemodynamic responses after isosorbide nitrate therapy in patients with coronary artery disease. *Am J Cardiol* 1985; **56**: 390–5.

97   Strauer BE. Isosorbide dinstrate: Its action on myocardial contractility in comparison with nitroglycerin. *Int J Clin Pharm Ther Toxicol* 1982; **66**: 321–7.

98   Lablanche JM, Delforge MR, Tilmant PY, *et al.* Effects hemodynamiques et coronaires du dinitrate d'isosorbide: Comparaison entre les voies d'injection intracoronaire en intraveineuse. *Arch Mal Coeur* 1982; **75**: 303–16.

99   Thomas AC, Davies MJ, Dilly S, Dilly N, Franc F. Potential errors in the estimation of coronary arterial stenosis from clinical arteriography with reference to the shape of the coronary arterial lumen. *Br Heart J* 1986; **55**: 129–39.

100   Dehmer GJ, Popma JJ, van den Berg EK, *et al.* Reduction in the rate of early restenosis after coronary angioplasty by a diet supplemented with n-3 fatty acids. *N Engl J Med* 1988; **319**: 733–40.

101   Lesperance J, Hudon G, White CW, Laurier J, Waters D. Comparison by quantitative angiographic assessment of coronary stenoses of one view showing the severest narrowing to two orthogonal views. *Am J Cardiol* 1989; **64**: 462–5.

102   Loaldi A, Polese A, Montorsi P, *et al.* Comparison of nifedipine, propranolol and isosorbide dinitrate on angiographic progression and regression of coronary arterial narrowings in angina pectoris. *Am J Cardiol* 1989; **64**: 433–9.

103   Hudon G, Lesperance J, Waters D. Reproducibility of quantitative angiographic measurements under different conditions: in search of a gold standard. *Circulation* 1990; **82**: III-617 (abstract).

104   Reiber JH, van Eldik Helleman P, Kooijman CJ, Tijssen JG, Serruys PW. How critical is frame selection in quantitative coronary angiographic studies? *Eur Heart J* 1989; **10 (Suppl)**: F54–59.

105   Herrington DM, Siebes M, Walford GD. Sources of error in quantitative coronary angiography. *Cathet Cardiovasc Diagn* 1993; **29**: 314–21.

106   Gurley JC, Nissen SE, Booth DC, DeMaria AN. Influence of operator- and patient-dependent variables on the suitability of automated quantitative coronary arteriography for routine clinical use. *J Am Coll Cardiol* 1992; **19**: 1237–43.

107   Umans VAWM, Beatt KJ, Rensing BJWM, Hermans WRM, de Feyter PJ, Serruys PW. Comparative quantitative angiographic analysis of directional coronary atherectomy and balloon coronary angioplasty. *Am J Cardiol* 1991; **68**: 1556–63.

108   Cusma JT, Fortin DF, Spero LA, Groshong BR, Bashore TM. Which media are most likely to solve the archival problem? *Int J Card Imaging* 1994; **10**: 165–75.

109   Nissen SE, Pepine CJ, Bashore TM, *et al.* Cardiac angiography without cine film: erecting a 'Tower of Babel' in the cardiac catheterization laboratory. *J Am Coll Cardiol* 1994; **24**: 834–7.

110   Koning G, van Meurs BA, Haas H, Reiber JH. Effect of data compression on quantitative coronary measurements. *Cathet Cardiovasc Diagn* 1995; **34**: 175–85.

111   Group ACC/ACR/NEMA Ad Hoc. American College of Cardiology, American College of Radiology and Industry develop standard for digital transfer of angiographic images. *J Am Coll Cardiol* 1995; **25**: 800–2.

112   Nissen SE. Evolution of the filmless cardiac angiography suite: promise and perils of the evolving digital era. *Am J Cardiol* 1996; **78**: 41–4.

113   Simon R, Brennecke R, Heiss O, Meier B, Reiber H, Zeelenberg C. Report of the ESC Task Force on digital imaging in cardiology. *European Heart J* 1994; **15**: 1332–4.

114   Brogan WC III, Popma JJ, Pichard AD, *et al.* Rotational coronary atherectomy after unsuccessful coronary balloon angioplasty. *Am J Cardiol* 1993; **71**: 794–8.

115   Israel DH, Marmur JD, Sanborn TA. Excimer laser-facilitated balloon angioplasty of a nondilatable lesion. *J Am Coll Cardiol* 1991; **18**: 1118–19.

116 Popma JJ, Bashore T. Qualitative and quantitative angiography. In: Topol E (ed.). *Interventional Cardiology* (Philadelphia: WB Saunders, 1993): 1058–62, vol 2.

117 Hermans WRM, Rensing BJ, Strauss BH, Serruys PW. Methodological problems related to the quantitative assessment of stretch, elastic recoil, and balloon-artery ratio. *Cathet Cardiovasc Diagn* 1992; **25**: 174–85.

118 Hjemdahl-Monsen CE, Ambrose JA, Borrico S, et al. Angiographic patterns of balloon inflation during percutaneous transluminal coronary angioplasty: role of pressure-diameter curves in studying distensibility and elasticity of the stenotic lesion and the mechanism of dilatation. *J Am Coll Cardiol* 1990; **16**: 569–75.

119 Hanet C, Wijns W, Michel X, Schroeder E. Influence of balloon size and stenosis morphology on immediate and delayed elastic recoil after percutaneous transluminal coronary angioplasty. *J Am Coll Cardiol* 1991; **18**: 506–11.

120 Rensing BJ, Hermans WRM, Beatt KJ, et al. Quantitative angiographic assessment of elastic recoil after percutaneous transluminal coronary angioplasty. *Am J Cardiol* 1990; **66**: 1039–44.

121 Rensing BJ, Hermans WR, Strauss BH, Serruys PW. Regional differences in elastic recoil after percutaneous transluminal coronary angioplasty: a quantitative angiographic study. *J Am Coll Cardiol* 1991; **17**: 34B–38B.

122 Rensing BJ, Hermans WRM, Vos J, et al. Angiographic risk factors of luminal narrowing after coronary balloon angioplasty using balloon measurements to reflect stretch and elastic recoil at the dilatation site. *Am J Cardiol* 1992; **69**: 584–91.

123 Parisi AF, Frolland ED, Hartigan P. A comparison of angioplasty with medical therapy in the treatment of single vessel coronary artery disease. *N Engl J Med* 1992; **326**: 10–16.

124 Rensing BJ, Hermans WRM, Deckers JW, de Feyter PJ, Tijssen JGP, Serruys PW. Lumen narrowing after percutaneous transluminal coronary balloon angioplasty follows a near Gaussian distribution: a quantitative angiographic study in 1,445 successfully dilated lesions. *J Am Coll Cardiol* 1992; **19**: 939–45.

125 Schatz RA, Penn IM, Baim DS, et al. STent REstenosis Study (STRESS): analysis of in-hospital results. *Circulation* 1993; **88**: I-594 (abstract).

126 Serruys PW, Macaya C, de Jaegere P, et al. Interim analysis of the benestent-trial. *Circulation* 1993; **88**: I-594 (abstract).

127 Gould KL. Percent diameter stenosis: battered gold standard, pernicious relic or clinical practicality? *J Am Coll Cardiol* 1988; **11**: 886–8.

128 Vogel RA. Assessing stenosis significance by coronary arteriography: are the best variables good enough? *J Am Coll Cardiol* 1988; **12**: 692–3.

129 Beatt KJ, Serruys PW, Hugenholtz PG. Restenosis after coronary angioplasty: new standards for clinical studies. *J Am Coll Cardiol* 1990; **15**: 491–8.

130 Grondin CM, Dyra I, Pasternac A, Campeau L, Bourassa MG, Lesperance J. Discrepancies between cineangiographic and postmortem findings in patients with coronary artery disease and recent myocardial revascularization. *Circulation* 1974; **49**: 703–8.

131 Popma JJ, Chuang YC, Sweet LC, Syed R, Leon MB. Clinical and angiographic predictors of target lesion revascularization after new device angioplasty. *Circulation* 1993; **88**: I-150 (abstract).

132 Serruys PW, Luijten HE, Beatt KJ, et al. Incidence of restenosis after successful coronary angioplasty: a time-related phenomenon. A quantitative angiographic study in 342 consecutive patients at 1, 2, 3, and 4 months. *Circulation* 1988; **77**: 361–71.

133 Nobuyoshi M, Kimura T, Nosaka H, et al. Restenosis after successful percutaneous transluminal coronary angioplasty: Serial angiographic follow-up of 229 patients. *J Am Coll Cardiol* 1988; **12**: 616–23.

134 Friedrich SP, Gordon PC, Leidig GA, et al. Clinical events following interventional devices are determined by time-dependent hazards. *Circulation* 1992; **86**: I-785 (abstract).

135 Gruentzig AR, King SB, Schlumpf M, Siegenthaler W. Long-term follow-up after percutaneous transluminal coronary angioplasty: the early Zurich experience. *N Engl J Med* 1987; **316**: 1127–32.

136 Weintraub WS, Ghazzal ZMAB, Cohen CL, et al. Clinical implications of late proven patency after successful coronary angioplasty. *Circulation* 1991; **84**: 572–82.

137 Rosen DR, Cannon RO, Watson RM, et al. Three year anatomic, functional and clinical follow-up after successful percutaneous transluminal coronary angioplasty. *J Am Coll Cardiol* 1987; **9**: 1–7.

138 Stone GW, Ligon RW, Rutherford BD, McConahay DR, Hartzler GO. Short-term outcome and long-term follow-up following coronary angioplasty in the young patient: an 8 year experience. *Am Heart J* 1989; **118**: 873.

139 Corcos T, David PR, Val PG, et al. Failure of diltiazem to prevent restenosis after percutaneous transluminal coronary angioplasty. *Am Heart J* 1985; **109**: 926–31.

140 Group The Multicenter European Research Trial with Cilazapril. After Angioplasty to Prevent Transluminal Coronary Obstruction and Restenosis (MERCATOR) Study.

Does the new angiotensin converting enzyme inhibitor Cilazapril prevent restenosis after percutaneous transluminal coronary angioplasty? Results of the MERCATOR Study: A multicenter, randomized, double-blind placebo-controlled trial. *Circulation* 1992; **86**: 100–10.

141 Holmes DR, Vlietstra RE, Smith HC, *et al.* Restenosis after percutaneous transluminal coronary angioplasty (PTCA): a report from the PTCA Registry of the National Heart, Lung, and Blood Institute. *Am J Cardiol* 1984; **53**: 77C–81C.

142 Charron P, Montalescot G, Drobinski G, Grosgogeat Y, Thomas D. [Coronary restenosis: the cardiologist facing problems of definitions]. *Arch Mal Coeur Vaiss* 1995; **88**: 13–19.

143 Gould KL, Lipscomb K, Hamilton GW. Physiological basis for assessing critical coronary stenosis: instantaneous flow response and regional distribution during coronary hyperemia as measures of coronary flow reserve. *Am J Cardiol* 1974; **33**: 87–97.

144 Serruys PW, Rutsch W, Heyndrickx GR, *et al.* Prevention of restenosis after percutaneous transluminal coronary angioplasty with thromboxane A2-receptor blockade: a randomized, double-blind, placebo-controlled trial. *Circulation* 1991; **84**: 1568–80.

145 Carozza JP, Kuntz RE, Fishman RF, Baim DS. Restenosis following arterial injury in diabetics: an analysis of intimal hyperplasia following coronary stenting. *Ann Int Med* 1993; **118**: 344–9.

146 Bourassa MG, Lesperance J, Eastwood C, *et al.* Clinical physiologic, anatomic and procedural factors predictive of restenosis after percutaneous transluminal coronary angioplasty. *J Am Coll Cardiol* 1991; **18**: 368–76.

147 Fishman RF, Kuntz RE, Carozza JP jr, *et al.* Long-term results of directional coronary atherectomy: predictors of restenosis. *J Am Coll Cardiol* 1992; **20**: 1101–10.

148 Popma JJ, De Cesare NB, Pinkerton CA, *et al.* Quantitative analysis of factors influencing late lumen loss and restenosis after directional coronary atherectomy. *Am J Cardiol* 1993; **71**: 552–7.

149 Hirshfeld JW, Schwartz JS, Jugo R, *et al.* Restenosis after coronary angioplasty: a multivariate statistical model to relate lesion and procedure variables to restenosis. *J Am Coll Cardiol* 1991; **18**: 647–56.

150 Kuntz RE, Hinohara T, Robertson GC, Safian RD, Simpson JB, Baim DS. Influence of vessel selection on the observed restenosis rate after endoluminal stenting or directional atherectomy. *Am J Cardiol* 1992; **70**: 1101–8.

151 Carozza JP jr, Kuntz RE, Levine MJ, *et al.* Angiographic and clinical outcome of intracoronary stenting: Immediate and long-term results from a large single-center experience. *J Am Coll Cardiol* 1992; **20**: 328–37.

152 Umans VA, Hermans W, Foley DP, *et al.* Restenosis after directional coronary atherectomy and balloon angioplasty: comparative analysis based on matched lesions. *J Am Coll Cardiol* 1993; **21**: 1382–90.

153 Foley DP, Melkert R, Umans VA, *et al.* Differences in restenosis propensity of devices for transluminal coronary intervention. A quantitative angiographic comparison of balloon angioplasty, directional atherectomy, stent implantation and excimer laser angioplasty. CARPORT, MERCATOR, MARCATOR, PARK, and BENESTENT Trial Groups. *Eur Heart J* 1995; **16**: 1331–46.

154 Mintz GS, Kovach JA, Javier SP, Ditrano CJ, Leon MB. Geometric remodeling is the predominant mechanism of late lumen loss after coronary angioplasty. *Circulation* 1993; **88**: I-654 (abstract).

155 Umans VAWM, Strauss BH, Rensing BJWM, de Jaegere P, de Feyter PJ, Serruys PW. Comparative angiographic quantitative analysis of the immediate efficacy of coronary atherectomy with balloon angioplasty, stenting, and rotational ablation. *Am Heart J* 1991; **122**: 836–43.

156 Berdan LG, Califf RM. Restenosis: Does the six month angiogram tell the story? CAVEAT one year follow-up. *Circulation* 1993; **88**: I-595 (abstract).

157 Popma JJ, van den Berg EK, Dehmer GJ. Long-term outcome of patients with asymptomatic restenosis after percutaneous transluminal coronary angioplasty. *Am J Cardiol* 1988; **62**: 1298–9.

158 Hernandez RA, Macaya C, Iniguez A, *et al.* Midterm outcome of patients with asymptomatic restenosis after coronary balloon angioplasty. *J Am Coll Cardiol* 1992; **19**: 1402–9.

159 Laarman G, Luijten HE, van Zeyl LG, *et al.* Assessment of silent restenosis and long-term follow-up after successful angioplasty in single vessel coronary artery disease: the value of quantitative exercise electrocardiography and quantitative coronary angiography. *J Am Coll Cardiol* 1990; **16**: 578–85.

160 Piana RN, Kugelmass AD, Moscucci M, Ho KKL, Mansour K, Kuntz RE. Coronary restenosis rates defined by 6 month angiography compared to those defined by specific clinical events. *Circulation* 1993; **88**: I-654 (abstract).

161 Kugelmass AD, Piana RN, Moscucci M, Leidig G, Senerchia C, Baim DS. Optimal 'clinical' endpoints for detecting coronary restenosis: analysis using cumulative hazards for specific clinical events. *Circulation* 1993; **88**: I-655 (abstract).

28

The role of intravascular ultrasound in coronary stenting

Harald Mudra

Background

Intracoronary stenting has emerged as the most powerful tool in interventional catheter based therapy since the introduction in 1977 of coronary balloon angioplasty by Grüntzig et al.[1] This is mainly due to the better predictability and improved clinical outcome with stent placement as compared to plain balloon angioplasty.[2] However, it soon became apparent that these positive results of coronary stent placement were threatened by thrombosis of the prosthesis, causing life-threatening acute or subacute complications. Stent thrombosis occurred in up to 16.6% in emergency cases, despite combined anticoagulant therapy with aspirin, coumadin and dipyridamol.[3] Stenting for imminent or definite vessel occlusion, length of the stented lesion, incomplete coverage of the dissection, and small vessel diameter, turned out to be risk factors for subsequent stent thrombosis.[4,5] In two large randomized trials with elective stent placement in discrete relatively short lesions, subacute stent occlusion occurred in 3.4% and 3.5% of the patients, and an unacceptably high rate of bleeding and vascular complications of 7.3% and 13.5%, respectively, was documented.[6,7] Since these landmark studies were performed with the articulated Palmaz–Schatz 15 mm slotted tube stent (Cordis, a Johnson & Johnson Company), two major concepts evolved that, in parallel, yielded a dramatic improvement in clinical outcome. First, a modification of the anticoagulant treatment with the administration of ticlopidine, an inhibitor of the fibrinogen binding site of thrombocytes, in addition to aspirin without coumadin, resulted in both a substantial reduction of stent thromboses and a dramatic reduction of bleeding and vas-cular complications. As a result, the bleeding and complication rates are now comparable to those observed after balloon angioplasty.[4] Second, observations of stents by intravascular ultrasound (IVUS) revealed that most stents were, in fact, underexpanded.[8,9] It was the pioneering approach of Antonio Colombo[10] that translated these findings into the concept of high pressure balloon dilatation and optimal balloon sizing for optimizing stent apposition. Since both of these strategy changes took place simultaneously, it is not yet clear which of the two is most important. Most interventionalists have now changed from anticoagulant therapy to a combination of aspirin with a 4-week treatment course of ticlopidine. Because high pressure dilatation (≥ 14 atm) is now routinely performed, the role of IVUS is questioned by many interventionalists, and is often considered a merely 'scientific tool'.

Rationale for intravascular ultrasound

Despite the dramatic reduction of the absolute rate of sub-acute stent thromboses to below 2%, the exponential increase of stent implantations, together with the inclusion of more complex and acute cases, still represents a significant clinical problem because of the mortality and myocardial infarction rates of 25% and 33%, respectively.[4] This is even more of a problem, since most patients are discharged very early after stent placement and therefore experience this threatening complication most probably outside of the hospital environment.

The second major drawback of coronary stenting is the still significant restenosis rate. Restenosis rates in special subsets of coronary lesions, such as lesions in small vessels, long lesions or lesions causing acute myocardial infarction, are reported between 27% and 38%.[11,12] The rationale for the continuing use of IVUS in stent procedures is therefore to

- further reduce acute and subacute complications,
- reduce restenosis rates
- improve the cost benefit ratio of stent procedures, especially in lesions where a multidevice approach is used.

What is the unique ultrasound information during coronary stenting?

As a silhouette technique, coronary angiography has well known limitations. It is not able to assess diffuse coronary atherosclerosis, and it is limited in depicting eccentric and focal lesions like napkin-ring or ostial stenoses.[13] Furthermore, coronary angiography depends on the adequacy of projection planes to avoid foreshortening and can often only provide suboptimal views for the detection of bifurcational or ostial lesions. For quantitative measurements which can help to overcome interobserver variabilities associated with 'eye-balling', the dependency on a correct calibration is an inherent limitation of up-to-date quantitative coronary angiography (QCA) systems. As quantitative angiography currently is only able to measure single frames, IVUS allows projection-independent cross-sectional image planes and does not need an external calibration system. It is able to depict and quantitate accurately complex lumen morphologies, eccentric or focal lesions, and to differentiate true and false lumen clearly.[14] Moreover, IVUS can qualitatively and quantitatively analyze the vessel wall up to the adventitial (EEM) border, thereby allowing an assessment of absolute vessel dimensions as well as of plaque composition and plaque burden.

Because of these prerequisites, a precise assessment of the target lesion before stent placement and an optimal stent expansion according to the anatomy of the artery are feasible. Thus, maximal lumen gain with a minimized risk of vessel trauma because of uncontrolled oversizing of the stent can be achieved. However, the key questions in times of limited financial resources and increasing financial constraints are therefore threefold:

- Do these features of IVUS reduce the adverse event rate?
- Can IVUS contribute to restenosis reduction?
- Can IVUS be performed cost-effectively?

How and when is ultrasound performed in intracoronary stenting?

Today, a motorized pullback at a speed of 0.5 mm/s should be routinely performed to avoid any operator dependent inaccuracies owing to a too quick pullback with the risk of missing discrete lesions, and to optimize the reproducibility of the method. The image quality of both systems currently available is sufficient for clinically relevant purposes, the catheter diameter of 2.9–3.5 F allows the interrogation of virtually all relevant coronary segments. Intracoronary nitroglycerin should be administered before each pullback to avoid spasms and to guarantee reproducible lumen dimensions. The risk of IVUS is low but not zero.[15] Ischemic symptoms may occur during the imaging of tight lesions but are reversible after removal of the catheter. Even tight lesions can mostly be passed without predilation. If this is not the case, in our experience, this is a good indication for Rotablator treatment before stent placement.[16]

Intracoronary ultrasound before stent placement

Whenever IVUS is used in a stent procedure, it should be used before the first device activation, in order to maximize its potential benefit with regard to the earlier mentioned key questions. IVUS should be used first to assess access to the target lesion before predilation is performed, or before stent placement. In case of significant left main involvement not appreciated by angiography,[17] or diffuse proximal plaque formation with less distal disease, a change of the procedure towards bypass surgery might not only be less dangerous but also more cost-effective in the long-term.

The target lesion composition with respect to the echo reflectiveness of the plaque is assessed next, and may in some cases lead to a change of treatment before stenting. If there is a large amount of calcification present, which is not only a marker for a higher dissection rate but also for a limited lumen gain,[18] Rotablator application before stent placement yields a more predictable lumen gain.[19] Because the plaque burden present before stent placement seems to correlate with the restenosis rate,[20] debulking before stenting is currently under investigation. This ultrasound-guided synergistic approach of combining various angioplasty techniques is extremely important in high risk lesions like left main stenoses, or in ostial right coronary or venous graft lesions, both of which show high restenosis rates.[21]

An important and unique information of IVUS which cannot be obtained by angiography alone is the precise measurement of plaque burden within and around the target lesion. Because in most coronary segments an angiographically silent plaque burden is present, reflecting compensatory enlargement of the artery according to the Glagovian effect,[22,23] the ultrasound measurements result in larger balloon diameters chosen *a priori* for predilation, stent placement and optimization (Fig. 28.1). From the angiographic point of view, this different approach which would be judged as substantial oversizing, is not only safe even without following stent placement,[24] but frequently reduces the number of balloons necessary for the procedure and thereby potentially the procedural costs. Additional IVUS-specific information concerning the longitudinal plaque distribution may direct the optimal length of stent coverage. A more precise calculation of the lesion length – including adjacent segments with a pronounced plaque burden based on the longitudinal ultrasound display or simply on the lesion length – calculated from the duration of the pullback through the lesion is feasible. This can help to choose the optimal stent from a variety of currently available stent lengths and thus reduce the procedural costs.

IVUS following stent placement

After stent placement, an IVUS evaluation is always indicated if an angiographically unclear or ambiguous result is present. This is indicated by any haziness within the stent, which is possibly due to thrombus formation or to non-uniform stent expansion due to a focal lesion calcification. Sometimes angiographically visible dissections at the stent margins, usually treated with an additional stent, may be caused by a broken calcium shell as assessed by ultrasound. In this case, if an appropriate lumen dimension is present no further stent is needed. Conversely, pocket flaps which are present in about 16% of the procedures with optimal angiographic appearance,[25] usually are an ultrasound-based indication for additional stent placement if they prolapse into the lumen. Any plaque prolapse detected by ultrasound within the stent, predominantly occurring in coil stents, is also an indication for further stent placement (i.e. stent in stent). If a balloon catheter does not easily recross the stent, ultrasound occasionally reveals an unexpanded stent portion due to partial dislodgement of the stent from the balloon during placement. Because the unexpanded part of the stent can be located in an angiographically undiseased segment it may not be detected by angiography (Fig. 28.2).

Assessment of adequate stent expansion

Since the first reports of inadequate stent expansion were documented by IVUS numerous criteria for optimal stent expansion have been suggested. There is still no consensus

about these criteria since all are empiric and there is as yet no definite scientific base for a 'golden parameter'. Based on data derived from the observations of Glagov et al.,[26] which suggests a compensation for plaque formation by vessel enlargement up to a plaque burden of about 40% of the total vessel area, one criterion of optimal stent expansion is a minimal in-stent area of 60% of the total vessel area. This criterion is not easy to achieve because exaggerated plaque formation may be present, especially in right coronary arteries where targeting this criterion would result in an unphysiologically large lumen diameter. Criteria based on hemodynamic considerations which attempt to create a smooth lumen channel within the stented segment with minimal turbulence are more widely accepted and easier to reach. Besides, a perfect vessel tapering, especially in longer stented lesions with a gradual and continuous lumen decrease from the larger to the smaller reference segment, a minimal stent lumen area of 80 to 90% of the mean reference lumen area is established. In addition, a smooth inlet and outlet of the stent with a stent marginal area of 90–100% of the corresponding reference site has been proposed. Today, the ultrasound criteria generally accepted are those used in the MUSIC study (Table 28.1), which resulted in a low complication and restenosis rate.[27]

Table 28.1

MUSIC Study
– IVUS Criteria –

1. In-stent minimal LA ⩾90% of the average reference LA
   or
   ⩾100% of LA of the reference segment with the lowest LA

2. In case minimal in-stent LA reaches ⩾9.0 mm²:
   In-stent minimal LA ⩾80% of the average reference LA
   or
   ⩾90% of LA of the reference segment with the lowest LA

3. In-stent LA of proximal stent entrance ⩾90% of proximal reference LA

4. Complete apposition of the stent over its entire length against the vessel wall

5. Symmetric stent expansion defined by LD min/LD max ⩾0.7

LA, luminal area; LD, luminal diameter.

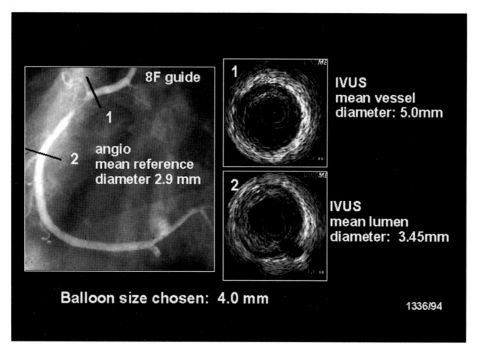

a

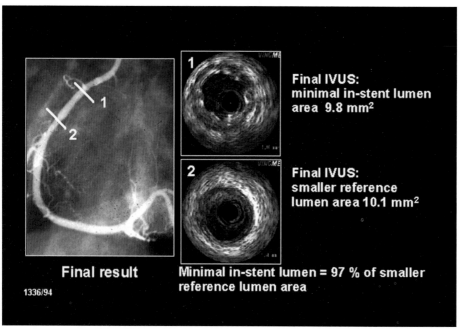

b

Figure 28.1

Target lesion for stent placement located in a proximal right coronary artery. (a) Based on the pre-interventional ultrasound assessment, a larger balloon diameter was chosen because an angiographically silent plaque burden was present at both reference sites (1 and 2). (b) The procedure could be performed with one single balloon catheter for predilation, stent placement and stent optimization according to the criteria of the MUSIC and OPTICUS studies.

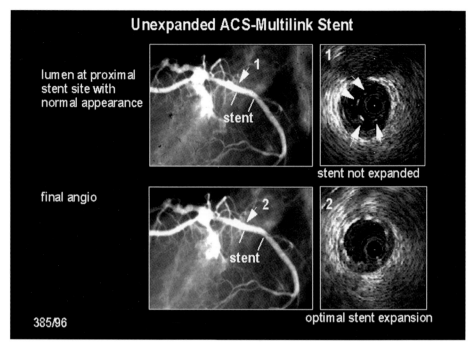

Figure 28.2
A stent placed in the circumflex artery could not be passed by a balloon catheter for routine post-stenting high pressure dilation. The reason could not be detected by angiography. Intravascular ultrasound revealed an underexpanded stent in its proximal portion with struts in the free lumen of the artery (white arrows, 1). The stent was apparently dislodged from the balloon catheter during the attempts to reach the target lesion. Based upon the ultrasound information the stent could be recrossed with a low profile balloon catheter and finally optimized (white arrows, 2).

Therefore, these criteria are currently used in numerous stent studies with different primary objectives like the WEST-II study, the TRAPIST study, the ERASER study and the OPTICUS study. The application of these criteria is potentially important in vessels smaller than 3.0 mm, where angiographic guidance alone neither yields a maximum lumen gain, or attempts to reach this target: oversizing the balloon incurs a substantial risk of persistent dissections. Other clinically important situations where accomplishing these ultrasound criteria is of potential benefit include:

- stenting of vital vessels,
- stenting in acute myocardial infarction,
- stenting of long coronary segments where an angiographic reference dimension is no longer available.

In a series of patients stented under ultrasound guidance and treated with a combined aspirin–ticlopidine antiplatelet therapy thereafter, a very low subacute occlusion rate of 0.8% was present in a variety of different indications for stenting.[10] The same group recently published data on a series of patients after angiographic guidance, receiving the same antiplatelet therapy with a subacute occlusion rate of 3.1%.[28] The application of ultrasound guidance together with a combined antiplatelet regimen of aspirin and ticlopidine currently seems to be the best way to avoid subacute stent closures and, therefore, represents the best choice for high risk patients.

Can ultrasound contribute to restenosis reduction?

Increasing evidence is available that ultrasound is a tool to reduce stent restenosis further. The Multicenter Ultrasound Stent in Coronary Artery Disease (MUSIC) trial, designed as a safety study to test the concept of ultrasound-guided stent optimization followed by aspirin treatment as the only antithrombotic therapy in patients with *de novo* lesions of less than 15 mm length, resulted in a 6-month angiographic restenosis rate of 7.8% and a target vessel revascularization

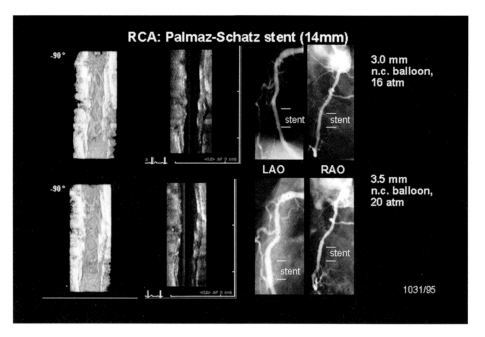

Figure 28.3
Intravascular ultrasound longitudinal display (ECG-triggered sagittal view and 3-D reconstruction) of a stented segment within a right coronary artery. Despite a perfect angiogram in two perpendicular views, ultrasound revealed suboptimal stent expansion which is most pronounced within the proximal and midportion of the stent. Redilation using higher pressure and a larger balloon diameter yields a result that meets the MUSIC and OPTICUS study criteria with an angiographic 'overdilation' (negative stenosis).

rate of 4.5%.[27] The lesion characteristics and reference segment diameters of this study were comparable to those of the BENESTENT-I and BENESTENT-II pilot studies being analyzed at the same institution, using the same angiographic algorithms. The restenosis rate of the MUSIC trial is markedly lower than that of both BENESTENT studies, with only a minimal additional acute lumen gain in angiography of 0.1 mm as compared to the BENESTENT-II pilot study where current stent techniques like high pressure application were also used (Fig. 28.3). Our single-center study – including consecutive patients with a variety of indications: multiple stents in 19% of the patients or restenosis as stent indication in 40% – yielded a restenosis rate of 15.3%.[29] Also in this study, the criteria of the MUSIC study were used and an average and maximal in-stent area stenosis of 7 ± 15% and 15 ± 14%, respectively, could be achieved. The physiological basis for these promising results, revitalizing the old concept of 'the bigger the better', is not yet fully understood. While there is a well-established positive correlation between acute gain and late loss in angiographically-guided stenting, which reflects the

increasing vessel response to larger overstretch,[30] this seems to be less valid after ultrasound guidance. This may be attributable to the precise sizing of the balloon diameters if ultrasound is used, which could result in a less traumatic stent optimization. A randomized multicenter trial, the OPTICUS study, will assess this hypothesis and may help to further elucidate the results of the MUSIC study.

References

1 Gruentzig AR, Senning A, Siegenthaler WE. Non-operative dilation of coronary artery stenosis: precutaneous transluminal angioplasty. *N Engl J Med* 1979; **301**: 61–8.

2 Ruygrok PN, Serruys PW. Intracoronary stenting. From concept to custom. *Circulation* 1996; **94**: 882–90.

3 Herrmann NC, Buchbinder M, Cleman MW, et al. Emergent use of balloon expandable coronary artery stenting for failed percutaneous transluminal coronary angioplasty. *Circulation* 1992; **86**: 812–19.

4   Karrillon GJ, Morice MC, Benveniste E, *et al.* Intracoronary stent implantation without ultrasound guidance and with replacement of conventional anticoagulation by antiplatelet therapy. *Circulation* 1996; **94**: 1519–27.

5   Moussa I, Di Mario C, Di Francesco L, Reimers B, Blengino S, Colombo A. Subacute stent thrombosis and the anticoagulation controversy: changes in drug therapy, operator technique, and the impact of intravascular ultrasound. *Am J Cardiol* 1997; **78 (Suppl 3A)**: 13–17.

6   Serruys PW, de Jaegere P, Kiemeneij F, *et al.* A comparison of balloon-expandable-stent implantation with balloon angioplasty in patients with coronary artery disease. *N Engl J Med* 1994; **331**: 489–95.

7   Fishman DL, Leon MB, Baim DS, *et al.* A randomized comparison of coronary stent placement and balloon angioplasty in the treatment of coronary artery disease. *N Engl J Med* 1994; **331**: 496–501.

8   Mudra H, Klauss V, Blasini R, *et al.* Ultrasound guidance of Palmaz–Schatz intracoronary stenting with a combined intravascular ultrasound balloon catheter. *Circulation* 1994; **90**: 1252–61.

9   Nakamura S, Colombo A, Gaglione A, *et al.* Intracoronary ultrasound observations during stent implantation. *Circulation* 1994; **89**: 2026–34.

10 Colombo A, Hall P, Nakamura S, *et al.* Intracoronary stenting without anticoagulation accomplished with intravascular ultrasound guidance. *Circulation* 1995; **91**: 1676–88.

11 Azar AJ, Detre K, Goldberg S, Kiemeneij F, Leon MB, Serruys PW. A meta-analysis on the clinical and angiographic outcomes of stent vs. PTCA in the different coronary vessel sizes in the BENESTENT-I and STRESS-1/2 trials. *Circulation* 1995; **92**: I-475 (abstract).

12 Schömig A, Neumann F-J, Walter H, *et al.* Coronary stent placement in patients with acute myocardial infarction: comparison of clinical and angiographic outcome after randomization to antiplatelet or anticoagulant therapy. *J Am Coll Cardiol* 1997; **29**: 28–34.

13 Nissen SE, Gurley JC, Grines CL, *et al.* Intravascular ultrasound assessment of lumen size and wall morphology in normal subjects and patients with coronary artery disease. *Circulation* 1991; **84**: 1087–99.

14 Topol EJ, Nissen SE. Our preoccupation with coronary luminology. The dissociation between clinical and angiographic findings in ischemic heart disease. *Circulation* 1995; **92**: 2333–42.

15 Hausmann D, Erbel R, Alibelli-Chemarin MJ, *et al.* The safety of intracoronary ultrasound: a multicenter survey of 2207 examinations. *Circulation* 1995; **91**: 623–30.

16 Mudra H, Henneke KH, Klauss V, Werner F, Regar E, Theisen K. Rotablation vor koronarer Stentimplantation: Ein sicher anwendbares Verfahren zur Maximierung des Lumengewinns in harten Läsionen. *Z Kardiol* 1996; **84 (Suppl 2)**: 75 (abstract)

17 Isner JM, Kishel J, Kent KM, Ronan JA Jr., Ross AM, Roberts WC. Accuracy of angiographic determination of left main coronary arterial narrowing. Angiographic – histologic correlative analysis in 28 patients. *Circulation* 1981; **63**: 1056–1064.

18 Fitzgerald PJ, Ports TA, Yock PG. Contribution of localized calcium deposits to dissection after angioplasty. An observational study using intravascular ultrasound. *Circulation* 1992; **86**: 64–70.

19 Mintz GS, Potkin BN, Keren G, *et al.* Intravascular ultrasound evaluation of the effect of rotational atherectomy in obstructive athereosclerotic coronary artery disease. *Circulation* 1992; **86**: 1383–93.

20 Moussa I, Di Mario C, Moses J, *et al.* The impact of preintervention plaque area determined by intravascular ultrasound on luminal renarrowing following coronary stenting. *Circulation* 1996; **94**: I-261 (abstract).

21 Mehran R, Mintz GS, Bucher TA, *et al.* Aorto-ostial instent restenosis: mechanisms, treatment, and results. A serial quantitative angiographic and intravascular ultrasound study. *Circulation* 1996; **94**: I-200 (abstract).

22 Glagov S, Weisenberg E, Zarins CK, Stankunavicius R, Kolettis GJ. Compensatory enlargement of human atherosclerotic coronary arteries. *N Engl J Med* 1987; **316**: 1371–5.

23 Mintz GS, Painter JA, Pichard AD, *et al.* Atherosclerosis in angiographically 'normal' coronary artery reference segments: an intravascular ultrasound study with clinical correlations. *J Am Coll Cardiol* 1995; **25**: 1479–85.

24 Stone GW, Hodgson JMcB, St Goar FG, *et al.* Improved procedural results of coronary angioplasty with intravascular ultrasound guided balloon sizing: the CLOUT pilot trial. *Circulation* 1997 (in press).

25 Metz JA, Mooney MR, Walter PD, *et al.* Significance of edge tears in coronary stenting: initial observations from the STRUT registry. *Circulation* 1995; **92**: I-546 (abstract).

26 Glagov S. Intimal hyperplasia, vascular remodeling, and the restenosis problem. *Circulation* 1994; **89**: 2888–91.

27 Mudra H, Sunamura M, Figulla H, *et al.* Six month clinical and angiographic outcome after IVUS guided stent implantation. *J Am Coll Cardiol* 1997; **29**: 171A (abstract)

28 Nakamura S, Hall P, Gaglione A, *et al.* High pressure assisted coronary stent implantation accomplished without

intravascular ultrasound guidance and subsequent anticoagulation. *J Am Coll Cardiol* 1997; **29**: 21–7.

29 Mudra H, Regar E, Klauss V, *et al.* Serial follow-up after optimized ultrasound-guided deployment of Palmaz–Schatz stents. In-stent neointimal proliferation without significant reference segment response. *Circulation* 1997; **95**: 363–70.

30 Kuntz RE, Baim DS. Defining coronary restenosis. Newer clinical and angiographic paradigms. *Circulation* 1993; **88**: 1310–23.

30

Lessons from coronary flow reserve in clinical practice

David Hasdai and Amir Lerman

Introduction

Clinicians are all too familiar with the difficult workup and management of patients with chest pain. Often times, the history, physical examination and data derived from ancillary diagnostic modalities alter the course of patient management, at times in conflicting directions. Take, for example, the case of a 55-year-old male presenting with exertional and emotional stress-induced chest pain in the preceding weeks. The patient has risk factors for coronary artery disease, including hypercholesterolemia, cigarette smoking and a family history of premature coronary artery disease. The physical examination and baseline electrocardiogram are both normal. Uncertain of the etiology of his chest discomfort, the attending physician refers the patient to a treadmill test; the patient completes 6.5 min of the Bruce protocol, at which time he develops his typical chest pain, accompanied by nondiagnostic electrocardiographic changes. The patient is then referred for diagnostic coronary angiography. There are three possible scenarios for such a patient during angiography. Coronary angiography may reveal either 1) nonsignificant coronary artery obstructive disease (<50% diameter stenosis of any epicardial coronary artery); 2) lesion/s of indeterminate significance (50% < percent diameter stenosis < 70%); or 3) significant narrowing of one or more epicardial coronary arteries (>70% diameter stenosis).

One must remember that the coronary angiogram is merely a 'road map' of the coronary epicardial tree, offering no information regarding the microcirculation, nor of the physiologic significance of obstructive/nonobstructive lesions. For example, do the findings of nonsignificant

obstructive coronary artery disease rule out a possible cardiac etiology for the patient's symptoms? What is the physiologic significance of indeterminate lesions? How can we assess lesions after coronary interventional procedures to discern whether the anatomic improvement is accompanied by physiologic improvement? The aim of this chapter is to outline the use of coronary flow reserve measurements within the cardiac catheterization laboratory to guide the management and therapy of patients with obstructive or nonobstructive coronary artery disease.

Coronary blood flow and flow reserve

Coronary blood flow (CBF) is autoregulated to meet the changing demands of the myocardium. The autoregulation of CBF remains nearly constant over a wide range of aortic pressure, by reducing or increasing vasomotor tone through the modulation of locally secreted and circulating neurohormones. When the demands of the myocardium are not met by the coronary circulation, myocardial ischemia may occur, often accompanied by angina.

At rest, myocardial demand is low, and accordingly CBF is at its lowest level. Coronary resistance vessels have a high basal vasomotor tone in this state. However, the normal physiologic response to an increase in myocardial demand is enhanced CBF,[1] which is achieved by vasodilation of epicardial and resistance vessels, mediated by endothelium-dependent and independent mechanisms.[2]

The ability to increase CBF by reducing vasomotor tone to meet myocardial demand is called coronary flow reserve (CFR). Normal individuals may increase CBF up to 6- to 8-fold to face the increased myocardial demand. In patho-physiologic states, CFR may be impaired, resulting in an imbalance between myocardial demand and blood flow. It is convenient to analyze the cause for impaired CFR based on the loci along the coronary artery tree which may adversely affect the modulation of CBF, as well as on the underlying pathophysiology (i.e. endothelium dependent or independent).

Impaired CFR based on abnormalities along the coronary artery tree

A simplistic approach to the understanding of factors affecting resting CBF and CFR is to divide the coronary circulation into three levels: epicardial arteries, resistance vessels and the ventricular wall. Abnormalities at one or more levels may lead to impaired CFR.

Epicardial arteries

Under physiologic conditions, the coronary perfusion pressure that determines CBF corresponds to aortic pressure. However, in the presence of epicardial coronary artery stenoses, the poststenotic coronary pressure determines the perfusion pressure. Coronary resistance vessels compensate for epicardial coronary artery stenoses upstream by vasodilating. By reducing the pressure downstream from the lesion, the perfusion pressure gradient across the lesion is maintained, allowing for the preservation of CBF. When the resistance vessels are maximally dilated, CBF may not be able to increase to face myocardial demand. The landmark work of Gould and Lipscomb[3] demonstrated that normal resting coronary flow is not altered by coronary artery stenosis of approximately 60% of the diameter. Compensatory vasodilatation of the distal coronary vascular bed maintains near-normal resting flow for lesions between 60 to 85% diameter stenosis but adaptive vasodilatation fails to compensate for lesions greater than 85% diameter stenosis. These important findings have served as the reference for our current definition of obstructive coronary artery disease. Thus, it is widely accepted that 70% or more stenosis of an epicardial artery constitutes significantly obstructive coronary artery disease.

Microvessels

Coronary microvessels may have reduced vasodilating abilities due to structural or functional abnormalities.[4–7] This

abnormality may entail an enhanced basal tone and/or the inability to decrease vasomotor tone during stress.

Left ventricular wall

Myocardial contraction affects the coronary circulation. Coronary vessels within the ventricular wall collapse during systole, as the extravascular tissue pressure exceeds intravascular pressure. During diastole, blood enters these vessels. The driving pressure for CBF is determined by the perfusion pressure gradient between the resistance vessels and the left ventricle during diastole. When left ventricular diastolic pressure is higher than arteriolar pressure or when diastole is significantly shortened (i.e. during tachycardia), CBF may rise insufficiently to meet myocardial demands.

Endothelium-dependent and independent CFR

Impaired CFR may also be the result of endothelium-dependent and independent mechanisms. Coronary vasomotor tone is regulated by an intricate balance between factors causing vasoconstriction and vasodilatation (Fig. 30.1). The coronary endothelium is an active paracrine organ involved in the control of coronary tone via release of vasoactive factors.[8] Under normal circumstances, coronary vasodilatation is mediated, at least in part, by the release of endothelium-derived relaxing factors (EDRF) or nitric oxide, which is released from the endothelial cells.[9,10] The endothelium is also involved in the production of vasoconstrictors, the most potent of which is endothelin.[11] Impaired endothelium-dependent CFR, often termed endothelial dysfunction, is clinically defined as an attenuated increase or a decrease in CBF in response to endothelium-dependent vasodilators (e.g. acetylcholine or substance P). Endothelial dysfunction may affect coronary epicardial arteries and/or microvessels. The precise mechanisms underlying endothelial dysfunction are not yet defined. However, recent observations suggest that endothelial dysfunction may involve an imbalance between vasodilator and vasoconstrictor agents released by the endothelium.[8] In particular, the basal and pharmacologically stimulated bioavailability of EDRF may be impaired in states of endothelial dysfunction,[12] whereas the activity of vasoconstrictor substances such as endothelin are increased.[13,14]

The endothelium plays an important role in the regulation of CBF in response to increased myocardial demand. EDRF is elaborated by the intact endothelium and mediates the increase in CBF in response to physical and mental stress.[15–17] This response is reproduced by the administration of acetylcholine.[15–17] Impaired endothelium-independent CFR refers to the inability of the vascular smooth muscle adequately

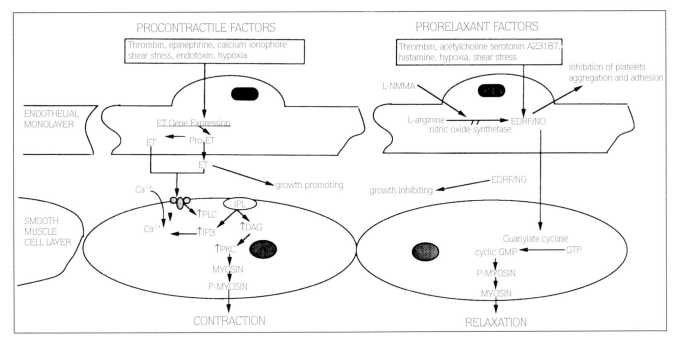

Figure 30.1

A schematic figure depicting the intricate balance between procontractile (ET = endothelin) and prorelaxant (EDRF = endothelium-derived relaxing factor, NO = nitric oxide) factors which regulate vasomotor tone. Several precontractile factors including thrombin, epinephrine, calcium ionophores A23187, shear stress, endotoxin and hypoxia are known to stimulate gene expression and release of ET. Mature ET binds to smooth muscle cell surface receptors and eventually induces the opening of voltage-sensitive plasma membrane calcium channels and activation of phospholipase C to liberate inositol triphosphate (IP_3) and diacylglycerol (DAG) from plasma membrane inositol phospholipids (IPL). IP_3 and DAG in turn promote Ca^{2+} release from intracellular stores and activation of protein kinase C (PKC), respectively. Calmodulin aids in the phosphorylation of myosin light heavy chains, a precondition for smooth muscle contraction. Similarly, prorelaxant factors including thrombin, acetylcholine, serotonin, calcium ionophore A23187, histamine, hypoxia and shear stress stimulate the release of EDRF, which is produced by L-arginine by the enzyme nitric oxide synthase. EDRF diffuses into the smooth muscle cell and stimulates soluble guanylate cyclase to convert GTP to cyclic GMP (cGMP). cGMP activates cGMP-dependent protein kinase and leads to dephosphorylation of myosin light chains and muscle cell relaxation. (Reproduced with permission from reference 8.)

to relax at the level of coronary epicardial arteries and/or microvessels to accommodate the increased flow needed to meet increased myocardial demand. Impaired endothelium-dependent coronary vasodilatation is associated with thallium scintigraphic defects suggestive of myocardial ischemia in response to exercise and mental stress.[15,16] Transient perfusion defects were observed in a substantial proportion of patients with acetylcholine-induced coronary epicardial vasoconstriction injected with thallium during peak acetylcholine infusion.[18]

Pharmacological assessment of CFR

Specific pharmacological tools are currently used to discern abnormalities in CFR. Pharmacological provocation of the coronary vasculature should be considered after other possible causes of impaired coronary circulation have been ruled out. For example, a patient with severe aortic stenosis might have reduced CBF and CFR due to abnormal perfusion pressure. Reduced CBF in this condition would reflect the impaired cardiac output, and not a structural or functional abnormality of the coronary vasculature. Likewise, a patient with severely increased left ventricular end-diastolic pressure or significant tachycardia is likely to have reduced CBF and CFR, as explained above.

Due to their unique modes of action, the drugs used in the catheterization laboratory aid in determining whether abnormalities in CFR are endothelium dependent or independent, and whether the impaired CFR involves coronary epicardial arteries or the microcirculation.

Endothelium-dependent mechanisms

Acetylcholine is a drug commonly used to evaluate endothelium-dependent vasomotor tone regulation. Stimulation of acetylcholine receptors produces a uniform endothelium-dependent dilatation of coronary vessels of all sizes.[19] Normal coronary endothelial function is characterized by coronary vasodilatation and an increase in CBF in response to acetylcholine. Endothelial dysfunction may be manifested by a significant attenuation of the increase in CBF in response to intracoronary acetylcholine, no change or even a decrease in CBF.[20]

Substance P is an alternative endothelium-dependent agent used by some clinicians, particularly in patients with moderate coronary artery disease.[21] The normal response to substance P is an increase in CBF. An abnormal response is an attenuated increase in CBF. In contrast to acetylcholine, the administration of substance P is not associated with coronary vasoconstriction; hence its relatively greater safety profile in patients with more advanced coronary artery disease.[21] Although both acetylcholine and substance P are used for the assessment of endothelium-dependent vasoreactivity, there are reports of a differential response to the two agents in patients with endothelial dysfunction.[22] Others have reported a good correlation between the two agents.[23]

Nonendothelial-dependent mechanisms

Nonendothelial-dependent mechanisms can be assessed using several drugs: adenosine, nitroglycerin and ergot alkaloids.

Adenosine

Adenosine is thought to act on the coronary vasculature via stimulation of the adenosine A2 receptor on smooth muscle cells.[24] At pharmacological doses, such as given in the cardiac catheterization laboratory, adenosine can cross the endothelial barrier and stimulate the receptor on the smooth muscle directly in an endothelium-independent mechanism.[25] Adenosine acts predominantly on vessels less

than 150 μm in diameter[24] and, therefore, mainly assesses changes in the coronary resistance vessels as reflected by changes in coronary flow. The administration of adenosine provides mainly an endothelium-independent evaluation of the coronary microvasculature (altered endothelium-dependent vasomotor regulation has been shown in response to the increase in flow induced by adenosine), and may reveal abnormal CFR even in the presence of normal epicardial endothelial function.

Papaverine and dipyridamole are alternative agents to adenosine. Although some investigators have reported variability in values of CFR using different pharmacological agents,[26,27] others have reported similar values.[28,29] These differences may be attributed, at least in part, to differences in doses and routes of administration of the different drugs. In contrast to the minimal effect of adenosine on epicardial arteries, papaverine may affect epicardial arteries; in fact, papaverine may even cause epicardial vasoconstriction after vascular injury.[30] In addition, papaverine may prolong the QT-interval, thus causing ventricular dysrrhythmias.[28] Adenosine may cause bradyarrhythmias including sinus bradycardia and atrioventricular block, facial flushing and bronchoconstriction. Due to the short half-life of adenosine, the duration of these side-effects is very brief. In our experience of over 400 patients receiving intracoronary adenosine (24–42 μg), no significant side-effect has been recorded.

Nitroglycerin

Nonendothelial-dependent vascular responses can be assessed in the epicardial arteries by the administration of nitroglycerin. Nitroglycerin is a vasodilator which acts directly on vascular smooth muscle.[31] Since the coronary microvessels lack the enzyme needed to convert nitroglycerin to its active form nitric oxide, nitroglycerin produces a dose-related dilatation of coronary vessels larger than 200 μm in diameter, and has no effect on smaller coronary vessels.[24]

Ergot

Acetylcholine causes coronary vasoconstriction in the majority of patients with vasospastic angina, even in the presence of a normal response to substance P.[32,33] In the instance where variant or Prinzmetal's angina is still clinically suspected despite a normal endothelial response to acetylcholine and normal adenosine CFR, ergot alkaloids, such as ergonovine maleate or methacholine, may be administered. Ergot alkaloids are vasoconstrictors which act nonspecifically on the vascular smooth muscle cell. The mechanism of action is not fully understood and may involve the alpha-adrenergic and serotonin receptors on vascular smooth muscle.[34] Ergonovine testing is positive (i.e. causing vasoconstriction) in fewer than 5% of patients whose symptoms do not suggest variant angina.[35] In our laboratory, we administer methergine intravenously at escalating doses of 1, 2, 3 and 6 µg/kg for 3 min at each dose. Heart rate, blood pressure and the electrocardiogram should be closely monitored. Because the response may not be localized, online intracoronary monitoring of coronary hemodynamics of one epicardial artery may not be indicative of the coronary response, thus precluding the immediate cessation of drug infusion when CBF is compromised. The test is discontinued prematurely if the patient experiences severe chest pain or severe hypertension. We have to emphasize the risks involved when all three major epicardial arteries vasoconstrict in response to ergots, a condition which may be lethal if not readily reversed. Nitroglycerin should be readily available to reverse the vasospasm. At the conclusion of the final dose of methergine, coronary angiography is performed. Coronary spasm may be focal or diffuse. Contraindications to ergot infusion include hypertension, toxemia, pregnancy and ergot hypersensitivity.

Measurements

Measurement of changes in the epicardial diameter may be achieved by both qualitative and quantitative coronary angiography. Clearly, quantitative angiography provides a more objective and reproducible method of assessing change in coronary artery diameter. Another method of determining artery diameter, intravascular ultrasound, supplies a very sensitive tool to measure not only coronary artery diameter but also to provide a cross-sectional view of the intima, media and adventitia of the vessel, often exposing atherosclerosis not visible on angiography.[36] Moreover, intravascular ultrasound is probably the gold standard for excluding the presence of coronary atherosclerosis.[37]

Measurement of CBF has been attempted by several methods in the past, including coronary sinus thermodilution, gas clearance, and densimetric techniques and bulky intracoronary Doppler devices.[38] More recently, the availability of a 0.014 or a 0.018-inch intracoronary Doppler guidewire has made the measurement of CBF with good correlation to actual flow easily available in the cardiac catheterization laboratory.[39] CBF blood flow is calculated using the formula $\pi D^2 \times$ APV/8, where D represents the coronary diameter measured 5 mm distal to the tip of the Doppler wire (by quantitative angiography or intravascular ultrasound) and APV equals the average peak velocity from the Doppler tracing.[40] The CFR is calculated by the ratio of peak-to-baseline CBF in response to drug infusion or injection. When coronary artery diameter is presumed to remain unchanged in response to drug manipulation (i.e. adenosine injection), the CFR is calculated by the ratio of peak-to-baseline flow velocities (APV).

Minimally obstructive coronary artery disease

It is estimated that approximately 10–20% of patients undergoing coronary angiography due to angina pectoris have minimally obstructive coronary arteries. The patient with minimally obstructive coronary artery disease and angina pectoris poses a difficult and often frustrating challenge to the attending physician. The majority of these patients are severely debilitated by angina pectoris over many years, often with serious social, psychological and economical consequences.[41,42] The angina may be classic (associated with physical or mental stress and with relief of symptoms with rest or nitroglycerin) or atypical. Although these patients frequently have an abnormal noninvasive test for myocardial ischemia, they are often dismissed with a diagnosis of chest pain of noncardiac origin after their coronary angiogram is found to be either normal or to have only minimally obstructive lesions; they then often subsequently undergo extensive workups in search of gastrointestinal, psychiatric and other disorders. During follow-up, many of these patients continue to require multiple hospitilizations for chest pain, often with repeated coronary angiography procedures.[41,42]

In recent years, it has been recognized that changes in coronary vasomotor tone regulation may precede or accompany gross morphological changes of atherosclerosis.[43–45] Moreover, altered coronary vasomotor tone regulation may be the pathophysiologic basis for angina pectoris in these patients with minimally obstructive coronary artery disease or normal coronary arteries at the time of angiography. This altered vasomotor regulation cannot be appreciated by coronary angiography or intracoronary ultrasonography. Furthermore, impaired vasomotor regulation occurs in the presence or absence of visible atherosclerosis as discerned by intracoronary ultrasound,[46] and may involve the coronary microcirculation.[47] Known risk factors for atherosclerosis, such as diabetes, hypecholesterolemia, hypertension and smoking may be associated with altered coronary vasomotor regulation by altering the integrity of the endothelium,[46–53] resulting in endothelial dysfunction.

The following protocol is currently used in the authors' cardiac catheterization laboratory in assessing these patients (Fig. 30.2). Cardioactive medications are withheld 24 hours prior to the study, and diagnostic coronary angiography is performed without the administration of nitroglycerin to rule out obstructive coronary disease. The coronary circulation is then investigated in the following manner. First, a number 2.2 F Tracker coronary infusion catheter or an Ultrafuse catheter (SciMed Life System, Maple Grove, MN, USA) and 0.014-inch Doppler guidewire (Cardiometrics, Santa Anna, CA, USA) are inserted via a 7 F or 8 F guiding catheter into the left anterior descending coronary artery or the ischemia-related artery based on a

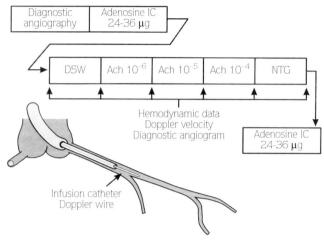

Figure 30.2
The current protocol in the authors' laboratory for the assessment of coronary endothelium-dependent and nonendothelium-dependent function. Adenosine is usually given as intracoronary (IC) boluses of 24–36 μg. In case of severe bradycardia we begin the test with 16 μg of adenosine. If no side-effects are observed with adenosine, and the CFR ratio is borderline, we often administer 42 μg of adenosine. Acetylcholine (Ach) is infused over 3 min at each dose. Following the last dose of acetylcholine, an intracoronary bolus injection of nitroglycerin (NTG) is given. Adenosine is given again after nitroglycerin to confirm the CFR ratio. D5W=Dextrose 5% in water

prior functional test. Secondly, baseline intracoronary Doppler readings and coronary angiography in the optimal projection are obtained. Thirdly, the nonendothelium-dependent CBF reserve ratio is determined by administering boluses of intracoronary adenosine (24–36 μg; solution of 6 mg adenosine in one liter of saline). Fourthly, in order to assess the endothelial function and endothelial-dependent CFR, intracoronary acetylcholine is administered. Graded concentrations of acetylcholine (10^{-6}, 10^{-5} and 10^{-4} M to achieve an intracoronary concentration of 10^{-8}, 10^{-7} and 10^{-6} M, respectively, assuming blood flow in the left anterior descending coronary artery of 80 mL/min) are infused intracoronary (at a rate of 1 ml/min) over 3–5 min, followed by a bolus injection of 200 μg of intracoronary nitroglycerin (volume of 2 ml). Fifthly, symptoms, hemodynamic data, electrocardiogram and Doppler velocities are recorded at the end of each infusion or bolus injection, followed by a selective coronary angiogram. The coronary angiograms are performed in the same projection as the baseline coronary angiogram. Measurements of CBF and CRF are performed as detailed above.

Interpretation of results

The regulation of CBF involves epicardial and resistance vessels in endothelial-dependent and nonendothelial-dependent mechanisms. Our clinical protocol evaluates endothelial-dependent (acetylcholine) and nonendothelial-dependent (adenosine, nitroglycerin) mechanisms, involving epicardial (acetylcholine, nitroglycerin) and resistance vessels (acetylcholine, adenosine). Based on prior studies, we consider an increase above 50% in CBF above baseline in response to acetylcholine (Fig. 30.3) and a CFR ratio above 2.5 in response to adenosine (Fig. 30.4) as being normal. Nitroglycerin normally causes profound vasodilatation and an increase in CBF without significant changes in flow velocities. Impaired coronary vasomotor tone regulation in patients with angina and minimally obstructive coronary artery disease may occur at one or several levels. Patients may manifest intact endothelium-dependent and nonendothelium-dependent responses, in which case they are given a diagnosis of normal vasomotor regulation. In our experience, only approximately 30% of patients with minimal coronary artery disease and angina have a normal response to pharmacological stimuli. This rate may vary among different laboratories based on referral bias. Patients with an abnormal response may manifest impaired endothelium-dependent responses to acetylcholine and/or impaired nonendothelium-dependent responses to adenosine. In our experience, the majority of the patients demonstrate coronary endothelial dysfunction, underscoring the ubiquity of this once unrecognized pathophysiological state. It must be emphasized that some patients have an impaired response to acetylcholine with an intact response to adenosine, or vice versa.

A patient with impaired response to acetylcholine and adenosine can be considered as having dysfunction of epicardial and resistance vessels involving endothelium-dependent and nonendothelium-dependent mechanisms. An abnormal response to adenosine with a normal response to acetylcholine indicates microvessel disease in a nonendothelium-dependent mechanism. An attenuated response to acetylcholine with a normal response to adenosine indicates endothelium-dependent disease. Last, a lack of response to nitroglycerin may suggest nonendothelium-dependent dysfunction of epicardial arteries.

Establishing the etiology of chest pain in patients with minimally obstructive coronary artery disease has important clinical implications. First, by determining the cause for their symptoms, the need for additional, costly workup may be avoided. Secondly, the association between risk factors for coronary artery disease and endothelial dysfunction may prompt the patient to pursue a risk-factor modification program. Indeed, endothelial dysfunction has been shown to be improved with lowering of cholesterol.[54] Last, new therapeutic approaches are currently being investigated for patients with endothelial dysfunction. For example, a recent

Intracoronary Doppler: the technique and clinical applications

Carlo Di Mario, Lucia Di Francesco, Yoshio Kobayashi, Tatsuro Akiyama, Gianni Cuman, Bernhard Reimers and Antonio Colombo

Introduction

Intracoronary Doppler is an established research technique to study the coronary flow dynamics in humans and its changes in the presence of various pathological conditions and, in particular, of coronary stenoses. Recent technical improvements have made this technique easily applicable during coronary interventions but still intracoronary Doppler is rarely used for clinical decision making. In this chapter we review the technique and clinical applications of intracoronary Doppler in order to establish the current indications to intracoronary Doppler in clinical practice.

Technique

Intracoronary Doppler probes

The last 10 years have seen rapid changes in intracoronary Doppler technology, with the progressive miniaturization of the transducers and refinement of signal analysis. The first intracoronary Doppler tracings with a percutaneous technique in humans were obtained in 1977 by Cole and Hartley, using a 20 MHz piezoelectric circular crystal mounted at the tip of a standard 8F Sones catheter.[1] A modification of this approach, with a crystal mounted caudally at the tip of a left Judkins catheter, has been more recently proposed by Kern et al.[2]

Selective measurements in the vessel of interest became possible with the development of intracoronary Doppler catheters which have a piezoelectric crystal mounted laterally or at the tip of flexible 3F catheters.[3,4] Although these catheters have been extensively used in research cardiac catheterization laboratories, the routine application of the technique in clinical practice started only with the development of Doppler probes mounted at the tip of coronary guidewires.[5] The currently available Doppler guidewires are flexible and steerable 0.014-inch or 0.018-inch guidewires with a tip-mounted 12 or 15 MHz piezoelectric ultrasound transducer. Because of their small diameter (0.37 mm or 0.46 mm for the 0.014-inch and 0.018-inch guidewires, respectively), the Doppler guidewire can be passed distal to coronary stenoses without creating significant flow obstruction. The forward-directed ultrasound beam diverges at 14° from the Doppler transducer. Maintained 5.2 mm beyond the transducer, the Doppler sample volume is distal to the area of distortion of the flow velocity profile which is induced by the Doppler guidewire and includes a large portion of the flow velocity profile.[6] A real-time spectral analyzer using on-line fast Fourier transformation provides a scrolling gray scale spectral display. The system software automatically tracks the instantaneous peak velocity and calculates on-line the average peak velocity over two consecutive beats.

The Doppler guidewire has been validated in straight tubes and canine coronary arteries by Doucette et al,[5] showing a linear correlation to absolute flow, which was measured by on-line electromagnetic flow meters.

Intracoronary Doppler examination

Technique of examination

Because of their small size, the Doppler guidewires can be used with standard diagnostic catheters. The insertion through guiding catheters facilitates manipulation of the Doppler guidewire and allows, if needed, immediate lesion treatment once the guidewire has passed distal to the stenosis for evaluation. In a recent multicenter study applying intracoronary Doppler during balloon angioplasty, the Doppler guidewire could be used as a primary wire to cross the stenosis in 289 of 297 patients (97%) and basal velocity measurements before balloon angioplasty could be obtained proximal and distal to the stenosis in 74% and 99% of patients, respectively.[7] In most cases (93%), the inability to measure flow velocity proximal to the stenosis was not due to technical failure but to a too proximal position of the lesion under evaluation.

The possibility of recording very high velocities (>4 m/s) allows the measurement of the velocity of the stenotic jet and the calculation of the percent area stenosis based on the continuity equation. The second method, already proposed using Doppler catheters for mild stenoses,[8] has been shown to be applicable with the Doppler guidewire in severe stenoses, yielding good correlation with independent measurements of stenosis severity with quantitative angiography.[9] Unfortunately, flow velocity tracings suitable for quantitative analysis are difficult to record in the stenotic segment because of misalignment of the guidewire with the stenotic jet and reduced intensity of the blood backscatter in segments with high shear stress, which leads to disaggregation of the red blood cell rouleaux.[10] The low success rate in the recording of flow velocity within the lesion has been recently confirmed in the large multicenter study DEBATE (Doppler Endpoints Balloon Angioplasty Trial Europe), in which high quality recordings of the stenotic jet were obtained in 12% and 22% of patients before and after balloon angioplasty, respectively.[7]

A setting in which the application of the continuity equation appears more feasible is the evaluation of the velocity changes within the stented segment in order to detect segments of residual lumen reduction requiring further stent expansion (Fig. 32.1), but the practical application of the technique requires further refinements in transducer technology.

Post-stenotic flow measurements

The tip of the Doppler guidewire should be advanced at least 2 cm distal to the stenosis to avoid recordings in segments of post-stenotic flow turbulence. The Doppler signal should be optimized by gentle rotation/advancement/withdrawal until an intense flow velocity envelope, with optimal automatic tracking of the systo-diastolic signal is obtained. To increase the reproducibility of measurements it is essential to maintain a fixed, maximally vasodilated vessel area at the site of measurement. An intracoronary injection of 100–300 mg of intracoronary nitroglycerin or 1–3 mg of isosorbide dinitrate can be used. Basal velocity should be recorded after stabilization of the signal (at least 2–3 min after injection of nitrates or contrast) and should be followed by the injection of a maximally vasodilating dose of papaverine or adenosine to measure coronary flow reserve. An automatic detection system is available to search for the peak hyperemic velocity and calculate and display the coronary flow reserve. Duplicate flow reserve measurements are highly recommended. Flow obstruction due to the guiding catheter engaged in the coronary ostium is rarely observed with the routine use of small (6–7F) guiding catheters but should be excluded with a careful monitoring of the pressure waveform during hyperemia (pressure damping).

The Doppler guidewire can be detached from the rotary connection and used to advance percutaneous transluminal coronary angioplasty (PTCA) balloons or other interventional devices. Afterwards, the wire can be reconnected to monitor the flow velocity changes during and immediately after PTCA and repeat the flow reserve assessment after treatment.

Assessment of coronary flow reserve

Rationale

The principle of flow reserve has been established by the original work of Gould, Lipscomb, and Hamilton.[11] The presence of a flow limiting stenosis in a major epicardial vessel generates a pressure drop across the stenotic lesion which is the result of viscous and turbulent resistances. Only for extremely severe stenoses (>90% diameter stenosis), however, the pressure drop at rest is such that a reduction in baseline velocity occurs. To study the effect of stenoses in the 40% to 90% diameter stenosis range, it is necessary to induce a complete vasodilatation of the distal resistance vessels, thereby unmasking the flow limitation induced by the epicardial stenosis.

In animal experiments, flow reserve discriminantly detects lesions of increasing severity.[11,12] Although the concept can be easily and accurately applied in an optimal physiological situation in humans,[13,14] it should be recognized that coronary flow reserve is influenced by several factors independent from the hydrodynamic characteristics of the stenotic lesion. Since flow reserve is a ratio, changes

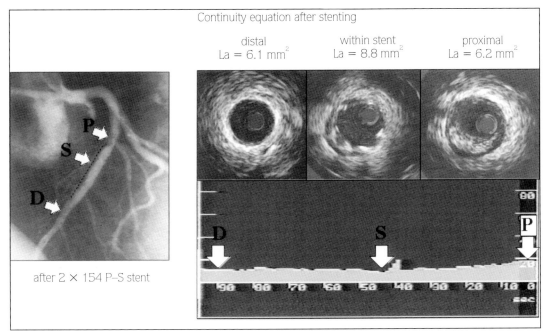

a

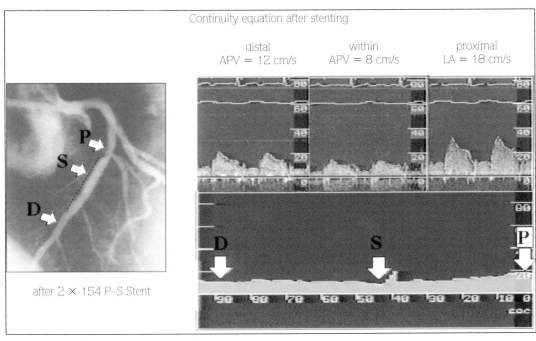

b

Fig. 32.1

(a) Left panel: angiographic result after implantation of two 14-mm Palmaz–Schatz (P–S) stents. Three ultrasonic cross-sections distal, within the stent, and proximal to the stent are shown and measured. Note that these three positions are also indicated in the velocity trend recorded during the pull-back of the Doppler guidewire. (b) Corresponding Doppler measurements. Note that a reduction in flow velocity occurs at the site of the increased lumen area within the stent. Note also the optimal recordings obtained throughout the pull-back with the exception of a minor artefact within the stent. APV = time-averaged peak velocity.

in resting flow without changes in hyperemic flow will considerably affect the result. Furthermore, factors such as heart rate, preload, myocardial hypertrophy or disease of the microvasculature,[15] which affect the hyperemic pressure flow relationship, would modify the flow reserve and thereby change the assessment of the severity of the coronary lesion under study.

Pharmacologic agents

An increase in coronary blood flow can be observed during reactive hyperemia induced by transluminal occlusion or by pharmacologically induced hyperemia. Widely used vasodilator agents are:

- dipyridamole,
- nitroglycerin,
- papaverine,
- adenosine.

The hyperosmolar ionic and low osmolar non-ionic contrast media cannot be used because they do not produce maximal vasodilatation. Likewise, the nitrates have a predominant effect on large conductance vessels and do not consistently induce a maximal flow increase. Continuous infusion of an adequate dose of dipyridamole results in maximal coronary vasodilation, but it has the disadvantage of a long duration of action. In dogs, the hyperemic response after an intracoronary bolus injection of adenosinetriphosphate or papaverine is of the same magnitude as that occurring after a 15-second occlusion of the coronary artery.[16] The dosage range of intracoronary papaverine needed to produce maximal coronary vasodilation has been established in humans by Wilson and White.[17] Papaverine in this dosage range (8–12 mg) produced a response equal to that of an intravenous infusion of dipyridamole in a dose of 0.56–0.84 mg/kg of body weight.

The coronary vasodilation after intravenous or intracoronary adenosine is of a comparable magnitude to that observed after papaverine, with the advantage that the time from intracoronary injection of adenosine to peak hyperemia, as well as the total duration of the hyperemic response, is about four times shorter.[18] Furthermore, intracoronary adenosine does not prolong the QT-interval, avoids the potentially dangerous ventricular arrhythmias observed after papaverine,[19] and does not induce significant changes in heart rate or blood pressure or side-effects. A continuous intravenous infusion of 140 µg/kg/min of adenosine also induces maximal coronary vasodilation but is associated with the presence of mild hypotension and bradycardia and the frequent development of flushing, chest discomfort, headache, dyspnea, and first to second degree atrioventricular block (<10%).[20] In view of the extremely high safety profile, the absence of side-effects to the patient and easiness of use, low dose intracoronary adenosine is the agent and route of administration of choice.

Normal range and correlation with perfusion scintigraphy

Intracoronary papaverine has been reported to increase coronary blood flow velocity four–six times the resting value in patients with normal coronary arteries.[13] In these series, however, a highly selected patient population was studied, with the exclusion of myocardial hypertrophy, previous myocardial infarction, or any other condition known to increase the baseline flow (anemia, hyperthyroidism, etc.).

In unselected patients undergoing percutaneous coronary interventions, coronary flow reserve, measured in arteries without hemodynamically significant coronary artery stenosis, was equal to 2.9±0.95, with a large individual variability (range 2.1–4.2).[21] Similar results have been obtained using intracoronary adenosine by the St Louis group in a large control group of 490 patients which included patients with chest pain and angiographically normal arteries, arteries without stenoses in patients with significant coronary artery disease, and cardiac transplant recipients.[22]

Various groups have investigated the correlation of coronary flow reserve measured with Doppler flow wires and Tl[201] or Tc[99]MIBI-SPECT. Myocardial perfusion scintigraphy assesses relative differences of myocardial perfusion in the territory of distribution of different arteries, but despite this basic difference a good clinical correlation was observed (Fig. 32.2). A cut-off value between 1.7 and 2.0 of coronary flow reserve can identify more than 90% of patients with abnormal scintigraphy.[23–27] To improve the diagnostic accuracy of the test and to identify false positive flow reserve measurements (normal scintigraphy with <2.0 flow reserve), the measurement of flow reserve in a second artery without significant stenoses has been advocated (relative flow reserve) (Fig. 32.3). A direct application of this method in the catheterization laboratory is cumbersome and not feasible in all patients, since it requires the presence of a normal artery for comparison.

Diastolic-to-systolic flow velocity ratio

In contrast with the flow characteristics of most arterial districts, coronary blood flow has a distinctive and unique phasic pattern, with a higher flow in diastole than in systole.

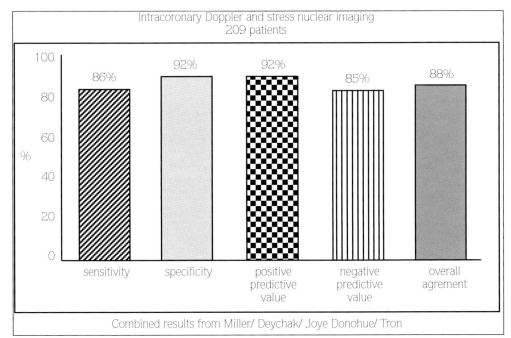

Intracoronary Doppler and stress nuclear imaging
209 patients

86% 92% 92% 85% 88%

sensitivity | specificity | positive predictive value | negative predictive value | overall agrement

Combined results from Miller/ Deychak/ Joye Donohue/ Tron

Fig. 32.2
Sensitivity, specificity, positive and negative predictive value and overall agreement of a metaanalysis of five studies.[23–27] Coronary flow reserve cut-off was 2.0[23–25] and 1.8.[26,27]

Squeezing of the capillary network owing to the increase in tissue pressure during myocardial contraction explains this phenomenon which characterizes the Doppler tracings obtained in the left coronary system or in the distal right coronary artery (RCA). In the proximal RCA, a similar amplitude of the systolic and diastolic components is observed because of the lower pressure which develops in the right ventricle.[28]

Experimental and intra-operative human studies have shown that the predominance of diastolic flow is decreased in the presence of a significant epicardial stenosis.[29,30] Similar flow patterns have been observed in arteries with significant stenoses, with a noticeable difference with the flow patterns recorded in normal arteries or in the same arteries after coronary angioplasty.[31–33] Unfortunately, the practical applicability of the diastolic-to-systolic velocity ratio in individual cases is limited by the large variability of this index, which is influenced by changes in myocardial contractility, the site of measurement[34] and measurements artefacts.

Proximal-to-distal ratio

A minor reduction in flow velocity is present from proximal to distal in normal coronary arteries, and is explained by the progressive reduction in the luminal cross-sectional area as the flow is distributed to side-branches along the proximal to distal vessel course. The gradual pattern of velocity decrease in epicardial normal arteries is drastically modified in the presence of a significant coronary stenosis which induces a reduction of post-stenotic velocity because of flow redistribution in the lower resistance branches proximal to the stenosis.

The ratio of proximal to distal flow velocity is significantly lower in normal arteries than in arteries with significant stenoses.[35] Based on clinical studies assessing the pressure gradient and the results of myocardial scintigraphy,[33,35] a cut-off value of 1.7 has been proposed to identify hemodynamically significant stenoses. Major limitations, however, are encountered in the practical use of this index. As previously reported, flow velocity proximal to the stenosis can be measured only in two-thirds of patients.[7] In the RCA or in bypass grafts, vessels characterized by an absence of important side-branches along the vessel course, no significant redistribution of flow occurs.[34]

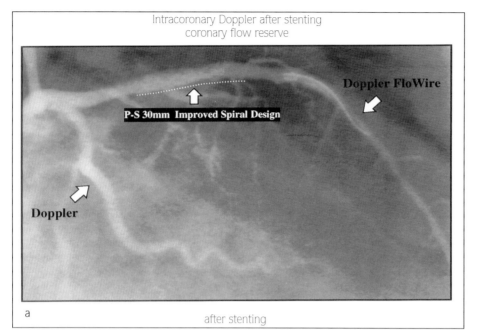

Intracoronary Doppler after stenting
coronary flow reserve

P-S 30mm Improved Spiral Design

Doppler FloWire

Doppler

a

after stenting

Fig. 32.3
(a) Angiographic result after elective stent implantation of a 30-mm long Palmaz–Schatz stent in the proximal left anterior descending coronary artery (LAD) after recanalization of a chronic total occlusion. Arrowheads indicate the position of the Doppler guidewire in the LAD and left circumflex arteries. (b) Coronary flow reserve (CRF) measured in the LAD after stenting. (c) Coronary flow reserve (CRF) in the left circumflex artery, untreated and without angiographically visible stenoses, used as a reference vessel. The calculated relative flow reserve (1.1) can be considered within normal limits (10% variability has been shown in measurements performed in all three major arteries in control normal subjects).
APV = time-averaged peak velocity.

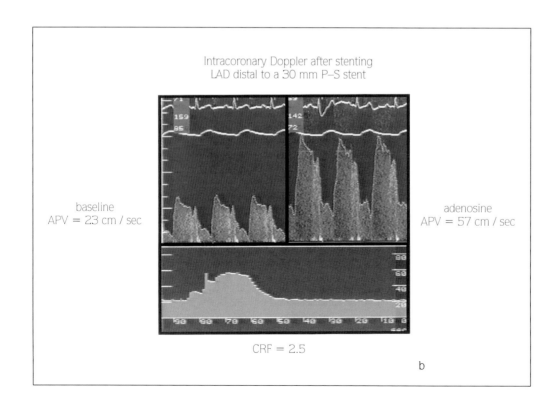

Intracoronary Doppler after stenting
LAD distal to a 30 mm P–S stent

baseline
APV = 23 cm / sec

adenosine
APV = 57 cm / sec

CRF = 2.5

b

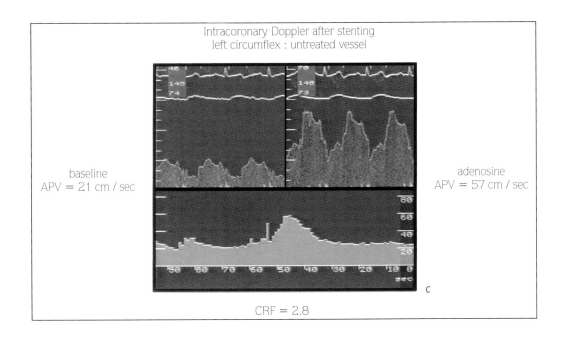

Intracoronary Doppler after stenting
left circumflex : untreated vessel

baseline
APV = 21 cm / sec

adenosine
APV = 57 cm / sec

c

CRF = 2.8

Clinical applications

Assessment of patients with chest pain and angiographically normal vessels

The presence of normal or near-normal coronary arteries in patients with typical chest pain and/or evidence of ischemia during non-invasive tests is observed in 10–20% of patients undergoing coronary angiography. When the presence of vasospasm or of significant non-angiographically-evident lesions (ostial or bifurcation lesions) is ruled out, the cause of the symptoms or of the signs of ischemia remains to be investigated. The presence of microvascular disease with flow reserve impairment has been proposed and flow reserve measurements can be performed to confirm this etiology.[36] Contradictory results have been reported: these are probably explained by differences in inclusion criteria and methodology.[37,38] The most recent large experience indicates that the flow velocity response in this population is heterogeneous and suggests the importance of assessing not only the flow velocity changes induced by endothelial independent vasodilators such as adenosine but also the endothelium-mediated response, which was impaired in a subset of these patients.[39,40] This assessment, however, has not been used for guidance of

new therapeutic strategies. Longitudinal studies are still missing and so cannot confirm the therapeutic and long-term prognostic value of these findings.

Transplant vasculopathy

Pathology reports describe transplant arteriopathy as a diffuse disease involving vessels smaller than 400 μm and potentially resulting in a reduction of maximal flow. The initial experience with Doppler catheters documented a normal flow reserve in these patients.[41] More recent studies using Doppler guidewires suggest that the maximal flow velocity increase in these patients is frequently impaired, with a dissociation between flow impairment and the presence and severity of the intimal thickening of the epicardial vessels, as assessed by intracoronary ultrasound.[42,43]

Intermediate stenosis

The clinical dilemma of lesions with a diameter reduction of 40% to 60% in multiple angiographic projections is a daily experience for the angiographer. At the time of catheterization rarely has the presence of ischemia in the distribution territory been unequivocally confirmed or ruled out by non-invasive tests. In particular, provocative tests are not performed in patients with unstable coronary syndromes who are directly referred to the catheterization laboratory based on electrocardiographic (ECG) abnormalities at rest. In patients with multivessel disease, the test most frequently performed (ECG during bicycle or treadmill stress test) is unable to identify the location of the ischemic area. Also more specific tests such as perfusion scintigraphy or stress-echocardiography are not always able to discriminate between the relative contributions of stenoses involving contiguous territories of distribution. The common practice with coronary artery bypass surgery (CABG) is to perform a revascularization as completely as possible, by treating arteries with intermediate stenoses since additional coronary anastomoses do not increase the surgical risk. Moreover, according to the worst case hypothesis (lesions hemodynamically not yet significant), a patent graft will have a preventive role in case of stenosis progression. With percutaneous interventions only hemodynamically significant lesions must be treated, because of the additional risk of multivessel treatment for immediate

complications and late restenosis. Further non-invasive investigations are thus required, precluding the possibility of an immediate percutaneous treatment at the time of the diagnostic procedure[44]—thus prolonging the in-hospital stay and adding further to treatment cost and patient discomfort.[45] A method which is able to establish the importance of an intermediate stenosis at the time of initial catheterization or angioplasty of the most severe vessel would be of great clinical usefulness. In a proportion of cases, the combination of quantitative angiography with intracoronary ultrasound (ICUS) may help to solve the clinical dilemma proposed by angiographically intermediate stenoses that remain ambiguous on a purely visual analysis of the angiogram; however, the most effective analysis of intermediate stenoses severity in the catheterization laboratory is made with functional investigations. As previously discussed, coronary flow reserve measured with intracoronary Doppler is well-correlated with the results of radioisotopic perfusion tests[23-27] and large clinical studies have reported the safety of deferring angioplasty based on the results of flow velocity measurements[46-48] (Fig. 32.4).

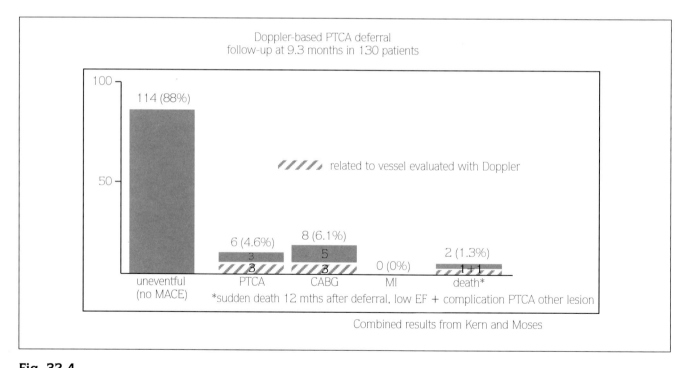

Fig. 32.4
Metaanalysis of two studies[46,47] including 130 patients in whom at least one lesion was not treated because of normal translesional velocity and/or pressure measurements. CABG, coronary artery bypass graft; MACE, major adverse cardiac events; MI, myocardial infarction; PTCA, percutaneous transluminal coronary angioplasty.

Applications during coronary interventions

Percutaneous transluminal balloon angioplasty

The angiographic evaluation of coronary interventions is limited by the presence of wall disruption so that the true lumen which is free for blood passage cannot be easily assessed. ICUS gives a better definition of presence and severity of wall disruption after angioplasty and has been instrumental in teaching interventional cardiologists that many cases of recurrent symptoms after PTCA were not due to restenosis but were the result of an insufficient initial lumen enlargement.[49] ICUS, however, requires the separate insertion of a new catheter and is not always able to determine whether the complex neolumen created by the dilatation is sufficient to normalize vascular conductance. Intracoronary Doppler is an appealing alternative since this

technique can precisely determine the functional severity of a coronary stenosis and can be easily integrated into a standard interventional procedure.

Balloon angioplasty improves the flow velocity parameters[32,33,50] but despite a good angiographic result an incomplete normalization is observed in a subset of patients. Hemodynamic changes during the procedure, microembolization, or transient or persistent changes of the distal microvascular response may explain part of this discrepancy, as indicated by the late normalization in some lesions.[51] In other cases, however, the abnormal flow response may reflect the persistence of a severe residual stenosis. A recently completed multicenter study has shown that a persistent impairment in flow reserve after PTCA is associated with a higher incidence of persistence or recurrence of angina or positive exercise test at 1 month[52] and of target lesion revascularization at 6 months (Fig. 32.5).[53] The combination of an optimal angiographic result (<35% diameter stenosis) and of a flow reserve equal or greater than 2.5 was associated with a favourable clinical outcome at 6 months (16% incidence of major

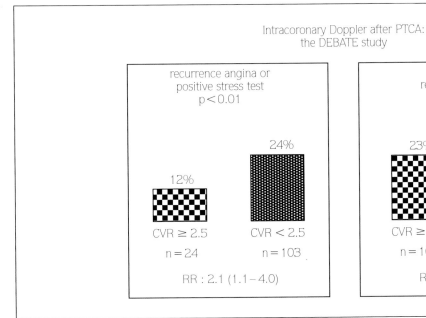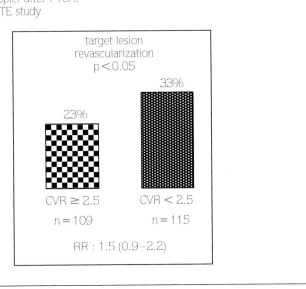

Fig. 32.5
Early (left panel) and six months (right panel) follow-up results in 224 patients enrolled in the DEBATE trial. Note that a coronary velocity reserve (CVR) ≥2.5 was predictive of a better immediate and long-term clinical outcome.
RR: relative risk (confidence intervals between brackets).

adverse cardiac events)[54]. Based on these observations, different groups are testing the hypothesis that the combination of angiographic and functional end-points can be used to identify the lesions with a worse prognosis after PTCA alone and which require additional treatment.[55] The absence of cyclic flow variations, a condition at risk for abrupt occlusion and the restoration of a normal flow velocity reserve almost exclude the development of immediate complications after PTCA,[56,57] suggesting the clinical relevance of these measurements in the case of long dissections or of suboptimal PTCA results which appear not to favour stent implantation (long lesions, small vessels).

Rotational and directional coronary atherectomy

Unlike balloon angioplasty, a flow velocity improvement is rarely observed after rotational atherectomy, because of persistent flow impairment despite optimal angiographic results and a regular circular lumen demonstrated with ultrasound. The microembolization of minute particles of plaque debris may explain this phenomenon, which limits the role of intracoronary Doppler for the assessment of the results for this specific intervention.[58] Similarly, the higher frequency of platelet emboli created by the repeated passes of the atherectomy cutter, which is responsible for the higher frequency of non-Q-wave myocardial infarction in comparison with PTCA, might explain the lower average flow reserve increase observed after atherectomy in comparison with PTCA.

Stent implantation

For stent implantation, intracoronary Doppler can be used to limit the treatment after balloon angioplasty to lesions with an insufficient functional recovery.[54,55] In selected patients, without factors impairing the peripheral coronary vascular resistances and after short balloon inflations at conventional pressures, a normalization of flow velocity reserve has been shown after stenting, with a large increase in comparison with the velocity reserve after balloon angioplasty alone.[59–61] When a large consecutive series is considered and repeated high pressure dilatations are performed in order to obtain an optimal stent expansion, lower flow velocity reserves are observed, with values below 2.0 in almost 30% of cases despite the complete absence of residual lumen stenosis as confirmed by ICUS.[62,63] Although a low flow reserve after stenting has been suggested as a predictive factor for restenosis based on anecdotal cases,[64] more recent larger experiences do not support this statement.[63]

Acute myocardial infarction

Flow velocity measurements do not correlate with angiographic TIMI flow or frame count to disappearance of contrast. In particular, a very low flow velocity is observed in the majority of patients with TIMI 2 flow, showing on average no difference with TIMI 1[65] and suggesting that an incomplete recanalization is responsible for the poor prognosis and limited recovery of left ventricular function in these cases.[66,67] Continuous monitoring of flow velocity with the Doppler guidewire confirms the restoration of blood flow after thrombolysis and the persistence of anterograde flow in the hours following thrombolysis.[68,69] Confirmation that a persistent flow impairment is present in many patients with angiographically successful thrombolysis is the flow velocity improvement observed after PTCA and stenting. In other patients, however, flow velocity remains low despite optimal treatment of the epicardial stenoses. An abnormal pattern of early systolic retrograde flow and prolonged diastolic flow velocity has been shown to be associated with the presence of a 'no reflow' phenomenon.[70]

Conclusion

The coronary Doppler guidewire is the first applicable method for the assessment of coronary stenosis severity in the everyday practice of a busy catheterization laboratory. For intermediate stenoses, post-stenotic Doppler flow reserve is well-correlated with the results of non-invasive nuclear stress tests, and has the potential to assess directly the functional severity of coronary stenoses in the catheterization laboratory. Despite the encouraging results of a large observational study after balloon angioplasty,[54] the rationale for using Doppler for decision-making during coronary interventions still needs to be established in prospective randomized trials. In individual cases (e.g. doubtful results after PTCA, especially if not ideal for stent implantation), it is current practice in many centers to use post-stenotic flow monitoring and measurement of flow reserve to exclude the persistence of a severe flow limitation and the risk of early occlusion.

Intracoronary Doppler has raised a new interest in the physiologic assessment of stenosis severity and stimulated the application of new methods of assessment such as fractional flow reserve,[71–78] an index based on post-stenotic pressure measurements during maximal hyperemia which can overcome many of the previously discussed limitations of velocity-based flow reserve:

- measurement variability,
- dependency on hemodynamic conditions at the time of measurement,[79,80]

- inability to differentiate flow impairment because of epicardial stenoses and microvascular disease.

When flexible and detachable pressure sensors become available, the complete assessment of translesional hemodynamics by velocity and pressure sensors[81] will offer new possibilities in the catheterization laboratory to improve diagnostic assessment and the treatment of coronary stenoses.

References

1   Hartley CJ, Cole JS. An ultrasonic pulsed Doppler system for measuring blood flow in small vessels. *J Applied Physiol* 1974; **37**: 626–32.

2   Kern MJ, Courtois M, Ludbrook P. A simplified method to measure coronary blood flow velocity in patients: validation and application of a new Judkins style Doppler tipped angiographic catheter. *Am Heart J* 1990; **120**: 1202–7.

3   Wilson RF, Laughlin DE, Ackell PH, et al. Transluminal, subselective measurement of coronary artery blood flow velocity and vasodilator reserve in man. *Circulation* 1985; **72**: 82–92.

4   Sibley DH, Millar H, Hartley CJ, Whitlow PL. Subselective measurement of coronary blood flow velocity using a steerable Doppler catheter. *J Am Coll Cardiol* 1986; **8**: 1332–40.

5   Doucette JW, Corl DP, Payne HP, et al. Validation of a Doppler guide wire for intravascular measurement of coronary artery flow velocity. *Circulation* 1992; **85**: 1899–911.

6   Tadaoka S, Kagiyama M, Hiramatsu O, et al. Accuracy of 20 MHz Doppler catheter coronary artery velocimetry for measurement of coronary blood flow velocity. *Cathet Cardiovasc Diagn* 1990; **19**: 205–13.

7   Di Mario C, Serruys PW, on behalf of the DEBATE Study Group: Doppler guide wire as a primary guide wire for PTCA. Feasibility, safety and continuous monitoring of the results. *Circulation* 1995; **92**: 1255 (abstract).

8   Nakatami S, Yamagishi M, Tamai J, Takaki H, Haze K, Miyatake K. Quantitative assessment of coronary artery stenosis by intravascular Doppler catheter technique. *Circulation* 1992; **85**: 1786–91.

9   Di Mario C, Meneveau N, Gil R, et al. Maximal blood flow velocity in severe coronary stenoses measured with a Doppler guidewire. *Am J Cardiol* 1993; **71**: 54D–61D.

10 Yuan YW, Shung KK. Ultrasonic backscatter from flowing whole blood. *J Acoust Soc Am* 1988; **84**: 52–8.

11 Gould KL, Lipscomb K, Hamilton GW. Physiologic basis for assessing critical coronary stenosis: instantaneous flow response and regional distribution during coronary hyperemia as measures of coronary flow reserve. *Am J Cardiol* 1974; **33**: 87–94.

12 Klocke FJ. Measurements of coronary flow reserve: defining pathophysiology versus making decisions about patient care. *Circulation* 1987; **76**: 245–53.

13 Wilson RF, Marcus ML, White CW. Prediction of the physiologic significance of coronary arterial lesions by quantitative lesion geometry in patients with limited coronary artery disease. *Circulation* 1987; **75**: 723–32.

14 Harrison DG, White CW, Hiratzkam LF, Eastha CL, Marcus ML. The value of lesional cross-sectional area determined by quantitative coronary angiography in assessing the physiologic significance of proximal left anterior descending coronary artery stenoses. *Circulation* 1984; **69**: 111–19.

15 Klocke FJ. Cognition in the era of technology: 'seeing the shades of gray'. *J Am Coll Cardiol* 1990; **16**: 763–9.

16 Bookstein JJ, Higgins CB. Comparative efficacy of coronary vasodilatory methods. *Investigational Radiology* 1977; **12**: 121–32.

17 Wilson RF, White CW. Intracoronary papaverine: an ideal coronary vasodilator for studies of the coronary circulation in conscious humans. *Circulation* 1986; **73**: 444–51.

18 Wilson RF, Wyche K, Christensen BV, Laxson DD. Effects of adenosine on human coronary arterial circulation. *Circulation* 1990; **82**: 1595–606.

19 Wilson RF, White CW. Serious ventricular dysrhythmias after intracoronary papaverine. *Am J Cardiol* 1988; **62**: 1301–5.

20 Kern MJ, Deligonul U, Aguirre F, Hilton TC. Intravenous adenosine: continuous infusion and low dose bolus administration for determination of coronary vasodilator reserve in patients with and without coronary artery disease. *J Am Coll Cardiol* 1991; **18**: 718–31.

21 Serruys PW, Di Mario C, Kern MJ. Intracoronary Doppler. In: Topol EJ (ed.). *Textbook of Interventional Cardiology* (Philadelphia: WB Saunders, 1994): 1324–404.

22 Kern MJ, Donohue TJ. Doppler assessment of coronary blood flow. *Am J Cardiol* 1996; **78**: 520–5.

23 Donohue TJ, Miller DD, Bach RG, et al. Correlation of poststenotic hyperemic coronary flow velocity and pressure with abnormal stress myocardial perfusion imaging in coronary artery disease. *Am J Cardiol* 1996; **77**: 948–54.

24 Miller DD, Donohue TJ, Younis LT, et al. Correlation of

pharmacological ^{99m}Tc-SestaMIBI myocardial perfusion imaging with post-stenotic coronary flow reserve in patients with angiographically intermediate artery stenoses. *Circulation* 1994; **89**: 2150–60.

25 Tron C, Donohue TJ, Bach RG, *et al.* Comparison of pressure-derived fractional flow reserve with poststenotic coronary flow velocity reserve for prediction of stress myocardial perfusion imaging results. *Am Heart J* 1995; **130**: 723–33.

26 Joye JD, Schulman DS, Lasorda D, *et al.* Intracoronary Doppler guide wire versus stress single photon emission computed tomographic Thallium-201 imaging in assessment of intermediate coronary stenoses. *J Am Coll Cardiol* 1994; **24**: 940–7.

27 Deychak YA, Segal J, Reiner SR, *et al.* Doppler guide wire flow velocity indexes measured distal to coronary stenoses associated with reversible thallium perfusion defects. *Am Heart J* 1995; **129**: 219–27.

28 Sabistom DC jr, Gregg DE. Effect of cardiac contraction on coronary blood flow. *Circulation* 1957; **15**: 14–23.

29 Kajiya F, Ogasawara Y, Tsujioka K. Evaluation of human coronary blood flow with an 80 channel 20 MHz pulsed Doppler velocimeter and zero-cross and Fourier transform methods during cardiac surgery. *Circulation* 1986; **74 (Suppl III)**: III-53–III-59.

30 Kajiya F, Ogasawara Y, Tsujioka K. Analysis of flow characteristics in post-stenotic regions of the human coronary artery during bypass graft surgery. *Circulation* 1987; **76**: 1092–7.

31 Ofili EO, Labovitz AJ, Kern MJ. Coronary flow dynamics in normal and diseased artery. *Am J Cardiol* 1993; **71**: 3D–9D.

32 Segal J, Kern MJ, Scott NA. Alteration of phasic coronary artery flow velocity in human during percutaneous coronary angioplasty. *J Am Coll Cardiol* 1992; **20**: 276–86.

33 Ofili EO, Kern MJ, Labovitz AJ, *et al.* Analysis of coronary blood flow velocity dynamics in angiographically normal and stenosed arteries before and after endolumen enlargement by angioplasty. *J Am Coll Cardiol* 1993; **21**: 308–16.

34 Heller LI, Silver KH, Vilegas BJ, Balcom SH, Weiner BH. Blood flow velocity in the right coronary artery: assessment before and after angioplasty. *J Am Coll Cardiol* 1994; **24**: 1012–17.

35 Donohue TJ, Kern MJ, Aguirre FV, Ofili EO. Assessing the hemodynamic significance of coronary artery stenosis: analysis of translesional pressure-flow velocity relationship in patients. *J Am Coll Cardiol* 1993; **22**: 449–58.

36 Cannon RO, Schenke WH, Leon MB, Rosing DR, Urquhart J, Epstein SE. Limited coronary flow reserve after

dipyridamole in patients with ergonovine-induced coronary vasoconstriction. *Circulation* 1987; **75**: 163–74.

37 Chauhan A, Mullins PA, Petch MC, Schofield PM. Is coronary flow reserve in response to papaverine really normal in syndrome X? *Circulation* 1994; **89**: 1998–2004.

38 Rosen SD, Uren NG, Kaski JC, Tousoulis D, Davis GJ, Camici PG. Coronary vasodilator reserve, pain perception, and sex in patients with syndrome X. *Circulation* 1994; **90**: 50–60.

39 Erbel R, Ge A, Bockisch A, *et al.* Value of intracoronary ultrasound and Doppler in the differentiation of angiographically normal coronary arteries: a prospective study in patients with angina pectoris. *Eur Heart J* 1996; **17**: 880–9.

40 Quyyumi AA, Cannon RO III, Panza JA, Diodati JG, Epstein SE. Endothelial dysfunction in patients with chest pain and normal coronary arteries. *Circulation* 1992; **86**: 1864–71.

41 McGinn AL, Wilson RF, Oliver MT, Homans DC, White CW. Coronary vasodilator reserve after human orthotopic cardiac transplantation. *Circulation* 1988; **78**: 1200–9.

42 Wolford T, Kern MJ. Assessment of transplant arteriopathy by intracoronary two-dimensional ultrasound imaging and coronary flow velocity. *Cathet Cardiovasc Diagn* 1995; **35**: 335–42.

43 Caracciolo EA, Wolford TL, Underwood RD, *et al.* Influence of intimal thickening on coronary blood flow responses in orthotopic heart transplant recipients. *Circulation* 1995; **92 (Suppl II)**: II-182–II-190.

44 Hill JA. Single-stage coronary angiography and angioplasty: a new standard? *Am J Cardiol* 1995; **75**: 75–6.

45 Joye JD, Cates CU, Farah T, *et al.* Cost analysis of intracoronary doppler determination of lesion significance: preliminary results of the PEACH study. *J Invasive Cardiol* 1995; **7**: 22A (abstract).

46 Kern MJ, Donohue TJ, Aguirre FV, *et al.* Clinical outcome of deferring angioplasty in patients with normal translesional pressure-flow velocity measurements. *J Am Coll Cardiol* 1995; **25**: 178–87.

47 Moses JW, Shaknovich A, Kreps EM, Undemir C, Lieberman SM. Clinical follow-up of intermediate coronary lesions not hemodynamically significant by doppler flow wire criteria. *Circulation* 1994; I-227 (abstract).

48 Deychak YA, Segal G, Reiner JS, Nachnani S. Doppler guidewire-derived coronary flow reserve distal to intermediate stenosis used in clinical decision making regarding interventional therapy. *Am Heart J* 1994; **128**: 178–81.

49 Nakamura S, Mahon DJ, Maheswaran B, Gutfinger DE, Colombo A, Tobis JM. An explanation for discrepancy

between angiographic and intravascular ultrasound measurements after percutaneous transluminal coronary angioplasty. *J Am Coll Cardiol* 1995; **25**: 633–9.

50 Serruys PW, Di Mario C, Meneveau N, *et al*. Intracoronary pressure and flow velocity from sensor tip guidewires. A new methodological comprehensive approach for the assessment of coronary hemodynamics before and after interventions. *Am J Cardiol* 1993; **71**: 41D–53D.

51 Wilson RF, Johnson MR, Marcus ML, *et al*. The effect of coronary angioplasty on coronary blood flow reserve. *Circulation* 1988; **71**: 873–85.

52 Sunamura M, Di Mario C, Piek JJ, *et al*. Intracoronary Doppler guidewire during angioplasty. Results of the second interim analysis. In: de Feyter PJ, Di Mario C, Serruys PW (eds). *Quantitative Coronary Imaging* (Delft: Barjesteh, Meeuwes & Co, 1995): 267–80.

53 Serruys PW, Di Mario C, on behalf of the DEBATE Study Group. Are flow velocity measurements after PTCA predictive of recurrence of angina or of positive exercise stress test early after balloon angioplasty? *Circulation* 1995; **92**: 1257 (abstract).

54 Serruys PW, Di Mario C. Prognostic value of coronary flow velocity and diameter stenosis in assessing the short and long term outcome of balloon angioplasty: the DEBATE Study. *Circulation* 1996; **34**: I-317 (abstract).

55 Di Mario C, Muramatsu T, Moses J, *et al*. on behalf of the DESTINI-CRF Study Group. Aggressive dilatation strategy to optimize the angiographic and functional PTCA result: preliminary results of the DESTINI study. *Eur Heart J* 1997; in press (abstract).

56 Anderson HV, Kirkeeide R, Stuart Y, Smalling RW, Heibing J, Willerson T. Coronary artery flow monitoring following coronary interventions. *Am J Cardiol* 1993; **71**: 62D–69D.

57 Sunamura M, Di Mario C, Serruys PW, on behalf of the DEBATE Study Group. Cyclic flow variations after angioplasty: a rare phenomenon predictive of immediate complications. *Am Heart J* 1996; **132**: 960–8.

58 Kumar K, Dorros G, Jain A, *et al*. Coronary flow measurements following rotational ablation (atherectomy). *Am J Cardiol* 1994; **32**: 97 (abstract).

59 Ge J, Erbel R, Zamorano J, *et al*. Improvement of coronary morphology and blood flow after stenting. *Int J Cardiovasc Imaging* 1995; **11**: 81–7.

60 Verna E, Gil R, Di Mario C, Sunamura M, Gurne O, Porenta G, on behalf of the DEBATE Study Group. Does coronary stenting following angioplasty improve distal coronary flow reserve? *Circulation* 1995; **92**: I-551.

61 Haude M, Baumgart D, Caspari G, Erbel R. Does adjunct coronary stenting in comparison to balloon angioplasty

have an impact on Doppler flow velocity parameters? *Circulation* 1995; **92**: I-547 (abstract).

62 Vrints CJ, Claeys MJ, Bosmans J, Snoeck JP. Coronary stenting after suboptimal PTCA does not lead to normalization of distal coronary flow reserve. *Circulation* 1996; **94**: I-135 (abstract).

63 Di Francesco L, Di Mario C, Reimers B, *et al*. A low coronary flow reserve after stenting is not predictive of an adverse clinical outcome. *Eur Heart J* 1997; in press (abstract).

64 Hong MK, Wong SC, Mintz GS, *et al*. Can coronary flow parameters after stent placement predict restenosis? *Cathet Cardiovasc Diagn* 1995; **36**: 278–89.

65 Moore JA, Kern MJ, Donohue TJ, *et al*. Disparity of TIMI grade flow and directly measured coronary flow velocity during direct angioplasty for acute myocardial infarction. *Cathet Cardiovasc Diagn* 1994; **32**: 86 (abstract).

66 Karagounis L, Sorensen SG, Menlove RL, Moreno F, Anderson JL, for the TEAM-2 Investigators. Does Thrombolysis In Myocardial Infarction (TIMI) perfusion grade 2 represent a mostly patent artery or mostly occluded artery? Enzymatic and electrocardiographic evidence from the TEAM-2 study. *J Am Coll Cardiol* 1992; **19**: 1–10.

67 Keiman NS, White HD, Ohman EM, *et al*. for the GUSTO Investigators. Mortality within 24 hours of thrombolysis for myocardial infarction: the importance of early reperfusion. *Circulation* 1994; **90**: 2658–65.

68 Gershony G, Cishek MB, Galloway M. Intracoronary Doppler flow to monitor the results of selective saphenous vein graft thrombolytic therapy. *Cathet Cardiovasc Diagn* 1995; **35**: 277–81.

69 Tsunoda T, Nakamura M, Wakatsuki T, *et al*. Continuous monitoring of coronary flow velocity in acute myocardial infarction using Doppler guidewire. *Circulation* 1994; **90**: I-449 (abstract).

70 Iwakura K, Ito H, Takiuchi S, *et al*. Alteration in the coronary blood flow velocity pattern in patients with no reflow and reperfused acute myocardial infarction. *Circulation* 1996; **94**: 1261–75.

71 Pijls NHJ, van Son JAM, Kirkeeide RL, Bruyne BD, Gould KL. Experimental basis of determining maximum coronary, myocardial, and collateral blood flow by pressure measurements for assessing functional stenosis severity before and after percutaneous transluminal coronary angioplasty. *Circulation* 1993; **86**: 1354–67.

72 Pijls NHJ, Van Gelder B, Van der Voort P, *et al*. Fractional flow reserve: a useful index to evaluate the influence of an epicardial coronary stenosis on myocardial blood flow. *Circulation* 1995; **92**: 3183–93.

73   De Bruyne B, Paulus WJ, Pijls NHJ. Rationale and application of coronary transstenotic pressure gradient measurements. *Cathet Cardiovasc Diagn* 1994; **33**: 250–61.

74   De Bruyne B, Baudhuin T, Melin JA, *et al.* Coronary flow reserve calculated from pressure measurements in humans: validation with positron emission tomography. *Circulation* 1994; **89**: 1013–22.

75   De Bruyne B, Bartunek J, Sys SU, Heyndrickx GR. Relation between myocardial fractional flow reserve calculated from coronary pressure measurements and exercise-induced myocardial ischemia. *Circulation* 1995; **92**: 39–46.

76   Bartunek J, Sys SU, Heyndrickx GR, Pijls NH, De Bruyne B. Quantitative coronary angiography in predicting functional significance of stenoses in an unselected patient cohort. *J Am Coll Cardiol* 1995; **26**: 328–34.

77   Pijls NHJ, De Bruyne B, Peels K, *et al.* Measurement of fractional flow reserve to assess the functional severity of coronary-artery stenoses. *N Engl J Med* 1996; **334**: 1703–8.

78   Bartunek J, Marwick TH, Rodrigues AC, *et al.* Dobutamine-induced wall motion abnormalities: correlations with myocardial fractional flow reserve and quantitative coronary angiography. *J Am Coll Cardiol* 1996; **27**: 1429–36.

79   Di Mario C, Gil R, Serruys PW. Long-term reproducibility of intracoronary Doppler measurement. *Am J Cardiol* 1995; **75**: 1177–80.

80   De Bruyne B. Variability of invasive indices of coronary stenosis severity. In: de Bruyne B, PhD thesis: Coronary Pressure. From a Physiological Index to a Clinical Tool (University of Louvain Medical Press, 1995): 85–99.

81   Di Mario C, Gil R, de Feyter PJ, Schuurbiers JCH, Serruys PW. Utilization of translesional hemodynamics: comparison of pressure and flow methods in stenosis assessment in patients with coronary artery disease. *Cathet Cardiovasc Diagn* 1996; **38**: 189–201.

VII

Non-Coronary Interventions in the Adult

33

Peripheral angioplasty: a perspective for now and the future

Gerald Dorros and Michael R Jaff

Introduction

In 1964, Dotter percutaneously recanalized a popliteal arterial obstruction with coaxial catheters and this concept, refined by Gruentzig in 1973, developed into the balloon dilation technique now known as angioplasty. Angioplasty today, also described as endovascular surgery, is a primary therapeutic modality for the treatment of obstructed peripheral arteries, and holds promise to be the method for repairing aneurysmal disease and traumatic injury.

The objectives of angioplasty have been to:

- relieve ischemia as a result of lower extremity arteriosclerosis obliterans (LE ASO),

- repair aneurysms without open surgical procedures,

- utilize stent-grafts and covered stents to correct arterial tears, perforations, or dissections.

Correction of ischemia can produce relief of intermittent claudication, the most common clinical manifestation of LE ASO, ischemic rest pain, and promote ischemic wound healing. Often, angioplasty can limit the extent of amputation in patients with critical limb ischemia. Angioplasty of renal arteries is shown to improve renal blood flow, to facilitate control of hypertension and/or preserve renal function by preventing ischemic atrophy. These interventions (whether done with balloons, stents, catheters, or grafts) differ from those of traditional vascular surgery, since reconstruction is achieved with minimal morbidity, diminished hospitalization time, rapid return to work, significant cost effectiveness, and excellent long-term success. However, before any of these new therapeutic alternatives are employed, the physician must be aware of not only what they are, but also what is feasible, possible, and appropriate.[1-6]

Evaluation and diagnostic studies

Medical history

The physician's evaluation will determine the therapy and the timing of the intervention, either with medical therapy, surgery or angioplasty.[7-13] Eliciting the medical history of transient ischemic attacks (TIAs) and stroke, renal dysfunction, cardiac disease (coronary artery disease, congestive heart failure, myocardial infarction, angina pectoris) is a critical first step. Diabetes mellitus, hyperlipidemia, tobacco use, hypertension, and a family history of vascular disease must be included in the history. Intermittent claudication, lower extremity ulcers and non-healing wounds, gangrene, or ischemic rest pain must be covered in the evaluation of the patient with vascular disease.

Physical examination

The physical examination, detailing arterial pulses, presence of bruits, and appearance of and condition of the extremities (trophic changes, capillary filling time, venous filling time, ulcers, non-healing wounds, gangrene) enables a clearer focus upon what needs doing and how to accomplish it, especially with regard to arterial access. Objective noninvasive and invasive data further defines the extent of the disease. Extracranial carotid bifurcation disease requires duplex ultrasonography, magnetic resonance angiography (MRA), and occasionally, contrast angiography. Aneurysmal disease in the descending thoracic or infrarenal aorta requires careful analysis with contrast enhanced helical computerized tomographic (CT) scans. Arterial obliterative disease of the lower extremities requires a graded exercise treadmill test to determine quantitatively the distance traveled and the severity of claudication, establishing a baseline to be used as comparison with post-intervention studies. Color assisted duplex ultrasonography and ankle-brachial indices (ABIs) are mainstay noninvasive evaluations for these patients. Such studies enable accurate assessment of the patient with LE ASO and can clearly define the extent of the obliterative disease in critical limb ischemia patients.

Clinical management

The management of patients with LE ASO involves:

- protection of the limb from trauma,
- avoidance of vasoconstricting factors (beta-blockers, cold temperatures, elimination of smoking),
- control of hypertension, hyperlipidemia and diabetes,
- walking exercise programs,
- consideration to randomization into experimental claudication pharmaceutical trials.

Nevertheless, none of these therapies can relieve the impedance to arterial blood flow which can be achieved by angioplasty and/or surgery. In patients with lifestyle-limiting intermittent claudication or critical limb ischemia, aggressive revascularization is often required.

Arteriography

Assessment

Arteriography has been a key in the invasive assessment of the peripheral vascular patient. Arteriography delineates the obstructive lesion(s) causing the patient's symptoms, the extent and location of all lesions, and the feasibility of various interventional therapies. The digital imaging techniques (acquired and subtraction) and new mechanical freely moveable gantries provide freedom of views and has been crucial in the metamorphosis of standard surgery to percutaneous methods. In addition, the use of non-ionic contrast agents, carbon dioxide as a contrast agent, and helical CT and MRA has allowed acquisition of better

images in all types of patients, including those with severe renal dysfunction or with very poor lower extremity circulation.

Treatment

Assessment of those images, coupled with other data, permits determination of therapeutic choices. Fortunately, the multiple arterial access sites enable virtually all lesions to be treated with endovascular methods:

- the brachial and retrograde femoral approaches are applicable for renal, mesenteric, aorta, iliac, superficial femoral artery, profunda, and brachiocephalic lesions;
- a percutaneous femoral antegrade technique permits therapy of lesions in the femoropopliteal and tibioperoneal arteries;
- the retrograde popliteal approach permits successful angioplasty of occluded femoropopliteal arteries (especially cases in which the origin of the superficial femoral artery is occluded), and iliofemoral lesions;
- the contralateral femoral technique is helpful for disease involving the iliac and femoropopliteal arteries;
- distal common femoral or proximal superficial femoral artery lesions are best approached using the brachial, contralateral, or ipsilateral popliteal approach.

The overwhelming majority of therapies and adjunctive procedures can be accomplished through arterial entry holes of 6–9F (2–3 mm in diameter) which will allow transstenotic pressure gradient measurements, balloon angioplasty, stent deployment, atherectomy, aspiration, intra-arterial Doppler flow, and intravascular ultrasound (IVUS).[14–20]

Procedural success for obliterative disease has been measured by a significant decrease in the percent diameter stenosis, reduction of the transstenotic gradient, IVUS demonstration of a widely patent vessel, and improvement in post-procedural noninvasive studies. However, a truly successful procedure is one in which dilation of the critical stenosis (or stenoses) offers relief of the patient's clinical symptoms, such as improvement in pain-free walking distance, elimination of rest pain, healing of an ischemic ulcer, or limitation of the extent of amputation.

Percutaneous interventions

The accepted 'ideal' indications for peripheral balloon angioplasty are based upon both a physician's knowledge of the anatomic, pathologic, and physiologic considerations, the interventionist's skill level, and the available imaging systems and devices. In reality, peripheral angioplasty, complemented by stents, atherectomy, and occasionally thrombolysis, has enabled the vast majority of lesions, whether they be discrete stenoses, short occlusions, diffuse (>4 cm) occlusive lesions, long occlusions (including those ≥30 cm), ectatic vessels, heavily calcified lesions, and ulcerative lesions, to be successfully recanalized. In fact, subclavian stenoses or occlusions, and renal artery stenoses are best managed in more than 99% of cases with endovascular techniques, with few associated significant complications, especially when considering the surgical alternatives.

Successful dilatation of stenotic lesions throughout the peripheral vascular system can be attained in over 95% of cases, while occluded vessels have success rates varying with the length of occlusion (<5 cm long, 90–95%, to >30 cm long, 75–80%). Procedural failure is usually related to arterial tear or dissection, abrupt vessel occlusion, or inability to cross or to dilate a calcified occlusion. The balloon expandable and/or self-expanding stents have significantly improved the recanalization success of occluded vessels by eliminating flow limiting intimal flaps or severe dissections. The significant complications encountered are transient contrast-induced renal failure, large arterial access site hematomas that may require surgical evacuation, or access site pseudoaneurysms, which can frequently be treated with direct ultrasound-guided compression. Less frequently, arterial tear, distal embolization, and rarely, retroperitoneal hemorrhage, may occur, requiring rapid identification and correction. The need for urgent or emergent vascular bypass or unexpected amputation should be an unusual and rare occurrence. Death may occur and is usually related to the use of angioplasty in very sick patients who have extensive co-morbidities.

Focal and diffuse stenoses and short occlusions can be treated with balloon angioplasty. However, when an arterial tear occurs, or hemodynamic evidence of impedance to blood flow persists (persistent transstenotic pressure gradients), stents should be deployed to eliminate the problem and re-establish excellent blood flow. Long occlusions can be treated by balloon angioplasty, with or without thrombolytic therapy. Thrombolysis can precede balloon angioplasty so as to better define the obstructing lesion and reduce the extent of the angioplasty procedure. Ulcerated plaques or recurrent emboli are not contraindications to angioplasty, but stent(s) or stent graft(s) may be the preferred treatment, since neoendothelialization (if no stent covering were used) following the intimal injury from PTA relines the ulcerated plaque. Even arterial tears or perforations can be corrected by prolonged balloon inflation, or covered stents which maintain blood flow through the true lumen.

Aneurysms: diagnosis and treatment

For aneurysmal disease, especially of the infrarenal aorta and descending thoracic aorta, the best method of assessment is the contrast enhanced helical CT scan, which provides accurate measurements of the aortic diameter and aneurysm length, aneurysmal involvement of the iliac arteries, and occlusive disease or marked tortuosity of the iliofemoral arteries. The important difference between angiography and spiral CT is that angiography only supplies an image of the contrast enhanced lumen, and does not reflect the true size and extent of the aneurysm. The postprocedure CT scan defines procedural success, i.e. aneurysmal exclusion or any significant perigraft leakage, as does duplex ultrasonography. Aneurysm exclusion has been defined by the presence of an intact graft, no holes or perforations, and a tight seal at the proximal and distal ends of the graft. The graft ends should be in contact with the arterial wall (intima) without thrombus interposed between the intima and stent-graft.[21–23]

Summary

The advantages of percutaneous interventions are

- their excellent success rates,
- minimal morbidity and mortality,
- diminished length of hospitalization,
- minimal or absent recuperative period,
- decreased costs (remembering the early return to work),
- the small penalty for failure.

If endovascular therapy fails, the lesion usually remains unchanged, the patient's status remains the same, and the patient remains a 'viable' surgical candidate. Furthermore, percutaneous techniques may compliment vascular surgery by increasing inflow and/or outflow so that difficult surgical procedures can be performed more successfully.

During the 1990s, peripheral vascular interventional procedures have become a primary therapy for renal, brachiocephalic, iliofemoral, femoropopliteal, as well as tibioperoneal vessels, and will likely become the primary treatment for carotid and intracranial cerebral arterial disease. The use of endovascular techniques, employing stent grafts and covered stents (with autologous vein and synthetic materials), may well become the standard for the management of arterial aneurysmal disease, ruptures, or injuries to the vessel, and perhaps, obstructive disease as well. These procedures will be performed in outpatient settings, and will involve the use of balloons, stents, covered stents, and stent grafts, as well as adjunctive methods, such as platelet receptor antagonists, direct thrombin inhibitors, and endovascular brachytherapy.

References

1   Kannel WB. The demographics of claudication and the aging of the American population. *Vascular Medicine* 1996; **1**: 60–4.

2   Widlus DM, Osterman FA. Evaluation and percutaneous management of atherosclerotic peripheral vascular disease. *JAMA* 1989; **261**: 3148–54.

3   Hughson WG, Mann JI, Garrod A. Intermittent claudication: prevalence and risk factors. *BMJ* 1978; **1**: 1379–81.

4   Jonason T, Bergstrom R. Cessation of smoking in patients with intermittent claudication. Effects on the risk of peripheral vascular complications, myocardial infarction, and mortality. *Acta Med Scand* 1987; **221**: 253–60.

5   Orchard TJ, Strandness DE. Assessment of peripheral vascular disease in diabetes. Report and recommendations of an International workshop sponsored by the American Diabetes Association and the American Heart Association. *Circulation* 1993; **88**: 819–28.

6   Reiber GE, Pecoraro RE, Koepsell TD. Risk factors for amputation in patients with diabetes mellitus. A case-control study. *Ann Intern Med* 1992; **117**: 97–105.

7   Weitz JI, Byrne J, Clagett GP, et al. Diagnosis and treatment of chronic arterial insufficiency of the lower extremities: a critical review. *Circulation* 1996; **94**: 3026–49.

8   Gardner AW, Poehlman ET. Exercise rehabilitation programs for the treatment of claudication pain. A meta-analysis. *JAMA* 1995; **274**: 975–80.

9   Lindgarde F, Jeines R, Bjorkman H, et al. Conservative drug treatment in patients with moderately severe chronic occlusive peripheral arterial disease. *Circulation* 1989; **80**: 1549–56.

10   The European study group. Intravenous pentoxifylline for the treatment of chronic critical limb ischemia. *Eur J Vasc Endovasc Surg* 1995; **9**: 426–36.

11   DeWeese JA, Leather R, Porter J. Practice guidelines: lower extremity revascularization. *J Vasc Surg* 1993; **18**: 280–94.

12   Tunis SR, Bass EB, Steinberg EP. The use of angioplasty, bypass surgery, and amputation in the management of peripheral vascular disease. *N Engl J Med* 1991; **325**: 556–62.

13   Hallett JW. Trends in revascularization of the lower extremity. *Mayo Clin Proc* 1986; **61**: 369–76.

14   Martin EC. Percutaneous therapy in the management of aortoiliac disease. *Semin Vasc Surg* 1994; **7**: 17–27.

15   Fraser SCA, Aghiad AIM. Percutaneous transluminal angioplasty of the infrapopliteal vessels: the evidence. *Radiology* 1996; **200**: 33–43.

16   Stanley B, Teague B, Raptis S, et al. Efficacy of balloon angioplasty of the superficial femoral artery and popliteal artery in the relief of leg ischemia. *J Vasc Surg* 1996; **23**: 679–85.

17   Henry M, Amor M, Ethevenot G, et al. Palmaz stent placement in iliac and femoropopliteal arteries: primary and secondary patency in 310 patients with 2–4 year follow-up. *Radiology* 1995; **197**: 167–74.

18   Treiman GS, Ichikawa BS, Treiman RL, et al. Treatment of recurrent femoral or popliteal artery stenosis after percutaneous transluminal angioplasty. *J Vasc Surg* 1994; **20**: 577–87.

19   Blum U, Krumme B, Flugel P, et al. Treatment of ostial renal-artery stenoses with vascular endoprosthesis after unsuccessful balloon angioplasty. *N Engl J Med* 1997; **336**: 459–65.

20   Dorros G, Jaff M, Jain A, et al. Follow-up of primary Palmaz–Schatz stent placement for atherosclerotic renal artery stenosis. *Am J Cardiol* 1995; **75**: 1051–5.

21   Parodi JC. Endovascular repair of abdominal aortic aneurysms and other arterial lesions. *J Vasc Surg* 1995; **21**: 549–57.

22   Rozenblit A, Marin ML, Veith FJ, et al. Endovascular repair of abdominal aortic aneurysm: value of postoperative follow-up with helical CT. *AJR* 1995; **165**: 1473–9.

23   Marin ML, Veith FJ, Panetta TF, et al. Transluminally placed endovascular stented graft repair for arterial trauma. *J Vasc Surg* 1994; **20**: 466–73.

34

Tools in peripheral interventions

Michel Henry, Max Amor, Isabelle Henry, Gérard Ethevenot, and Kiril Tzvetanov

Introduction

Peripheral angioplasty has become a wide field, today representing the first therapy resource so far as peripheral arterial diseases are concerned. Balloon angioplasty was initially performed in large iliac arteries to treat simple and short lesions. Since then, numerous tools have been used, evaluated, abandoned or adopted so that they can be used to treat renal or femoral arteries with complex or long stenoses. Unlike in coronary diseases, many tools have been developed, thus widening the choice of access site arteries and the category of treated lesions. Access sites, creating a channel, widening and maintaining the lumen, prevention and treatment of the complications are all problems that can be tackled through instrumental or therapeutical means. Although surgery was originally considered the 'gold standard' of revascularization, angioplasty is now the method of preference.

Numerous tools requiring technical experience and skill may be used in peripheral angioplasty. While some of these tools are specific to peripheral angioplasty (covered stents, hydrophilic guide wires, etc.), others are also used at the coronary level.

We describe herein the main tools used in peripheral revascularization and treatment, highlighting the corresponding clinical applications and results.

Clinical and diagnostic tools

Peripheral arterial diseases may be detected using clinical tools, whereas invasive diagnostic tools enable the confirmation of the diagnosis and the evaluation of the extent of the lesions.

Clinical symptoms

Peripheral arterial diseases may be detected in different ways:

- intermittent claudication (worsening severity);
- acute or subacute ischemia requiring emergency treatment;
- blue-toe syndrome;
- sexual disorders;
- haphazardous discovery in an at-risk patient (diabetes, hypertension, smoking, hyperlipemia, etc.);
- severe hypertension resistant to medical therapy and/or renal insufficiency, implying a potential stenosis of the renal artery;
- tension asymmetry and vertigo syndrome, implying a potential lesion of the subclavian artery; and
- transient ischemic accident or constituted ischemic accident, implying a potential lesion of the carotid artery.

Diagnostic and postprocedure follow-up tools

Color echotomography Doppler and steady Doppler: These studies enable a global evaluation of the patient, looking for multiple localizations and evaluating the severity of the lesions. These techniques are now very useful not only for evaluation but also for postangioplasty therapeutical follow-up.

Angiography is the diagnostic method of preference, enabling a global arterial evaluation. It also enables the determination of an indication for angioplasty and therapeutic implications in cases of multiple lesions.

Spiral CT scan and magnetic resonance imaging are useful in the evaluation of aneurysmal diseases.

Lesion quantification and follow-up

In most cases, angiography enables us to study the characteristics of the lesion, to determine severity (stenosis, occlusion, etc.), morphology (ulceration, chronic dissection, intraluminal image, excentration, etc.), extension and calcification. Angiography monitors procedure. Multiple views and road-mapping ensure both the safety and success of the procedures.

Endovascular echography is performed to guide stent placement; it is also used to evaluate the results and to measure precisely arterial segments to enable the placement of endoprostheses (arterial aneurysm or abdominal aorta). Some centers still use angioscopy to detect thrombi as well as to evaluate the postprocedure results. Translesion gradient measurement, is a simultaneous measurement of the pressures below and above the lesion. Hemodynamical disorders may be detected through flow maps, which may help in the understanding of the mechanism of restenosis.

The different therapeutical instruments

Percutaneous endoluminal balloon angioplasty

Percutaneous endoluminal balloon angioplasty (PTCA) is the most commonly used method for peripheral artery interventions. It enables the correct enlargement of the arterial lumen by fracturing the atheromatous plaque and compressing it against the arterial wall (Fig. 34.1). The best indications for percutaneous endoluminal balloon angioplasty procedures without complementary procedures are short, concentric, slightly calcified lesions. It is used more frequently as an adjunct to other procedures. Hence it actually completes new techniques, thus widening its range of indications and improving its results.

Balloon angioplasty currently benefits from technological advancement in coronary angioplasty with regard to introducers, guiding catheters, the material and the profile of the balloons. Indeed, low-profile balloons, the small diameter shaft catheters and torque guidewires allow access to the majority of lesions and the treatment of small-caliber arteries such as lower limb arteries, while the 'kissing' technique (Fig. 34.2) enables the treatment of lesions at bifurcations.

Fibrous, calcified lesions may be dilated with high-pressure inflation balloons; compliant balloons improve the results. Numerous occlusions may be recanalized and rendered accessible to dilatation with hydrophilic guide wires. Long introducers (40–100 cm) enable guidewires, balloons and diverse instruments to be used for certain lesions from a remote access site, thus enabling angioplasties which were not previously possible.

A good knowledge of the different access sites (contralateral, humeral, popliteal) widens the range of balloon angioplasty indications. The primary success rate of balloon angioplasty has greatly improved over the last few years, with a success rate of 95–100% for stenoses and 85–90% for occlusions. Morgenstern et al.[1] report a success rate of 95% for occlusions from 1 to 4 cm long and of 86% for occlusions from 5 to 10 cm long.

The long-term results depend on the quality of the angioplasty. One should try to obtain the best result possible, with no residual stenosis or dissection. Not only does the restenosis rate depend on the result but it also depends on other factors such as location, length, characteristics of the lesion and artery size.

It has been demonstrated that the restenosis rate after percutaneous transluminal angioplasty (PTA) is significantly higher when a residual stenosis with pressure gradients still exists.[2] Long-term patency is 75% when the arterial lumen is smooth, 66% when it is irregular at the femoral level, 80% for short lesions and 55% for long lesions.[3,4] Complex lesions (long, irregular, ulcerated) have poor results.

Capek et al.[5] report success rates of 93% for stenoses and 82% for occlusions. Long-term results are better at the iliac level than at the femoropopliteal level. Tegtmeyer et al.[6] report a primary patency of 86% at the iliac level on a 7.5-year follow-up, and a secondary patency of 92%, while Van Andel et al.[7] report 90% at 7 years. At the femoropopliteal level, Capek et al.[5] report the following patencies: at 1 year, 91%; at 2 years, 61%; at 5 years, 58%.

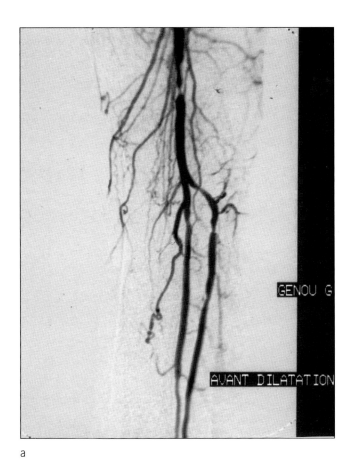

a

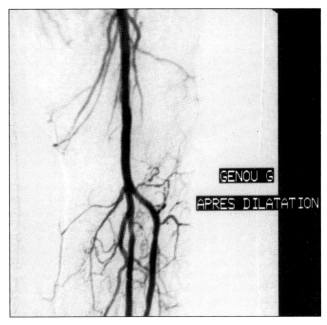

b

Figure 34.1
(a) Popliteal and anterior tibial stenoses. (b) Result after balloon angioplasty alone.

Krepel et al.[8] report 70% at 5 years, and 60% at 7 years; Vogelzang[2] reports 49% at 5 years and 35% at 10 years. Becker et al.[9] on a total of 4034 angioplasties, report a patency of 67% at 4–5 years, ranging from 54 to 73%. According to Johnston,[10] the long-term patency depends on the flow below. Darcy[11] discusses Johnston's conclusions, since those results come from relative data and techniques dating back to 1978–86. Therefore, the development of new angioplasty techniques, as well as the experience of the operators, should improve these results.

Recent occlusion recanalization techniques

Recanalization with the Fogarty sheath is the most commonly used technique: it has proved to be efficient in treating acute occlusions, especially embolic occlusions. However, it is not as efficient for the treatment of throm-

boses in atheromatous arteries which are difficult to cross and prone to complications (dissections, spasms, distal embolisms),[12,13] which may lead to parietal lesions and lesions in distal arteries.

In order to cope with these problems, several techniques have been developed, including fibrinolysis, thromboaspiration and mechanical thrombectomy.

Fibrinolysis

In situ fibrinolysis should be preferred to general fibrinolysis. *In situ* fibrinolysis consists of placing a catheter in contact with or within the thrombus, either by ipsilateral or contralateral access, and in perfusing the fibrinolytic medium. The fibrinolytic medium may be urokinase (Fig. 34.3), following MacNamara's protocol,[14] who associates heparin and a high dose of urokinase (4000 units/min, until the artery is patent, then 2000/min until lysis is complete) with an average success rate of 88%. Other protocols may be used with lower doses[15] and recombinant t-PA may be

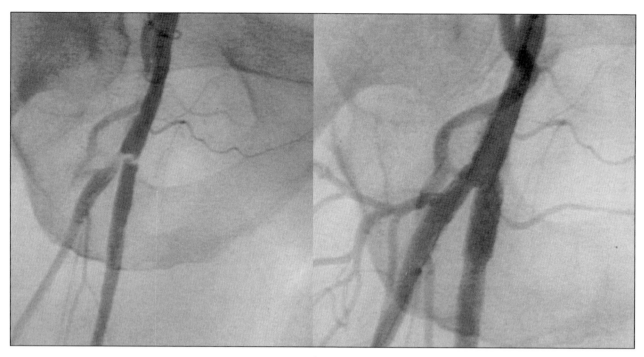

a   b

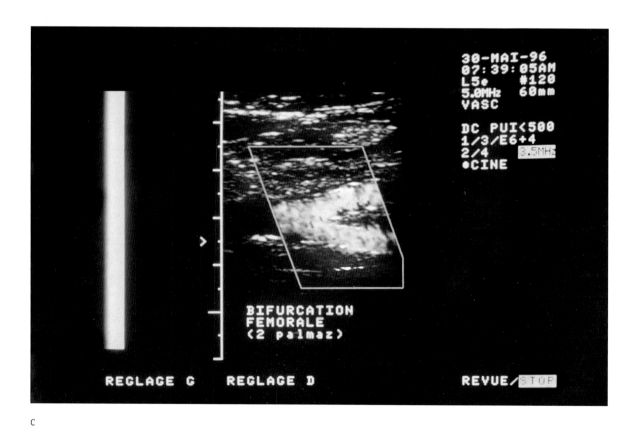

c

Figure 34.2

(a) Deep femoral ostial artery and right superficial femoral artery stenosis. (b) Result after 'kissing' angioplasty and placement of two Palmaz stents. (c) Echodoppler control showing the two stents.

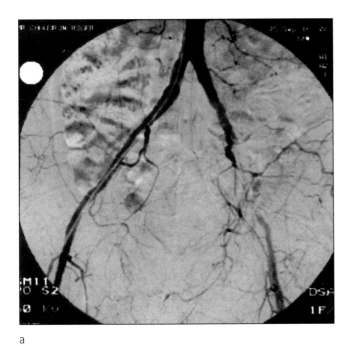

a

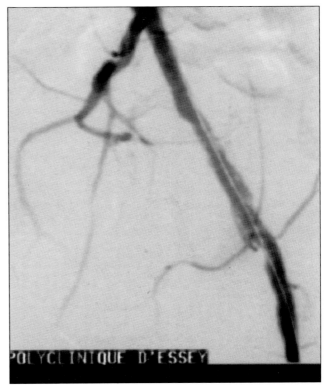

b

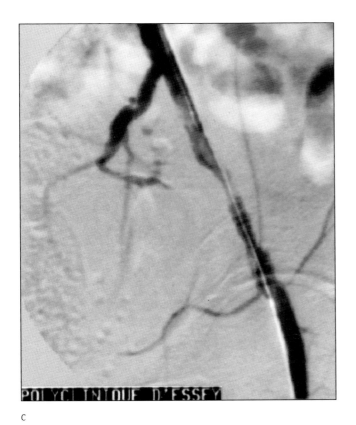

c

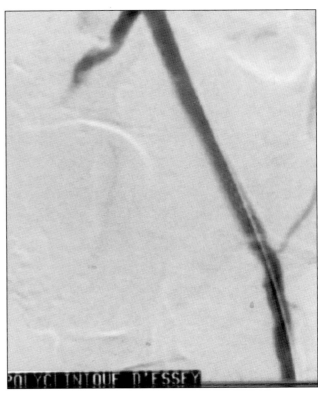

d

Figure 34.3
(a) Recent left external iliac thrombosis.   (b) Result after balloon angioplasty.   (c) 24-hour treatment through fibrinolytic drugs (urokinase).   (d) Placement of a covered stent (Corvita).

preferred to urokinase. Specific catheters have been developed, increasing local fibrinolysis through contact between thrombus and thrombolytic medium—for instance, multi-purpose catheters[16,17] and occlusion balloon catheters which are placed on both parts of the thrombus facilitating the thrombolysis at this level,[18] as well as catheters enabling pulsed injections under urokinase pressures.[19–21] Not only does fibrinolysis recanalize vascular accesses but it also recanalizes collateral branches.[22,23]

Several factors limit fibrinolysis, thus minimizing its indications in case of acute ischemia: it is effective within 4–48 hours; its side-effects, such as hemorrages; and its cost. Percutaneous mechanical techniques have therefore been developed in the last few years which are meant to recanalize arteries in very shot timespans and at lower costs.

Thromboaspiration

With this method the obstructing material is aspirated, after fragmentation or not. A syringe is placed at the distal end of a large lumen catheter and placed in contact with the thrombus. A negative pressure which is generated by the 'Venturi' effect, withdraws the thrombus. Large lumen introducers and removable media line valves make the procedure easier and improve its results.

There are many indications to this technique:

- Distal embolisms of cardiac or atheromatous origin (lesion lying above, ulcerated embolic plaques, aneurysms, etc.).

- Embolisms of iatrogenic origin secondary to an arterial catheterization, more especially arterial recanalization of a lesion lying above.

- Acute thrombosis on an underlying atheromatous lesion. Thromboaspiration may be performed at first intention, removing the thrombogenic part of the occlusion and thus avoiding migration of an embolus during angioplasty.

- Acute thrombosis of bypass grafts.

- Postangioplasty acute thrombosis at the site of the procedure itself.

Thromboaspiration may be performed alone or in association with local fibrinolysis.[24] In this case fibrinolysis is then quicker and more efficient. It may also be used as an adjunct to thromboaspiration. Thromboaspiration can be improved or completed by mechanical thrombectomy techniques. These are then used to fragment the thrombotic material and free the arterial wall, thus enabling aspiration.[25–30]

Mechanical thrombectomy

Several types of catheters may be used in mechanical thrombectomy.

'Vortex' effect catheters. A negative pressure is applied at the end of the catheter in order to attract and reduce the thrombotic material in contact. This type of catheter does not enable the aspiration of the fragmented material. The devices available are the Amplatz catheter,[31–34] the Kensey catheter, the Schmitz–Rode and Günther catheters and the Thrombolizer catheter. These catheters seem efficient in the treatment of recent thromboses, bypass thromboses or arteriovenous fistulas. However, their rigidity and the fact that they cannot be used on a guiding catheter make their use somewhat aggressive for the arterial wall, implying the risk of perforation, and they cannot be used through contralateral access. Moreover, since there is no aspiration device, there is a risk of distal embolism, and it therefore often requires an adjunct fibrinolytic treatment.

Ultrasound catheters[35,36] enable lysis of the clots. However, their rigidity limits their applications.

'Venturi' effect catheters. These double lumen catheters enable the injection of saline solution under pressure through an opening situated at its extremity, orientating the retrograde jet towards a larger central lumen. Clots are fragmented under the jet's pressure without threatening the arterial wall; thrombotic material is aspirated through the 'Venturi' effect. The large lumen allows the passage of a guide wire, thus avoiding any false position or arterial perforation, and it also allows the injection of saline solution. Permanent aspiration of the thrombotic material avoids distal embolism. The use of a compression device beneath also enable the reduction of the distal flow, limiting the risks of distal embolisms.

There are three types of 'Venturi' effect: the Hydrolyser[37–39] (Fig. 34.4), the Thrombektomat and the AngioJet, which requires a special injector whereas the other two devices benefit from functioning with the usual angioplasty injector. These three catheters are soft enough to be used through the contralateral access site and may be used on a guide wire. They seem to be particularly efficient in case of a thrombosis of less than 15 days. The Hydrolyser and the Thrombektomat are efficient in vessels from 5 to 10 mm in diameter, while the AngioJet seems to be more efficient in small-caliber vessels, from 6 to 7 mm. These catheters are easy to use, simple and quick. An arterial recanalization may be performed within 15–20 min, which enables treatment of threatening acute ischemias.

All these mechanical thrombectomy devices may be used alone or in association with other techniques, such as thromboaspiration, to withdraw the remaining clots, or with interventional techniques, such as balloon angioplasty, sometimes completed by placement of stents to treat the origin of the occlusion.

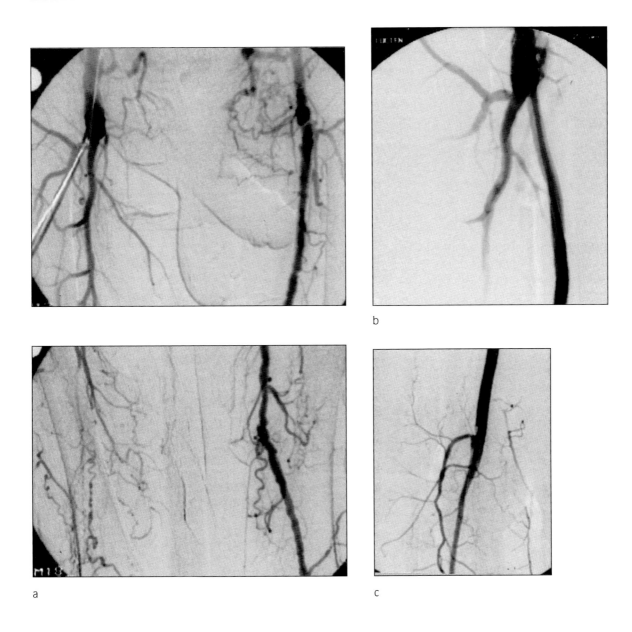

Figure 34.4
(a) Right femoropopliteal bypass thrombosis. (b) Placement of a Palmaz stent at the proximal anastomosis. (c) Result after recanalization with the Hydrolyser.

To conclude, these techniques are particularly efficient, quick, easy to use and less expensive than fibrinolysis. They should be used more often at first intention to treat recent occlusions, be it at the iliac or femoro-distal level. In case of failure, fibrinolysis or Fogarty techniques may always be referred to. 'Venturi' effect catheters seem particularly easy to use and are reliable; the AngioJet is better adapted to small-caliber arteries.

Chronic occlusion recanalization techniques

Mechanical devices (hydrophilic guidewires) should be used at first intention enabling the recanalization of numerous occlusions. Long iliac or superficial femoral occlusions may be recanalized, using the contralateral or popliteal access sites. These approaches may also be used in case of failure through the usual anterograde femoral or ipsilateral retrograde routes. Placement of the guidewires is made easier by hydrophilic sheaths, which maintain the guidewires in the intended direction. In case of failure, laser techniques may be used.[40,41] Laser fibers may be used either on a guidewire, bringing the fiber in contact with the lesion, or isolated, without guidewire. In this case, there is a risk of perforation with local bleeding.

Fibers may be placed more easily into the obturator due to the associated hydrophilic guidewire/laser fiber/'step-by-step' technique, thus improving the success rates. The authors currently consider that about 90% of occlusions may be treated through these techniques. However, the success rate still depends on localization, age, length and calcification of the lesion.

Any recanalization should be followed by balloon angioplasty. In case of calcification, rotational atherectomy should be performed prior to balloon angioplasty. Covered or noncovered stents tend to be more often used after balloon angioplasty, depending on the localization and the length of the lesion.

Atherectomy techniques

Atherectomy techniques tend to be used less often since the long-term results are not better than those obtained with angioplasty alone. Moreover, adjunct balloon angioplasty is often required owing to the caliber of the different devices used:

- The Simpson catheter.[42,43] The indications for this catheter are limited to stenoses located on segments of arteries with little or no tortuosity, and with little calcification. Specific indications for its use are: short excentrated lesions, soft elastic stenoses, bypass stenoses, stenoses inside endoprostheses, embolic ulcerated stenoses with suspected thrombus, withdrawal of dissection flaps and ostial stenoses at bifurcations.

- The TEC (Transluminal Extraction Catheter).[44,45] This catheter allows fragment aspiration and may therefore be indicated for bypass stenoses (old, degenerated grafts) in which thrombotic material is most often located.

- Atherectomy devices such as Pull Back have limited indications.

- The diameter of the Redha Cut may be brought to 8–9 mm, and may therefore be used in iliac arteries without adjunct angioplasty.

Pulverization or rotational ablation techniques: the Rotablator[46,47]

This well-known device consists of a burr (sizes range from 1.25 to 3 mm diameter for percutaneous peripheral use) which is mounted on a very thin guidewire (0.009-inch). This device is quite useful, and sometimes necessary, for fibrous and more specifically calcified lesions. The artery is then 'cleaned' and its compliance is modified, allowing better balloon angioplasty results under low pressures, without significant dissections. The best indications are:

- Long femoral and popliteal calcified lesions.

- Long calcified lesions which cannot be crossed with a balloon.

- Lower-limb calcified lesions (limb salvage) and the improvement of long-term patencies of bypasses and of iliofemoropopliteal angioplasties.

- Lesions at arterial bifurcations (Fig. 34.5).

- Ostial calcified lesions.

- Tortuous lesions. Flexibility and ease of use of the devices enable the practitioner to have access to stenoses which could not be accessed otherwise.

- Bypasses and endoprostheses stenoses may be successfully treated.

In a published series[48] reporting 212 lesions in 150 patients treated with this technique, 50% of the lesions were located below the knee. The authors have obtained an immediate success rate of 97%. Most of the complications (spasms, thromboses, etc.) were treated through interventional techniques. Remote results were satisfactory owing to the lesions since the restenosis rate was 24% globally, 36% at the femoral level and 21% at the distal level. The restenosis rate depends on the length of the lesion treated, the limit being, as far as the authors are concerned, 7 cm. For longer lesions, the restenosis rate is too high. These unique devices deserve a place in the list when choosing from the interventional treatment instruments available. We have extended our indications for Rotablator to renal ostial tight calcified stenoses. Thirteen patients were successfully treated with this technique, completed by balloon angioplasty and stent placement.[48a]

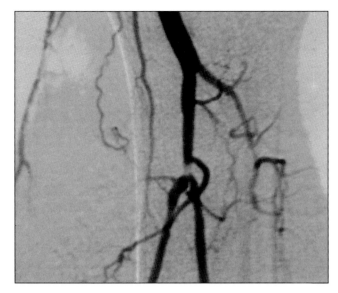

a

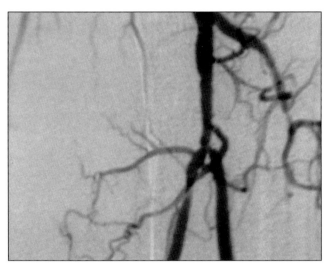

b

Figure 34.5
(a) Tibioperoneal trunk stenosis. (b) Treatment with Rotablator. Good result.

Stents

Stenting has been widely developed over the last few years. Endoprostheses have been placed in any artery greater than 3 mm in diameter. Several types of stents are available. Noncovered prostheses are shape memory prostheses (InStent, Memotherm, Cragg stent); and balloon-expandable stents (Strecker stent, Palmaz stent, AVE stent). There are also covered prostheses (stent grafts) with material outside (Cragg Endopro System 1/Passager), with material inside (Corvita), and co-knitted stents. The

main characteristics of the stents are summarized in Table 34.1.

Indications for stent placement are open to controversy. Some think they are wide,[49,50,55] others think they are limited.[57,58] The indications include:

- postangioplasty residual stenosis, stenosis greater than 30% with pressure gradient higher than 5 mmHg;
- stenoses which cannot be dilated (rigid, elastic stenoses);
- dissection following angioplasty procedure, which may lead to occlusion or flow reduction. This enables a considerable reduction in acute complications of angioplasty.
- restenosis: the stent would have an effect on 'remodeling'.

Beyond these general indications, covered stents and stent grafts have their own indications for aneurysms, arteriovenous fistulas, perforations and arterial ruptures, and they may be traumatic of iatrogenic (postangioplasty).

The choice of the stent depends on several factors:

- *Length of the lesion.* Whereas noncovered stents give good results for short lesions (<8 cm, and more especially <5 cm), the results are not so good for longer lesions. In this case, the authors recommended the placement of covered stents, provided there are no large collateral branches or division branches that could be threatened as well in this type of lesion—more especially at the femoral level.
- *Nature of the lesion.* A rigid stent with a good radial force is better indicated for a calcified lesion, whereas a covered stent will better suit an ulcerated lesion with embolic risks.
- *Localization of the lesion.* Some stents may be placed very precisely at bifurcations (Palmaz, AVE) (Fig. 34.2).
- *Lesions in tortuous arteries or at a bifurcation* are best treated with soft stents (InStent—Figs 34.6 and 34.7—and AVE, Wallstent etc.).

Table 34.2 summarizes the different indications for stents and Table 34.3 summarizes the choice of stent in relation to the access site, depending on the localization and on the nature of the lesion. With experience, complications linked with stent placement are rare (loss of a stent, false positioning). Primary stenting is indicated for occlusive lesions since it avoids embolic migrations.[49]

Acute stent thromboses are currently rare as long as stents are well deployed, owing to high-pressure balloons and well adapted antiaggregant protocols (ticlopidine 250 mg/day, aspirin 250 mg/day for 1 month, associated with low molecular weight heparin for 8 days and aspirin 250 days thereafter).

Table 34.1 Principal stent characteristics.

	Palmaz Cordis, a Johnson & Johnson Company	AVE Arterial Vascular Engineering, Inc.	Strecker Catholic University Leuven	Wallstent Schneider (Europe) AG	InStent Medtronic InStent	Memotherm BARD Inc.	Endopro/ Passager Boston Scientific Corp	Corvita Schneider (Europe) AG
Self-expanding	−	−	−	+	+	+	+	+
Balloon expandable	+	+	+	−	−	−	−	−
Diameter with balloon	+	+	−	−	−	−	−	−
Removability	−	−	+	−	+	−	−	−
Flexibility	−	+	+	+	+	+	+	+
Radiopacity	+	+	+	±	+	±	+	+
Delivery device	−	−	−	+	+	+	+	+
Minimum introducer size	6Fr	8F	7Fr	7Fr	8Fr	8Fr	7Fr	7F
Precise placement	+ +	+	+	±	±	±	+	+
Protective sheath	No	No	No	Yes	Yes	Yes	Yes	Yes

Notes: + = Characteristic of the stent
+ + = Obviously characteristic of the stent
± = More or less characteristic of the stent
− = Uncharacteristic of the stent

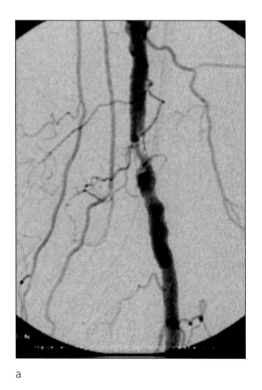
a

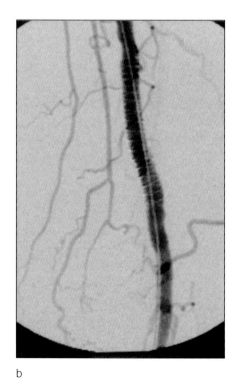
b

Figure 34.6
(a) Upper-right popliteal artery tight ulcerated stenosis. (b) Result after angioplasty and placement of an InStent stent.

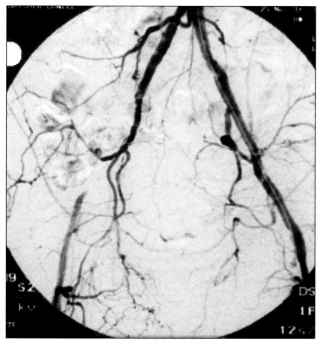

a

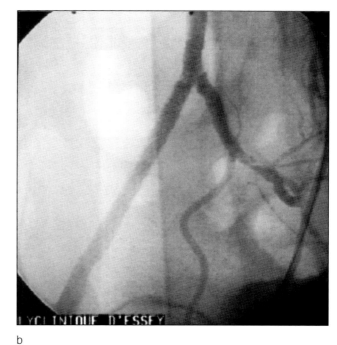

b

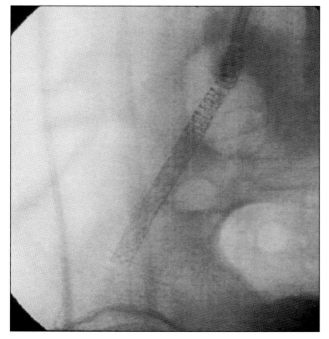

c

Figure 34.7
(a) Right external iliac occlusion. Internal iliac stenosis.
(b) Result after recanalization through contralateral approach.
Internal iliac artery angioplasty. Placement of a Medium Spiral
stent in the external iliac artery and (c) of an InStent stent at the
bifurcation to preserve the origin of the internal iliac artery
treated by angioplasty.

Table 34.2 Indications for specific stents.

	Palmaz	AVE	Strecker	Wallstent	InStent	Memotherm	Endopro	Corvita
Tortuous arteries	−	+	+	+	+	+	+	+
Calcifications	+	+	±	−	−	−	±	±
Ostium	+	+	±	−	−	−	±	±
Joint	±	+	+	+	++	+	+	+
Long lesions >8 cm	±	±	+	+	−	−	+	+
Collateral branches	±	+	±	+	++	±	−	−
Aneurysm	−	−	−	−	−	−	+	+

Notes: + = Good indication
++ = Excellent indication
± = More or less an indication
− = Bad indication

Table 34.3 Type of stent according to the entry port..

	Palmaz	AVE	Strecker	Wallstent	InStent	Memotherm	Endopro	Corvita
Femoral ipsilateral	+	+	+	+	+	+	+	+
Contralateral	+	+	+	+	±	±	±	+
Brachial	+	+	±	+	−	±	±	+
Popliteal	+	+	+	+	+	+	+	+

Notes: + = Approach may be used
± = Approach may be discussed
− = Approach cannot be used

Stents experience

It seems that stent placement has improved mid and long-term angioplasty results. The authors' experience with different stents is detailed below.

The Palmaz stent[50]

In a series of 310 patients (184 in the iliac artery, 126 in the femoral artery) and over a 4-year follow-up period, the following results were obtained. The average 6-month restenosis rate for all lesions in the series was 4.8%. This rate increased as interventions descended the arterial sys-

tem: 0.5% for iliac artery lesions, 4% for upper femoral artery lesions, 10% for middle femoral artery lesions, and 18% for lesions in the lower third of the femoral artery and 20% for lesions in the popliteal artery. When we combined the results for the iliac artery with those from the upper and middle saphenofemoral artery (SFA), the restenosis rate was significantly higher for occlusions than for stenoses (11% vs. 1.8%; $p < 0.02$). However, this distinction between stenoses and occlusions was curiously absent for lower SFA and popliteal arteries (22% vs. 16%). The restenosis rate was not significantly affected by the lesion length (<3 cm vs. >3 cm). However, statistically significant differences were found when we looked at the number of stents placed (1 vs. more than 1; $p < 0.05$) and the

treatment with a thrombosuction catheter. *Radiology* 1996; **198**: 49–53.

40 Henry M, Beron R, Chastel A, *et al*. Place de l'angioplastie laser dans la prise en charge des artériopathies périphériques. A propos de 79 cas. *J Mal Vasc* 1990; **15**: 326–31.

41 Lammer J, Pilger E, Karnel F, *et al*. Femoropopliteal laser recanalization. A multicenter study. *Radiology* 1990; **30**: 45–9.

42 Ariani M, Fishbein MC, Chae JS, *et al*. Peripheral artery atherectomy: description of technique and report of initial results. *Radiology* 1988; **169**: 677–80.

43 Simpson JB, Selmon MR, Robertson GC, *et al*. Transluminal atherectomy for occlusive peripheral vascular disease. *Am J Cardiol* 1988; **61**: 96G–101G.

44 Graor RA. Transluminal atherectomy for occlusion peripheral vascular disease. *J Am Coll Cardiol* 1989; **170**: 391–4.

45 Von Polnitz A, Nerlich A, Berger J, *et al*. Percutaneous peripheral atherectomy: angiographic and clinical follow-up of 60 patients. *J Am Coll Cardiol* 1990; **15**: 682–8.

46 Henry M, Amor M, Ethevenot G, *et al*. Percutaneous peripheral rotational ablation using the Rotablator: immediate and mid-term results. Single center experience concerning 146 lesions treated. *Int Angiol* 1993; **12**: 231–44.

47 Ahn SS, Eton D, Yeatman LR, *et al*. Intraoperative peripheral rotary atherectomy: early and late clinical results. *Ann Vasc Surg* 1992; **6**: 272–80.

48 Henry M, Amor M, Ethevenot G, *et al*. Percutaneous peripheral atherectomy using the Rotablator: a single-center experience. *J Endovasc Surg* 1995; **2**: 51–66.

48a Henry M, Amor M, Henry I. Stent placement in the renal artery: three-year experience with the Palmaz stent. *JVIR* 1996; **7**: 343–50.

49 Vorwerk D, Guenther RW, Shurmann K, *et al*. Primary stent placement for chronic iliac artery occlusions: follow-up results in 103 cases. *Radiology* 1995; **194**: 745–9.

50 Henry M, Amor M, Ethevenot G, *et al*. Palmaz stent placement in iliac and femoropopliteal arteries: primary and secondary patency in 310 patients with 2–4 year follow-up. *Radiology* 1995; **197**: 167–74.

51 Henry M, Amor M, Beyar R, *et al*. Clinical experience with a new Nitinol self-expanding stent in peripheral arteries. *J Endovasc Surg* 1996; **3**: 369–79.

52 Henry M, Amor M, Porte JM, *et al*. Endoluminal bypass grafting in leg arteries with the Cragg Endopro System 1. A series of 142 patients. *Circulation* 1996; **94 (Suppl I)**: I-619.

53 Henry M, Amor M, Porte JM, *et al*. Endoluminal bypass grafting in leg arteries with the Cragg Endopro System 1. A series of 142 patients. *Radiology* 1996; **201 (Suppl)**: 244 (abstract).

54 Henry M, Amor M, Cragg A, *et al*. Occlusive and aneurysmal peripheral arterial disease: assessment of a stent-graft system. *Radiology* 1996; **201**: 717–24.

55 Vorwerk D, Günther RW, Bohndorf K, *et al*. Self-expanding vascular endoprostheses in the treatment of peripheral arteries: appraisal of a 2-year experience. *Radiology* 1989; **173**: 106.

56 Sapoval M, Long AM, Raynaud, AC, *et al*. Femoropopliteal stent placement: long term results. *Radiology* 1992; **184**: 833–9.

57 Joffre F, Rousseau H, Chemall R. Self-expandable intravascular stent: long-term results in the iliac and superficial femoral artery. In: Maynar M, Castaneda-Zuniga R, Joffre F (eds). *Percutaneous Revascularization Techniques* (New York: Thieme Medical, 1993): 301–6.

58 Martin EC, Katzen BT, Benenati JF, *et al*. Multicenter trial of the Wallstent in the iliac and femoral arteries. *J Vasc Interven Radiol* 1995; **6**: 843–9.

59 Henry M, Amor M, Porte JM, *et al*. Initial experience with the Corvita endoluminal graft in peripheral arteries. *Circulation* 1996; **94 (Suppl I)**: I-87.

35

Peripheral stenting for the cardiologist

Richard R Heuser

Introduction

Peripheral vascular disease: an overview

Peripheral vascular disease (PVD) is a common and disabling malady, and patients seeking treatment may turn to cardiologists to direct their care. The age-adjusted prevalence of peripheral arterial disease in the US population approaches 12%.[1] Occlusion of peripheral arteries has a variety of clinical consequences including:

- pain with walking (claudication),
- pain at rest
- tissue destruction in the distal limbs.

Amputation of a portion of the lower extremity is sometimes indicated in those with advanced disease. PVD also manifests itself in the renal and brachiocephalic arteries. The severity of symptomatic and asymptomatic carotid artery disease in patients with PVD has been recently assessed, and routine carotid ultrasound screening of 373 consecutive patients (mean age 70 ± 10 years) with category 1 or greater PVD revealed 25% of the study cohort were surgical candidates; an additional 9% of patients were potential candidates for enrollment into the North American Symptomatic Carotid Endarterectomy Trial and European Carotid Surgery Trial (NASCET).[2] PVD has been linked with an increased risk of mortality—results of a study of 2,871 consecutive patients discharged after coronary artery bypass graft surgery (CABG) indicates that even after successful myocardial revascularization, patients with PVD faced substantially higher mortality rates.[3]

Treatment options

Conventional treatment of PVD has included medical management and, inevitably, surgical bypass. Therapeutic agents like pentoxifylline, ticlopidine, aspirin and dipyridamole are sometimes given to patients newly diagnosed with mild PVD, but mechanical intervention is indicated in more severe, symptomatic disease. The advent of catheter-based therapies has profoundly altered the treatment of PVD. Treatment of occlusive disease with angioplasty has revolutionized therapeutic alternatives for patients with PVD. More recent advances in interventional cardiology have led to a variety of new medical devices that aid in the treatment of vascular disease.

Stents are proving to be one of the most exciting interventional technologies and have significantly impacted the outcome of endoluminal treatment and expanded therapeutic options in the arteries and veins. Stenting has been used with great success to improve luminal diameter and restore flow in occluded arteries. The results have quickly eclipsed those seen with laser and atherectomy procedures.

Stenting has been used successfully to correct arterial obliterative lesions in the iliac arteries and is associated with a lower restenosis rate as compared with balloon angioplasty.[4] Dilatation of an artery with balloon angioplasty may injure the arterial lumen and produce a rough, irregular surface with small areas of dissection. The current theory of restenosis suggests a myoproliferative response to this injury, resulting in subsequent intimal hyperplasia and a rapid cellular proliferation that leads to stenosis.[5] Stenting may prevent injury to the lumen[4] and reduce the potential for hyperplasia and restenosis; the likelihood of plaque disruption and embolization may also be reduced.

The use of stents in the brachiocephalic region has become more prevalent in the last several years and may offer an alternative to surgical revascularization. Transthoracic and extrathoracic revascularization procedures carry a 4–11% morbidity rate and a 0–5% mortality rate.[6–10]

There are now more than 20 different types of stents; the majority have been designed for use in the coronary arteries, are still in clinical trials, and have not yet been approved for use in the USA. The market for these devices appears infinite. Although current estimates indicate 15% of today's percutaneous procedures include stents, that percentage is expected to quadruple by the year 2000.

A review of devices, access, imaging techniques, and a discussion of clinical results and complications is provided.

Stents

Stents are a technology in motion; new designs that reflect lessons learned with earlier devices are being developed by a variety of manufacturers. The process of bringing a stent to market is long. Laboratory tests are vital in determining the safety of a stent; important study parameters include the measurement of radial strength, recoil resistance, and metal stress and fatigue. A series of preclinical and clinical studies culminating in a randomized trial are necessary to ensure safety and efficacy and win approval from the US Food & Drug Administration (FDA). Currently the stents used in peripheral interventions include the Palmaz (Cordis, a Johnson & Johnson Co, Warren NJ, USA) and the Wallstent (Schneider-USA, Minneapolis MN, USA).

Palmaz stent

The Palmaz stent is a stainless steel tube designed with multiple rows of staggered rectangular slots that assumes a diamond-shape when expanded, reducing to 10% the amount of metal in contact with the luminal surface. The Palmaz stent is available in varying lengths from 10–39 mm with expansion ranges of 4–18 mm. Its longitudinal rigidity and large diameter make it ideally suited for straight vessels like the distal aorta, the renal and the iliac arteries, and end-to-end graft anastomoses.

The Wallstent

The Wallstent is a cylindrical device constructed by braiding multiple stainless steel monofilaments. The Wallstent is flexible, compliant, and self-expanding. It is ideal for delivery through curved arteries, and in vessels subject to flexion from adjacent joints or structures. The Wallstent comes in a variety of lengths ranging from 50–150 mm and in diameters from 5–10 mm. The latest configuration of the self-expanding Wallstent is a stainless steel mesh mounted on a low-profile delivery catheter with an outside diameter of 1.57 mm.

Access

The site of arterial access is of great importance in successful peripheral intervention. Proper site selection often dictates the ease of the procedure and may decrease the potential for complications.

Iliac and femoral access

Iliac and femoral access are most frequently obtained via a femoral artery puncture just below the inguinal ligament (a detailed description of the most commonly used approach—retrograde femoral—is provided in the section entitled, 'Brachiocephalic access'). Approaches include the contralateral and ipsilateral. The contralateral approach requires a puncture opposite the anatomic target lesion. Advancement of the catheter may be retrograde or antegrade depending on the location of the lesion. The antegrade approach is indicated for lesions in the superficial femoral artery, popliteal artery, and trifurcation vessels. This advancement approach allows a stronger push for penetration across tight stenoses or occlusions, but may be less familiar than retrograde advancement and requires additional practice to master. Popliteal access is still more complex and is used infrequently by most interventionists. It requires an ipsilateral or contralateral approach for injection of dye to identify the popliteal artery and may be used to gain access to the superficial femoral artery. Brachial or axillary approaches may be employed in patients with interrupted aortas and for those with lesions of the superficial femoral artery or profunda when an antegrade femoral approach is contraindicated.

Complications

Puncture of an artery may result in significant hemorrhage, and site compression may be difficult in areas with little underlying bone. Although punctures may heal spontaneously, significant plaque formation may result. One of the most common complications of percutaneous intervention is the development of a hematoma at the puncture site. Peripheral vascular intervention procedures require larger catheters than those employed in the coronary arteries, and the likelihood of hematoma is increased in this setting. Hematomas generally occur early on in the procedure and are usually discovered and brought under control without operative intervention. Small to medium-sized hematomas usually resolve spontaneously within a few days of the procedure.

Pseudoaneurysms occur when a puncture site in the artery fails to close, and a communication between the artery and the soft surrounding tissue results. Surgical repair or compression under duplex observation may be required to correct the problem. Arteriovenous fistulas are formed when a puncture results in a small channel where the artery bridges the vein; blood then flows from the artery into the vein. There is no simple way to prevent this complication, but it is certainly related to the skill and experience of the operator.

Brachiocephalic access

In general, most interventionists are familiar and comfortable with the retrograde femoral access method. This type of access has replaced the direct carotid stick for angiographic visualization of the arch, cervical, and intracranial arterial system.

Procedure

Patients who are to undergo brachiocephalic access procedures should be pretreated with ticlopidine (250 mg bid) and aspirin (325 mg bid) for 48 hours prior to the intervention. Selection of the common femoral artery should take into consideration the condition of the iliac artery. The side with the less tortuous and stenotic iliac artery should be used. Placement of a 9F sheath in the femoral artery and a 6F sheath in the femoral vein (for administration of intravenous heparin and fluids and possibly, a temporary pacer) are the first steps in the access procedure.

After an activated clotting time of 200 seconds is obtained, access to the carotid artery may be achieved by use of a small bore (5F or 6F) diagnostic neuroradiology catheter; a 0.038-inch guidewire may be used to place the catheter in the origin of the appropriate vessel. Prior to entrance to the common carotid should include a careful flush of saline should be performed to eradicate any debris, and an angiogram should be performed to identify the bifurcation and origin of the external carotid.

Roadmapping at this time allows repositioning of the guidewire within the diagnostic catheter. The 0.038-inch

guidewire and the diagnostic catheter should be advanced into the common carotid, and the guidewire should then be replaced with an exchange length wire. At the Arizona Heart Institute, we have used the extra stiff 0.038-inch Amplatz (Cook, Bloomington IN) wires with good results.

The diagnostic catheter should be removed once the tip of the exchange wire is placed within the distal external carotid. A 9F guiding catheter (Cordis, Miami FL) should be placed and advanced slowly into the common carotid. Once the guiding catheter is positioned below the bifurcation, the guidewire should be removed and the catheter back-flushed through the Tuohey–Borst adapter. Contrast is then injected to determine the dimensions of the artery and the nature and length of the lesion.

An appropriately sized balloon should be selected for predilation, and a stent should be chosen and mounted on another balloon in preparation for delivery. The lesion itself may be crossed with a soft, steerable 0.018-inch extra-support guidewire, and the predilation balloon should be passed to the lesion.

After confirmation that atropine has been administered, the balloon should be inflated with several short inflations. High pressure inflations are not generally used when intravascular ultrasound (IVUS) guidance is employed. A small bolus of contrast should be injected to assess the angioplasty result. The balloon with stent should then be passed to the lesion, and a second contrast injection should be administered to confirm the proper location: patient movement is always a possibility. The stent should be deployed with a short balloon inflation.

The balloon catheter should be used for a wire exchange in order to accommodate the 0.018-inch wire for the IVUS catheter. If IVUS analysis confirms perfect deployment, a final control angiogram should be performed. In cases in which the IVUS image indicates incomplete stent deployment, additional dilation with a larger balloon(s) should be performed until stent–wall apposition is adequate throughout. The guiding catheter should then be withdrawn into the descending thoracic aorta and a short sheath should be substituted in the groin.

Post-procedure

The patient should be transferred to the intensive care unit for observation and duplex scanning. When the patient's activated clotting time has returned to normal, the groin sheath should be removed. All carotid stent patients should have their antiplatelet therapy (ticlopidine [250 mg bid] and aspirin [325 mg bid]) restarted following the procedure. No postprocedural anticoagulation is necessary. Neurologic changes should be reported immediately, with neurology consultation and appropriate studies initiated as required. Computed tomography (CT) should be used to assess any suspected embolic event. The majority of the patients may be discharged the day following the procedure.

Complications

Many of the same complications described in the section on iliac and femoral access are seen with brachiocephalic stenting. However, particularly in stenting of the carotids, the potential for more serious or even life-threatening complications such as a transient ischemic attack (TIA) or stroke certainly exists. This arterial territory is unusual among the peripheral vessels, and interventionists certainly recognize the complications in these vessels may yield far more serious consequences than the same events in the kidneys or limbs.[11]

Imaging techniques

Angioscopy

Angioscopic imaging has afforded a unique view of lesion morphology and has value in assessing the etiology of restenosis after interventional therapy. Post-stent dissection, bulging of tissue into the lumen at the stent articulation site, gaps between stents, and thrombus—an important risk factor in the mechanism of stent restenosis—are easily seen via angioscopy, enabling immediate treatment decisions. In the coronary arteries, angioscopic data has motivated changes in therapy or guided the selection of treatment before and after stent deployment in more than half of the patients studied.[12–14]

Intravascular ultrasound

Angioscopic techniques, however, cannot quantify minimal disease or define lesion architecture and composition. The use of IVUS is supplanting contrast angiography and angioscopy in the evaluation of stent deployment. In patients with peripheral vascular disease, IVUS is most frequently used following percutaneous transluminal angioplasty (PTCA), intravascular stenting, atherectomy, and in the deployment of endoluminal grafts (ELGs).[15–18] IVUS enables interventionists to obtain high-resolution, real-time images that delineate irregularities and other structures inside the lumen and on the vessel wall and surrounding tissues. Clear depictions of calcification, dissection, and stent positioning are virtually unrivaled by any diagnostic method. IVUS also allows reproducible measurements of lumen diameter and cross-sectional areas for baseline, post-treatment, and follow-up evaluation of therapeutic effectiveness.

Clinical experience with peripheral stenting

Stenting in the iliac and femoral arteries

In the USA, stents are currently approved for use in the iliac artery. Results of stenting in this vessel have been encouraging, while success in the femoral arteries has been less consistent. As the first approved device the Palmaz stent has seen extensive use in both the iliac and femoral arteries. The self-expanding Wallstent has also been a popular choice in the extremities. The long-term efficacy of iliac artery stent placement with the Palmaz stent was recently reported.[19] A total of 83 patients underwent 108 iliac artery stent placements; 80 of the patients were followed clinically for a mean of 25.8 months (range 1–70 months). Thirty patients were followed with angiography for a mean of 10.4 months (range 1–48 months). Six different categories of ischemic rankings were defined, and improvement leading to a minimum of one category of advancement was defined as clinical success. Clinical success was 98.9% immediately after the procedure and 86.2% at 48 months. A primary patency rate of 87.5% was demonstrated arteriographically at the latest follow-up period; there were five occlusions (12.5%) and two restenoses (5.0%). The overall complication rate was 9.7%, and 30-day mortality was 1.2%. Based on long-term clinical and angiographic follow-up the authors concluded that iliac artery stent placement for treatment of limb ischemia was safe.

The results of an FDA phase II multicenter trial of the Wallstent in the iliac and femoral arteries were reported in 1995.[20] A total of 225 patients (mean age 64.2 years, range 32–88 years) entered the trial. Iliac and femoral stents were placed in 140 and 90 patients, respectively. Five patients required stent placement in both the iliac and femoral arteries. Clinical patency was measured with clinical and hemodynamic studies and life-table analysis according to the Rutherford scale was performed. Angiographic patency at 6 months in the iliac was 93%, and primary clinical patency was 81% and 71% at 1 and 2 years, respectively. Secondary clinical patency was 91% at 1 year and 86% at 2 years. Results in the femoral system were less favorable with a 6-month angiographic patency of 80% and a primary clinical patency of 61% and 49% at 1 and 2 years, respectively. Secondary patency was 84% at 1 year and 72% at 2 years. Major and minor complications occurred more frequently in stenting the femoral artery. Overall, major complications (hematoma, pseudoaneurysm, arteriovenous fistula, distal embolus, acute thrombosis, cerebrovascular and other hemorrhagic complications) were seen in 9.3% of patients. Minor complications were seen in 11.3% of all patients. The results of stenting with the Wallstent in the iliac and femoral were very similar to those seen with the Palmaz stent. The authors concluded that the Wallstent was a viable option for patients with unsatisfactory angioplasty procedures, particularly in the iliac artery.

Stenting in the brachiocephalic arteries

Proximal lesions

Successful stenting of lesions in the subclavian and innominate arteries is described in several series reports.[21–23] At the Arizona Heart Institute, we have performed hundreds of brachiocephalic interventions for treatment of stenoses and recurrent lesions,[21] and our implantation success has reached 100% for stent placement in the subclavian and innominate arteries. Palmaz stents have been implanted in the majority; Wallstents and Strecker stents (Boston Scientific, Watertown MA, USA) have been used less frequently. Percutaneous access was normally gained through the brachial artery. In some cases, the presence of ulcerated lesions has led to the use of primary deployment to prevent embolic consequences. In a follow-up period that spanned 4 years, duplex Doppler scans and/or arteriography confirmed patency in the majority of cases.

Others have demonstrated excellent results with primary stent deployment in the subclavian artery as well.[22,23] Palmaz stent implantation was successfully performed in 27 consecutive patients with 31 obstructed subclavian arteries.[22] A total of 50 stents were successfully deployed using the brachial ($n = 7$), femoral ($n = 16$), or combined ($n = 8$) approach. The percent diameter stenosis improved from $85 \pm 12\%$ to $6 \pm 7\%$ ($p < 0.001$). Peak and mean translesion gradients decreased, respectively, from 56 ± 35 mmHg to 3 ± 4 mmHg ($p < 0.01$), and 29 ± 18 mmHg to 2 ± 2 mmHg ($p < 0.01$). Complications were minor and procedural; one stent migration was treated uneventfully with deployment in the right external iliac artery, and two brachial arteries required repair. The investigators concluded that primary subclavian artery stent deployment was 100% successful in the immediate restoration of pulsatile flow.

In another series, primary stenting with Palmaz stents in 33 patients with lesions of the subclavian (31) and innominate arteries (2) resulted in technical success in 31 patients.[23] Thirty of the 32 stented arteries (97%) were patent over a follow-up period of up to 2 years. Complications in this series included:

- asymptomatic vertebral artery occlusion (1),
- entry site hematoma or pseudoaneurysm (4),
- distal embolization (1).

The investigators concluded that endovascular repair of symptomatic lesions in the subclavian and innominate arteries was a viable alternative to standard surgical repair.

Cervical lesions

At the Arizona Heart Institute, a total of 109 patients were treated successfully with 129 stents (128 Palmaz, 1 Wallstent).[11] Lesions meeting the treatment criteria were in the proximal common ($n = 3$), mid common ($n = 12$), distal common ($n = 8$), internal ($n = 92$), and external ($n = 2$) carotid arteries. Seven patients had bilateral internal carotid artery (ICA) stenoses, and 17 patients were treated for post-surgical recurrent disease. Minor complications in this series included four cases of spasm (successfully treated with papaverine); one flow-limiting dissection (stented); and six access site problems. There were seven strokes (2 major, 5 reversible) (6.4%) and five minor transient events (4.5%) that resolved within 24 hours. Three patients were converted to endarterectomy (2.7%) prior to discharge; one stroke patient expired (0.9%), and another patient died of an unrelated cardiac event in-hospital. In the 30-day post-procedural period, two ICA stents occluded (patients asymptomatic). Clinical success at 30 days (no technical failure, death, endarterectomy, stroke, or occlusion) was 89.1% (98/110). Life-table analysis showed an 89% cumulative primary patency rate.

Based on this early experience, we have concluded that carotid stenting appears feasible from a technical standpoint and results in good midterm patency. However, the incidence of neurological sequelae is clearly a serious problem; technical enhancements and a more aggressive antiplatelet regimen warrant further study.

Summary and conclusions

The last two decades have brought exciting changes in the management of peripheral vascular disease. Percutaneous intervention with angioplasty paved the way for innovative advances in device design and manufacture, and a variety of stents are now making their way through bench and clinical testing. Several stents are currently FDA-approved and in common use for treatment of peripheral lesions. Stents have shown efficacy in the treatment of peripheral lesions of the extremities: results in the iliac artery have been very encouraging. More recently, stents have been used to treat occlusions and stenotic lesions in the brachiocephalic vessels. Results in proximal and cervical lesions have been promising with impressive technical success rates and midterm patency. Complications are rarely seen with stenting in the proximal vessels, but stenting in the cervical region presents the operator with a greater challenge given the fragile and sensitive nature of the tissue these vessels supply. The complications seen in stenting these vessels are often catastrophic in nature, and interventionists must continue to seek ways to minimize their occurrence. The use of innovative imaging techniques like IVUS may provide the interventionist with important information about lesion morphology and appropriate stent placement. IVUS should be considered indispensable in complex and sensitive procedures such as carotid artery stenting.

Successful stenting is dependent on choosing a device appropriate to lesion type and location and, moreover, in knowing when *not* to stent. Ongoing trials are providing valuable information regarding the efficacy of different stents in various settings and are evaluating the utility of covered stents and ELGs in diffuse lesions. Ultimately, one must accept the idea that stenting is a technique-sensitive technology proven most appropriate for use by interventionists performing a large volume of cases in adequately equipped facilities.

References

1   Isner JM, Walsh K, Symes J, *et al.* Arterial gene transfer for therapeutic angiogenesis in patients with peripheral artery disease. *Hum Gene Ther* 1996; **7**: 959–88.

2   Alexandrova NA, Gibson WC, Norris JW, Maggisano R. Carotid artery stenosis in peripheral vascular disease. *J Vasc Surg* 1996; **23**: 645–9.

3   Birkmeyer JD, Quinton HB, O'Connor NJ, *et al.* The effect of peripheral vascular disease on long-term mortality after coronary artery bypass surgery. *Arch Surg* 1996; **131**: 316–21.

4   Richter GM, Roeren TH, Noeldge G, *et al.* Initial long-term results of a randomized 5-year study; iliac stent implantation versus PTA. *Vasa Suppl* 1992; **35**: 192–3.

5   Bourne EE, Kumpe DA. Percutaneous transluminal angioplasty and transcatheter embolization: fundamental considerations. In: Rutherford RB (ed.). *Vascular Surgery*, 3rd edn (Philadelphia: WB Saunders, 1989): 328–34.

6   Smith JM, Koury HI, Hafner CD, Welling RE. Subclavian steal syndrome. A review of 59 consecutive cases. *J Cardiovasc Surg* 1994; **35**: 11–14.

7   Branchereau A, Magnan PE, Espinoza H, Bartoli JM. Subclavian artery stenosis: Hemodynamic aspects and surgical outcome. *J Cardiovasc Surg* 1991; **32**: 604–12.

8   Mingoli A, Feldhaus RJ, Farina C, Schultz RD, Cavallero A. Comparative results of carotid-subclavian bypass and axillo-axillary bypass in patients with symptomatic subclavian diseaes. *Eur J Vasc Surg* 1992; **6**: 26–30.

9   Diethrich EB, Garrett HE, Ameriso J, Crawford ES, el-Bayar M, DeBakey ME. Occlusive disease of the common carotid

10 and subclavian arteries treated by carotid-subclavian bypass. Analysis of 125 cases. *Am J Surg* 1967; **114**: 800–8.

10 Criado FJ. Extrathoracic management of aortic arch syndrome. *Br J Surg* 1982; **69 (Suppl)**: S45–S51.

11 Diethrich EB, Ndiaye M, Reid DB. Stenting in the carotid artery: initial experience in 110 patients. *J Endovasc Surg* 1996; **3**: 42–62.

12 Tierstein PS, Schatz RA, Rocha-Singh KJ. Coronary stenting with angioscopic guidance. *J Am Coll Cardiol* 1992; **19**: 223A (abstract).

13 Strumpf RK, Heuser RR, Eagen JT. Angioscopy: a valuable tool in the deployment and evaluation of intracoronary stents. *Am Heart J* 1993; **126**: 1204–10.

14 Senneff MJ, Schatz RA, Tierstein PS. The clinical utility of angioscopy during intracoronary stent implantation. *J Interven Cardiol* 1994; **7**: 181–6.

15 Gussenhoven EJ, van der Lugt A, Pasterkamp G, *et al.* Intravascular ultrasound predictors of outcome after peripheral balloon angioplasty. *Eur J Vasc Endovasc Surg* 1995; **10**: 279–88.

16 Cavaye DM, Diethrich EB, Santiago OJ, Kopchok GE, Laas TE, White RA. Intravascular ultrasound imaging: an essential component of angioplasty assessment and vascular stent deployment. *Int Angiol* 1993; **12**: 212–20.

17 Katzen BT, Benenati JF, Becker GJ, *et al.* Role of intravascular ultrasound in peripheral atherectomy and stent deployment. *Circulation* 1991; **84**: 2152 (abstract).

18 White RA, Scoccianti M, Back M, Kopchok G, Donayre C. Innovations in vascular imaging; arteriography, three-dimensional CT scans, and two- and three-dimensional intravascular ultrasound evaluation of an abdominal aortic aneurysm. *Ann Vasc Surg* 1994; **8**: 285–9.

19 Murphy KD, Encarnacion CE, Le VA, Palmaz JC. Iliac artery stent placement with the Palmaz stent. *J Vasc Intervent Radiol* 1995; **6**: 321–9.

20 Martin EC, Katzen BT, Benenati JF, *et al.* Multicenter trial of the Wallstent in the iliac and femoral arteries. *J Vasc Intervent Radiol* 1995; **6**: 843–9.

21 Diethrich EB. Initial experience with stenting in the innominate, subclavian, and carotid arteries. *J Endovasc Surg* 1995; **2**: 196–221.

22 Kumar K, Dorros G, Bates M, *et al.* Primary stent deployment in occlusive subclavian artery disease. *Cathet and Cardiovasc Diagn* 1995; **34**: 281–5.

23 Sullivan TM, Bacharach M, Childs MB. PTA and primary stenting of the subclavian and innominate arteries. *Circulation* 1995; **92**: I-383 (abstract).

36

The use of stent grafts in arterial pathologies: an overview after review of 147 clinical cases

Juan Carlos Parodi

Introduction

This chapter deals with the development and evolution of an endovascular treatment created as an alternative solution to the abdominal aortic aneurysms (AAAs) in patients with such a prohibitive risk that they might not afford conventional surgery.[1-3] We analyze its very new application to the thoracic descending aorta, to a dissection of the ascending thoracic aorta, as well as to all arterial-venous fistulae and false aneurysms repaired by this means.

The system combines the use of arterial grafts and stents for arterial repair. It is noticeable that the improvement of all auxiliary diagnostic methods has led to a more accurate definition of the images as well as the enhancement of the number of cases the surgeon has to solve.

We also refer to the minor and deadly complications, and the elective treatment and the low postoperative mortality rate at respected medical centers. Still, the pathology associated to AAA in increasingly older patients has augmented mortality up to 60%[4] when related to aortic aneurysm surgery. Our procedure is based upon the replacement of all sutures; and, by stents, to fix the proximal and distal ends of the graft to the normal arterial wall in the AAA obstructive pathologies. A-V fistulas are occluded by stents previously covered by autologous saphenous vein or else a predilated poly-tetra-flouroethylene (PTFE) graft. This system is supported by experimental trials which demonstrated that stents can act by friction against the arterial wall, fixing the graft by its edges in the appropriate place with the aid of radioscopy. The device could be applied owing to the development of an endoluminal implantation graft consisting of a modified Palmaz' stent which seized a very soft Dacron graft. They were both opened by means of a balloon carried by a catheter placed in the axis of the system. When insufflated from the free end, the balloon would push them both radially against the arterial wall, deploying them to its maximum. In this way, a watertight seal was created to exclude the aneurysm completely with no leakage.

Today, new metallic alloys are available and, since the beginning of 1996, we are implanting a new device provided with a self-expandable stent where the balloon is electively used and generally, corrects or improves the watertight seal.

The arterial approach is made with an 18F (ID) introducer, through the femoral artery. The arteriotomy is a very small one. The device is advanced over the guiding wire, and then positioned and deployed under fluoroscopy guidance. In these cases, the approach is not only femoral but also brachial, to direct a guidewire between the arm and the isolated iliac branch of the device, and to make its connection possible with the corresponding stump in the main body of the graft.

Material and methods

Stent graft device

A teflon 18F (ID) sheath, 45 cm in length with a hemostatic valve closure in the operator end contains the balloon catheter, consisting of a 9F polyethylene shaft and one or two nylon balloons, 3.5 cm in length, and either 30, 25 or

16 mm in diameter. The assembly contains one or two balloon-expandable stents (in case of two balloons, either two aortic stents or an aortic and an iliac stent). A thin-walled, crimped-knitted Dacron graft was sutured to the stents, overlapping one half of the length of the stent.

The graft is a thin-walled (0.2 mm) weft-knitted graft with compliant ends (45%) to allow expansion of the stent. The diameters of the grafts are 18 and 20 mm when tubular grafts are applied and 18 and 8 mm when tapered grafts for aortoiliac position are needed. For thoracic aorta application, a 25 mm diameter graft was utilized. Figure 36.1 shows the components of the endovascular device.

The balloon catheter we currently used (Balt Company, Paris, France) was constructed of nylon material and had some degree of compliance. This compliance allowed us to use only two balloon sizes (25 and 30 mm in diameter).

For aortoiliac grafting either a double balloon (25 and 12 mm in diameter) or two independent balloons are used. Since the beginning of 1996, we have been using our new Vanguard device, provided with self-expandable stent grafts. They are introduced in a closed position with the aid of cold saline solution which is infused through a lateral lure lock. Once in place, the covering sheath is drawn back, setting the stent graft free in place with the aid of warm saline solution through the lateral pathway.

In cases where arteriovenous fistulas or false aneurysms were treated, a covered stent was constructed by means of covering the stent with an expandable Dacron graft or a preexpanded PTFE graft; on two occasions the stent was covered with autogenous vein because of the risk of infection. The only case of false aneurysm of the internal carotid was treated by a vein-covered stent with the intention of providing a less thrombogenic surface.

We introduced the self-expandable stent to our device in the beginning of 1996; this was a Stentor Nitinol Mintech model. Soon after, we tried our Vanguard, manufactured by Boston Scientific following our directions for the design.

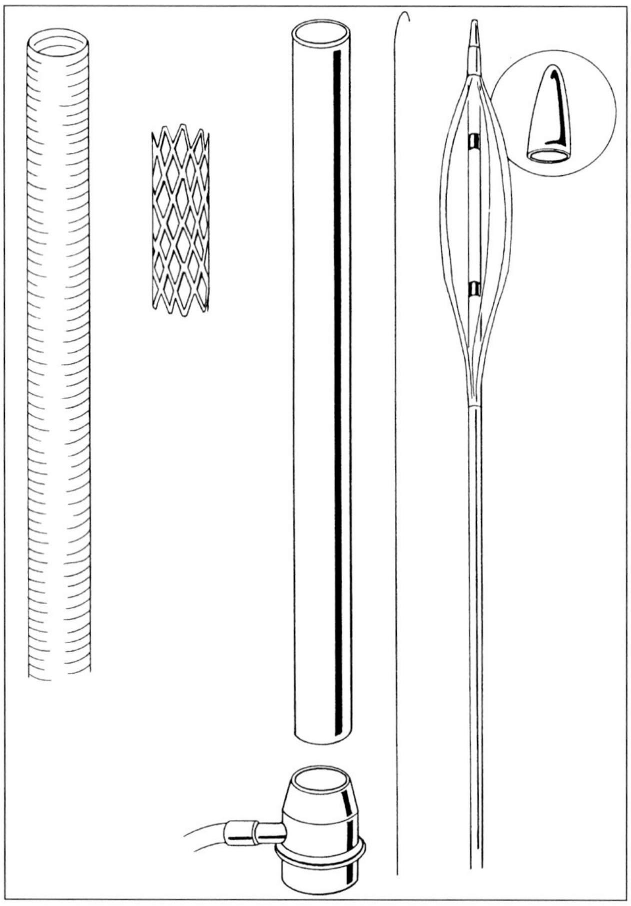

Procedure

The procedure[5] is briefly described. Every patient, and a close relative, signed a written informed consent form. Under local or epidural anesthesia the patient is prepared and draped as for a standard AAA resection. In the three cases in which the thoracic aneurysm was treated, general anesthesia was utilized. A small incision is developed over the chosen common femoral artery. Usually the straighter and wider artery is selected for access. A soft-tipped guidewire is advanced in the aorta up to the level of the diaphragm; over the wire a pigtail diagnostic catheter is placed inside the lumen of the aorta with the tip located proximal to the renal arteries. The first injection of 30 cc of contrast media is performed. The pigtail catheter has radio-opaque markers engraved on its surface every 2 cm to facilitate lengths and diameter measurements using quantitative angiography.

The target areas are defined from previously obtained images, i.e. angiography and computed tomography (CT) scans. Today the most accurate means of sizing is the three-dimensional (3D) reconstruction of a contrasted CT scan, which lets us appreciate the kinks and axial deviations. These are the proximal neck of the aneurysm and distal cuff, if the latter exists, or the common iliac artery in the case of absence of the distal cuff.

The preloaded sheath containing the stent and graft mounted on a balloon is placed inside the lumen of the aneurysm under fluoroscopic guidance (Fig. 36.2).

Once in place, the sheath is removed and the cranial balloon is inflated with a diluted solution of ionic contrast

Figure 36.1
The graft-stent combination is mounted on a valvuloplasty balloon and placed under fluoroscopy through the sheath introduced through femoral arteriotomy.

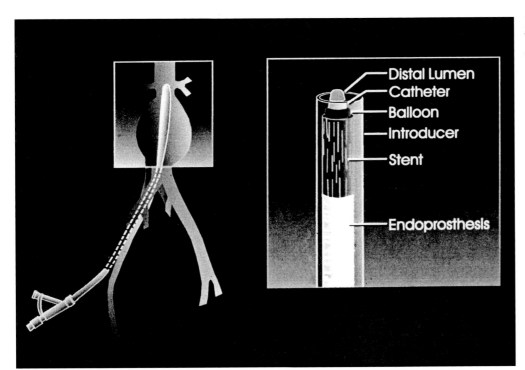

Figure 36.2
The elements comprising the
endovascular device.

media (we discarded the nonionic contrast media because of the potential problem of crystallization) and saline. The balloon is kept inflated for 1 min and then gently deflated. Before proceeding with balloon inflation the main blood pressure is dropped using nitroglycerin solution. Blood pressure is kept at 70 mm of mercury during balloon inflation.

The size of the balloon is selected beforehand according to the diameter of the neck of the aneurysm measured in the previous angiogram and CT scan.

After securing the proximal stent, the second stent is placed. In some cases, when a double balloon device was used, the second balloon (either aortic or iliac) is positioned at the appropriate level and inflated deploying the second stent. A final angiogram is performed. The contralateral common iliac artery is then occluded by means of the use of an occluding stent graft. Blood flow from the femoro-femoral bypass perfuses the internal iliac artery in a retrograde fashion (Fig. 36.3).

A new device composed of self-expandable stents with thermal memory, and covered by very thin polyester grafts, has been used by us since the beginning of 1996. Twelve patients have received this new graft for the repair of aneurysms. Both a femoral and a brachial approach are needed. The device is introduced through a femoral artery to place the aortoiliac body of the graft and a guidewire is introduced downwards, from the arm, to reach the puncture of the contralateral femoral artery. This will lead to the isolated femoral branch of the graft all the way up. By this

means the assembly of both parts of the stent graft is completed.

A total of 106 patients with abdominal aortic aneurysms were treated from September 1990 to December 1996. Table 36.1 summarizes the associated pathologic conditions of the patients threatened. Three patients were admitted with the diagnosis of blue-toe syndrome with the source of the thrombus being an AAA. The size of the aneurysm at the time of treatment was more than 5 cm in diameter in 69 patients. Two patients had small aneurysms that caused microembolization—the reason they were included in this therapeutic group. The third patient with an aneurysm of less than 5 cm had a bilateral carotid endarterectomy and coronary bypass surgery the same year. It was decided to have his 4.5 cm AAA treated by the endoluminal method; sizes ranged from 3.8 cm to 12 cm. The last 16 cases, included in a clinical trial in Europe, had AAA of diameters ranging from 3.8 to 5 cm.

One patient had a type A dissecting aneurysm at the site of cannulation after coronary bypass which was treated surgically by replacing a segment of the ascending aorta with a Dacron graft. A few days after the procedure the patient developed a new flap of dissection starting from the distal aortic suture, and a rupture of the descending aorta. A covered stent (Dacron) was implanted at the suture line, effectively closing the false lumen.

A 68-year-old female was treated for a thoracic abdominal aneurysm with a stent graft; the aneurysm did not involve visceral branches. In addition, a descending thoracic

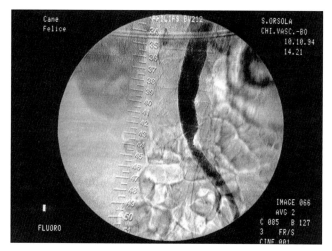

a

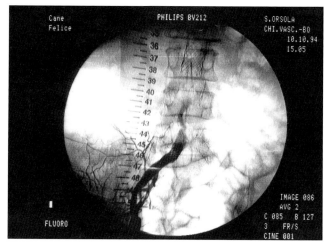

b

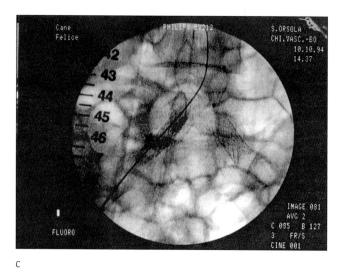

c

Figure 36.3
Aortoiliac graft in place. Balloon occlusion of the contralateral iliac artery and femoro-femoral bypass.

Table 36.1 Associated pathologic conditions.

Severe chronic heart disease	53 Patients
Acute myocardial infarction	23 Patients
Severe pulmonary insufficiency	26 Patients (three oxygen dependent)
Renal insufficiency	6 Patients (two on dialysis)
Acute hemorrhagic cerebral infarction	1 Patient
Two previous strokes	10 Patients
Hostile abdomen	2 Patients
Cirrhosis ascitis GI bleeding	2 Patients
Mild pulmonary insufficiency	12 Patients
Intermittent claudication	33 Patients
DIC	1 Patient
Pre-existing atheroembolism	3 Patients

aneurysm was treated in an inoperable 74-year-old patient. Patients treated for other conditions (A-V fistulas and FA) are described later.

Demographics (patients with aneurysms)

A total of 100 men and 6 women were treated for abdominal aneurysms. Average age was 78 years (range: 57–100 years). Nine patients were over 80 years. All three cases of thoracic aorta were men. All patients had at least one associated morbid condition (Table 36.1). Eight patients were considered to be an acceptable risk and were to be treated with the standard surgery but were included as volunteers. Thirty-one patients were clearly in the high-risk group and 24 were considered inoperable by at least two well-recognized vascular surgeons. The procedures performed are shown in Table 36.2.

Acute results

Seventy-nine of the 109 (73%) procedures for AAA exclusion were considered successful. Definition of a successful procedure includes complete exclusion of the aneurysm with restoration of the normal blood flow. The stent graft should be in contact with normal intima, since sealing in an area covered with laminated thrombus is usually incomplete and temporary.

Patients with successful procedures recovered rapidly, eating the next morning and walking within 24–48 hr after the procedure. Typically they were discharged from the hospital after 3 or 4 days. Thirty out of the 109 (27%) procedures were considered as initial failures. Five of the 30 failures were correctable using endoluminal treatment, but because of the prohibitive risk of this group of patients, additional treatment was not attempted at that time.

Failures and complications

One case of misplacement of the proximal stent was treated by standard surgical procedure. The patient survived and did well.

Four cases of proximal leak occurred. In one patient with minimal leak, the size of the aneurysm decreased in spite of the leak and it disappeared in a few weeks. This patient died 6 months after the procedure of an unrelated cause. The second and third patients had an important leak. One died after 7 months of cardiac insufficiency and the remaining two patients died of a ruptured aneurysm 2 and 7 months after the procedure, respectively. Every case of leak is considered a failure.

One case of incomplete deployment of the proximal stent resulted in migration of the graft. Because of this failure, the patient was treated by standard AAA resection. Liver cirrhosis, ascitis and gastrointestinal bleeding were the indication for endoluminal treatment. The patient survived the operation but died of abnormal bleeding the next day.

Seven patients had distal leaks. In one patient, the leak

Table 36.2 Procedures performed in aneurysms.

Aortoaortic graft with one stent (proximal)	8 Procedures
Aortoaortic graft with two stents (both ends)	43 Procedures
Aortoiliac graft	46 Procedures*
Aorto-bi-iliac graft	12 Procedures
Ilioiliac graft	4 Procedures**
Total procedures	113
Total of patients	110

Notes:

*One secondary procedure was performed after a late failure of an aortoaortic graft.

**In two patients a simultaneous aortoaortic and ilioiliac graft was used to treat an AAA and a common iliac aneurysm. In one patient the common iliac aneurysm was repaired one week later. One patient had an isolated common iliac artery.

persisted for 3 weeks and subsided. In a second patient, the leak persisted, although minimal. This patient died of pulmonary and cardiac insufficiency 8 months later.

Three patients had massive microembolization after difficult procedures applied in large and tortuous aneurysms. These procedures ended with massive microembolization and the patients died, after developing disseminated intravascular coagulopathy (DIC) and multiple organ failure. One additional patient died suddenly after 2 days. The post-mortem examination disclosed intestinal ischemia and renal infarcts, probably related to embolization during the procedure.

Incomplete deployment of the distal stent occurred in one patient. Attempts to open the stent with different balloons failed and the procedure was converted to an open procedure. Operative mortality (within 30 days) was 9%. Causes of death were massive microembolization (3), visceral embolization (1), pulmonary embolism (1), pulmonary insufficiency (1), myocardial infarction (1) and coagulopathy (1).

In addition to the above-mentioned complications that caused the procedure to fail, we had some others that could be solved at the time of occurrence (Table 36.3). In 8 of the 106 aortic abdominal procedures, both renal artery ostias were covered with the stent. The graft attached to the stent was placed distal to the renal arteries. None of these patients developed renal insufficiency and color duplex of the renal arteries were normal. They are repeated every 6 months. Three balloon dilatations of the iliac arteries were performed in the series before inserting the stent-graft device; two common femoral aneurysms were corrected surgically at the time of the procedure and four common iliac temporary conduits with a 10 mm tubular Dacron graft were constructed to permit access to the aorta in the presence of very tortuous and stenotic iliac arteries.

Three patients had iliac artery injury during the procedure due to difficult access. Iliac arteries were calcified and very tortuous. Two patients required a surgical solution for the complication and one patient was treated with an endovascular stent graft.

Long-term results

The average follow-up period was 32 months with a range between 1 and 60 months. All patients were followed by clinical examination, color duplex studies every 6 months and CT scans once a year. Angiograms were performed in some patients and in each one in whom the color duplex and/or CT scan indicated or suggested any sign of leak into the aneurysmal sac (incomplete sealing), dilatation or any change when compared with the study performed immediately after the procedure.

One patient developed a distal aortic dilatation after 18 months of the initial procedure. The distal stent was placed too distally of the aortic bifurcation and in contact with a mural thrombus and not with the normal aortic wall. This complication was corrected by adding a short segment of graft, performing a surgical anastomosis between the old graft and the aortic bifurcation. The patient recovered uneventfully.

Four patients who had only the proximal stent deployed developed a distal reflux with shrinkage of the graft 8, 18, 24 and 29 months after the procedure. Two patients underwent an additional procedure to correct this complication (insertion of a covered stent at the distal end) completely sealing the leak in one, and leaving a minimal leak in the second patient (it was impossible with our current resources to obtain the expected result). One patient is ready to have additional treatment and the fourth declined undergoing any further procedures.

One patient who had an aortoiliac graft implanted two

Table 36.3 Complications (failures treated separately).

Groin hematoma	2 Patients
Proximal leak (treated with a covered stent)	4 Patients
Injury to the external iliac artery (sutured)	3 Patients
Minimal distal microembolization treated by intra-arterial injection of prostaglandin	3 Patients
Distal leak (treated with covered stent)	7 Patients
Incomplete deployment of distal stent	1 Patient
Incomplete deployment of proximal stent	1 Patient

years previously developed a distal leak. The iliac artery in which the distal stent was implanted was aneurysmal and the stent was anchored at the point of a ring of normal caliber in the middle of the common iliac artery. The aneurysm increased in size and a leak was created. An attempt to seal the leak failed.

Four patients with aortoaortic graft with two stents developed a distal leak after 12 and 16 months. The reason for this change could not be explained. The possible causes considered were dilatation of the neck and lysis of the thrombus when the stent graft was improperly positioned—being the end of the graft in contact with the thrombus and not the arterial wall.

Two patients died 13 and 24 months respectively after the procedure, affected by a carcinoma of the colon. An additional patient died after being admitted to the clinic because of cardiac failure and respiratory insufficiency 8 months after the initial procedure. Two patients died of cardiac insufficiency 6 and 7 months after the procedure. One patient with proximal leak (failure) died of a ruptured AAA two months after an unsuccessful procedure. One patient who had a late failure, 16 months after the procedured (distal leak after an aortoaortic graft) sustained a ruptured aneurysm and died. One patient was readmitted to the clinic 3 months after the initial procedure with pulmonary edema and was discharged one week later.

One patient developed a subdural hematoma 3 months after the initial treatment, but recovered after draining the hematoma surgically. The hematoma was probably caused by a small trauma since our patients did not receive any specific medication after the treatment, not even antiplatelet drugs.

Sixty-four percent of the patients of the initial group and 84% of the initially successful group of patients had good results after the primary procedure until the last clinical visit or until the moment of death due to unrelated causes.

Only one patient with an aortoiliac procedure had a late failure (distal reflux into the aneurysmal sac). Initial results of aortoiliac procedures were inferior when compared with aortoaortic procedures, due to the larger profile of the introducer needed for its deployment that generated inconveniences with access. However, late results were more favorable with the aortoiliac procedure. Most of the complications were correctable by additional endoluminal procedures.

Arteriovenous fistulas: Six patients were treated using the covered stent procedure. The first patient had a subclavian arteriovenous fistula that developed 2 years after a gunshot wound. The patient had a favorable outcome after implantation of a Dacron-covered stent.

The second patient had a common iliac-inferior vena cava fistula caused by an accident during laparoscopic surgery. A percutaneous stent graft was applied from the ipsilateral common femoral artery.

The third patient was referred to us to solve an A-V fistula between the abdominal aorta and the inferior vena cava. The patient had sustained a gunshot wound several months before and underwent four surgical attempts to treat multiple lesions in the abdomen including the A-V fistula. The endoluminal procedure was performed under local anesthesia. A 3.5-cm covered stent was deployed covering the communication, interrupting effectively the flow through the fistula. The patient was discharged the next day. An additional patient who was admitted because of an aortocava fistula was treated successfully in the same way.

The sixth patient treated for an A-V fistula was a young female injured by a gunshot in her right thigh. An A-V fistula between the superficial femoral artery and vein was diagnosed. A covered stent was applied at the site of the fistula percutaneously using a 14F sheath applied anterogradely through the common femoral artery.

Infected femoral false aneurysm: One patient was admitted with an infected false aneurysm of the common femoral artery caused by a coronary stenting procedure performed 10 days before. This patient suffered from renal insufficiency and unstable angina. A stent covered with autologous vein was deployed through the superficial femoral artery. Expansion of the false aneurysm subsided and the cavity was debrided and drained. A 30-year-old male who sustained a gunshot wound in the right supraclavicular region developed an A-V fistula between the subclavian artery and vein, and a false aneurysm of the thyrocervical branch of the subclavian artery. A detachable balloon occluded the false aneurysm of the branch and a Dacron-covered stent occluded the abnormal communication between the artery and vein.

A 20-year-old male, suffering from AIDS, was admitted to the clinic with a false aneurysm of the common carotid artery near its take-off from the innominate trunk. A covered stent using an autologous vein was deployed covering the orifice of the carotid artery.

Another vascular trauma case we treated was of a 38-year-old patient who had sustained a neck trauma in the past and who had developed, probably related to a carotid dissection, a false aneurysm at the level of the base of the skull. This patient had five episodes of cerebral ischemia with resulting cerebral infarcts depicted in the CT scan; the last two episodes of cerebral ischemia occurred during oral anticoagulation treatment. The patient was treated using a vein-covered Palmaz stent, and experienced no further episodes of cerebral ischemia; the false aneurysm was effectively excluded. After 18 months the patient interrupted oral anticoagulation and the day after developed an hemispheric transient ischemia attack (TIA), arteriogram depicted an external compression of the Palmaz stent at the level of the base of the skull. All the procedures to treat trauma cases with the exception of this last patient were successful.

Two patients were treated for common iliac aneurysms,

one patient had an AAA treated simultaneously. Both procedures were successful in the short- and long-term.

Three patients with aortic occlusive disease underwent aortic stent angioplasty.

Discussion

After 109 procedures for treating aneurysms and 38 for other applications (A-V fistulas, false aneurysms, occlusive disease), some preliminary conclusions can be made. The procedure is feasible and, when successfully applied, has the great attraction of simplicity. The application of covered stents in trauma cases appears to be a main application of this method since it transforms a complicated and potentially dangerous procedure into a simple and safe one. Stenosis can be defined as the only potential long-term complication. In the near future stent grafts could eventually be used in acute injuries of the vessel, both in civil or war conditions, to temporarily stop blood loss.

This procedure can be combined with endovascular control of bleeding of secondary branches using detachable balloons, coils, occluding stents or the injection of fluids that become solid inside the body when body temperature is reached. This procedure has proved to be useful in injuries to vessels, such as the subclavian artery, that represent a real challenge even to the experienced surgeon.

In treatment of aortic aneurysms, there were, however, more problems than initially could be predicted. The procedure is simple in theory, but there are several details that should be taken care of before moving ahead with the widespread use of the method.

Diameter and length measurement

Measurement of diameters and lengths are crucial. We learnt with experience how to obtain reliable data using enhanced CT scan, quantitative angiography and 3D reconstruction using MR or CT scan images. Intraluminal measurement and some geometric calculations helped us to obtain reasonably reliable data. Understanding that elongation occurs as dilatation of the aorta develops and also that elongation occurs in different planes allowed us to calculate more accurately the actual length of the artery.

It appears that the final answer with regard to measurements will come from computer image processing using 3D reconstruction of spiral CT or MRI scans and, probably, a simulation program of insertion of a stent-graft device. In the meantime, we prefer to overestimate the length instead of underestimate it, since graft in excess can be accommodated by the 'accordion mechanism' allowed by the crimping of the graft. Based on our own experience, such kinking could be solved by placement of an inner stent at that level.

Access problems

Access problems accounted for several difficulties to be overcome. Narrow, stenotic and tortuous iliac arteries were responsible for these difficulties. The rigid stent and the large diameter of the sheath needed for the implantation represented a drawback from the beginning. We overcame some of these problems by modifying the device and using different maneuvers during the procedure. Reducing the diameter of the sheath to 18F was a remarkable advance towards the ideal device.

The use of an extra-stiff wire, the 'pulldown' maneuver and sometimes implantation of a temporary conduit on the common iliac artery were also useful resources to overcome some of these problems. The pulldown maneuver consists of dissecting free the common femoral and external iliac arteries, just lifting the inguinal ligament up, and using blunt dissection, reaching the iliac bifurcation from the groin. Small branches should be divided between suture ligatures. When the arteries are free, and pulling the artery gently towards the feet of the patient, the tortuous artery becomes staighter making the introduction of the sheath possible.

Our findings dictate, that in some groups of patients a tubular graft would be applicable. When the distal aortic cuff is not present, an aorto-bi-iliac graft has to be used as advocated by Chuter.[6] In addition, when the angle between the iliac arteries becomes larger than 90°, an aortoiliac graft should be used, placing a femoro-femoral bypass. We foresee that the three systems available will be applicable in patients with AAA. Small and medium-sized AAAs will benefit with an aortoaortic system, large aneurysms with aorto-bi-iliac or aortoiliac systems with the addition of a femoro-femoral bypass and exclusion of the contralateral common iliac artery.

We believe, at this stage, that endoluminal treatment of AAA will be applicable in patients with large or symptomatic aneurysm in whom the standard surgical graft replacement represents a prohibitive operative risk. The best solution for these patients will be the aortoiliac procedure since most of them have tortuous and often aneurysmatic iliac arteries. Frequently, the axis of both common iliac arteries defines an angle in excess of 100°, making the placement of a bifurcated graft impossible.

The issue of arterial dilatation should be addressed. We still do not know what the impact will be of a stent embedded in the vessel wall, in terms of prevention of future dilatation. In the mean time we have elected to treat high-risk patients with large or symptomatic aneurysms. We believe that only well controlled limited trials involving young patients with small aneurysms should be conducted due to the uncertain long-term results of the endoluminal treatment of AAA.

The extraperitoneal laparoscopic approach seems not to be very difficult and perhaps will represent a step forward eventually to treat young patients with AAA with a long life expectancy, without the compromise of the stent-graft attachment due to arterial dilatation.

Anchoring mechanism

Balloon-expandable stents, because of their high radial force, appear to be the ideal device as an anchoring mechanism. This is probably true for the time of implant and shortly after. The diameter of arteries increases with time. In addition, the effect of a stent producing an internal radial force would produce further dilatation.

We experienced one problem when the stent was incompletely deployed (one case of stent migration). Intraluminal ultrasound will be the ideal way to check for completeness of stent deployment. In this regard, the pioneer work of Cavaye and White[7] indicates that intraluminal ultrasound should be almost mandatory as a completion study after finishing a stent-graft implantation. In our modest experience with this method, abnormalities were found with intraluminal ultrasound that were not detected with digital angiogram. As predicated by Cavaye and White, ultrasound real-time imaging during stent deployment will probably be a requirement in the future, to obtain reliable results. An ultrasound probe can be placed in one of the lumens of the balloon catheter and positioned at the level of the balloon. In our opinion, having experienced many difficulties, this will be one of the most striking new developments to improve the endoluminal technique to treat AAA.

In regard to the use of a modification of the Palmaz stent as an anchoring system, it should be said that clinical results utilizing the Palmaz stent in occlusive disease cannot be compared with the reaction of the arterial tissue to this new application. Arteries in patients with AAA are usually dilated, not stenotic, and its wall is very often thinner than that of the normal arteries and much thinner than the atherosclerotic artery. We do not know the reaction of the thin-walled artery. It should also be emphasized that this segment of the artery with a normal, or near normal, diameter has some biochemical changes such as enhanced activity of elastase and collagenase that make the situation more unpredictable. Most probably the next generation of stents will have an intermediate radial force which will be enough to anchor the graft properly but, on the other hand, do not produce dilatation of the artery.

Using an extraperitoneal laparoscopic approach in pigs, we placed a tape around the aorta close to the renal arteries in order to create external banding and prevent dilatation of the artery. The tape is a polyethylene mesh with wide-open interstices to avoid decubitus when compressing the arterial wall with the stent inside.

Microembolization

We consider microembolization to be the most serious problem with this procedure. We were able to solve almost all the complications except microembolization. This complication occurred four times in our experience; three of the four cases resulted in death. In the remaining case, discrete microembolization of the right foot was successfully treated with intra-arterially administration of prostaglandin EI.

The three cases resulting in massive microembolization were technically difficult procedures in patients with large aneurysms. In one case visceral ischemia was found in the post-mortem examination. In this last case technical problems occurred during the procedure in relation to inappropriate balloon sizing.

A third case of embolization occurred, also after a complex situation created by a technical failure of the balloons used in the procedure. The patient died suddenly, 48 hr after the procedure. Post-mortem examination disclosed visceral embolization.

Reviewing our cases of embolization it is clear that large and tortuous aneurysms pose an increased potential incidence of embolization which is probably due to two factors:

1 On advancing the guidewire from the femoral artery into the aorta and then into the proximal neck, the operator will negotiate it inside a large and tortuous chamber coated with friable material. Sometimes it is difficult to get the guidewire inside the proximal neck, since from within the cavity of the aneurysm, the orifice of the proximal neck is very often small. Such maneuvers could eventually cause dislodgement of particles of the laminated thrombus. Thus, it is advisable in cases of large aneurysms with wide lumens to insert the guidewire percutaneously from the brachial artery.

2 Very often miscalculation of the length of the aneurysm created the necessity to change the device, or to use a complementary procedure such as implanting a third covered stent to increase the length of the device or cover a leak. The more intravascular manipulation performed, the greater the risk for dislodgement of particles from the aortic wall.

What can be done to prevent microembolization? In cases of large aneurysms with large lumens, the soft-tipped guidewire should be introduced from the brachial artery distal wise and recovered from the common femoral artery that has been chosen in advance.

Care should be taken to measure the length and diameters of the arteries precisely and to perform a simple well planned procedure.

After successfully treating patients who were admitted due to spontaneous visceral and distal embolization, we can say that, even in the presence of friable thrombus in the lumen of the AAA, endoluminal treatment can be performed safely.

Future considerations

It is clear that this new development has represented a different and new challenge for the medical industry. How do we foresee the future in terms of the ideal device to be utilized in endoluminal treatment of aneurysms?

Anchoring mechanism

The balloon-expandable stent we are using seems to be the ideal way to obtain a dependable fixation of the graft. A computer projection study of the stress load to the stent struts during the foreseeable lifespan of an average patient suggested that the fatigue limit of the stent will not be approached.

A flexible stent will be needed to be able to negotiate tortuous iliac arteries. Hooks are probably not needed and dangerous. Self-expandable spring-loaded stents are, in general, weaker in terms of radial force and do not accommodate to irregular lumens. In addition, if made of multiple parts, micromotion between metal surfaces disrupts protective oxide films, allowing the area to corrode rapidly, leading to mechanical failure. One should keep in mind that this device should last intact for the lifespan of the patient.

Self-expanding spring-loaded stents made of nitinol with thermal memory deserve independent comment. This stent has a combination of two forces that, when interacting, create a stronger force. Radial force in self-expandable stents depends on the strength and diameter of the wire, among other characteristics. If, in addition to this mechanism, a second force generated by thermal memory of the metal produces a secondary expansion of the stent as soon as the given temperature is reached, the final hoop stress is/will be almost comparable with a strong, one piece, balloon-expandable stent.

Graft

Either Dacron or PTFE could be used for grafts. A thin wall is needed as is the crimping in the case of Dacron or the stretch ability if PTFE is used. Crimping is needed to obtain a kink-resistant graft.

Balloons

Balloons should be partially compliant, scratch resistant, reinforced to prevent rupture and wrapped in such a way that rotation does/will not take place or at least should not be significant. A rigid, noncompliant balloon could be an inconvenience in dealing with patients with irregular lumens. In those cases gaps between the stent and arterial wall could generate thrombus and leaks between the graft and arterial lumen.

Preprocedure studies

Preprocedure studies should include CT scans (slices every 5 mm or less and 3D reconstruction) and angiography. Spiral CT scan, when available, would represent a significant advantage. MR angiography with additional software may be/can be the procedure of choice in the future.

Imaging

During the procedure high-resolution fluoroscopy is needed. Road-mapping seems advantageous. Intravascular ultrasound (IVUS) proved to be very useful to assess completeness of stent deployment. We have used IVUS in two instances. The second time, IVUS allowed to detect and solve a graft fold in the iliac artery that was missed in the arteriogram. Speculation can be made in regard to imaging in endovascular stent-graft treatment of AAA and occlusive disease in the near future. It will be possible to complete the procedure without using any x-ray method. MR imaging and ultrasound could, eventually, cover all the needs, providing that new developments now in research are completed, without irradiating the patient and the attending staff.

Conclusions

We still have some basic doubts about the procedure we are proposing. Long-term stent-graft interaction is one of our main concerns. Stent edges could cause damage to the graft through direct mechanical action or through a material fatigue mechanism. As the stent and graft are covered by tissue in a few weeks, the potential impact of this possible damage will probably be without clinical importance. What is unquestionable is that the device should be designed to last, achieving aneurysm exclusion and maintaining flow throughout the lifetime of the patient.

A second main concern is the tissue reaction after the endovascular treatment of AAA. It is known[8] that both the composition and mechanical properties of AAA are different from those of nonaneurysmal aortas. The aneurysms are stiffer, and the volume fractions of collagen and ground substance are increased, whereas the volume fractions of elastin and muscle are decreased in aneurysms.

The changes in diameter of the neck of the aneurysm after stent implantation are unknown. Intimal hyperplasia develops over the stent, with some atrophy of the media and reaction of the adventitia. These changes and the presence of the stent itself forming part of the architecture of the arterial wall will probably prevent dilatation of the aneurism, then reducing the tension on the arterial wall.

It should be emphasized that watertight sealing between the arterial wall and the stent-graft unit should be obtained from the first moment. The lack of a leak into the aneurysmal sac injecting contrast media should not be considered as a primary success. A graft and stent in contact with a thrombus can temporarily seal, but not for a long time. The thrombus dissolves and a leak appears in few weeks or months. Endovascular ultrasound and or CT scanning with contrast media can tell for sure the completeness of stent deployment. Both ends of the graft should be in contact and sealed with the arterial wall, and not with the thrombus, to consider the result acceptable. X-ray images during procedures should be interpreted through a reconstruction of the actual aneurysm based on CT scans taken in small slices (5 mm or less). A clear definition on where the thrombus starts and finishes will allow the placement of stents in the appropriate site.

Spontaneous embolization is the second complication of AAA in number and importance. Embolization takes place when a thrombus becomes friable and the mural thrombus suffers a dissection. Usually, microthrombi migrate to the extremities and, also in a retrograde fashion, to the visceral arteries, mainly the renal arteries. In our experience, these very sick patients can be treated endoluminally. Providing that great care is taken to prevent rupture and damage of this friable material while the procedure is performed, thrombus can be effectively excluded, interrupting the shower of microemboli. We treated three patients affected by spontaneous microembolization with this method, associating intra-arterial prostaglandin E1 injection to control distal tissue damage.[9]

The relationship between stented grafts and microembolization deserves special comment. Microembolization is the most dreadful complication of the use of stented grafts for endoluminal treatment of AAA. On the other hand, endoluminal exclusion of AAAs is an emerging tool to treat microembolization from aneurysms.

At first glance, it seems unreasonable to use a therapy for a condition that can be caused by the proposed technique. The explanation for this is that aneurysms that embolize spontaneously are usually small. Small aneurysms have straight iliac arteries and aneurysms are usually nontortuous. Conversely, aneurysms that caused microembolization during endoluminal treatment were, in our experience, very large and tortuous and the iliac arteries were elongated. All these characteristics created technical difficulties in performing the endoluminal exclusion of the aneurysm. In 109 procedures of endoluminal treatment of AAA, massive microembolization occurred in four (3.6%) and mild unilateral microembolization in one (0.9%).

In spite of our encouraging results, we are aware of the necessity to perform controlled trials with a significant number of patients followed over a long period of time, before introducing the endoluminal treatment in clinical practice. In the mean time, experience should be concentrated in a few centers with the appropriate equipment, and a skilled group of surgeons and interventional radiologists or cardiologists with experience in interventional vascular procedures.

A word of caution should be given. We are finding new abnormalities among the groups of patients treated by us, as much as 3 years after performing, what we considered, a successful procedure. Before this procedure can be offered to the community as an alternative treatment for AAA, however, a clear, unremarkable long-term experience should be available to be presented to the medical community.

Regarding other applications of the stent-graft combination, treatment of arteriovenous fistulas appears to be a simple and effective application of the principle, saving time and preventing bleeding and peripheral nerve injuries. Treatment of false aneurysms in a nonaccessible place is also a very promising application, as it is a vascular trauma. Arterial dissections, mostly aortic dissections, will probably be efficiently treated endoluminally, interrupting the flow through intimal tearing. One of our cases showed how promising this approach could be. The development of an 'internal bypass' after balloon dilatation is an appealing idea in view of the failure of balloon dilatation in long stenosis or occlusions. In theory, isolating the inner surface of the treated artery will eventually prevent the interaction between the damaged intima and the circulating elements and substances of the blood. Our initial experience on treating thoracic aneurysms (one resulting in a type A dissection, a descending thoracic and a thoracoabdominal aneurysm with no compromise of the visceral arteries) indicates that the procedure is simpler than treating AAA and very promising.

Summary

Between September 1990 and December 1996, 148 patients were treated with transluminally placed endovascular grafts: 106 had abdominal aortic aneurysms (AAAs), 4 had iliac artery aneurysms (3 in association with AAAs), 3 had thoracic aneurysms, 8 had iliac occlusive disease and 25 had vascular injuries in various locations of the arterial tree.

Additionally, 3 patients with occlusive aortic disease were treated with single stents implanted in the aorta. The AAAs were excluded from the blood flow with a device composed of a balloon-expandable stent (modification of the Palmaz stent) attached to a Dacron graft designed to expand at both ends of the accompanying stent extension. By the end of 1995, the authors began to implant bifurcated grafts but had technical problems that led them to combine it with a Corvita stent to complete the procedure successfully. Those cases were considered as 'initial failures'. At the beginning of 1996, this device was changed to a self-expandable balloon stent-graft model but the final results are not yet available as the follow-up is less than 12 months. An 18F sheath containing the stent-graft device was introduced through a small cut-down in the common femoral artery and advanced under fluoroscopic guidance. Color duplex, contrast-enhanced computed tomography (CT) scanning and angiography were performed before the procedure and every 6 months. (Arteriography was performed once during the follow-up period and whenever other studies disclosed an abnormal finding.) A total of 106 patients (100 men and 6 women) with an AAA were treated: 51 patients underwent an aortoaortic procedure (8 patients had only a proximal stent implanted and 43 had proximal and distal stents). Forty-six patients were treated by implanting an aortoiliac graft, completing the procedure with a femoro-femoral bypass. The contralateral common iliac artery was occluded by means of an occluding stent; 12 aorto-bi-iliac procedures were performed and 4 ilioiliacs. The longest follow-up was 60 months and the shortest 1 month. Initial success was obtained in 84% of the aortoaortic cases and in 75% of the aortoiliac procedures. Long-term follow-up (>12 months) disclosed 78% success for the aortoaortic cases and 90% for the aortoiliac procedures. Late failures included distal aortic dilatation, distal leak into the aneurysmal cavity and proximal leak into the aneurysm. They completed 113 procedures in 110 patients. One type A dissecting aneurysm and two descending thoracic aneurysms were successfully treated by the endovascular technique. All trauma cases included false aneurysms (common carotid, subclavian, common femoral arteries) and arteriovenous fistulas (subclavian, aortocava, common iliaccava and superficial femoral artery and vein).

The authors concluded that stent-graft combination devices appear to be an alternative for treating vascular trauma and aneurysms. Initial success for treating AAA is almost 100%, and late success in aortoiliac cases is also high (90%) for aortoaotic reconstruction. However, late failures are frequent and require further evaluation in relation to a persistent increase in the diameter of the proximal neck and distal cuff.

References

1   Melton NJ, Bickerstaff LK, Hollier LH, et al. Changing incidence of abdominal aortic aneurysms: a population based study. Am J Epidemiol 1984; **120**: 379–86.

2   Brown OW, Hollier LH, Pairolero PC, et al. Abdominal aortic aneurysm and coronary artery disease: a reassessment. Arch Surg 1981; **116**: 1484–8.

3   Karmody AL, Leather RP, Goldman M, et al. The current position of non resection treatment for abdominal aortic aneurysms. Surgery 1983; **94**: 591–7.

4   McCombs RP, Roberts B. Acute renal failure after resection of abdominal aortic aneurysm. Surg Gynecol & Obstet 1979; **148**: 175–9.

5   Parodi JC, Palmaz JC, Barone HD. Transfemoral intraluminal graft implantation for abdominal aortic aneurysms. Ann Vasc Surg 1991; **5**: 491–9.

6   Chuter T, Donayre C, Wendt G. Bifurcated endovascular graft insertion for abdominal aortic aneurysms. Preliminary case reports. Surg Endosc 1994; **8**: 800–2. In: Greenhalgh, RM (ed.). Vascular and Endovascular Surgical Techniques, 3rd ed (Philadelphia, PA: WB Saunders, 1994): 92.

7   Cavaye DM, White RA. Intraluminal ultrasound and the management of peripheral vascular disease. In: Whittemore AD, et al, Advances in Vascular Surgery Volume 1 (St Louis: Mosby Yearbook, Inc, 1993): 137–56.

8   He CM, Roach MR. The compostion and mechanical properties of abdominal aortic aneurysms. J Vasc Surg 1994; **20**: 6–13.

9   Parodi J. Use of intra-arterial injection of prostaglandin E1 in the blue toe syndrome. In: Yao, J. Ischemic Extremity: Advances in Treatment (Norwalk CT: Appleton and Lange, 1996): 325–31.

37

Balloon mitral valvuloplasty: a single Israeli center experience

Yoav Turgeman and Tiberio Rosenfeld

Introduction

Since the introduction of percutaneous transvenous balloon mitral valvuloplasty (BMV) by Inoue et al.[1] in 1984, extensive clinical trials have established this procedure as an effective and safe alternative to surgical commissurotomy among selected patients with rheumatic mitral stenosis.[2-7] As the mechanism of BMV is similar to closed mitral commissurotomy, mainly commissural splitting,[8,9] their rate of success is comparable.[10,11] More redent studies have shown that the long-term results of BMV are equivalent to open mitral commissurotomy.[12] In contrast to the western countries where rheumatic fever has shown a steady decline, BMV has been extensively studied in the Far East, the Mediterranean, eastern Europe and South Africa.[13] Over the years, technical modalities and procedure-related equipment have been greatly improved. At the same time, while the indications were continuously expanded, the limitations of BMV have been quite well defined.[14] This chapter provides a report of the author's experience with BMV and a review of the literature.

Methods

Patients

Since March 1990, 185 patients with significant rheumatic mitral stenosis were referred to the authors' institute for preprocedure evaluation. The group included 165 females (89%) and 20 males (11%), mean age was 39 (12 years;

range 16–82). While 122 (66%) patients were in functional capacity (FC) III and/or IV (New York Heart Association [NYHA]) there were no patients in FC I. Twelve patients (6%) had an associated mild to moderate aortic regurgitation, 21 (11%) were after previous mitral valve surgery, 37 (20%) had chronic atrial fibrillation and three were pregnant.

All the patients with chronic or recurrent atrial tachyarrhythmias including history of embolic events were treated by warfarin for 6 weeks before the procedure.

Noninvasive preprocedure evaluation

Physical examination

Physical examination was concentrated on the clinical criteria for valvular pliability, the presence of additional valvular lesions, degree of pulmonary hypertension and severe chest deformities that have a significant meaning while performing trans-septal puncture.[15]

Echocardiography

Transthoracic: A comprehensive two-dimensional (2D) color Doppler study was undertaken in order to define diastolic gradient, pressure half-time and planimetric mitral valve areas; valvular and subvalvular components morphology; commissural pathoanatomy; and preprocedure mitral regurgitation.

The 'Wilkins' echocardiographic score[16] was used only as a rough parameter for patient selection; however, we did not perform the procedure among highly deformed valves with a score ≥12.

Transesophageal: Since 1993 all the candidates underwent preprocedure transesophageal echocardiography looking for the presence of left atrial thrombi, providing a better understanding of the leaflet and subvalvular components morphology and functional inter-relations.

Fluoroscopy

Fluoroscopy is used for determining the degree of valvular calcification. As a rule, we did not perform valvular balloon dilatation of heavily calcific mitral valves, unless an absolute contraindication for surgery was present.

Invasive protocol

Hemodynamic assessment

Conventional left and right heart studies before and immediately after valvular dilatation were performed through the left groin. Pre- and postprocedure angiographic mitral regurgitation were assessed in the 30° right anterior oblique view. Candidates with preprocedure >II/IV angiographic mitral regurgitation of Seller classification[17] were excluded. We used left ventriculography in 3% (5) of our patients during the procedure, in order to assess deterioration of valvular regurgitation. Coronary angiography was performed routinely among candidates over 40 years of age.

Left-to-right shunt at the atrial level was detected by oximetry. Pulmonary saturation greater than right atrial saturation, in more than 7%, was considered as a marker for the presence of shunt.[18]

Cardiac output was measured by thermodilution and assumed by Fick's principle. Postvalvuloplasty measurements were undertaken while trans-septal puncture was occluded either by balloon system or shaft catheter.[19] Mitral valve area was calculated according to Gorlin's formula,[20] except in the presence of significant angiographic mitral regurgitation.

Trans-septal puncture and interatrial septal dilatation

A standard adult Brochkenbrough needle and an 8F Mullins sheath (USCI Billerica MA, USA) were used for trans-septal puncture. Atrial puncture was carried out in the left lateral position guided by the classical landmarks of fluoroscopy[21] and monitored by continuous pressure recording.

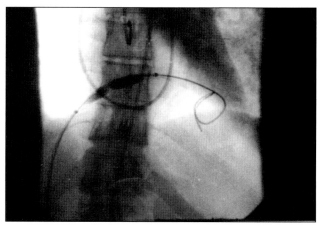

a

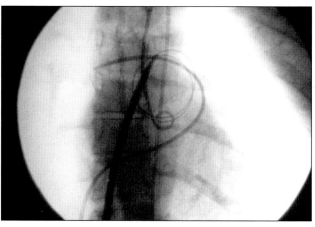

b

Fig. 37.1
Interatrial septal dilatation by (a) 8 mm (Mansfield) balloon and (b) 14F Inoue (Torray) rigid dilator.

In our initial experience, using the stiff over-the-wire balloon systems, interatrial septal dilatation was undertaken by 6–8 mm balloons (Mansfield [Boston Scientific, Mansfield MA, USA]). For the last four years we have used the Inoue 14 F rigid dilator (Torray [Industries Inc, Tokyo, Japan]) for this purpose (Fig. 37.1). Postinteratrial septal dilatation, 5000 units of heparin was given intravenously.

Valvular dilatation: right-sided transvenous antegrade approach

During the first 2 years of the authors' initial experience we used bifoil or trefoil (Schneider [Europe] AG, Bülach, Switzerland, or Mansfield) over-the-wire single-shaft multi-balloon systems (Fig. 37.2) in a group of 52 patients. The

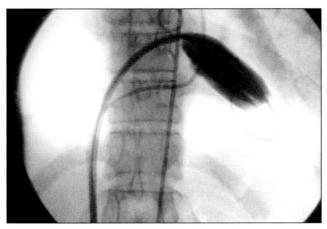

a

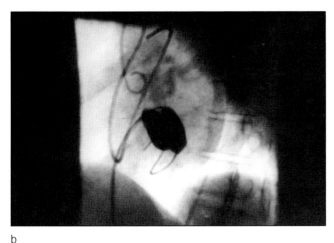

b

Fig. 37.2
Over-the-wire single-shaft multiballoon systems. (a) Trifoil
3 × 15 mm; (b) bifoil 2 × 19 mm.

bifoil systems consisted of 2 × 17 mm and 2 × 19 mm (Schneider), and 18 × 20 mm and 20 × 20 mm pigtail-ended (Mansfield) balloons. The trifoil systems were 3 × 12 mm and 3 × 15 mm (Schneider). These systems needed the presence of a stiff backup wire in the left ventricle with potentially hazardous complications. Our group had no previous experience with the dual-shaft double-balloon technique.

During the last 4 years we have used the Inoue balloon system (Torray, Japan) which has several advantages in comparison to the over-the-wire systems.[22] Since the distal part of the balloon is, as a first step, inflated by using the balloon floating principle and steering stylet to cross the valve, there is no need for the presence of a stiff backup wire in the left ventricle. The balloon structure enables the user to increase balloon diameter gradually, i.e. the step-wise inflation technique.

Generally, we performed the first inflation 2–4 mm less than the preprocedure-determined diameter. This system has rapid inflation and deflation times and also enables us to follow left atrial pressure dynamics immediately after every inflation. For an adult, balloon size was selected according to patient height.[23] A 26-mm balloon was selected for patients 160 cm tall or shorter, a 28-mm balloon for 160–180 cm tall and a 30-mm balloon for patients over 180 cm tall.

Principles of dilatation

After crossing the valve with the balloon tip floating in the left ventricular cavity, the distal part is further inflated and the balloon is then pulled back towards the mitral anulus. Inflation pressure is then continuously increased in the mid and proximal segments of the balloon system until the central waist of the balloon system disappears (Fig. 37.3).

Monitoring the procedure

In our first 3 years of experience we used both fluoroscopy and hemodynamic parameters as a guide for procedure monitoring. Balloon position, disappearance of waist and crossing the valve with a large inflated balloon were used as fluoroscopic monitoring markers.

Several patients underwent repeat left ventricular angiography during the procedure in order to assess mitral regurgitation severity. Hemodynamic monitoring landmarks were mean left atrial pressure level, waveform dynamics, diastolic gradient reduction and calculated Gorlin valve area.

Due to the fact that multiple pitfalls may accompany the hemodynamic assessment of this group, during the last three years we found transthoracic Doppler echocardiography to be a very useful tool for monitoring the stepwise inflation technique, particularly concerning postinflation commissural morphology, and either appearance or deterioration of mitral regurgitation.[24]

Miscellaneous

Definitions

Optimal valvular dilatation was considered when we found both an increase in mitral valve area of more than 25% and a final valve area greater than 1.5 cm[2]. Suboptimal results were achieved when there was an increase in valve area of more than 25% but a final valve area less than 1.5 cm[2].[25]

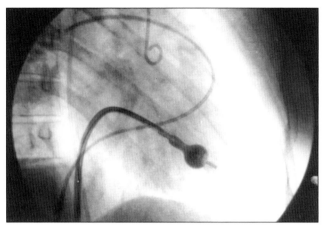

a

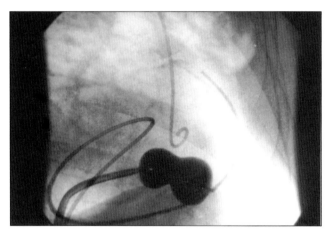

b

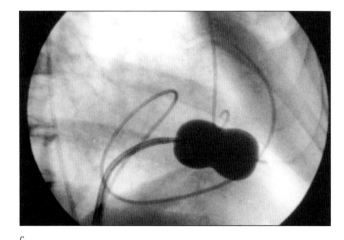

c

Fig. 37.3
Three stages of Inoue balloon dilatation.   (a) Distal segment inflation.   (b) Partial inflation at annular level.   (c) Complete inflation, disappearance of balloon waist.

Indication for procedure termination

The procedure was terminated if:

- there was a mitral valve area greater than 1.5 cm², without major complications;

- opening of at least one of the mitral commissures was demonstrated by 2D echocardiography; and

- appearance or an increase of significant mitral regurgitation occurred.

Clinical and echocardiographic follow-up

Clinical follow-up was undertaken every 6 months after the procedure. At every visit functional capacity (FC) (NYHA) determination and physical assessment, including transthoracic echo-Doppler, were performed in order to assess mitral valve area and evaluate restenosis. A decrease of more than 25% from immediate postvalvotomy mitral valve area with an absolute area of less than 1.5 cm² was used as a criterion for restenosis.[26]

Results
Exclusion of patients

Fifteen patients (8%) were initially excluded for the following reasons:

- Ten patients showed left atrial thrombi on transesophageal echocardiography.

- Two patients were found to suffer from significant mitral regurgitation based on clinical and color Doppler examinations.

- One patient showed significant submitral calcification.

- Two patients were excluded after the first hemodynamic evaluation due to the presence of additional congenital cardiac disorders. In one patient, interruption of the inferior vena cava with Azygos continuity occurred when we were unable to perform transseptal puncture by the classical technique. In the second patient, an extracardiac left-to-right shunt between the left lower pulmonary vein and the left brachiocephalic vein was present.

Technical failures

The authors attempted BMV in 170 patients. However, we terminated the procedure technically in only 168 patients and, therefore, our technical failure rate is 1%. In our initial experience we could not propagate the balloon system towards the left ventricle in one patient due to stiff backup wire instability. Recently, we could not dilate the interatrial septum in another patient, due to repeated rapid atrial tachyarrhythmias followed by severe hypotension which was terminated only by recurrent direct current (DC) shocks.

There was no failure related to the trans-septal puncture technique.

Six other patients suffered from major complications during the procedure; four had cardiac tamponade and two had severe (IV/IV) angiographic mitral regurgitation, making our procedural success rate 162/170 = 95%.

significant stenotic valve. This unique group was found to have a relatively mild reduced left ventricular ejection fraction (44% ± 6), low cardiac index (2 ± 0.3 L/min/M^2) and a high systemic vascular resistance (2150 ± 353) dyn-sec-cm^{-5}, associated with inferobasal hypokinesis by left ventriculography. Discrepancies between immediate hemodynamic and echocardiographic results were noticed in 26% of our patients. We noticed that when a single commissure was successfully split during the procedure the final valve area was always greater than 1.5 cm^2. Based on initial echocardiographic assessments we noticed optimal results among 118 patients (73%), where the final mitral valve area was greater than 1.5 cm^2, while 44 patients (27%) had suboptimal results with a mitral valve area of less than 1.5 cm^2 at the end of the procedure.

Immediate hemodynamic and echocardiographic results

Successful valvular dilatation brought immediate hemodynamic improvement as can be seen from Fig. 37.4. Increased mitral valve area was associated with a reduction of mean diastolic gradient, improved cardiac output and reduction of pulmonary artery systolic pressure.

Fourteen percent of our patients showed preprocedure low diastolic gradient (<10 mmHg) in the presence of

Subgroup analysis

Adults over 50 years of age

Thirty-six patients (21%) were over the age of 50 years, the oldest one being 82 years of age. All were in FC III or IV. Although postvalvotomy mean mitral valve area was 1.6 ± 0.3 cm^2 the percentage of optimal results among this group was 65% compared to 78% in the youngest group. Only two patients from the elderly group had major

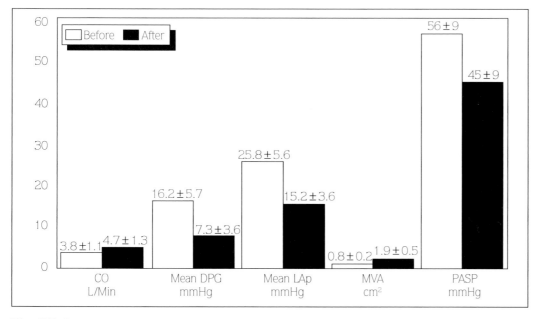

Fig. 37.4
Immediate hemodynamic improvement after valvular dilatation. (CO = cardiac output, DPG = diastolic pressure gradient, LAp = left atrial pressure, MVA = mitral valve area, PASP = pulmonary artery systolic pressure.)

cardiac complications; one had severe angiographic mitral regurgitation and the other developed cardiac tamponade during the procedure.

Postmitral valve surgery

Twenty-one candidates for BMV were postmitral valve surgery: 18 were after closed and 3 were after open mitral commissurotomy. BMV was undertaken at 13 ± 6 yr after surgery. Mean age was 48 ± 9 yr, 6/21 had chronic atrial fibrillation and 4/21 suffered from an associated mild to moderate aortic valve disease. Eighty percent were in FC III or IV and their mean echo score was 9 ± 2. Mitral valve area increased among this group from 0.9 ± 0.2 to 1.5 ± 0.3 cm^2. Thirteen patients (62%) had optimal results and six patients (28%) had suboptimal results. Among this group we noticed two major complications: one patient suffered from cardiac tamponade and another had severe mitral regurgitation, immediately postvalvuloplasty which was treated by urgent mitral valve replacement.

Pregnant women

BMV was performed in three pregnant women with a mean gestational age of 26 ± 4 weeks. All were in FC III or IV, under combined beta-blockers and diuretics. Protection of the fetus was maintained by a large lead cover placed below the diaphragm. In these cases we did not perform right heart study or left ventriculography.

The only time we used fluoroscopy in these cases was for trans-septal puncture and crossing the stenotic mitral valve. The mean fluoroscopic time was 13 (4 min). Balloon inflation, positioning and deflation were guided by transthoracic echocardiography. The mean mitral valve area increased from 0.9 (0.2–1.7; 0.2 cm^2). There were no major complications in this group. All patients delivered normal infants at a mean gestational age of 36 ± 3 weeks).

Initial experience versus late experience

Several differences were noticed when we compared the results from the initial two years of our experience using the 'over-the-wire system' to the last four years, when using the 'Inoue balloon system':

- The mean duration time of the procedure was shortened from 130 ± 15 to 45 ± 15 min.

- An increase of 20% in the immediate mitral valve area was noticed in the last four years, as compared to the initial period, 1.8 ± 0.5 vs. 1.5 ± 0.3 cm^2, respectively ($p < 0.05$).

- There was a significant difference in major complication rates between the two periods.

Major complications

Major complications were tamponade in 2%, severe mitral regurgitation in 3% and ASD in 4% of the patients.

Although we performed BMV in-hospital without an on-site surgical backup team there were no procedural-related deaths during our 6 years of balloon mitral dilatation program. However, 15 of the 168 patients (9%) have developed major complications during the last 6 years. Four patients suffered from cardiac tamponade when we used the stiff backup wires in the left ventricle and another five patients had III–IV/IV mitral regurgitation, immediately post-dilatation. Only 5/9 of these patients were referred for urgent surgery. One patient from the tamponade group stabilized and was treated conservatively, due to the appearance of left hemiparesis after pericardiocentesis. No patient with III/IV mitral regurgitation required urgent surgery. There were no other cases of cardiac tamponade or IV/IV mitral regurgitation since the introduction of the Inoue balloon system using the stepwise dilatation technique guided by echocardiography. However, we did see a mild increment in the mitral regurgitation rate among 65% of our patients who underwent successful commissural splitting.

Twenty-six patients (15%) had left-to-right shunt at the atrial level, post-BMV detected by oximetry. However, only in 6/26 (23%) was the Qp/Qs higher than 1.5/1. All the significant left-to-right shunts were created in the first 2 years, when we used the stiff wires and separate balloons for interatrial septal dilatation. No significant left-to-right shunt at the atrial level was detected when using the Inoue balloon system.

Clinical follow-up

Mean clinical follow-up of 42 (7 months) showed that the vast majority of patients (97%) were either in FC I or II (Fig. 37.5), while four patients were in FC III. We could not find any patient in FC IV. Seven patients underwent mitral valve replacement during the follow-up period; 4/7 had initially suboptimal results and 3/7 suffered from III/IV mitral regurgitation immediately after BMV. No clinical deterioration or need for surgery among the acquired ASD group was noticed during follow-up.

Three patients underwent a repeated procedure by the Inoue balloon system, where the first dilatation was performed by the old over-the-wire systems. During follow-up only one noncardiac-related death was reported.

Echocardiographic follow-up

Eighty percent of our patients had at least two transthoracic echocardiographic examinations during the follow-

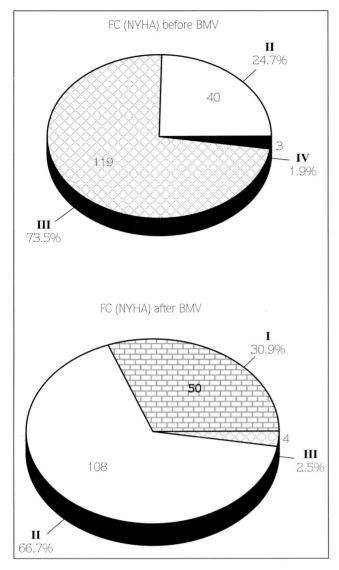

Fig. 37.5

FC (NYHA) (a) before and (b) after balloon mitral valvuloplasty (BMV).

up period. Some 126/154 patients (82%) had a mitral valve area greater than 1.5 cm², while 28/154 (18%) fulfilled the echocardiographic criterion of restenosis, i.e. more than a 25% decrease in mitral valve area compared to initial post-valvotomy results with a final valve area of less than 1.5 cm². Twenty-one patients from this group (75%)

belonged to the immediate postvalvotomy suboptimal results. One of the interesting observations during repeated echocardiographic studies at the first 2 years of follow-up was a mild decrease in mitral valve area, i.e. 0.1–0.2 cm² with no relation to the restenosis phenomenon (Fig. 37.6).

Discussion

Over the last 13 years BMV has established itself as an attractive alternative for selected patients suffering from rheumatic valvular mitral stenosis. To date, thousands of patients worldwide have been treated with this technique. Data are available from a large number of centers[27,28] for a wide range of patient populations with different valve morphologies,[29–31] including multicenter studies.[32,33]

Mechanism

Multiple observations have indicated that commissural splitting is the main contribution to the valvular dilatation procedure.[8,9,34] However, Reifart et al. and others[35,36] proposed that calcific noduli fracture or anular stretching may contribute to the valvular dilatation process. Our observation, during the follow-up period, of a mild reduction of valvular area without restenosis may indicate that acute anular stretching is a possible contribution to the early hemodynamic results.

Technique

Over the years, different groups have published different approaches, i.e. transvenous antegrade versus transarterial retrograde approaches. In the transarterial approaches there are two possibilities depending on whether or not trans-septal puncture is performed. In the 'Babic technique' a wire is delivered through a trans-septal catheter into the left ventricle, and later on snared and exteriorized via the contralateral artery.[37] Stefanides et al.[38] developed a special preshaped device that enabled the propagation of the wire retrogradely to the left atrium without trans-septal puncture. Most of the involved groups perform BMV today by using the transvenous retrograde approach, which requires a trans-septal puncture. As a result, there has been a revival of the trans-septal technique worldwide.[39] Similar to other groups (mainly the French one) we would like to emphasize that in the last 2 years, transthoracic echocardiography is more frequently used among patients with deformed

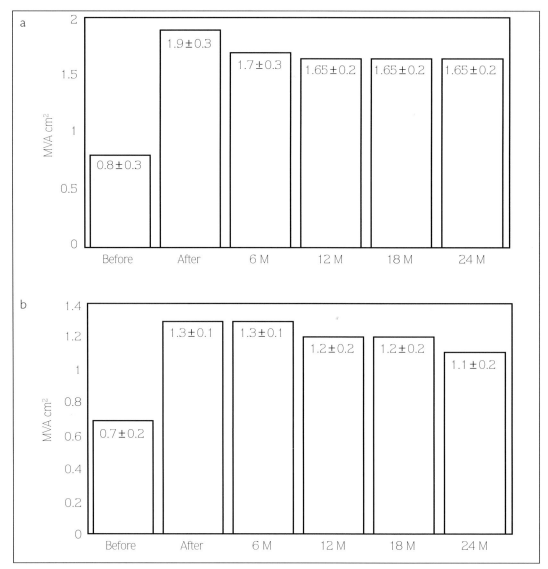

Fig. 37.6
Mild decrease in mitral valve area (MVA) during two years for follow-up among   (a) optimal and   (b) suboptimal immediate results.

valves, mainly to monitor and/or determine termination of the procedure.[40] After 6 years of a valvuloplasty program we did not find transesophageal echocardiography to be an essential or additive tool during the procedure.

Balloons

Most groups started to perform the procedure by using single large or double-balloon techniques and, later on, shifted to the Inoue system. In the authors' institute we began to use the single-shaft multiballoon system, and over the last 4 years we have used the Inoue system. In our initial experience with the single-shaft system we noticed that the complication rate was higher, procedure time was longer and the mean postvalvoplasty mitral valve area was 15% lower, as compared to the second phase of our experience using the Inoue balloon. As with other interventional techniques, we do believe that part of these differences belong to the learning curve phenomenon.[41] There are several advantages of the Inoue balloon compared to the over-the-wire system:

- There are no wires in the left ventricle and therefore the rate of ventricular perforation is minimal.

- The lack of wires enables the monitoring of immediate and continuous hemodynamic parameters during the procedure.

- This system enables use of the stepwise inflation technique in order to achieve maximal valvular dilatation with the smallest possible balloon diameter.

Immediate hemodynamic results

Similar to previous published data,[42,43] most of our patients demonstrated hemodynamic improvement immediately after the procedure. We must emphasize that our group is relatively highly selective, with the initial selection generally undertaken by the referring physicians. For the entire group, 73% of the patients had a postprocedure mitral valve area greater than 1.5 cm^2. However, if we concentrate on the immediate results in the second phase of our experience, using the Inoue system, we notice optimal results among 82% of our patients. This success rate is comparable to the reported data of the mitral valve surgery series.[44,45]

Complications

Antegrade transvenous BMV, which involves the transseptal procedure, has several potential cardiac and extracardiac complications.[46] These are

- mechanical cardiac complications, including tamponade, severe mitral regurgitation and left-to-right shunt at the atrial level; and

- extracardiac complications that may be related to embolic phenomena and vascular damage, following the use of large-caliber catheter devices.

We would like to emphasize that 86% (13/15) of our mechanical complications occurred during our first 2 years of experience when using the stiff backup wire system. However, in the last 3 years, using both the Inoue balloon system and the stepwise inflation technique guided by echocardiography, we saw no mechanical cardiac event. Our major complication rate for the whole group is similar to the published data in the literature (Table 37.1). Urgent surgery is indicated only for the patients with hemopericardium and/or the appearance of grade IV/IV mitral regurgitation.

No patient with grade III/IV mitral regurgitation or significant ASD (Qp/Qs > 1.5/1) needed early or urgent surgical intervention.

Major embolic events and periprocedural death rates that have been reported are 0–3.3% and 0–3%, respec-

Table 37.1 Complications of percutaneous mitral valvuloplasty.

Ref.	Patients	Mortality (%)	Embolism (%)	IV/IV MR (%)	ASD (%)	Tamponade (%)
MGH	570	0.5	1.0	1.4	16	1.0
LL	238	1.0	1.0	1.0	2	1.2
BI	146	1.7	1.7	1.7	19	3.0
M-Heart	73	2.7	4.0	2.0	18	6.0
MC	120	1.0	1.0	1.5	—	2.0
Tenon	600	0.5	3.3	3.8	—	4.0
Afula	162	0.0	0.0	1.0	4	2.0

Notes:
MGH = Massachusetts General Hospital. LL = Loma Linda. BI = Beit Israel. MC = Mayo Clinic. M-Heart = Multicenter valvuloplasty registry.

tively. During the 6 years of our BMV program, these complications have not occurred.

Restenosis

As long as the definition for restenosis was based on clinical criteria a very wide range of this phenomenon (2–60%) was reported after mitral valve commissurotomy.[47] However, 10 years of echocardiographic follow-up postsurgical commissurotomy[48] has indicated that the restenosis rate is close to 27%. Most data focusing on restenosis after BMV are based on serial echocardiographic studies.[49] However, there is no single definition for restenosis based on echocardiography. When we used strict criteria (i.e. a decrease in mitral valve area of more than 25% relative to the initial result and an area of less than 1.5 cm^2), only 28 patients (18%) fulfilled these parameters. Two thirds of these patients belonged initially to the suboptimal dilatation group, and 75% of them were performed during our initial experience, where we used the over-the-wire systems. Similar to Nakatani et al.'s report,[50] we noticed that the time-related changes in mitral valve area are most probably due to anular recoil after dilatation. This phenomenon does not carry any relationship to the long-term restenosis rate.

Conclusion

After 6 years of an active BMV program and based on hundreds of procedures, we may conclude that BMV is a safe and beneficial procedure for most of the patients with pliable mitral stenosis. The immediate and mid-term results are encouraging and the complication rate is low. Therefore, it can be performed in relatively large-volume centers, without an ultimate need for an on-site surgical backup team.

References

1 Inoue K, Owaki T, Nakamura T, Kitamura F, Myamoto N. Clinical application of transvenous mitral commissurotomy by new balloon catheter. J Thorac Cardiovasc Surg 1984; **87**: 394–402.

2 Lock JE, Kalilullah M, Shirvastava S, Bahl V, Keane JF. Percutaneous catheter commissurotomy in rheumatic mitral stenosis. N Engl J Med 1985; **313**: 1515–18.

3 Palacios I, Block PC, Brandi S, et al. Percutaneous balloon valvotomy for patients with severe mitral stenosis. Circulation 1987; **75**: 778–84.

4 Vahanian A, Michel PL, Cormier B, et al. Results of percutaneous mitral commissurotomy in 200 patients. Am J Cardiol 1989; **63**: 847–52.

5 Al Zaibag M, Al Kasab SA, Al Fagig MR. Percutaneous double balloon mitral valvotomy for rheumatic mitral stenosis. Lancet 1986; **I**: 757–61.

6 McKay CR, Kawanishi DT, Rahimtoola SH. Catheter balloon valvuloplasty of the mitral valve in adults using balloon technique. J Am Med Assoc 1987; **257**: 1753–61.

7 Al Zaibag M, Al Kasab SA, Al Fagig MR. Percutaneous double balloon mitral valvotomy for rheumatic mitral stenosis. Lancet 1986; **I**: 757–61.

8 Inoue K, Nakamura T, Kitamura F, Miyamoto N. Nonoperative mitral commissurotomy by a new balloon catheter. Jpn Circ J 1982; **46**: 877 (abstract).

9 Block PC, Palacios IF, Jacobs ML, Fallon JT. Mechanism of percutaneous mitral valvotomy. Am J Cardiol 1987; **59**: 178–9.

10 Patel JJ, Shama D, Mitha AS, et al. Balloon valvuloplasty versus closed commissurotomy for pliable mitral stenosis: a prospective hemodynamic study. J Am Coll Cardiol 1991; **18**: 1318–22.

11 Arora R, Mohan N, Kalra SG, Nigam M. Immediate and long-term results of balloon and surgical closed mitral valvotomy: a randomized comparative study. Am Heart J 1993; **125**: 1991–4.

12 Farhat BM, Ayari M, Betbout F, et al. Percutaneous balloon versus surgical closed and open mitral commissurotomy. J Am Coll Cardiol 1993; **21**: 428A.

13 Cheng TO. Percutaneous balloon mitral valvuloplasty: are Chinese and western experiences comparable? Cathet Cardiovasc Diagn 1994; **31**: 23–8.

14 Vahanian A, Acar J. Mitral valvuloplasty: the French experience. In Topol EJ (ed.). Textbook of Interventional Cardiology (Philadelphia, PA: WB Saunders, 1994): 1206–25.

15 Baim DS, Grossman W. Percutaneous approach and transseptal catheterization. In: Grossman W (ed.). Cardiac Catheterization and Angiography (Philadelphia, PA: Lea & Febiger, 1986): 71–5.

16 Wilkins GT, Weyman AE, Abascal VM. Percutaneous mitral valvotomy. An analysis of echocardiographic variables related to outcome and mechanism of dilatation. Br Heart J 1988; **60**: 299–308.

17 Seller RD, Levy MJ, Amplatz K, Lillehei CW. Retrograde cardioangiography in acquired heart disease: technique, indications and interpretation of 100 cases. Am J Cardiol 1964; **14**: 437–47.

18 Anthan EM, Marsh JD, Green LH, Grossman W. Blood oxygen measurements in the assessment of left-to-right shunts: a critical appraisal in methodology. *Am J Cardiol* 1980; **46**: 265–71.

19 Petrossian GA, Tuzcu EM, Ziskind AA, Block PC, Palacios IF. Atrial septal occlusion improves the accuracy of mitral valve area determination following balloon mitral valvotomy. *Cath Cardiovasc Diag* 1991; **22**: 21–4.

20 Grossman W. Hemodynamic principles. In: Grossman W (ed.). *Cardiac Catheterization and Angiography* (Philadelphia, PA: Lea & Febiger, 1986): 101–17.

21 Rocha P, Berland J, Rigaud M, et al. Fluoroscopic guidance in transseptal left heart catheterization for percutaneous mitral balloon valvotomy. *Cath Cardiovasc Diag* 1991; **23**: 172–6.

22 Inoue K, Hung JS. Percutaneous transvenous mitral commissurotomy: the Far East experience. In Topol EJ (ed.). *Textbook of Interventional Cardiology* (Philadelphia, PA: WB Saunders, 1994): 1226–42.

23 Feldman T. Hemodynamic results, clinical outcome, and complications of Inoue balloon mitral commissurotomy. *Cath Cardiovasc Diag* 1994; **2**: 2–7.

24 Vahanian A, Michel PL, Cormier B. A prospective evaluation of stepwise mitral balloon dilatation using the Inoue technique. *Circulation* 1991; **84 (Suppl II)**: II-27 (abstract).

25 Abascal VM, Wilkins GT, O'Shea JP, et al. Prediction of successful outcome in 130 patients undergoing balloon mitral valvotomy. *Circulation* 1990; **82**: 448–56.

26 Lefervere T, Bonan R, Serra A, et al. Percutaneous mitral valvuloplasty in surgical high risk patients. *J Am Coll Cardiol* 1991; **17**: 348–54.

27 Tuzcu EM, Block PC, Palacios IF. Comparison of early versus late experience with percutaneous mitral balloon valvuloplasty. *J Am Coll Cardiol* 1991; **17**: 1121–4.

28 Ruiz CE, Allen JW, Law FYK. Percutaneous double balloon valvotomy for severe rheumatic mitral stenosis. *Am J Cardiol* 1990; **65**: 473–7.

29 Shrivastava S, Chandra YV, Krishnamoorthy KM, Radhakrishnan S. Mitral valvotomy with the Inoue balloon in juvenile rheumatic mitral stenosis. *Am J Cardiol* 1995; **76**: 404–6.

30 Palacios IF, Lock JE, Keane JF, et al. Percutaneous transvenous balloon valvotomy in patient with severe calcific mitral stenosis. *J Am Coll Cardiol* 1986; **7**: 1416–19.

31 Yoshida Y, Kubo S, Tamaki S, Inoue K. Percutaneous transvenous mitral commissurotomy for mitral stenosis patients with markedly severe mitral valve deformity: immediate results and long-term clinical outcome. *Am J Cardiol* 1995; **76**: 406–8.

32 The National Heart, Lung and Blood Institute Balloon Valvuloplasty Registry. Complication and mortality of percutaneous balloon mitral commissurotomy. *Circulation* 1992; **85**: 2014–24.

33 Petit J, Vahanian A, Michel PL, et al. Percutaneous mitral valvotomy: French Cooperative Study: 114 patients. *Circulation* 1987; **76 (Suppl IV)**: IV-496 (abstract).

34 Ribeiro PA, Zaibag M, Rajendarn V, et al. Mechanism of mitral valve area increase by in vivo single and double balloon mitral valvotomy. *Am J Cardiol* 1988; **62**: 264–8.

35 Reifart N, Nowak B, Baykutt D, et al. Experimental balloon valvuloplasty of fibrotic and calcific mitral valves. *Circulation* 1990; **81**: 1105–11.

36 McKay RG, Lock JE, Safian RD, et al. Balloon dilatation of mitral stenosis in adults patients: postmortem and percutaneous mitral valvuloplasty studies. *J Am Coll Cardiol* 1987; **9**: 723–31.

37 Babic UU, Pejcic P, Djurisic Z, et al. Percutaneous transarterial balloon valvuloplasty for mitral valve stenosis. *Am J Cardiol* 1992; **70**: 553–4.

38 Stefanidis C, Stratos C, Pitsavos C, et al. Retrograde nontransseptal balloon mitral valvuloplasty: immediate and long term follow-up. *Circulation* 1992; **85**: 1760–7.

39 Turgeman Y, Suleiman K, Bloch L, Rosenfeld T. Transseptal left heart catheterization: an old invasive technique with new applications. *Harefua* 1995; **129**: 14–16.

40 Cormier B. Echo monitoring during percutaneous mitral commissurotomy. *Proc First Course of 'Balloon mitral valvuloplasty in practice' Paris* (2), 1996.

41 Rihal CS, Nishimura RA, Holmes DR jr. Percutaneous balloon mitral commissurotomy: the learning curve. *Am Heart J* 1991; **122**: 1750–6.

42 Hung JS, Chen MS, Wu JJ, et al. Short and long term results of catheter balloon percutaneous transvenous mitral commissurotomy. *Am J Cardiol* 1991; **67**: 854–62.

43 Vahanian A, Michel PL, Cormier B, et al. Immediate and mid-term results of percutaneous mitral commissurotomy. *Eur Heart J* 1991; **12 (Suppl B)**: 84–9.

44 Ellis FH, Kirklin JW, Parker RL, et al. Mitral commissurotomy—an overall appraisal of clinical and hemodynamic results. *Arch Int Med* 1954; **94**: 774–84.

45 Feigenbaum H, Linback RE, Nasser WK. Hemodynamic studies before and after mitral instrumental commissurotomy. *Circulation* 1968; **38**: 261–76.

46   Shawi FA, Domanski MJ, Yackee JM, *et al.* Left ventricular rupture complicating percutaneous cardiopulmonary bypass support. *Cathet Cardiovasc Diagn* 1990; **21**: 26–7.

47   Arora K, Khalilluah M, Gupta MP, Padmavati S. Mitral restenosis incidence and epidemiology. *Indian Heart J* 1978; **30**: 265–8.

48   Heger JJ, Wann IS, Weyman AE, *et al.* Long term change in mitral valve area after successful mitral commissurotomy. *Circulation* 1979; **59**: 443–8.

49   Desidri A, Vanderperon O, Serra A, *et al.* Long-term (9–33 months) echo-cardiographic follow-up after successful percutaneous mitral commissurotomy. *Am J Cardiol* 1992; **69**: 1602–6.

50   Nakatani S, Nagata S, Beppu S, *et al.* Time related changes in mitral valve area after balloon mitral valvuloplasty assessed by Doppler continuity equation method. *Circulation* 1988; **78**: II-487.

VIII

Pediatric Interventions

38

Interventional pediatric cardiology: an overview

Lee Benson and David Nykanen

Introduction

Over the past decade, the focus of the pediatric catheterization laboratory has changed from primarily a diagnostic modality to a conduit for therapeutics. Although the first application of catheter interventions was described over 43 years ago by Rubio-Alvarez,[1] it was not until 1966, when Rashkind and Miller[2] described the technique for percutaneous creation of an atrial septal defect in the setting of complete transposition of the great arteries, that such catheter maneuvers decisively impacted patient management.[3–12]

Such interventions may be corrective, reparative or palliative (Table 38.1). Lesions that are amenable to repair include typical dome-shaped pulmonary valve stenoses, recoarctation of the aorta and the persistently patent arterial duct (beyond the newborn period). Newer approaches may extend this list to selected patients with atrial and muscular ventricular septal defects. Palliation can be accomplished in lieu of surgery, or as an adjunct in a staged approach to patient care. Lesions amenable to such palliation include aortic stenosis, residual postoperative systemic or venous obstructions, native coarctation of the aorta, stenotic prosthetic tissue valves and congenital pulmonary arteriovenous fistulae. Catheter therapies may also be applied as adjuncts to surgery and include embolization to systemic-to-pulmonary arterial collaterals, surgically created systemic-to-pulmonary shunts, venous obstructions, interatrial communications and peripheral pulmonary atrial stenosis. Therapeutic interventions, like cardiac surgery, have three principal objectives: improvement and/or preservation of cardiac function, improvement in longevity and

Table 38.1 Catheter therapeutics.

Lesions amenable to repair	Lesions amenable to palliation	Lesions amenable to palliation or an adjunct to surgery
Pulmonary stenosis	Aortic valve stenosis	Systemic-to-pulmonary collaterals or shunts
Recurrent coarctation of the aorta	Postoperative systemic or venous obstructions	Venous obstructions (systemic or pulmonary)
Persistent patent arterial duct	Native coarctation of the aorta	Interatrial communications
Atrial septal defects	Obstructed prosthetic tissue valves	Peripheral pulmonary stenosis
Muscular ventricular septal defects	Pulmonary arteriovenous fistulae	

maintenance or improvement in the quality of life. When these ends are met, interventional catheterization obviates surgical morbidity and mortality. Unsuccessful outcomes, including complications and nondefinitive outcomes, may in part yield to experience and improvements in technique.[13]

Dilatation of vascular lesions

Mechanism of dilatation

Histologically, vascular stenoses present a spectrum from normal to exaggerated medial or intimal hyperplasia with alterations in the proportions of elastin, collagen and smooth muscle,[14-16] with those lesions acquired after surgery having additional mural and perivascular fibroses.[17,18] In this setting, successful angioplasty results in longitudinal or oblique intimal or medial tears[16-19] with organization of intramural hemorrhage and scar formation the mode of healing. Neoendothelialization is complete in 3–6 weeks while areas of mural thinning within the scar may predispose to aneurysm formation.[18] Postoperatively, perivascular fibrosus may reinforce the outer vessel wall and lessen balloon angioplasty risk, although this has not been confirmed. Several months must be allowed after surgery to afford complete tissue granulation and to avoid transmedial tears during the catheter intervention.[20]

Dilatation of pulmonary artery stenosis

Stenosis of the proximal pulmonary arteries or their branches may occur as a primary congenital lesion (isolated or as a component of Fallot's tetralogy) or a residua of surgical repairs or shunts. As such, they may lead to maldistribution of pulmonary blood flow, right heart failure and right ventricular hypertension, and are a significant cause of mortality after biventricular repair or the creation of an atrial-dependent circulation. Surgical approaches have been of limited success in addressing this lesion and approaches are frequently confined to the proximal branches.[21-23]

Indications for pulmonary angioplasty (Table 38.2) include near systemic or suprasystemic right (pulmonary) ventricular pressures, decreased flow to affected segments of the lung, pulmonary hypertension in nonaffected lung segments receiving increased flow, symptoms of exercise intolerance or dyspnoea and significant angiographic stenosis in the preoperative patient considered for further operative intervention.

The technique of angioplasty is well described in the literature. Once the stenosis has been identified, the lesions

Table 38.2 Indications for dilatation of stenotic pulmonary arteries.

- Symptoms, i.e. exercise intolerance, dyspnoea, right heart failure
- Near systemic or suprasystemic right ventricular pressures
- Decreased segmental pulmonary perfusion
- Elevated pulmonary pressures in nonaffected lung segments
- Stenosis in the preoperative patient for future surgical repair

and adjacent vessels are measured using a reference grid or catheter to correct for angiographic magnification. Access to the vessel may be from the native outflow tract or surgically created connection with consideration given to the reliability of pulmonary blood flow during the procedure. The lesion is crossed and a wire positioned distally for catheter exchanges. A balloon catheter is chosen whose diameter is 3–5 times the diameter of the minimal stenosis, taking into account the size of the vessel proximal and distal as well as the size of the patient. The lengths of the balloon and taper are determined by the characteristics of the vessel being dilated in an effort to avoid creating a distal aneurysm within normal vessel. The catheter is advanced over the wire and positioned so that the balloon straddles the lesion. Inflations, using dilute contrast media, are monitored with an intraballoon pressure manometer, which may vary depending on the size of the balloon catheter employed. Dilatation is followed by hemodynamic measurements. While many different methods have been used for postdilatation studies, a power injection over a wire will yield the most informative angiogram. It is not safe to advance a wire across a newly dilated vessel as the tip may result in a dissection or rupture of the artery; hence, maintaining wire position for catheter exchanges is of paramount importance.

Balloon dilatation is clinically well tolerated and should be considered as an initial form of intervention. It carries a low morbidity risk and 1–2% mortality.[20] Although angiographic improvement in vessel caliber (>50% increase in vessel diameter) can be achieved in half the patients,[24-28] restenosis is common (15–20%)[29,30] and long-term clinical benefit is achieved in less than 35% of patients (Tables 38.3 and 38.4).[29] The procedure has been applied in supravalvular pulmonary stenosis, seen after the arterial switch procedure, with little clinical improvement.[31]

Table 38.3 Morphological criteria for a successful balloon dilatation of stenotic pulmonary arteries.

- Stenosis diameter increase of >50% from predilatation size
- Stenosis diameter increase to >75% of adjacent vessel
- A >20% increase in pulmonary perfusion from predilatation flow
- A >20% reduction in right ventricular to systemic pressure ratio

Table 38.4 Clinical criteria for a successful balloon dilatation of stenotic pulmonary arteries.

- Allows a surgical repair on a previously inoperable patient
- Avoids a surgical intervention on the vessel
- Symptomatic relief, i.e. improved exercise tolerance, weight gain

Dilatation of coarctation of the aorta

Coarctation of the aorta may lead to profound heart failure in the newborn. In the older patient, systemic hypertension, vascular and myocardial sequelae predispose to endarteritis, aneurysms and dissection.[32-34] Surgery is recommended before the age of 2 years to lessen the incidence of persistent hypertension.[34] The incidence of reoperation (10–30%) in patients repaired in early infancy (particularly the newborn period) is significantly higher than those repaired over 1 year of age.[35-37] Surgery for recurrent coarctation is difficult and has an associated increased morbidity.[38,39] Percutaneous balloon angioplasty is the 'treatment of choice' in restenosis after surgical repair, irrespective of surgical technique.[40]

Balloon angioplasty can also be used as an alternative to surgical management for unoperated (so-called native)

coarctation. It has been performed in this setting in all age groups, and avoids thoracotomy. Its advantages are many, but complications have been reported at the site of dilatation and there have been a few reported deaths due to vessel rupture or arrhythmia.[41]

The application of the technique in unoperated coarctation is not universal, and many centers today still consider it experimental.[42] However, it is being offered to patients as an alternative in increasing numbers.[43-45] There is no clear consensus as to which patient dilatation is most appropriate. In one early series,[46] balloon dilatation was only performed if an associated cardiac defect would preclude successful surgical repair of both lesions, or the patient was thought to be 'high risk'. Most investigators today would suggest that such patients would be surgical candidates for repair rather than angioplasty. Initial studies also suggested that long tubular lesions were the best angioplasty candidates,[46] but subsequent studies[47,48] have shown that such lesions and nondiscrete obstructions are not as amenable as more localized lesions. Finally, some investigators[45] found that very severe (<3 mm in diameter) lesions were associated with higher residual peak systolic gradients.

The minimal systolic gradient for intervention is also still debated. Some centers advocate a peak systolic gradient at cardiac catheterization of 25–30 mmHg,[48,49] but this is not generally accepted. In other centers a systolic blood pressure of greater than the 97th percentile for age, uncontrolled hypertension on medication or congestive heart failure have been suggested (Table 38.5).[50] Generally accepted criteria today would include an anatomically discrete lesion, upper extremity hypertension and a resting gradient of at least 20 mmHg. Some centers, including the Hospital for Sick Children, Toronto, limit application to patients over 1 year of age to avoid arterial injury in the small infant and the known discouraging results in neonates.[51] There are other investigators however, who have found such angioplasty techniques useful in the newborn.[52-55]

To yield optimal results, the choice of catheter, the size

Table 38.5 Criteria for balloon dilatation of unoperated coarctation of the aorta.

- Discrete lesion, without transverse arch hypoplasia
- Upper extremity hypertension
- Resting arm to leg systolic gradient ≥20 mmHg

of balloon, the type of shaft and balloon shape should be taken into consideration.[56] Vascular access varies, although some investigators feel that bilateral femoral arterial cannulation is helpful to monitor intravascular pressures across the lesion. The pre- and postintervention angiograms and angioplasty are obtained from retrograde arterial cannulation sites. In the authors' institution, a transeptal atrial puncture is performed and a balloon-tipped catheter floated to the ascending aorta, and used for angiography and pressure monitoring, avoiding initial arterial cannulation if the obstruction appears a poor dilatation candidate. Sequential angiographic assessment without removing the retrograde arterial catheter. If dilated, can also be performed, lessening arterial trauma.

Systemic heparin sulfate is administered, at a dose of 150 IU/kg following arterial entry. Aortography is obtained from the transeptal catheter in the lateral and 15° left anterior oblique projection. Occasionally, to profile the lesion better, owing to overlap of the isthmus on the descending aorta, a caudal tilt is employed.

No single standard for arch measurements is available to choose the diameter of the dilatating balloon catheter. Some authors measure the isthmus just above the coarctation, the coarctation itself or the descending aorta at the level of the diaphragm. If an isthmic measurement is made, a balloon diameter equal to, or 1 mm less than, that of the isthmus is used. Others suggest using balloons 2–3 times the diameter of the coarctation, or 1–2 mm less than the descending aorta. There is no supportive data of the superiority of one set of measurements over another. The Multicenter Valvuloplasty and Angioplasty of Congenital Anomalies registry (VACA)[56] tabulated follow-up data from 92 dilated patients. The ratio of balloon diameter to coarctation size varied greatly (range 1.1–5.5) while residual pressure gradients were less (<10 mmHg) when ratios of 2.9–3.2 were employed. At the Hospital for Sick Children, Toronto, the initial balloon diameter is chosen to be equal to or within 1 or 2 mm of the aorta at the level of the left subclavian artery, and not to exceed the diameter of the aorta at the diaphragm. Short inflation times are employed (5–10 sec) but repeated (2–4 times) before repeat aortography is obtained. If no significant change in the lesion is noted, the next larger balloon is used within the guidelines as above.

The results of the VACA registry confirm[56] that native coarctations of the aorta could be effectively dilated. Early restenosis is an important problem, primarily in the newborn when isthmic and/or transverse arch hypoplasia coexist. In the neonate, however, the procedure may have a palliative role where a short-term benefit may be anticipated to provide for metabolic and hemodynamic relief, allowing more elective surgical repair at an older age.[57,58] Up to 80% of patients undergoing balloon angioplasty over 1 year of age have been reported to have a good initial outcome (systolic gradient < 20 mmHg), while 20–30% of patients may have a hemodynamically poor result or develop aneurysms (6%) at the dilatation site.

Complication rates appear to be higher in younger patients, particularly vascular injury,[59] but aneurysm formation appears less. Aneurysm rates have been estimated at 5–7% in carefully studied series.[44] There is, however, no relationship between the balloon size and coarctation diameter and the risk of aneurysm formation.[56] As such, the risk may relate more to intrinsic aortic wall issues rather than the technique itself. Unsuccessful balloon angioplasties do not preclude low-risk successful surgical interventions.[60]

Finally, endovascular stent prosthesis, such as used in pulmonary artery stenoses, may avoid many of the disadvantages imposed by balloon angioplasty (see below). The application in the older adolescent and adult is preliminary, but early results appear excellent and follow upon extensive earlier experimental work.[61] Issues pertinent to such prosthetic implantations in the thoracic aorta, however, need further study.[62]

Dilatation of systemic and pulmonary obstructions

Systemic and pulmonary venous obstructions can occur after atrial switch procedures. Baffle stenosis can result in venous congestion, pulmonary edema, reduced exercise tolerance and heart failure. Balloon angioplasty appears to be the initial treatment modality based upon several centers' experience.[63–65] The criteria for balloon intervention are the same as for surgery.

Pulmonary vein stenosis, on the other hand, whether congenital or surgically acquired, has had generally disappointing results, either nondilatable or developing early restenosis.[65,66] These stenoses can appear discrete with intimal hyperplasia and fibrosis, but frequently, and not apparent angiographically, long vessel segments are involved that complicate local attempts at repair. Surgical approaches have had similar high restenosis rates. The application of endovascular stents[67,68] appears promising although such implants have also had a high restenosis rate. The implantation of a covered stent may avoid such problems, but concerns over redilatation and enlargement with patient growth limit their ultimate effectiveness. Long segment lesions and the timing of intervention in terms of their progressive nature interplay in affecting outcome.

Dilatation of miscellaneous lesions

Balloon dilatation has been applied in the setting of fibromuscular dysplasia and Takayasu's arteritis with partial success.[69] Aortopulmonary collaterals, in the setting of pulmonary atresia and ventricular septal defect, have also been successfully dilated. A number of reports have noted improvement in oxygen saturation in dilatation of stenotic surgically created aortopulmonary shunts.[70,71] The potential application of endovascular stents may be useful in these situations.

Dilatation of valvular lesions

Typical valvular stenoses are characterized by fused, partially absent or underdeveloped commissures with small eccentric orifices. Echocardiographic,[72] intraoperative[73–75] and post-mortem examinations[76] have documented commissural splitting as the mechanism of dilatation, often with complete separation of the previously fused leaflets. Extracommissural tears and avulsions of the valve leaflets may occur as the disruptions develop along areas of least resistance[72,77] and result in various degrees of valve insufficiency, more likely in unicommisural valves.[78] Pulmonary valve dilatation has been shown to be safely accomplished with balloons larger than 20–40% of the valve anulus[72,79,80] while aortic valve dilatations are tolerated best with balloons no larger than 10% of the anulus diameter.[81,82] Residual gradients and the degree of insufficiency remain unchanged in follow-up.[83]

Dilatation of pulmonary valve stenosis

Severe pulmonary valve stenosis may lead to right heart failure and cyanosis if an atrial defect is present. Dynamic infundibular muscular obstruction is common, particularly in long-standing and severe lesions.[84] Surgical mortality for pulmonary valvotomy is less than 10% for patients under 2 years and less than 0.5% in older individuals.[85] Gradients below 25 mmHg are found in 81% of surgically treated patients 5 years and more after surgery. Pulmonary insufficiency is present in 50% of patients but infrequently the cause of clinical symptoms.

Rubio-Alvarez et al.[1] initially described the technique by which pulmonary valve stenosis could be relieved by a catheter technique. Twenty-one years later Semb,[86] using an inflated balloon-tipped catheter, ruptured a stenotic valve when withdrawn from the main pulmonary artery to the right ventricle, reducing the outflow gradient. However, it was the introduction of the static balloon dilatation by Kan et al.[87] which fostered the application of this therapeutic modality to a greater audience. The technique has, over the decade, become the 'treatment of choice' for pulmonary valve stenosis at any age and with any valve morphology.[88–119]

Table 38.6 Indications for balloon dilatation of valvar pulmonary stenosis.

- Pulmonary valve systolic peak-to-peak gradient >40 mmHg
- Cyanosis in the neonate with any gradient and clear valve stenosis on echocardiography
- Absence of fixed subvalvar pulmonary obstruction
- Absence of anular hypoplasia
- Right heart failure

The safety and efficacy of the technique in infants, children and adolescents have been confirmed by numerous studies summarized by McCrindle and Kan.[90] Indications for intervention in these age groups, with or without symptoms, is a transvalvar gradient above 40 mmHg in the absence of fixed subpulmonary obstruction or additional lesions which need surgical attention (Table 38.6). This has been applied successfully in all forms of pulmonary valve obstructive morphologies (see below), after endocarditis and in cyanotic congenital heart disease.[120,121]

The procedure is not technically difficult but depends upon high-quality angiography for valve location and definition. A number of different protocols have been found successful.[122,123] Generally, a right ventriculogram is performed using a 25° cranial tilt (we also add 10° left anterior obliquity) with 90° lateral projections. The valve anulus is measured from the valve hinge points, in the lateral projection. A 5F right coronary artery catheter is used to cross the valve with a floppy guide and directed to the left pulmonary artery (or through the arterial duct into the aorta in neonates). An exchange wire (0.035-inch) is placed through this catheter, over which a single balloon, 2 or 3 cm in length, is positioned to straddle the valve. The balloon diameter chosen is generally 30–40% larger than the measured anulus, and it is inflated several times until the 'waist' of the stenotic valve is no longer visualized. Hemodynamics and angiography are then repeated.

Morphological changes in valve mobility can be seen angiographically, as well as alterations in flow dynamics, subpulmonary valve function (dynamic subpulmonary stenosis) and the presence of any pulmonary artery tears (rare).[124,125] When the pulmonary valve diameter is too large (>18 mm), two 'kissing' balloons, placed to straddle the valve are required. In this case, the combined diameters of the two balloons should be 50–60% larger than the measured valve anulus. The balloons distort the valve in an elliptical configuration with a gap between the balloons, allowing blood to reach the pulmonary circulation.

Hypotension from right ventricular outflow tract obstruction is less common in this situation, but its technical requirements (i.e. a second balloon) far outweigh the marginal benefit.

Acute and long-term studies[74,90,91,102,103,126,127] have uniformly attested to the efficacy of the procedure with persistence of valve gradient reduction in the majority of patients to nonhemodynamically significant levels. Unsuccessful results were generally due to inability to cross the valve or valve dysplasia (obstructive, but with little commissural fusion).[88] In the latter situation, however, the degree of valve fusion is difficult to define (where its lack would predict failure).[128] In such situations, in the absence of a hypoplastic anulus (which itself is obstructive) and perhaps the finding of a dilated main pulmonary artery, dilatation should be attempted.[126,129–134] Major complications outside the neonatal period are few and are summarized by Stanger et al.[88] from the VACA registry.

The application of the technique in the neonate is technically more demanding. Early studies found traversing the hypoplastic infundibulum problematic,[135] but with the use of a right coronary artery curve, traversing the valve has been simplified. Additional maneuvers to help achieve the dilatation include placement of the guidewire into the aorta (through the patent arterial duct) for increased guide control, and in some situations the use of graduated balloon diameters.[136,137–149] Acute and medium-term results have generally been as encouraging as in older patients, although in some the smaller noncompliant right ventricle may not be adequate for maintaining a normal pulmonary blood flow, requiring prolonged support with prostanoids or placement of an arterial shunt.[136] Morphological follow-up studies have confirmed that the thickened pulmonary valves mature from their dysplastic appearance, and the anulus and right ventricular cavities grow.[136] Those newborns with the most profound (hypoplastic) right heart maldevelopment will require additional sources of pulmonary blood flow.[137,145,147] The experience in adults similarly reflects the technical simplicity and hemodynamic improvement seen in the pediatric age group.[150–153]

Balloon angioplasty of the pulmonary valve has similarly been applied in children with complex forms of cyanotic heart disease, such as Fallot's tetralogy, with some success in improving systemic oxygenation. The first reported attempts to relieve outflow tract obstruction in the setting of Fallot's tetralogy were by Labadidi and colleagues in 1983.[74,75] Concern over induced avulsion of the pulmonary valve leaflets after dilatation dampered the initial enthusiasm. However, subsequent investigations into the clinical impact of this form of intervention[154–166] have established this approach as effective in providing improvement in pulmonary blood flow, such that early surgical palliation can be avoided or postponed. The dilatation is approached in the same manner as that for critical pulmonary valve stenosis (with intact ventricular septum) in the newborn.[163,166]

Temporary arterial desaturation occurs during balloon inflation but generally rapidly recovers. Maintenance of arterial blood pressure and circulating blood volume helps modify the extent of right to left shunting.[158] The use of general anesthesia during the procedure may give better overall procedural control.

The impact on the clinical course has been encouraging with the majority of patients attaining and maintaining an increase in arterial oxygen saturation and avoiding a surgical aortopulmonary shunt. Alterations in outflow tract morphology have been more variable, ranging from no change in anular dimensions or pulmonary artery sizes[161] to significant improvements[159,160,162] in follow-up. Similarly, the need for transanular patch outflow tract reconstruction also varied among the series reported. There appears to be no relationship with outcome (i.e. anular or pulmonary artery growth) with dilating balloon diameter or initial anatomic substrate. With such varied results, institutional prerogatives and operator-related variables have a strong impact on outcome results. The application of such techniques to a wide variety of pulmonary outflow tract obstruction lesions can, in many patients, avoid surgical palliation (shunts) if the patient is not a candidate for primary repair.

Dilatation of the aortic valve

Aortic stenosis can precipitate ventricular failure and subendocardial ischemia. Severe stenosis is associated with a 19% risk of sudden death,[167] and the lesion is often progressive.[168] Surgical therapy beyond infancy carries less than a 2% mortality.[169] In large referral centers, mortality for newborns and infants is 10–15%.[170,171] Actuarial survival after surgical valvotomy is 87% at 10 years and 82% at 20 years,[172] with a late mortality risk at 0.4% per year[169,172,173] for patients with significant residual disease. Mortality from reoperation ranges from 0 to 18% (mean 12%), with an actuarial probability of reoperation of 19% at 15 years, and 35% at 20 years.[172] Restenosis is more frequent after surgery in infancy. Surgery does not prevent endocarditis[172] and valve incompetence is induced in 40–50% of patients.[170,174,175] Balloon dilatation of the aortic valve was first reported by Lababidi.[176,177] A number of other reports followed[178–192] substantiating this approach as an effective form of intermediate-term palliation. Indications for intervention are the same as for surgery: a peak-to-peak systolic gradient of 80 mmHg or greater irrespective of symptoms or a gradient of 50 mmHg or greater with symptoms or electrocardiographic abnormalities at rest or with exercise (Table 38.7). A reduction in the transaortic gradient of 50–60% is generally achieved. The presence of moderate or greater valve insufficiency is a relative contraindication, although worsening of the degree of regurgitation is not inevitable. Patients with mixed disease but dominant

Table 38.7 Indications for balloon dilatation of aortic valve stenosis.

- Resting peak-to-peak systolic gradient >80 mmHg
- Resting peak-to-peak systolic gradient >50 mmHg with ECG changes or clinical symptoms
- Absence of significant aortic insufficiency

stenosis, where valve replacement is the only surgical option, might benefit from attempted valve dilatation as even moderate to severe regurgitation may be well tolerated for many years. Angiography is performed to profile the aortic valve anulus best. This may be accomplished in the 30° right anterior oblique and left lateral axial projections from both aortic and left ventricular injections. Aortography also angiographically defines the degree of regurgitation, if present.[193] The aortogram allows identification of the direction of the hemodynamic orifice (jet of unopacified blood) and helps in guiding the catheter across the valve. Finally, the location of the aortic valve plane can be used during the dilatation to assure that the dilating balloon straddles the aortic valve anulus. The left ventriculogram allows assessment of ventricular form and function, but importantly shows to best advantage the hinge points of the aortic valve leaflets, from which the diameter of the valve can be measured.

One,[78] two[180,182,190] or three[194] balloons can be used— the effective dilating diameter not greater than the diameter of the valve anulus[180,190,195,196] or a combination of balloons whose combined circumference is not larger than the circumference of the measured anulus. A simple rule of thumb for using two balloons (of any balloon diameter combinations) is to choose balloons whose combined diameters are 1.3 times the aortic valve anulus. These two balloons together will have a circumference equivalent to the measured anulus. With the availability of low-profile balloon catheters, we generally use single balloons unless the anulus diameter is larger than 20 mm. The catheters are guided retrogradely over wires placed across the valve into the left ventricular cavity. Placement of a guidewire through the small eccentric hemodynamic orifice in aortic valve stenosis can be difficult, and a variety of catheter shapes (right coronary artery, pigtail, multipurpose) and wires are often required.[197] To circumvent such difficulties, some workers have utilized a transseptal approach, floating a balloon across the valve from the left ventricle and exteriorizing a wire from the femoral artery forming a femoral vein–femoral artery loop[198] or antigrade snaring of the

guidewire.[199] The mechanism of increase in the hemodynamic orifice was investigated by Walls et al.[75] by observations made at surgery, where tearing of the valve raphe, leaflets and avulsion were all encountered.

Complications during and immediately after the procedure have been remarkably minimal. Deaths have been reported[78,179,186,200–205] often related to aortic rupture[186,203,205] or occlusion of the outflow in critical stenosis,[201–203] perforation of the valve or avulsion,[186] exanguination from a disrupted arterial vessel[186] or ventricular fibrillation.[204] Aortic insufficiency is a serious complication but may not occur or only increase by 1 or 2 grades in the majority.[78,181,183,185,200,201] Induction of severe aortic regurgitation is rare. Rocchini and colleagues[186] reported the VACA registry data and noted an incidence of life-threatening events to be 5%, with complications generally greater in young and smaller patients. Arterial compromise represented the most often encountered adverse event particularly in children under 10 kg and especially in the neonate.[206,207] Because of the potential for arterial injury in the neonate, balloon dilatation has been performed via a carotid artery countdown,[208,209] the umbilical artery[209] axillary cutdown[210] or antigrade delivery of the balloon placed across the atrial septum,[211] with similar hemodynamic results as retrograde arterial approaches.

Neonates and infants presenting with severe congestive heart failure almost always have a unicommissural aortic valve.[78,212] In spite of the apparent unfavorable anatomic appearance due to dysplasia of the valve apparatus, the results of balloon dilatation appear satisfactory in this setting with relief of most of the transaortic gradient[78,189,201,208,210,213–216] and induction of generally no more than mild to moderate aortic insufficiency.[216] These results can probably be related to the morphological characteristics of the unicuspid valve, since the condition results from fusion of the valve cushions in early valvogenesis. The presence of two raphe anchor the valve leaflets following tearing, preventing incompetence.

The results of the procedure have been generally favorable[179–186,188–190,217–220] with an expected acute reduction in valve gradient of approximately 60%. Follow-up studies of intermediate term[78,179,184,185,187,200,220,221] report persistent gradient reduction in the majority, although a few have been above 50 mmHg. Restenosis appears to occur no more frequently than after surgical valvotomy.[222–229] Application of the technique after surgical valvotomy has also resulted in similar gradient reductions.[78,182,183,219]

Dilatation of subaortic stenosis

Similar to other forms of left ventricular outflow tract obstruction, balloon dilatation has been applied to subaortic stenosis in attempts to reduce the hemodynamic obstruction. A number of investigators have attempted balloon dilatation in subaortic fixed obstruction both in childhood[230-241] and in adults.[241-244] Although initially applied in the setting of both a 'thin' discrete obstructing lesion and a more prominent thicker ridge-like obstruction, it has become clear that recurrence was the norm when the latter obstruction was dilated.[231,235] When limited to the more discrete (<2 mm) membrane-like lesions, the reported acute hemodynamic results are excellent, although elimination of the gradient not usual. Limited follow-up studies[230-237] would suggest the persistence of outflow gradients in the range of 15–30 mmHg in the majority. The technique for dilatation is similar to that of balloon dilatation of valve aortic stenosis (see above), with balloon diameters equal to, or 1–2 mm larger than, the aortic valve anulus.[230,232,234] The development of, or increase in, aortic insufficiency has not been a significant procedural occurrence. When there is coexistent aortic valve stenosis, larger diameter balloons should, however, be avoided. The mechanism of gradient reduction is by tearing the subaortic membrane. Complications are similar to that in aortic valve stenosis valvuloplasty. However, controversy surrounds the application of this therapeutic modality.[245,246] That this lesion, although apparently discrete, may involve the mitral valve, can adhere to the ventricular surface of the aortic valve and forms a complex obstruction involving the outlet septum makes the use of this procedure less appealing. The well-known progressive nature of the obstruction, and its not uncommon recurrence (postsurgical intervention), makes wide surgical excision (myotomy and myectomy) more attractive alternative. Indeed, the gradients themselves are usually not severe (as in aortic valve stenosis). The timing of intervention is targeted to prevent the development of aortic valve thickening[247] and insufficiency, rather than a primary hemodynamic intervention.

Dilatation of bioprosthetic valves

Bioprosthetic valves (bovine or porcine) have a high failure rate in children and adolescents (>40%) at 3–5 years[248,249] after implantation. Valve failure is characterized by calcification of the commissures and within leaflets, often with leaflet tears and ulcerations.[250] Case reports of balloon dilatation of such valves[251,252] have resulted in an average 40% gradient reduction with increased valve incompetence in the majority.[253] In selected cases, reduction in gradient can defer surgery until an adult-sized implantation can be achieved.

Closure of extracardiac and intracardiac communications

Transcatheter closure of cardiovascular communications can be accomplished with implantation of occluding devices or materials to promote clot formation, with subsequent ingrowth of fibrous tissue. A variety of embolization materials are available.[254]

Ethanol, acrylates and small particles of polyvinyl alcohol are used to obliterate arteriolar end-arteries with diameters under 2 mm. Ethanol (96 vol/%) causes immediate vascular occlusion, dehydration and necroses, while tissue adhesives form an instant spongy plug upon injection into the target vessels. Care must be taken to avoid malembolization into nontargeted vessels by overflow. Polyvinyl alcohol sponge particles are flushed selectively through wedge catheters into the target vessels. They do not result in permanent occlusion and can be resorbed,[254] and as such are mainly used for temporary flow control, protecting vulnerable beds during embolization.

Detachable balloons

Detachable silicone balloons with various inflated diameters (2–9 mm) can be delivered while attached to 2 or 3F catheters through guide delivery systems. The balloons are flow directed to the target and are inflated with isotonic contrast material where the balloons eventually become embedded in fibrous tissue. If premature deflation occurs, the balloon can migrate distally. If inflation is sustained for more than 10 days, permanent occlusion occurs in 90% of the vessels.[255]

Ivalon plugs for occlusion of the persistently patent arterial duct

Transfemoral closure of the ductus arteriosus can be accomplished with a conical plug of Ivalon polyvinyl alcohol sponge.[256] The plug is precut 20–40% below the aortic end of the ductus, allowing it to become securely wedged in the ductal ampulla. The femoral artery must be at least the size of the ductus to accommodate the plug. It is inserted through a sheath and positioned via a wire loop extending from the femoral artery to the femoral vein. The plug, once positioned, is subsequently invaded by fibrous tissue. Due to the size of the introducer system, its application is limited to adolescents and adults. Arterial complication, plug embolization and dislodgement can occur.[257,258]

Rashkind double umbrella occluder

The double umbrella Rashkind occluder (Bard Inc., Billerica, MA, USA) is made of two opposing spring-loaded polyurethane foam umbrellas, in 12 mm (ductus < 4 mm) and 17 mm (ductus 4–8 mm) diameters. The device is folded into a delivery catheter which is guided to the ductus from a transvenous approach with a long sheath.[259] Complete occlusion is frequent (45% acutely), but small residual shunts require several weeks or months for complete flow obliteration. Residual shunt rate is 6–8% at 3 years.[260] Embolization to pulmonary and systemic vessels has been reported[261–263] but catheter retrieval is frequently possible. The Rashkind double umbrella can be used to close ductus in children as small as 10 kg, the major limitation in the very small child being the development of left pulmonary artery stenosis.[261,264] In the large ductus (>8 mm) large umbrella occluders (Lock Clamshell, Bard Inc., Billerica, MA, USA) have been used successfully.[263]

Gianturco steel coils

Gianturco coils (Cook Inc., Bloomington, IN, USA) are helical, flexible stainless-steel springs wrapped with Dacron stands. The straightened coil can be inserted into a 4F catheter and upon extrusion takes on the helical shape, with diameters of 2, 3, 5, 8 or 12 mm. The chosen coil should be 20–40% larger than the vessel to be occluded. Thrombosis occurs within 10 minutes and eventually the coil is embedded with fibrous tissue. These devices are easy to use, but can malembolize if flow control is not utilized. Utilizing embolization spring coils, Cambier et al.[265] reported successful occlusion of small ductal communications (<2.5 mm) using a retrograde approach in three or four children. Lloyd et al.[266] and Moore et al.[267] expanded the early experience with this technique to larger ductus, noting the approach effective and simple, not technically demanding, and performable in an outpatient setting.

Septal occluders

Modification of the Rashkind ductal double umbrella has evolved into an occluder that can be placed in selected atrial or ventricular defects.[268,269] The double occluder device consists of two opposing Dacron umbrellas that fold in opposite directions. The center spring hinges allow the device to fold back flat on the opposite aspect of the septum around the defect to be closed. Transesophageal 2D and 3D echocardiography has been found useful during device placement to visualize the atrial defect.[270] The device can be used to close defects up to 22 mm in diameter. Placement requires the use of an 11F guide. Experimental studies have found the Dacron fabric to be enmeshed in fibrous tissue, adherent to the septum and endothelialized by 1 month.[268] A single-sided occluder that is positioned against the left atrial septal wall and fixed with a countervailing arm on the right atrial wall is also under clinical investigation,[271] as are nitinol wire and fabric devices.[272]

Several morphological studies have addressed the feasibility of transcatheter occlusion of the ostium secundum atrial septal defect.[273,274] Considerable variation in the morphology has been found, including: defects situated in the superior or inferior aspect of the fossa ovalis; those with an attenuated posterior limbus of the atrial septum; subtotal absence of the septum; or complete or partial fenestration of the defect, in addition to the most commonly observed central muscular-type defect. With such noted variability in form, from 50 to 68% of such 'ostium secundum' defects will be judged suitable for closure. Thus, while angiographic definition is important during the procedure, to delineate the region of the atrial septum, it is inadequate to detail the size of the defect and extent of the muscular rim. The former can be estimated by balloon sizing during fluoroscopy (or echocardiography). During this procedure, an easily deformable balloon is withdrawn through the defect, creating a 'waist' which can be measured to define a 'stretched' defect diameter. The details of the morphology regarding the position of the defect within the septum and adequacy of the septal rim can only be determined from echocardiography, with the most sensitive being transesophageal approaches.[275,276]

In addition to the secundum atrial septal defect, several additional atrial lesions have been approached with transcatheter techniques for closure. These defects include the baffle fenestration after a modified Fontan operation (see below) and the patent foramen ovale after presumed paradoxical embolism.[277]

Closure of aortopulmonary collaterals

Aortopulmonary collaterals arise most often directly from the aorta and supply parts of the lung, either directly or as a dual supply with normally connected central pulmonary arteries. These vessels are thin walled and have segments of stenosis and dilatation. Although an additional source of pulmonary blood supply, they complicate surgical repair and postoperative management. Ligation is recommended at the time of corrective surgery, but this can be a technically difficult and time-consuming undertaking, and at times impossible from a median sternotomy.[278] A number of centers routinely occlude these vessels preoperatively with either steel coils or detachable balloons. The vessel must be test occluded to assure adequate arterial saturations, and angiographic confirmation that the distal lung has central pulmonary artery supply.[279] Complications from the procedure include malembolization into the pulmonary artery with or without pulmonary infarction or other clinical problems. From several reported series,[279-289] complete occlusion was accomplished in 73%, and subtotal or partial occlusion in 25%, with a 2% failure rate. In cyanotic patients, before surgical correction, arterial oxygen saturation decreased an average of 5% (1–15%). An average of three coils (1–8 coils) per vessel were required. Recanalization was found in 10% of previously completely occluded vessels while late occlusion can occur in subtotally occluded vessels.[279]

Closure of arteriovenous malformations

Systemic and pulmonary arteriovenous malformations can lead to cyanoses and heart failure. These thin-walled fistulae are prone to aneurysmal formation and rupture. Surgical approaches consist of local or partial resection of the organ. Transcatheter embolization has been well established as a first line of therapy, particularly in multiple lesions. The complication rate is low in the 100 published procedures.[286] Segmental pulmonary infarctions and embolization have occurred.[287] Using coils and detachable balloons, the feeding vessel can be completely occluded in 80–90% of cases,[286] with a 13% recurrence. In hepatic and pulmonary arteriovenous malformations, feeding vessels frequently reopen or further abnormal vessels recruited.

Closure of surgical systemic to pulmonary shunts

Surgical shunts that attempt to provide a reliable source of pulmonary blood flow are most often constructed of Gore-Tex (Gore & Associates, Flagstaff AZ, USA) between the subclavian and pulmonary arteries, and infrequently from the ascending aorta to pulmonary artery (central shunt). Transcatheter shunt closure is preferable if closure is the sole indication for surgery or to simplify surgery if arterial saturations can be maintained by another source of pulmonary blood flow. This is particularly true for left-sided shunts which are difficult to close surgically. The only complication is malembolization into the pulmonary arteries[279] which can be retrieved during catheterization. Both coils

and balloons have been employed. Distal balloon occlusion during delivery will reduce the rate of malembolization. A Rashkind umbrella can be used in selected instances. In the reported series,[279,288,289] 53% complete closure was achieved, with subtotal to partial occlusion in 40% and no occlusion in 7%. No recanalizations were found on follow-up.

Ventricular septal defects

Ventricular defects can lead to congestive heart failure and pulmonary hypertension. Defect size and location can vary and in some may have a muscular or fibrous rim. Closure is recommended for defects with heart failure, pulmonary hypertension, large shunts with failure to thrive or previous endocarditis. The surgical mortality is low, 2–8% in infancy and less than 1% over 2 years of age.[290] With apical or multiple muscular defects, surgical mortality is increased,[291] particularly when a left ventriculotomy is required. Long-term follow-up studies have noted that 35% of such patients have left ventricular dysfunction.[292] Transcatheter closure was attempted in three children with congenital defects using a Rashkind ductal occluder.[293] Although shunt reduction or complete closure occurred, it was clear that the device design was not appropriate. Subsequent investigations using the clam-shell design in 12 patients[294] have defined this approach as useful in selected patients.

Patients with isolated lesions may undergo percutaneous closure as a single procedure, or those with additional defects or lesions requiring surgical repair have the muscular or apical defect closed in the catheterization laboratory preoperatively.[294] In small infants percutaneous closure may prove impractical (<4 kg). Therefore a combined surgical approach with device closure placed through the tricuspid valve, while bypass is performed in the operating room.

The fenestrated Fontan

Ventricular dysfunction, an increased pulmonary vascular resistance and pulmonary artery distortion contribute to increased mortality after creation of an atrial-dependent pulmonary circulation. Fenestration of the intra-atrial baffle has been suggested to allow maintenance of cardiac output, and although systemic hypoxemia persists, shunting across the fenestration limits increases in right atrial pressure. Subsequent transcatheter closure of the defect can then be undertaken electively, if test balloon occlusion of the defect results in acceptable hemodynamics (right atrial mean pressure < 15 mmHg and maintenance of cardiac output).[295] If the procedure is performed later than 2 months after surgery, balloon angioplasty of the pulmonary arteries may be undertaken at the same procedure if required.

Endovascular stents

Various intravascular stent devices have been developed to provide a framework to resist the elastic recoil in vascular stenoses after balloon angioplasty.[296] A variety of designs and materials has been tested in experimental and clinical settings, including a spring-mesh self-expanding stent fitted over a balloon catheter, and temperature-dependent memory metals (nitinol) which expand at body temperatures. The most promising design, and one with clinical application in children,[297] is an expandable stainless-steel design mounted on a balloon. The stent is available in three sizes, expandable from 4 to 18 mm. It retains its size and shape after balloon expansion and can be further enlarged with increasing balloon diameters. Fibrin deposition and subsequent proliferation of neoendothelial cells integrate the stent into the arterial wall. Metal struts protruding into the lumen remain uncovered, and side-branches off the stented lumen remain patent. Stented vessels demonstrate medial thinning and intimal proliferation.[297,298] Implantation requires placement of 10 or 11F long sheaths across the stenotic segments for access to the balloon-loaded stent. In the one clinical trial,[297] 45 stents were placed in 30 patients, 0.2–30.2 years old. Twenty-three patients had branch pulmonary artery stenosis. Thirty-six (80%) of the stents were placed successfully and reduced pressure gradients from 50 to 15 mmHg. Five patients had atrial surgery, three had obstructed Fontans, one had a superior vena cava–right atrial junction after sinus venous surgery and one occurred after a Glenn shunt. Atrial stents reduced pressure gradients from 10 to 2 mmHg. Two stents migrated during implantation and one required surgical removal. Long-term anticoagulant or antithrombotic therapy may be required in selected cases.

Many of the issues associated with evaluation of pulmonary arteries for angioplasty also contribute to the lack of agreement as to the indications for stent implantation. In general the lesion must be a candidate for balloon dilatation and the stenoses should first fail conventional angioplasty. The lesion should also be demonstrated to be at least partially distensible. One notable exception is the stenosis associated with a fresh suture line where one cannot safely overdilate. In this situation, stent implantation used as postoperative 'rescue' therapy can be safely accomplished by utilizing a balloon size that does not exceed the caliber of the vessel on either side of the obstruction.[298]

The technique of implantation has been well described in the pulmonary arterial system. Implantations are performed under general anesthesia with antibiotic prophylac-

tic precautions and heparin sulfate administered. The lesion is assessed hemodynamically and angiographically. Emphasis is placed on obtaining angiographic projections that profile the stenosis utilizing a biplane axial angiographic system. Following angiography an extra stiff wire is positioned across the stenosis for catheter exchanges. For most work in the pulmonary arterial system and depending on the size of the stent to be implanted, a long 7–11F sheath fitted with a bleed-back tap and side-arm is introduced across the stenosis. For smaller patients, a premounted articulated coronary stent may be used instead. If not premounted, the stent can be crimped carefully by hand on to the delivery balloon, taking care that the underlying balloon is not punctured while ensuring that the stent is secure. The balloon and stent are then guided over the wire, through the sheath to the stenotic area. Alternatively, it has been found helpful to premount the balloon/stent complex in the sheath and advance the entire apparatus across the stenosis as a single unit, using the tip of the balloon catheter as the dilator for the sheath. Once in position the sheath is withdrawn over the balloon catheter to expose the stent. Positioning of the stent can be confirmed by a hand injection of contrast into the side-arm access of the sheath. If satisfactory position is confirmed, the balloon is inflated slowly while avoiding movement of the stent relative to the vessel. Once implanted the balloon is deflated and withdrawn, leaving the expanded stent *in situ*. Angiography is repeated to confirm and document the stent position. The patient is maintained on low-dose (10 IU/kg/h) heparin for 24 hours followed by low-dose aspirin (3–5 mg/kg/day) for 6 months. Anticoagulation with warfarin is considered if the stent has been implanted in a low-flow circulation or if a very small stent has been implanted. Occasionally, more than one stent may be required in the same vessel due to a long segment stenosis. In this situation the stents are serially placed with overlapping of the ends (about 0.5–1 cm). While the majority of reported implantations have been achieved in the catheterization laboratory, some have been implanted intraoperatively under direct vision[299,300] It is important to consider that stents may shorten with overinflation.

The most extensively reported device in pediatric applications has been the stainless-steel balloon-expandable design (Cordis, a Johnson & Johnson Co, Warren, NJ, USA). Intermediate follow-up has noted persistence of the hemodynamic profile created at implant confirming that the device not only can be safely placed and achieves gradient reduction with angiographic improvement but also maintains hemodynamic improvement.[301] Mean follow-up was 11 months (range 3–27 months) with no thromboses detected and no deaths attributed to the stent. Twenty-five patients underwent recatheterization from 1 day to 24 months (mean 8.6 months) following implantation. Only one had significant restenosis, which responded well to redilatation. Many, however, had a layer of presumed intimal proliferation within the stent. The pattern of proliferation was such that the internal lumen of the stent was no smaller than the adjacent vessel. Redilatation to expand the stent further was possible. A similar experience was reported[302] with a follow-up of 55 stents in 42 patients (6.1 ± 4.7 years) for a median of 15 months, with a higher incidence of significant intraluminal narrowing (29 of 42 patients) reflecting perhaps a longer follow-up interval. Such luminal ingrowth tended to occur at the site of vessel diameter mismatch and redilatation was possible. In a further study specifically addressing the issue of restenosis within devices (in the pulmonary arterial system), restenosis was found to occur with an incidence of approximately 3% at a mean of 13 months postimplantation; this too was amenable to redilatation or restenting.[305] It has also been suggested that stents can be enlarged safely with further dilatation from both the animal and clinical experience, a feature that becomes important to the growing child.[303–305]

Another issue associated with stent implantation is the fate of side vessels crossed by the stent. A recent study of small coronary vessels indicated that the incidence of decreased flow to branch vessels approximated 10%.[306] In a recently reported investigation, 12 side-branches were crossed with decreased perfusion in 7.[302] Acute decreases in flow may be related to spasm, thrombus formation, dissection and the so-called 'snow-plow' effect.[306–308] Experimental evidence suggests that the observed decrease in flow is not due to endothelial growth occlusion of the area between stent struts.[309,310] As a general principle, however, it is best to choose a stent that will not result in crossing side-branches, if at all possible. If a branch must be crossed, then it is best to straddle the branch completely with the stent.

Stented conduits

While the use of right ventricular-to-pulmonary conduits are central to successful surgical corrections of a number of congenital heart malformations, functioning conduit life has been disappointing.[311] While pulmonary insufficiency has been frequent, most often conduit stenosis is the indication for replacement. A number of factors contribute to conduit deterioration and include external compression, calcification, kinking and development of a fibrotic intimal peel. In addition, conduit dysfunction is more likely in the younger implant when, because of patient size, they 'outgrow' the conduit outflow diameters. Balloon-expandable stents have been employed to reduce such stenotic lesions[312–316] in attempts to prolong conduit lifespan and postpone surgical reintervention. Angiography is best performed in cranial and lateral projections, with or without a slight left anterior oblique rotation to open the left pulmonary artery. Prior to implantation, balloon dilatation is performed to assure the

conduit is distensible. This is particularly important when extensive calcification within the conduit wall is present. The stent should be long enough to seat throughout the conduit length (usually 3 cm) to avoid malpositioning and proximal migration. For proximal narrowings, the stent may, in part, appear to be free within the right ventricular cavity. Usually, it is still within the proximal extension of the conduit to the right ventricular free wall (the so-called Dacron extension). While this does not appear to result in difficulties,[316] care must be taken to avoid the implant from being in direct contact with beating muscle, which can result in stent fatigue and fracture. Finally, proximity of anomalous coronary arteries to the potential area of conduit stenting needs to be considered to avoid vessel compression.[317] Pulmonary insufficiency is inevitable, but in the intermediate term is well tolerated.[315,316]

Complications

Arterial complications are not uncommon after systemic balloon angioplasties or valvuloplasties, and have been recorded to be as high as 45% of procedures.[206,207] Acute thrombosis is most common, and is related to catheter profile and patient size.[206,318] Infrequently, complete or incomplete disruption or arterial tears can occur. The arterial tear created by catheter insertion results in a hemostatic thrombus which, if large enough, may occlude the vessel. In addition, arterial spasm may lead to stasis of blood and thrombus formation. Presently, use of heparinization protocols or thrombolytic therapy frequently leads to restoration of normal flow.[319] Potential adverse sequelae include decreased growth of the affected limb leading to leg-length inequality, vascular insufficiency and, of some importance, loss of arterial access for future diagnostic or interventional procedures. Because balloon intervention for left-sided lesions has only recently (since the mid-1980s) been widely applied, little long-term data are present to reflect accurately the incidence of this complication. From the multi-center registry[88] the incidence of transient pulse loss for aortic balloon valvuloplasties was 12% of 204 procedures, 2.5% persistent pulse loss (after medical therapy) and 30% requiring surgical intervention.[320,321] Of 141 angioplasties for native coarctation of the aorta, 10% had arterial complication, 30% of which required surgical intervention. Balloon angioplasty for recurrent coarctation reported from the same registry documented 8.5% transient pulse loss, 40% requiring surgical thrombectomy.[40,322] A review of the reported incidence of transient or persistent pulse loss by Rothman[322] summarized the acute incidences from a number of centers. The cumulative incidences of a persistent decrease of absence of leg pulses were only 4%, although systematic evaluation of pulses was not applied. Transarterial balloon procedures are generally effective and carry a small risk of significant arterial injury. The advent of low-profile catheters and increasing operator skills can lessen the incidence of such problems.

Summary

Catheter therapies have evolved to become an important component in the treatment algorithm used for patients with cardiovascular illnesses. The cumulative experience with balloon dilatation of valvular and vascular lesions has demonstrated their low morbidity and mortality with short-term results similar to surgery. Balloon dilatation is the currently accepted therapy for valvular pulmonary stenosis, pulmonary artery stenosis, recurrent coarctation, congenital valvular aortic stenosis and intra-atrial baffle obstruction. Various devices are available for closure of intra- and extracardiac lesions. Transcatheter occlusion of aortopulmonary collaterals, arteriovenous malformations and the ductus arteriosus is well established. Embolization of surgical shunts is possible in selected patients. Nonsurgical closure of atrial and ventricular defects has entered clinical trials with promising early results. Improvements in existing procedures and implementation of new concepts will solidify the role of catheter therapy for congenital and acquired defects.

References

1 Rubio-Alvarez V, Limon-Larson R. Treatment of pulmonary valvular stenosis and tricuspid stenosis with a modified cardiac catheter. *Program Abst II Second World Congress on Cardiology*, Washington, DC 1954: 205.

2 Rashkind WJ, Miller WW. Creation of an atrial septal defect without thoracotomy. *J Am Med Assoc* 1966; **196**: 991–2.

3 Lock JE, Keane JF, Fellows KE. Interventional cardiac catheterization. In: Macartney, FJ (ed.). *Congenital Heart Diseases* (Lancaster: MTP Press, 1986): 163–82.

4 Rashkind WJ. Transcatheter treatment of congenital heart disease. *Circulation* 1983; **67**: 711–16.

5 Rashkind WJ, Gibson J Jr. Interventional cardiac catheterization in congenital heart disease. *Int J Cardiol* 1985; **7**: 1–11.

6 Lock JE, Keane JF, Fellows KE. *Diagnostic and Interventional Catheterization in Congenital Heart Disease* (Boston, MA: Martinus Nijhoff, 1987).

7 Lock JE, Keane JF, Fellows KE. The use of catheter intervention procedures for congenital heart disease. *J Am Coll Cardiol* 1986; **7**: 1420–6.

8 Baker EJ. Valvoplasty, angioplasty and embolotherapy in congenital heart disease. *Int J Cardiol* 1986; **12**: 139–45.

9 Rashkind WJ. A glance forward: closure of cardiac defects without surgery. In: Graham G. Rossi E (eds). *Heart Disease in Infants and Children* (London: Edward Arnold, 1980): 249.

10 Radtka W, Lock J. Balloon dilatation. *Pediatr Clin North Am* 1990; **37**: 193–213.

11 Beekman RH 3rd. Pediatric cardiology: a specialty comes of age. *J Interv Cardiol* 1995; **8**: 447–605.

12 Rao PS, (ed.). Cardiac interventions in the pediatric patient. *J Invas Cardiol* 1996; **8**: 278–349.

13 Jarmakani JM, Isabel-Jones J. Cardiac catheterization as a therapeutic intervention. In: Perloff J, Child J, (eds). *Congenital Heart Disease in Adults* (Philadelphia, PA: WB Saunders, 1991): 224.

14 Balis JU, Chan AS, Conen PE. Morphogenesis of human aortic coarctation. *Exp Mol Pathol* 1967; **6**: 25.

15 Dunnill MS. Histology of the aorta in coarctation. *J Pathol Bacteriol* 1959; **78**: 203.

16 Edwards BS, Lucas RV, Lock JE, et al. Morphologic changes in the pulmonary arteries after percutaneous balloon angioplasty for pulmonary arterial stenosis. *Circulation* 1985; **71**: 195–201.

17 Lock JE, Niemi T, Einzig S, et al. Transvenous angioplasty of experimental branch pulmonary artery stenosis in newborn lambs. *Circulation* 1981; **64**: 886–93.

18 Brandt B, Marvin WJ, Rose EF, et al. Surgical treatment of coarctation of the aorta after balloon angioplasty. *J Thorac Cardiovasc Surg* 1987; **94**: 715–19.

19 Lock JE, Niemi T, Burke B, et al. Transcutaneous angioplasty of experimental aortic coarctation. *Circulation* 1982; **66**: 1280–6.

20 Fellows KE, Radtke W, Keane JF, et al. Acute complications of catheter therapy for congenital heart disease. *Am J Cardiol* 1987; **60**: 679–83.

21 Cohn LH, Sanders JH, Collins JJ. Surgical treatment of congenital unilateral pulmonary arterial stenosis with contralateral pulmonary hypertension. *Am J Cardiol* 1976; **38**: 257–60.

22 Fuster V, McGoon DC, Kennedy MA, et al. Long-term evaluation (12–22 years) of open heart surgery for tetralogy of Fallot. *Am J Cardiol* 1980; **46**: 635–42.

23 Gill CC, Moddie DS, McGoon DC. Staged surgical management of pulmonary atresia with dimuitive pulmonary arteries. *J Thorac Cardiovasc Surg* 1977; **73**: 436–42.

24 Lock JE, Castaneda-Zuniga WR, Fuhrman BP, *et al.* Balloon dilatation angioplasty of hypoplastic and stenotic pulmonary arteries. *Circulation* 1983; **67**: 962–7.

25 Ring JC, Bass JL, Marvin W, *et al.* Management of congenital stenosis of a branch pulmonary artery with balloon dilatation angioplasty. *J Thorac Cardiovasc Surgery* 1985; **90**: 35–44.

26 Rocchini AP, Kveselis DA, Crowley D, *et al.* Percutaneous balloon valvuloplasty for treatment of congenital pulmonary valvular stenosis in children. *J Am Coll Cardiol* 1984; **3**: 1005–12.

27 Kan JS, Marvin WJ, Bass JL, *et al.* Balloon angioplasty of branch pulmonary artery stenosis: results from the valvuloplasty and angioplasty of congenital anomalies registry. *Am J Cardiol* 1990; **65**: 798–801.

28 D'Orsogna L, Sandor EGS, Culham JAG, *et al.* Successful balloon angioplasty of peripheral pulmonary stenosis in Williams' syndrome. *Am Heart J* 1987; **114**: 647–8.

29 Hosking MCK, Thomaidis C, Hamilton R, *et al.* Clinical impact of balloon angioplasty for branch pulmonary artery stenoses. *Am J Coll Cardiol* 1992; **69**: 1467–70.

30 Rothman A, Perry SB, Keane JF, *et al.* Early results and follow-up of balloon angioplasty for branch pulmonary artery stenoses. *J Am Coll Cardiol* 1990; **15**: 1109–17.

31 Saxena A, Fong LV, Ogilvie BC, *et al.* Use of balloon dilatation to treat supravalvar pulmonary stenosis developing after anatomical correction for complete transposition. *Br Heart J* 1990; **64**: 151–3.

32 Abbott ME. Coarctation of the aorta of the adult type. II. A statistical study and historical retrospect of 200 recorded cases, with autopsy, of stenosis or obliteration of the descending arch in subjects above the age of two years. *Am Heart J* 1928; **3**: 392–574.

33 Reifenstein GH, Levine SA, Gross RE. Coarctation of the aorta. A review of 104 autopsied cases of the 'adult type', 2 years of age or older. *Am Heart J* 1947; **33**: 146.

34 Liberthson RR, Pennington DG, Jacobs ML, *et al.* Coarctation of the aorta: review of 234 patients and clarification of management problems. *Am J Cardiol* 1979; **43**: 835–40.

35 Hubbell MM, O'Brien RG, Krovetz LJ, *et al.* Status of patients 5 or more years after correction of coarctation of the aorta over age one year. *Circulation* 1979; **60**: 74–80.

36 Beekman RH, Rocchini AP, Behrendt DM, *et al.* Long-term outcome after repair of coarctation in infancy: subclavian

angioplasty does not reduce the need for reoperation. *J Am Coll Cardiol* 1986; **8**: 1406–11.

37 Ziemer G, Jonas RA, Perry SB, *et al.* Surgery for coarctation of the aorta in the neonate. *Circulation* 1986; **74 (Suppl)**: I-25.

38 Brewer LA, Fosburg RG, Molder GA, *et al.* Spinal cord complications following surgery for coarctation of the aorta. *J Thorac Cardiovasc Surg* 1972; **64**: 368–81.

39 Cerilli J, Lauridsen P. Reoperation for coarctation of the aorta. *Acta Chir Scand* 1965; **129**: 391.

40 Hellenbrand WS, Allen MD, Golinko RJ, Hagler M, Lutin W, Kan J. Balloon angioplasty for aortic recoarctation: results of the valvuloplasty and angioplasty of congenital anomalies registry. *Am J Cardiol* 1990; **65**: 793–7.

41 Rao PS. Balloon dilatation of aortic coarctation: a review. *Clin Cardiol* 1989; **12**: 618–28.

42 Roberts DH, Bellamy CM, Ramsdale DR. Fatal aortic rupture during balloon dilatation of recoarctation. *Am Heart J* 1993; **125**: 1181–2.

43 Rao PS, Galal O, Smith PA, Wilson AD. Five- to nine-year follow-up results of balloon angioplasty of native aortic coarctation in infants and children. *J Am Coll Cardiol* 1996; **27**: 462–70.

44 Mendelsohn AM. Balloon angioplasty for native coarctation of the aorta. *J Interven Cardiol* 1996; **8**: 487–508.

45 Rao PS, Chopra PS. Role of balloon angioplasty in the treatment of coarctation. *Ann Thorac Surg* 1991; **52**: 621–31.

46 Lock JE, Bass JL, Amplatz K, Fuhrman BP, Castaneda-Zuniga WR. Balloon dilatation angioplasty of aortic coarctations in infants and children. *Circulation* 1983; **68**: 109–16.

47 Tyagi S, Arora R, Kaul UA, *et al.* Balloon angioplasty of native coarctation of the aorta in adolescents and young adults. *Am Heart J* 1992; **123**: 674–80.

48 Beekman RH, Rocchini AP, Dick McDonald, *et al.* Percutaneous balloon angioplasty for native coarctation of the aorta. *J Am Coll Cardiol* 1987; **10**: 1078–84.

49 Mendelsohn AM, Lloyd TR, Crowley DC, *et al.* Late follow-up of balloon angioplasty in children with a native coarctation of the aorta. *Am J Cardiol* 1994; **74**: 696–700.

50 Rao PS, Solymar L. Tranductal balloon angioplasty for coarctation of the aorta in the neonate; preliminary observations. *Am Heart J* 1988; **116**: 1558–62.

51 Redington AN, Booth P, Shore DF, *et al.* Primary balloon

ovalis atrial septal defects (secundum); feasibility for transcutaneous closure with the clam-shell device. *Br Heart J* 1993; **69**: 52–5.

274 Ferreira SMAG, Ho SY, Anderson RH. Morphological study of defects of the atrial septum within the oval fossa: implications for transcatheter closure of left-to-right shunts. *Br Heart J* 1992; **67**: 316–20.

275 Boutin C, Musewe NN, Smallhorn JF, et al. Echocardiographic follow-up of atrial septal defect after catheter closure by double-umbrella device. *Circulation* 1993; **88**: 621–7.

276 Rosenfeld HM, van der Velde ME, Sanders SP, et al. Echocardiographic predictors of candidacy for successful transcatheter atrial septal defect closure. *Cath Cardiovasc Diagn* 1995; **34**: 29–34.

277 Bridges ND, Hellenbrand W, Latson L, et al. Transcatheter closure of patent foramen ovale after presumed paradoxical embolism. *Circulation* 192; **86**: 1902–8.

278 McGoon D, Baird DK, Davis GD. Surgical management of large bronchial collateral arteries with pulmonary stenosis or atresia. *Circulation* 1975; **52**: 109–18.

279 Perry SB, Radtke W, Fellows KE, et al. Coil embolization to occlude aortopulmonary collateral vessels and shunts in patients with congenital heart disease. *J Am Coll Cardiol* 1989; **13**: 100–8.

280 Dickinson DF, Galloway RW, Massey R, et al. Scimitar syndrome in infancy. Role of embolization of systemic arterial supply to right lung. *Br Heart J* 1982; **47**: 468–72.

281 Furhrman BP, Bass JL, Castaneda-Zuniga W, et al. Coil embolization of congenital thoracic vascular anomalies in infants and children. *Circulation* 1984; **70**: 285–9.

282 Grinnell VS, Mehringer CM, Hieshima BG, et al. Transaortic occlusion of collateral arteries to the lung by detachable valved balloons in a patient with tetralogy of Fallot. *Circulation* 1982; **65**: 1276–8.

283 Lock JE, Cockerham JT, Keane JF, et al. Transcatheter umbrella closure of congenital heart defects. *Circulation* 1987; **75**: 593–9.

284 Yamamoto S, Nozawa T, Aizawa T, et al. Transcatheter embolization of bronchial collateral arteries prior to intracardiac operation for tetralogy of Fallot. *J Thorac Cardiovasc Surg* 1979; **78**: 739–41.

285 Zuberbuhler JR, Dankner R, Zoltun R, et al. Tissue adhesive closure of aortic-pulmonary communications. *Am Heart J* 1974; **88**: 41–6.

286 Terry PB, White RI jr, Barth KH, et al. Pulmonary arteriovenous malformation: physiologic observations and results of therapeutic balloon embolization. *N Engl J Med* 1983; **308**: 1197–200.

287 Barth KH, White RI, Kaufman SL, et al. Embolotherapy of pulmonary arteriovenous malformations with detachable balloons. *Radiology* 1982; **142**: 599–606.

288 Culham JAG, Izukawa T, Burns JE, et al. Embolization of a Blalock–Taussig shunt in a child. *Am J Reontgenol* 1981; **137**: 413–15.

289 Morag B, Rubinstein ZJ, Smolinsky A, et al. Percutaneous closure of a Blalock–Taussig shunt. *Cardiovasc Intervent Radiol* 1984; **7**: 218–20.

290 Stark J, De Leval M. *Surgery for Congenital Heart Defects* (London: Grune & Stratton, 1983): 283.

291 Kirklin JW, Barratt-Boyes BG. *Cardiac Surgery: Morphology, Diagnostic Criteria, Natural History, Techniques, Results, and Indications* (New York: Wiley, 1986): 637–41.

292 Hanna B, Colan SD, Bridges ND, Mayer JE, Castaneda A. Clinical and myocardial status after left ventriculotomy for ventricular defect closure. *J Am Coll Cardiol* **17 (Suppl)**: 110A (abstract).

293 Lock JE, Block PC, McKay RG, et al. Transcatheter closure of ventricular septal defects. *Circulation* 1988; **78**: 361–8.

294 Bridges ND, Pery SB, Keane JF, et al. Preoperative transcatheter closure of congenital muscular ventricular septal defects. *N Engl J Med* 1991; **324**: 1313–27.

295 Bridges ND, Lock JE, Castaneda AR. Baffle fenestration with subsequent transcatheter closure: modification of the Fontan operation for patients at increased risk. *Circulation* 1990; **82**: 1681–9.

296 Palmaz JC, Sibbit RR, Reuter SR, et al. Expandable intraluminal graft: preliminary study. *Radiology* 1985; **156**: 73–7.

297 Mullins CE, O'Laughlin MP, Vick W III, et al. Implantation of balloon-expandable intravascular grafts by catheterization in pulmonary arteries and systemic veins. *Circulation* 1988; **77**: 188–99.

298 Hatai Y, Nykanen DG, Williams WG, Freedom RM, Benson LN. The clinical impact of percutaneous balloon expandable endovascular stents in the management of early postoperative vascular obstruction. *Cardiol Young* 1996; **6**: 48–53.

299 Mendelsohn AM, Bove EL, Lupinetti FM, et al. Intraoperative and percutaneous stenting of congenital pulmonary artery and vein stenosis. *Circulation* 1993; **88**: II-210–17.

300 Coles JC, Yemets I, Najm HK, et al. Experience with repair of congenital heart defects using adjunctive endovascular devices. *J Thorac Cardiovasc Surg* 1995; **110**: 1513–20.

301 O'Laughlin MP, Perry SB, Lock JE, Mullins CE. Use of endovascular stents in congenital heart disease. *Circulation* 1991; **83**: 1923–39.

302 Fogelman R, Nykanen D, Smallhorn JF, McCrindle BW, Freedom RM, Benson LN. Endovascular stents in the pulmonary circulation. Clinical impact on management and medium-term follow-up. *Circulation* 1995; **92**: 881–5.

303 Grifka RG, Vick GW, O'Laughlin MP, et al. Balloon expandable intravascular stents: aortic implantation and late further dilatation in growing mini-pigs. *Am Heart J* 1993; **126**: 979–84.

304 Morrow WR, Palmaz JC, Tio FO, Ehler WJ, Van DA, Mullins CE. Re-expansion of balloon-expandable stents after growth. *J Am Coll Cardiol* 1993; **22**: 2007–13.

305 Ing FF, Grifka RG, Nihill MR, Mullins CE. Repeat dilatation of intravascular stents in congenital heart defects. *Circulation* 1995; **92**: 893–7.

306 Iniguez A, Macaya C, Alfonso F, Giocolea J, Hernandez R, Zarco P. Early angiographic changes of side branches arising from a Palmaz–Schatz stented coronary segment: results and clinical implications. *J Am Coll Cardiol* 1994; **23**: 911–15.

307 Vetrovec GW, Cowley MJ, Wolfgang TC, Ducey KC. Effects of percutaneous transluminal coronary angioplasty on lesion-associated branches. *Am Heart J* 1985; **109**: 921–5.

308 Arora RR, Raymond RE, Dimas AP, Bhadwar K, Simpfendorfer C. Side branch occlusion during coronary angioplasty: incidence, angiographic characteristics and outcome. *Cathet Cardiovasc Diagn* 1989; **18**: 210–12.

309 Benson LN, Hamilton F, Dasmahapatra H, Rabinowitch M, Coles JC, Freedom RM. Percutaneous implantation of a balloon-expandable endoprosthesis for pulmonary artery stenosis: an experimental study. *J Am Coll Cardiol* 1991; **18**: 1303–8.

310 Schatz RA, Palmaz JC, Tio FO, Garcia F, Garcia O, Reuter SR. Balloon-expandable intracoronary stents in the adult dog. *Circulation* 1987; **76**: 450–7.

311 Razzouk AJ, Williams WG, Cleveland DC, et al. Surgical connections from ventricle to pulmonary artery: compari- son of four types of valval implants. *Circulation* 1992; **86**: II-154–II-158.

312 Hosking MC, Benson LN, Makanishi T, Burrows PE, Williams WG, Freedom RM. Intravascular stent prosthesis for right ventricular outflow obstruction. *J Am Coll Cardiol* 1992; **20**: 373–80.

313 O'Laughlin MP, Slack MC, Grifka RG, Perry SB, Lock JE, Mullins CE. Implantation and intermediate-term follow-up stents in congenital heart disease. *Circulation* 1993; **88**: 605–14.

314 Almagor Y, Prevosti LG, Bartorelli AL, et al. Balloon expandable stent implantation in stenotic right heart valved conduits. *J Am Coll Cardiol* 1990; **16**: 1310–14.

315 Powell AJ, Lock JE, Keane JF, et al. Prolongation of RV-PA conduit life span by percutaneous stent implantation: intermediate-term results. *Circulation* 1995; **92**: 3282–8.

316 Hayes AM, Nykanen DG, Smallhorn JS, Williams WG, Freedom RM, Benson LN. Balloon expandable stents in the palliation of right heart conduit obstruction. *Cardiol Young* 1997 (in press).

317 O'Laughlin MP. Balloon expandable stenting in pediatric cardiology. *J Intervent Cardiol* 1995; **8**: 463–75.

318 Franken EA jr, Girud D, Segurira FW, Smith WL, Hurwitz R, Smith JA. Femoral artery spasm in children: catheter size is the principal cause. *Am J Roentgen* 1982; **128**: 295–8.

319 Ino T, Benson LN, Freedom RM, Barker GA, Zipursky A, Rowe RD. Thrombolytic therapy for femoral artery thrombosis following pediatric cardiac catheterization. *Am Heart J* 1988; **115**: 633–9.

320 Allen HD, Mullins CS. Results of the Valvuloplasty and Angioplasty of Congenital Anomalies registry. *Am J Cardiol* 1990; **65**: 772–4.

321 Rocchini AP, Beekman RH, Ben Shacker G, Benson L, Schwartz D, Kan JS. Balloon aortic valvuloplasty: results of the Valvuloplasty and Angioplasty of Congenital Anomalies registry. *Am J Cardiol* 1990; **65**: 784–9.

322 Rothman A. Arterial complications of interventional cardiac catheterization in patients with CHD. *Circulation* 1990; **82**: 1868–971.

39

Transcatheter closure of patent ductus arteriosus as a pathfinder for interventional pediatric cardiology

Benjamin Zeevi

Introduction

Isolated patent ductus arteriosus (PDA) occurs in 1 in 2000–10 000 live full-term infants and accounts for about 2.4–10% of congenital heart diseases.[1,2] The constriction failure is probably due to a significant structural abnormality.

What lesion could be simpler than a patent duct? Traditionally, PDA was identified by detection of a continuous murmur beneath the clavicle with a plain stethoscope; it was usually repaired immediately after diagnosis by a simple surgical technique. Though closure is clearly indicated in the presence of a large left-to-right shunt and associated congestive heart failure, most clinicians also recommend closure of small PDAs to prevent bacterial endocarditis,[3] which remains a risk even in our antibiotic era.[4] The introduction of color Doppler echocardiography has led to the detection of subclinical ('silent') ducts, which may certainly have been overlooked in the past without the patient suffering any damage.

Surgical ligation or division remains the gold standard for treatment of PDA. Nevertheless, with the advent of interventional cardiology, much effort has gone into the development of percutaneous transcatheter methods in order to shorten hospitalization and recovery time and to prevent a permanent scar.

Ductus arteriosus was the first congenital heart defect to be treated surgically,[5] and again it has served as the pioneer defect in launching the transcatheter technique.[6] Porstmann et al.[6] were the first to use transcatheter closure for PDA in 1967, and in 1971 this group reported the results in 62 patients using an arterial approach and an Ivalon plug.[7] Despite the 90% success rate, the need for large arterial catheters (12–27F) and the cut-down method precluded the use of this technique in children. It is still used in adults in selected centers in Germany and Japan.[8–11] Recently, Schrader (pers. comm.) developed a new Ivalon plug (SKS-plug) for transvenous insertion through an 8–12F sheath which has been used successfully in 14 children, aged 1–12 years.

In 1979, Rashkind and Cuaso[12] demonstrated the successful transarterial closure of a PDA in a 3.5 kg infant using a specially designed occluder device. Further modification of this device led to the development of the Rashkind double umbrella occluder, which allows either a transvenous or a transarterial approach to the ductus. The newer model became available for clinical trials in 1981,[13] and it was for years the most widely used and the most thoroughly investigated system.[14–16] Recently, for reasons of cost, inavailability and inconvenience, new devices have been introduced. Most of these are still in the preliminary stages of investigation and are discussed later in this chapter.

The Rashkind double umbrella device

Reports of results with the Rashkind umbrella device have been good: learning curves are minimized and embolization is rare (0.5–4.3%) (Fig. 39.1).[15,17,18] However, the system has several disadvantages, particularly the size of the device and of its delivery system (8 to 11F), which prevents its use in

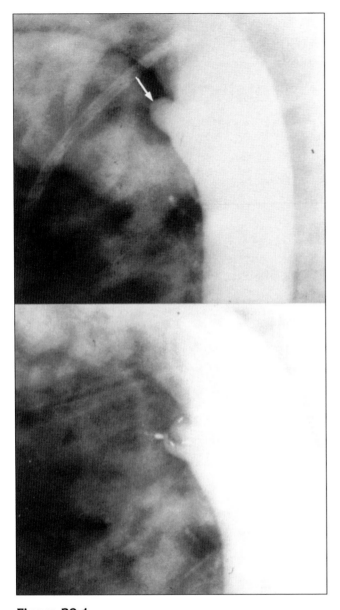

Figure 39.1

Still frames in the lateral projection demonstrating transcatheter closure of patent ductus arteriosus with a 12 mm Rashkind double umbrella device. Upper frame: angiogram of the descending aorta revealing a small type A patent duct measuring 2 mm at its narrowest diameter (arrow). Lower frame: angiogram of the descending aorta demonstrating complete closure of the duct by the double umbrella.

small infants (≤7 kg) and makes introduction difficult in very small patent arterial ducts. Some authors have suggested special techniques for the closure of a small PDA[19–21] and a very large PDA.[22] The front-loading technique enables delivery of the double umbrella through a smaller long sheath and successful closure of PDA even in

small infants.[23,24] The single transvenous catheter approach has been suggested to reduce the risk of arterial cannulation and radiation exposure.[25]

The second major problem with the Rashkind device is the high (21–34%) postimplantation mid-term residual patency rate on color Doppler echocardiography, at 6 months to 1 year after placement of a single device. On longer follow-up of 30–40 months, the rate of residual leaks remains 4–12%, even after placement of a second device.[14–18] Most leaks are due to malpositioning and inappropriate size of the occluder.[14,15,17,26]

The majority of residual leaks following successful implantation are very tiny, inaudible and appear as a low-velocity flame on color-flow mapping. Such low velocity is associated with only a negligible risk of endocarditis. Moreover, many of the leaks close spontaneously on longer follow-up.[14–18,24,27] The importance of this kind of small persistent residual flow after implantation of the Rashkind device is a matter of debate. Some authors argue that any amount of flow in the presence of a foreign body carries a risk of infective endocarditis and should be treated by implantation of a second device or an occluding spring coil once the chance of spontaneous closure becomes small.[15] Others believe[28–30] that the residual flow detected only by color Doppler echocardiography but not accompanied by a continuous murmur can be safely ignored, and that a second device or occluding spring coil should be offered only to those patients with residual patency and a continuous murmur[14,17,27,31–34] (Fig. 39.2). This recommendation is based on the fact that there have been no reported instances of late endocarditis in the subgroup without continuous murmur.[28–30] There seems to be agreement, however, that antibiotic prophylaxis for dental and other procedures is indicated in all patients with residual flow.

Hemolysis following percutaneous closure of a PDA is rare, and occurs in the presence of major leaks. Affected patients require early intervention, either surgery,[35] transcatheter removal of the device[36] or closure of the residual leak by a second device or spring coil.[14,15,37,38]

Concern has been expressed regarding possible encroachment of the occluder arms into the left pulmonary artery, leading to stenosis[14,20,39,40] and protrusion of the device into the aorta.[39,40] Pulsed Doppler-estimated branch obstruction is usually mild, but the long-term effect on the integrity of the left pulmonary artery and the risk of significant stenosis are unknown (Fig. 39.3).

Other rare complications have been described and their significance is not yet clear. These include recanalization of a previously completely occluded PDA,[41,42] acute thrombosis in the device[43] and material integrity problems, such as arm fractures and solder corrosion.[44]

The Rashkind device is very expensive, and to reduce the cost of the procedure, outpatient transcatheter occlusion of the PDA has been attempted and proven to be safe and effective.[45,46]

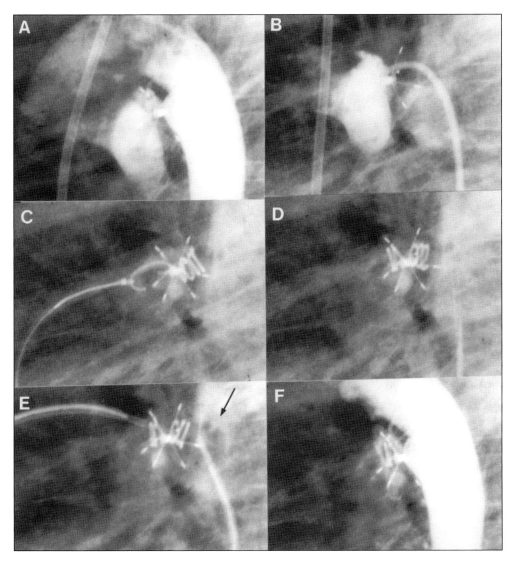

Figure 39.2
Still frames in the lateral projection demonstrating the steps of closure of residual leak, following 17 mm Rashkind double umbrella closure of patent ductus arteriosus, with coil and snare. (a) Angiogram of the descending aorta revealing a moderate residual leak through the duct at the upper border of the 17 mm double umbrella. (b) A Berenstein catheter crossing the duct in retrograde fashion to the pulmonary trunk. (c) The snare is still secured to the distal end of the coil while the aortic loops are coiled in the aortic ampulla. (d) Release of the snare from the coil revealing the good position of the coil loops on both sides of the double umbrella. (e) Balloon 'tampondade' of the aortic ampulla (arrow) as well as the pulmonary side of the duct in order to enhance elimination of residual flow. (f) Angiogram of the descending aorta demonstrating complete closure of the duct.

In adults with possible calcification of the ductus, surgical correction may be technically more difficult, requiring crossclamping of the aorta, which is associated with increased risk and longer recovery time. The safety and efficacy of transcatheter PDA closure in the adult, including some patients with pulmonary hypertension, congestive heart failure and calcified PDA have been demonstrated. The results are similar to those in children, with an occlusion rate of 86% on follow-up; clinically, 94% no longer had a continuous murmur.[47-50]

After transcatheter occlusion of the arterial duct with the Rashkind umbrella became a routine procedure in

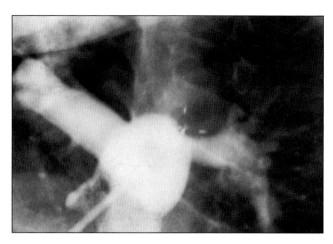

Figure 39.3
Angiogram of the main pulmonary artery in the cranial and left anterior oblique projection demonstrating mild proximal left pulmonary artery stenosis caused by the Rashkind double umbrella device.

many centers, the device was adapted, in an imaginative way, for closure of various other congenital or postoperative cardiovascular defects of different shapes and sizes.[51–53] This development has had a tremendous impact on interventional pediatric cardiology. The device has been successfully applied for occlusion of coronary artery fistulae,[54] closure of patent foramen ovale or small atrial septal defects,[51–54,56–58] surgical systemic-to-pulmonary arterial shunts,[51,57] atrial communication following a fenestrated Fontan operation,[58,59] venous connections after a Glenn operation,[51] left superior or inferior vena cava to the left atrium,[51] aortopulmonary collaterals,[52] valvular and paravalvular leaks,[60] ventricular septal defects (congenital, perimembranous or muscular),[52,61–64] residual postoperative ventricular septal defects[63] or ventricular septal defects complicating acute myocardial infarction when surgery was impossible,[65] native or residual aortopulmonary window[66,67] and ruptured aneurysm of sinus of Valsalva.[68] This experience has also yielded several important recommendations that have important implications for other transcatheter closure techniques, such as sizing defects with a balloon-tipped catheter and using the shortest, most direct and most perpendicular approach to the defect.

Some investigators have modified the Rashkind double umbrella by placing a gentle bend in the arms[52,58,62] for improved appositioning within the septum. The long-term effect, however, is unknown, and bending the arms may cause stress fractures.[44] This technique is not yet suitable for routine use, and all such procedures have been performed with special informed consent using investigational protocols. The technology of the Rashkind umbrella has also been applied by Dr Lock and the engineers at USCI to develop the Lock clamshell umbrella for closure of certain congenital heart defects.[55,59,64]

Additional devices

Other devices have been used in a relatively small number of patients, especially those with large or anatomically unfavorable PDAs deemed unsuitable for transcatheter closure with the Rashkind double umbrella, such as PDAs that are long and tubular or short and virtual windows. These devices include the adjustable buttoned device,[69–72] the clam-shell septal umbrella,[73] the Babic device[74] and the Bottalo occluder.[75] Some of them are no longer available,[73] and others are available only for clinical trials at a limited number of centers.[72]

The Rashkind double umbrella device, too, has become unavailable for use in the USA. This has prompted the use of the occluding spring coil.[76] Gianturco spring coils have been widely used for vessel occlusion for many years[77,78] and are now used in patients with small to medium-sized PDA or with residual PDA after surgery or implantation of the Rashkind device.[76,79–90] Spring coils have several advantages over the umbrella device: insertion is very simple and easy to learn and teach; the coils can be introduced via a 4 or 5F catheter and can therefore be employed in small infants; and most importantly, they are inexpensive compared to other devices (less than 10% of the cost of the Rashkind umbrella). In recent years, there have been several reports describing the successful use of occluding spring coils for percutaneous closure of small and medium-sized PDAs up to 5.2 mm in diameter,[76,79–87] and the technique is rapidly gaining popularity. Many authors now insert the spring coil as an outpatient procedure.

During the procedure, it is important that the cardiologist place the coil securely within the duct. This requires that the coil helical diameter be at least double the minimum ductal diameter and of a sufficient length for three or more loops, so that the high flow across the PDA will not dislodge the device.[79–87] Some teams advocate an arterial approach to occlude the duct,[76–81] but coils can also be delivered transvenously.[82] Although immediate residual leaks on the day of the procedure can be high (21–41%),[79,80,85] spontaneous closure of small residual shunts has been noted on follow-up color Doppler echocardiograms, with complete occlusion rates approaching 97%.[79–87] In most PDAs with a narrowest diameter 2.5 mm or less, a single coil is sufficient. In larger PDAs, the use of two to five coils has been described in the initial procedure[82] or in a second procedure to achieve definitive closure.[85,88]

In most of the cases in which there was embolization of the coils to the pulmonary artery, especially in the early experience, the coils were usually easily retrieved. In cases of embolization when retrieval was impossible, resulting in obstruction of a small pulmonary artery branch, the coil has been left in place without the risk of major complications.[78,83,86]

Owing to the early, relatively high rate of embolization with the spring coils, Sommer et al.[81] used a small goose-neck nitinol snare to hold and manipulate the coil as it is delivered from the arterial side of the patent arterial duct. This technique improves the control of the coil, the accuracy of its placement and the complete occlusion rate. In addition, it can be used to reposition or even retrieve a suboptimally positioned coil.[81,84,86,87]

Our group has used transcatheter coil occlusion in 75 PDA patients, with application of the snare in 68 of them. We found a 4% rate of residual leaks on repeat color Doppler imaging at a mean follow-up of 12.5 months, all in patients in whom the snare was not used (Fig. 39.4). We believe that the snare improves complete occlusion by pulling and compressing the coil loops into the aortic ampulla. There is however, one report in which snaring and manipulation of the coil resulted in wire fatigue and fracture.[91] Another tested technique that prevents coil embolization is the biopsy forceps delivery.[92]

Comparing the results of percutaneous closure of small PDAs, between the Rashkind double umbrella device and the occluding spring coil has demonstrated that coils are more effective and result in fewer residual leaks.[93–95] No instance of late coil migration, thromboembolism, endocarditis, coarctation of the aorta or significant acquired left pulmonary artery stenosis has been noted.[82–86,96] Recanalization of successful coil-occluded PDA,[97] as well as hemolysis,[98,99] have been reported.

Besides the spring coil, new developments include the Cook detachable PDA coil[100–102] and the Duct occluder Pfm coil.[103,104] The former is not yet available in the USA, and the latter is still undergoing a clinical trial in Europe. Both carry a much lower risk of embolization because the release is much more controlled than with the classic spring coil. If necessary, the detachable coil can be repositioned or withdrawn. Initial reports show excellent results and good feasibility even in infants weighing less than 5 kg.[100]

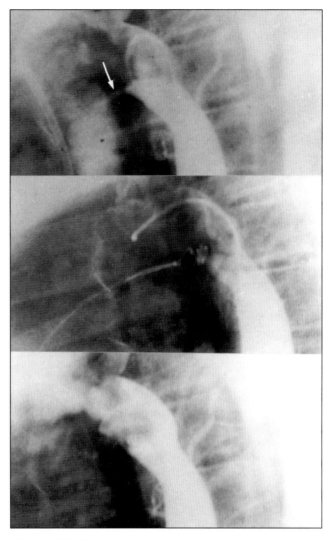

Figure 39.4
Still frames in the lateral projection demonstrating closure of patent ductus arteriosus with coil and snare. Upper frame: angiogram of the descending aorta revealing a small type E patent duct measuring 1.5 mm at its narrowest diameter (arrow). Middle frame: angiogram of the descending aorta demonstrating that the snare is still secured to the distal end of the coil while the aortic loops are well coiled in the aortic ampulla. Lower frame: angiogram of the descending aorta demonstrating complete closure of the duct.

Devices vs. surgery

How does the use of these devices compare with the gold standard of surgery in terms of efficacy and cost? For many years, PDA was closed surgically with near zero risk of death, although occasionally complications such as bleeding, damage to the recurrent laryngeal nerve and persistent residual shunts occurred. A recent multi-institutional study of resource utilization for the Rashkind PDA occluder concluded that surgical closure of isolated PDA was more effective and less costly than transcatheter closure.[105] However, several important points must be remembered. First, this study compared the results of the first years of experience with transcatheter occlusion with 60 years of experience with surgery. On review of the first 107 patients in whom an uninfected ductus had been treated surgically in the largest American centers, the success rate was only 76%.[106,107] The rate of residual patency gradually decreased to 0.4% by the 1970s.[108] Secondly, efficacy was judged on the basis of auscultation alone, rather than by the more objective method of color Doppler echocardiography.[109] Thirdly, the mean follow-up period was 2 months, which may not be enough time for complete closure to occur in patients who receive occluders. According to later results with color Doppler, the residual patency rate after surgical ligation is 6–23%,[110–112] i.e., probably no lower than the rate (about 4–6%) observed on longer follow-up after transcatheter occlusion. It is also clear today that complete occlusion can only be achieved if the duct is divided rather than ligated, though some surgeons still prefer ligation.

Comparison of hospital costs between transcatheter coil occlusion and surgery has demonstrated a marked savings for the former.[113] With the cumulative effects of time, competition and new technology, catheter occlusion of PDA should become even cheaper and more effective.

Although there are no randomized comparative clinical trials, based on the published literature and our experience, coil occlusion may be best suited for closure of small to medium-sized PDAs. Which method is preferable for a large PDA is not yet clear. Clinical trials on larger patient populations along with long-term follow-up are necessary to support these recommendations further. This debate is clearly not yet over.

If we judge surgery and transcatheter occlusion in the same light, there is sufficient evidence of both safety and efficacy to recommend the transcatheter technique as an alternative to surgery, and in the minds of most patients, it will be the procedure of choice. To the average patient, the prospect of outpatient closure of the ductus through a small skin nick in the groin with minimal recovery time outweighs the uncertainty of the long-term results when compared to the prospect of thoracic surgery with its attendant perioperative incisional pain, long hospitalization and permanent scar.

As Dr Kachaner stated,[114] we must be aware that interventional pediatric cardiology is still suffering from a growth crisis. We will continue to develop and use new interventions, but with care, concern, caution and judicious, meticulous adherence to protocols so that the 'device will not be lost'.

References

1   Mitchell SC, Korones SB, Berendes HW. Congenital heart disease in 56,109 births: incidence and natural history. *Circulation* 1971; **43**: 323–32.

2   Perry LW, Neill CA, Ferencz C, Rubin JD, Coffredo CA. Infants with congenital heart disease. The cases. In: Ferencz C, Rubin JD, Coffredo CA, Magee CA (eds). *Epidemiology of Congenital Heart Disease: The Baltimore–Washington Infant Heart Study 1981–1989* (Mount Kisco, NY: Futura, 1993): 33–61.

3   Campbell M. Natural history of persistent ductus arteriosus. *Br Heart J* 1968; **30**: 4–13.

4   Johnson DH, Rosenthal A, Nadas AS. A forty-year review of bacterial endocarditis in infancy and childhood. *Circulation* 1975; **51**: 581–8.

5   Gross RE, Hubbard JP. Surgical ligation of a patent ductus arteriosus. *J Am Med Assoc* 1939; **112**: 729–31.

6   Porstmann W, Wierny L, Warnke H. Der Verschluss des D.a.p. Ohne thorakotomie (I Mitheliung). *Thorax Chirurgie* 1967; **15**: 199.

7   Porstmann W, Wierny L, Warnke H, Gerstberger G, Romaniuk PA. Catheter closure of patent ductus arteriosus. *Radiol Clin North Am* 1971; **9**: 203–18.

8   Sato K, Fujino M, Kozuka T, *et al*. Transfemoral plug closure of patent ductus arteriosus. *Circulation* 1975; **51**: 337–41.

9   Schrader R, Kneissl GD, Sievert H, Bussmann WD, Kaltenbach M. Nonoperative closure of the patent ductus arteriosus: the Frankfurt experience. *J Interven Cardiol* 1992; **5**: 89–98.

10   Wierny L, Plass R, Porstmann W. Transluminal closure of patent ductus arteriosus: long-term results of 208 cases treated without thoracotomy. *Cardiovasc Interven Radiol* 1986; **4**: 279–85.

11   Takamiya M. Experience of 135 consecutive cases treated by Porstmann's method (plug closure of PDA) and present status of this method in Japan. *Radiol Diagn* 1987; **28**: 463–4.

12   Rashkind WJ, Cuaso CC. Transcatheter closure of patent ductus arteriosus. *Pediatr Cardiol* 1979; **1**: 3–7.

13   Rashkind WJ, Mullins CE, Hellenbrand WE, Tait MA. Nonsurgical closure of patent ductus arteriosus: clinical application of the Rashkind PDA occluder system. *Circulation* 1987; **75**: 583–92.

14   Hosking MC, Benson LN, Musewe N, Dyck JD, Freedom RM. Transcatheter occlusion of the persistently patent ductus arteriosus: forty month follow-up and prevalence of residual shunting. *Circulation* 1991; **94**: 2313–17.

15   Tynan M. Transcatheter occlusion of persistent arterial duct: report of the European Registry. *Lancet* 1992; **40**: 1062–6.

16   Khan MA, Yousef SA, Mullins CE, Sawyer W. Experience with 205 procedures of transcatheter closure of ductus arteriosus in 182 patients with special reference to residual shunts and long-term follow-up. *J Thorac Cardiovasc Surg* 1992; **104**: 1721–7.

17   Magee A, Stumper O, Burns J, Godman M. Medium-term follow-up of residual shunting and potential complications after transcatheter occlusion of the ductus arteriosus. *Br Heart J* 1994; **71**: 63–9.

18   Mullins CE, O'Laughlin MP. Therapeutic cardiac catheterization. In: Emmanuoilides GC, Allen HD, Riemenschneider TA, Gutgesell HP (eds). *Heart Disease in Infants, Children and Adolescents* (Baltimore, MD: Williams & Wilkins, 1995): 439–52.

19   Benson LN, Dyck J, Hecht B. Technique for closure of the small patent ductus arteriosus using the Rashkind occluder. *Cathet Cardiovasc Diagn* 1988; **14**: 82–4.

20   Nykanen DG, Hayes AM, Benson LN, Freedom RM. Transcatheter patent ductus arteriosus occlusion: application in the small child. *J Am Coll Cardiol* 1994; **23**: 1666–70.

21   Benson LN, Freedom RM. Balloon dilatation of the very small ductus arteriosus in preparation for transcatheter occlusion. *Cathet Cardiovasc Diagn* 1989; **18**: 48–9.

22   Sievert H, Moor T, Ensslen R, Spies H, Schefer D. Transcatheter closure of oversized persistent ductus arteriosus by simultaneous delivery of two Rashkind umbrella devices. *Cathet Cardiovasc Diagn* 1995; **36**: 251–4.

23   Perry SB, Lock JE. Front-loading of double-umbrella devices, a new technique for umbrella delivery for closing cardiovascular defects. *Am J Cardiol* 1992; **70**: 917–20.

24   Gatzoulis MA, Rigby ML, Redington AN. Umbrella occlusion of persistent arterial duct in children under two years. *Br Heart J* 1994; **72**: 364–7.

25   Abrams SE, Walsh KP, McDonald EA, Boothroyd AE. Single catheter approach for occlusion of a patent arterial duct with a Rashkind double umbrella. *Br Heart J* 1995; **74**: 300–4.

26   Vitiello R, Benson LN, Musewe NN, Freedom RM. Factors influencing the persistence of shunting within 24 hours of catheter occlusion of the ductus arteriosus. *Br Heart J* 1991; **65**: 211–12.

27   Musewe NN, Benson LN, Smallhorn JF, Freedom RM. Two-dimensional echocardiographic and color flow Doppler evaluation of ductal occlusion with the Rashkind prosthesis. *Circulation* 1989; **80**: 1706–10.

28   Latson LA. Residual shunts after transcatheter closure of patent ductus arteriosus: a major concern or benign 'techno-malady'. *Circulation* 1991; **84**: 2591–3.

29   Lloyd TR, Beekman RH III. Clinically silent patent ductus arteriosus. *Am Heart J* 1994; **127**: 1664 (letter).

30   Rao PS. Which method to use for transcatheter occlusion of patent ductus arteriosus? *Cathet Cardiovasc Diagn* 1996; **39**: 49–51.

31   Hijazi ZM, Geggel RL, Al-Fadley F. Transcatheter closure of residual patent ductus arteriosus shunting after the Rashkind occluder device using single or multiple Gianturco coils. *Cathet Cardiovasc Diagn* 1995; **34**: 255–8.

32   Hosking MC, Benson LN, Musewe N, Freedom RM. Reocclusion for persistent shunting after catheter placement of the Rashkind patent ductus arteriosus occluder. *Can J Cardiol* 1989; **5**: 340–2.

33   Huggon LC, Tabatabaei AH, Qureshi SA, Baker EJ, Tynan M. Use of a second transcatheter Rashkind arterial duct occluder for persistent flow after implantation of the first device. Indications and results. *Br Heart J* 1993; **69**: 544–50.

34   Moore JW, George L, Kirkpatrick SE. Closure of residual patent ductus arteriosus with occluding spring coil after implant of a Rashkind occluder. *Am Heart J* 1991; **127**: 943–5.

35   Chisholm JC, Salmon AP, Keeton BR, Webber SA, Monro JL. Persistent hemolysis after transcatheter occlusion of a patent ductus arteriosus. Surgical ligation of the duct over the occlusion device. *Pediatr Cardiol* 1995; **16**: 194–6.

36   Grifra RG, O'Laughlin MP, Mullins CE. Late transcatheter removal of a Rashkind PDA occlusion device for persistent hemolysis using a modified transseptal sheath. *Cathet Cardiovasc Diagn* 1992; **25**: 140–2.

37   Hayes AM, Redington AN, Rigby L. Severe haemolysis after transcatheter duct occlusion: a non-surgical remedy. *Br Heart J* 1992; **67**: 321–4.

38   Qureshi SA, Huggon LC. Hemolysis associated with umbrella occlusion of the arterial duct. *Pediatr Cardiol* 1995; **16**: 101–2 (letter).

39   Fadley F, Halees Z, Galal O, Kumar N, Wilson N. Left pulmonary artery stenosis. A serious complication of transcatheter occlusion of the persistent arterial duct. *Lancet* 1993; **341**: 559–60.

40   Ottenkamp J, Hess J, Talsma MD, Buis-Liem TN. Protrusion of the device: a complication of catheter closure of patent ductus arteriosus. *Br Heart J* 1992; **68**: 301–3.

41   Bjornstad PG, Smevik B. Recanalization of the arterial duct after initial total occlusion with a Rashkind umbrella. *Cardiol Young* 1995; **5**: 98–9.

42   Galal O, Abbag F, Fadley F, Redington A. Reopening of an

arterial duct after total occlusion with the Rashkind double umbrella device. *Cathet Cardiovasc Diagn* 1993; **33**: 132–4.

43 DeMoor M, Abbag F, Al Fadley F, Galal O. Thrombosis on the Rashkind double umbrella device: a complication of PDA occlusion. *Cathet Cardiovasc Diagn* 1996; **38**: 186–8.

44 Bard International Inc. Update information regarding the Bard PDA umbrella. (Letter) 1995.

45 Wessel DL, Keane JE, Parness I, Lock JE. Outpatient closure of the ductus arteriosus. *Circulation* 1988; **77**: 1068–71.

46 Galal O, Abbag F, Redington A, Szurman P, Oufi J. Transcatheter closure of the patent arterial duct as a day-care procedure. *Cardiol Young* 1995; **5**: 48–50.

47 Harrison DA, Benson LN, Lazzam C, Walters JE, Siu S, McLoughlin PR. Percutaneous catheter closure of the persistently patent ductus arteriosus in the adult. *Am J Cardiol* 1996; **77**: 1094–7.

48 Vita JA, Bittl JA, Selwyn AP, Lock JE. Transcatheter closure of a calcified patent ductus arteriosus in an elderly man. *J Am Coll Cardiol* 1988; **12**: 1382–5.

49 Bonhoeffer P, Borghia A, Onorato E, Carminati M. Transfemoral closure of patent ductus arteriosus in adult patients. *Int J Cardiol* 1993; **39**: 181–6.

50 Schenck MH, O'Laughlin MP, Rokey R, Ludomirsky A, Mullins CE. Transcatheter occlusion of patent ductus arteriosus in adults. *Am J Cardiol* 1993; **72**: 591–5.

51 Lock JE, Cockerham JT, Keane JF, Finley JP, Wakely PE, Fellows KE. Transcatheter umbrella closure of congenital heart defects. *Circulation* 1987; **75**: 593–9.

52 Redington AN, Rigby ML. Novel uses of the Rashkind double umbrella in adults and children with congenital heart disease. *Br Heart J* 1993; **69**: 47–51.

53 Mandell VS, Nimkin K, Hoffer FA, Bridges ND. Devices for transcatheter closure of intracardiac defects. *Am J Roentgenol* 1993; **160**: 179–83.

54 Perry SB, Rome JJ, Keane JF, Baim DS, Lock JE. Transcatheter closure of coronary artery fistulas. *J Am Coll Cardiol* 1992; **20**: 205–9.

55 Rome JJ, Keane JF, Perry SB, Spevak PJ, Lock JE. Double-umbrella closure of atrial defects. Initial clinical applications. *Circulation* 1990; **82**: 751–8.

56 Harrison DA, Benson LN, Cusimano RJ, McLaughlin PR. Right-to-left shunt following repair of partial anomalous pulmonary venous connection. A novel use of the Rashkind double-umbrella occlusion device. *Cathet Cardiovasc Diagn* 1994; **33**: 356–60.

57 Haude C, Zahn EM, Benson LN. Transcatheter closure of Blalock–Taussig shunts with a modified Rashkind umbrella delivery system. *Br Heart J* 1993; **69**: 56–8.

58 Redington AN, Rigby ML. Transcatheter closure of interatrial communications with a modified umbrella device. *Br Heart J* 1994; **72**: 372–7.

59 Bridges ND, Lock JE, Castaneda AR. Baffle fenestration with subsequent transcatheter closure: modification of the Fontan procedure for patients at increased risk. *Circulation* 1990; **82**: 1681–9.

60 Hourihan M, Perry SB, Mandell VS, *et al.* Transcatheter closure of valvular and paravalvular leaks. *J Am Coll Cardiol* 1992; **20**: 1371–7.

61 Bridges ND, Lock JE. Transcatheter closure of ventricular septal defects. *Prog Pediatr Cardiol* 1992; **1**: 72–7.

62 Rigby ML, Redington AN. Primary transcatheter umbrella closure of perimembranous ventricular septal defect. *Br Heart J* 1994; **72**: 368–71.

63 O'Laughlin MP, Mullins CE. Transcatheter occlusion of ventricular septal defect. *Cathet Cardiovasc Diagn* 1989; **17**: 175–9.

64 Bridges ND, Perry SB, Keane JF, *et al.* Preoperative transcatheter closure of congenital muscular ventricular septal defects. *N Engl J Med* 1991; **324**: 1312–17.

65 Lock JE, Block PC, McKay RG, Baim DS, Keane JF. Transcatheter closure of ventricular septal defect. *Circulation* 1988; **78**: 361–8.

66 Stamato T, Benson LN, Smallhorn JF, Freedom RM. Transcatheter closure of an aortopulmonary window with a modified double umbrella occlusion system. *Cathet Cardiovasc Diagn* 1995; **35**: 165–7.

67 Gildein HP, Mocellin R. Catheter closure of a residual aortopulmonary window after corrective surgery. *Cardiol Young* 1995; **5**: 96–7.

68 Cullen S, Somerville J, Redington A. Transcatheter closure of a ruptured aneurysm of the sinus of Valsalva. *Br Heart J* 1994; **71**: 479–80.

69 Rao PS, Wilson AD, Sideris EB, Chopra PS. Transcatheter closure of patent ductus arteriosus with buttoned device: first successful clinical application in a child. *Am Heart J* 1991; **121**: 1799–802.

70 Rao PS, Sideris EB, Haddad J, *et al.* Transcatheter occlusion of a patent ductus arteriosus with adjustable buttoned device. Initial clinical experience. *Circulation* 1993; **88**: 1119–26.

71 Lochan R, Rao PS, Samal SK, Khanna AR, Mani GR, Grover

DN. Transcatheter closure of patent ductus arteriosus with an adjustable buttoned device in an adult patient. *Am Heart J* 1994; **127**: 941–3.

72 Rao PS, Haddad J, Rey C, *et al.* Follow-up results of transvenous occlusion of patent ductus arteriosus with the adjustable buttoned device. *J Am Coll Cardiol* 1995; **25**: 332.

73 Bridges ND, Perry SB, Parness I, Keane JF, Lock JE. Transcatheter closure of large patent ductus arteriosus with the clamshell septal umbrella. *J Am Coll Cardiol* 1991; **18**: 1297–302.

74 Babic UU, Grujucic J, Popovic Z, Djurisic Z, Vucinic M, Pejcic P. Double-umbrella device for transvenous closure of patent ductus arteriosus and atrial septal defect. First experience. *J Interven Cardiol* 1991; **4**: 283–94.

75 Verrin VE, Savelien SV, Kolody SM, Porkubovsky VI. Results of transcatheter closure of the patent ductus arteriosus with the Bottalo occluder. *J Am Coll Cardiol* 1993; **22**: 1509–14.

76 Cambier PA, Kirby WC, Worthan DC, Moore JW. Percutaneous closure of the small (≤2.5 mm) patent ductus arteriosus using coil embolization. *Am J Cardiol* 1992; **69**: 815–16.

77 Anderson JN, Wallace S, Gianturco C, Gerson LD. 'Mini' Gianturco stainless steel coils for transcatheter vascular occlusion. *Radiology* 1979; **132**: 301–3.

78 Perry SB, Radtke W, Fellows KE, Keane JF, Lock JE. Coil embolization to occlude aortopulmonary collateral vessels and shunts in patients with congenital heart disease. *J Am Coll Cardiol* 1989; **13**: 100–8.

79 Lloyd TR, Fedderly R, Mendelson AM, Sandhu SK, Beekman RH. Transcatheter occlusion of patent ductus arteriosus with Gianturco coils. *Circulation* 1993; **88**: 1412–20.

80 Moore JW, George L, Kirkpatrick SE, *et al.* Percutaneous closure of the small patent ductus arteriosus using occluding spring coils. *J Am Coll Cardiol* 1994; **23**: 759–65.

81 Sommer RJ, Cutierrez A, Lai WW, Parness IA. Use of preformed Nitinol snare to improve transcatheter coil delivery in occlusion of patent ductus arteriosus. *J Am Coll Cardiol* 1994; **74**: 836–9.

82 Hijazi ZM, Geggel RL. Results of anterograde transcatheter closure of patent ductus arteriosus using single or multiple Gianturco coils. *Am J Cardiol* 1994; **74**: 925–9.

83 Doyle TP, Hellenbrand WE. Percutaneous coil closure of the patent ductus arteriosus. *Am Coll Cardiol Curr J Rev* 1994; **3**: 47–9.

84 Ing FF, Bierman FZ. Percutaneous transcatheter coil occlu-

sion of the patent ductus arteriosus aided by the Nitinol snare: further observations. *Cardiovasc Interven Radiol* 1995; **18**: 222–6.

85 Shim D, Fedderly RT, Beekman RT, *et al.* Follow-up of coil occlusion of patent ductus arteriosus. *J Am Coll Cardiol* 1996; **28**: 207–11.

86 Zeevi B, Berant M, Bar-Mor G, Blieden LC. Percutaneous closure of small patent arterial ducts using occluding spring coils and a snare. *Cardiol Young* 1996; **6**: 327–31.

87 Ing FF, Laskari C, Bierman FZ. Additional aortopulmonary collaterals in patients referred for coil occlusion of a patent ductus arteriosus. *Cathet Cardiovasc Diagn* 1996; **37**: 5–8.

88 Moore JW. Repeat use of occluding spring coils to close residual patent ductus arteriosus. *Cathet Cardiovasc Diagn* 1995; **35**: 172–5.

89 Moore JW, George L, Kirkpatrick SE. Closure of residual patent ductus arteriosus with occluding spring coil after implant of a Rashkind occluder. *Am Heart J* 1994; **127**: 943–5.

90 Hijazi ZM, Geggel RL, Al-Fadley F. Transcatheter closure of residual patent ductus arteriosus shunting after the Rashkind occluder device using single or multiple Gianturco coils. *Cathet Cardiovasc Diagn* 1995; **36**: 255–8.

91 Justo RN, Nykanen DG, Benson LN. Unravelling of a Gianturco coil during reocclusion of a patent ductus arteriosus. *Cathet Cardiovasc Diagn* 1996; **36**: 184–5.

92 Hays MD, Hoyer MH, Galsow PF. New forceps delivery technique for coil occlusion of patent ductus arteriosus. *Am J Cardiol* 1996; **72**: 209–11.

93 Zeevi B, Berant M, Bar-Mor G, Blieden LC. Percutaneous closure of small patent ductus arteriosus: comparison of the Rashkind double-umbrella device and occluding spring coils. *Cathet Cardiovasc Diagn* 1996; **39**: 44–8.

94 Galal O, de Moor M, Al-Fadley F, Hijazi ZM. Transcatheter closure of the patent ductus arteriosus: comparison between the Rashkind occluder device and the anterograde Gianturco coil technique. *Am Heart J* 1996; **131**: 368–73.

95 Bulbul ZR, Fahey JT, Doyle TP, Hijazi ZM, Hellenbrand WE. Transcatheter closure of the patent ductus arteriosus. A comparative study between occluding coils and the Rashkind umbrella device. *Cath Cardiovasc Diagn* 1966; **39**: 355–63.

96 Carey LM, Vemilion RP, Shim D, Lloyd TR, Beekman RH, Ludomirsky A. Pulmonary artery size and flow disturbances after patent ductus arteriosus coil occlusion. *Am J Cardiol* 1996; **78**: 1307–9.

97 Radtke WAK. Safety and efficacy of transarterial occlusion of patent ductus arteriosus using Gianturco coils. *Cardiol Young* 1996; **6 (Suppl I)**: III-04 (abstract).

98 Henry G, Danilowicz D, Verma R. Severe hemolysis following partial coil-occlusion of patent ductus arteriosus. *Cath Cardiovasc Diagn* 1996; **39**: 410–12.

99 Shim D, Wechsler DS, Lloyd TR, Beekman RH. Hemolysis following coil embolization of a patent ductus arteriosus. *Cath Cardiovasc Diagn* 1996; **39**: 287–90.

100 Hazama K, Nakanishi T, Tsuji T, *et al.* Transcatheter occlusion of arterial duct with new detachable coils. *Cardiol Young* 1996; **6**: 332–6.

101 Tometzki AJP, Walsh KP, Arnold R, *et al.* Transcatheter occlusion of the patent ductus arteriosus with Cook detachable coils. *Cardiol Young* 1996; **6 (Suppl I)**: III-01 (abstract).

102 Uzun O, Hancock S, Parsons JM, Dickinson DF, Gibbs LL. Transcatheter occlusion of the arterial duct with Cook detachable coils: early experience. *Heart* 1996; **76**: 269–73.

103 Neub MB, Coe JY, Tio F, Le TP, Grabitz RG, Redel DA. Occlusion of the neonatal patent ductus arteriosus with a simple retrievable device. A feasibility study. *Cardiovasc Interven Radiol* 1996; **19**: 170–5.

104 Grabitz RG, Neuss MB, Coe JY, Handt S, Redel DA, von Bernuth G. A small interventional device to occlude persistently patent ductus arteriosus in neonates: evaluation in piglets. *J Am Coll Cardiol* 1996; **28**: 1024–30.

105 Gray DT, Fyler DC, Walker AM, Weinstein MC, Chalmers TC. Clinical outcomes and costs of the transcatheter as compared with surgical closure of patent ductus arteriosus. *N Engl J Med* 1993; **329**: 1517–23.

106 Shapiro MJ, Keys A. The prognosis of untreated patent ductus arteriosus and the results of surgical intervention—a clinical series of 50 cases and an analysis of 139 operations. *Am J Med Sci* 1943; **106**: 174–83.

107 Jones JC. Twenty-five years' experience with surgery of patent ductus arteriosus. *J Thorac Cardiovasc Surg* 1965; **50**: 149–56.

108 Panagopoulos HG, Tatooles CJ, Aberdeen E, Waterston DJ, Bonham-Carter RE. Patent ductus arteriosus in infants and children. *Thorax* 1971; **26**: 137–44.

109 Smallhorn JF, Huhta JC, Anderson RH, Macartney FJ. Suprasternal cross sectional echocardiography in assessment of patent ductus arteriosus. *Br Heart J* 1982; **48**: 321–30.

110 Musewe NN, Alexander DJ, Teshima I, Smallhorn JF, Freedom RM. Echocardiographic and color flow Doppler evaluation of ductal occlusion with the Rashkind prosthesis. *Circulation* 1989; **80**: 1706–10.

111 Sorenson KE, Kristensen B, Hansen OK. Frequency of occurrence of residual ductal flow after surgical ligation by color-flow mapping. *Am J Cardiol* 1991; **67**: 653–4.

112 Zucker N, Qureshi SA, Baker EJ, Deverall PB, Tynan M. Residual patency of the arterial duct subsequent to surgical ligation. *Cardiol Young* 1993; **3**: 216–19.

113 Fedderly RT, Beekman RH, Mosca PS, Bove EL, Lloyd TR. Comparison of hospital charges for closure of patent ductus arteriosus by surgery and by transcatheter coil occlusion. *Am J Cardiol* 1996; **77**: 776–8.

114 Kachaner J. Pediatric cardiology en route to the third millennium—un long Fleuvie Tranquille. *Cardiol Young* 1994; **4**: 315–19.

40

Transcatheter closure of atrial septal defects and patent foramen ovale: Angel Wings device

Ziyad M Hijazi and Gerald R Marx

Introduction

Atrial septal defects (ASD) account for about 7% of congenital heart disease.[1] Moderate to large-sized defects are associated with right ventricle volume overload, and rare cases may culminate in irreversible pulmonary vascular obstructive disease. Even smaller defects, such as the patent foramen ovale (PFO), may be associated with stroke-like episodes from paradoxical shunting. Hence closure of the PFO and ASD secundum is standard. Recently, both the PFO and secundum ASD are amenable for transcatheter closure.

The first attempt at transcatheter closure of an ASD was reported in 1976.[2] Since then, few devices have been evaluated with variable degrees of success. The Bard clamshell device (USCI, Billerica, MA, USA) was the most extensively evaluated. However, this device had a high incidence of arm fractures (42%) and a high incidence of residual shunt (44%).[3,4] This led to the development of a new device—Cardioseal™ septal Occluder (Nitinol Medical Technologies, Boston, MA, USA)—similar in design to the clam shell with strengthening of the arms to prevent fracture. Currently, it is being evaluated in a Food and Drug Administration (FDA) randomized trial. The second device undergoing clinical investigation is the buttoned device (Custom Medical Devices, Amarillo, TX, USA). The major drawbacks of this device are unbuttoning of the right and left atrial disks, which initially was as high as 10%. With improved design and experience, this rate has dropped to 1.1%. However, on long-term follow-up, the incidence of residual shunting across the defect has been reported as high as 34%, 28% and 20% at 6, 12 and 24 months, respectively.[5] Das et al.[6] developed a new self-centering device (Das-Angel Wings)—Microvena, Vadnais, MN, USA). Phase I has just been completed with good results[7,8] and an FDA randomized trial will start soon. Another device awaiting FDA approval for a clinical IDE trial is the ASDOS (atrial septum defect occluder system) device manufactured by Osypka (Dr Ing. Osypka Corp., Germany). This is a double umbrella device made of nitinol and polyurethane. The device is available in different sizes ranging from 20 to 60 mm (5 mm increments) requiring an 11F sheath for placement. Additionally, delivery of the device requires a simultaneous antegrade and retrograde approach, adding to the complexity of the procedure. The device has been used clinically[9,10] and the results of the initial phase have been encouraging.[11] The newest device which has just started phase I of an FDA IDE trial is the Amplatzer Septal Occluder (AGA Medical Corporation, Golden Valley, MN, USA). This device is constructed from 0.004 to 0.005-inch nitinol wires, tightly woven into two flat buttons with a 4 mm connecting waist (Fig. 40.1). The left atrial button is slightly bigger than the right atrial button. The device diameter corresponds to the diameter of the waist and it is available from 4 to 20 mm sizes with 1 mm increments. The prosthesis is filled with fluffy Dacron threads to enhance thrombogenicity. The device is connected to a delivery cable by a microscrew connection and withdrawn into a loader for introduction into the delivery catheter (6–7F). The most unique feature of this device is the ability to reposition the device after deployment of the left and right atrial disks, prior to device release. An animal trial demonstrated 100% closure rate at 3 months' follow-up.[12,13]

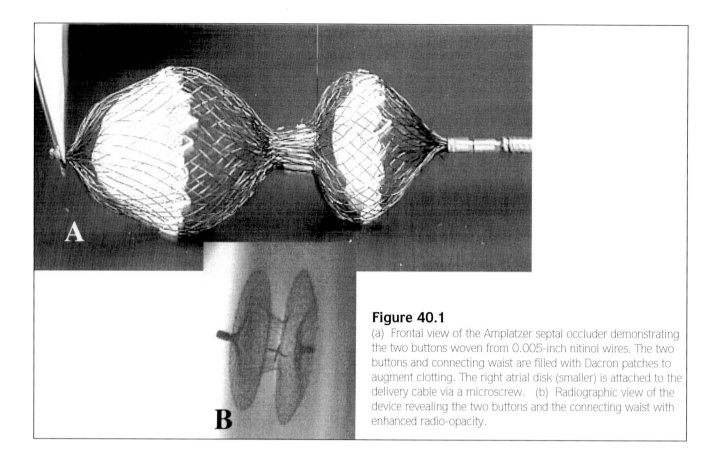

Figure 40.1
(a) Frontal view of the Amplatzer septal occluder demonstrating the two buttons woven from 0.005-inch nitinol wires. The two buttons and connecting waist are filled with Dacron patches to augment clotting. The right atrial disk (smaller) is attached to the delivery cable via a microscrew. (b) Radiographic view of the device revealing the two buttons and the connecting waist with enhanced radio-opacity.

Das-Angel wings device

This device consists of two square disks with the perimeter made of superelastic nitinol wire with radio-opaque marker wire of platinum. Each square has eight eyelets that function as torsion springs and permit the frame to be collapsed to load the device into the delivery catheter. The wire frame is covered by Dacron fabric. The two disks are attached to each other via a conjoint ring. This consists of a punched hole which is 50% of the right atrial disk fabric. The margin of this hole is sewn to the left atrial disk fabric (Fig. 40.2). The unique characteristic of the delivery system allows for precise placement. The device is available in different sizes including an 18, 22, 25, 30, 35 and 40 mm diameter (side-arm) requiring an 11–13F sheath for delivery from the venous route.

Preselection of patients

Phase I of the protocol consisted of patients with a secundum ASD (≤20 mm in diameter), or those with a PFO and an associated stroke episode. All patients underwent a transesophageal (TEE) echocardiogram for the accurate assessment of the defect size, and rims surrounding the defect. The atrial septum was interrogated with a multiplane probe, and the largest diameter was measured online with electronic calipers. The rims surrounding the defect were then assessed. The superior anterior rim was the distance from the defect to the aortic wall measured from a transverse plane at the level of the aortic valve (Fig. 40.3). The inferior-anterior rim was measured at the level of the tricuspid valve (Fig. 40.3). The longitudinal view was employed to measure the superior posterior rim as the distance from the defect to the superior vena cava, and the posterior-inferior rim was the distance from the defect to the inferior vena cava (Fig. 40.3). If the defect diameter was

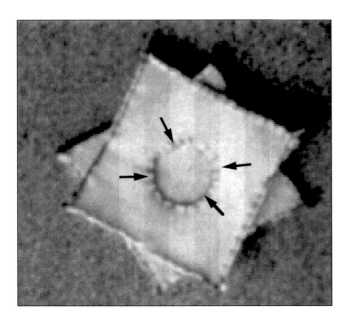

Figure 40.2
The Das-Angel Wings device which consists of two square disks attached in the middle by the conjoint ring (arrows).

20 mm or less and the individual rims were larger than 5 mm, the patient was considered for the use of the Angel Wings device. From both two (2D) and three-dimensional (3D) imaging the authors noticed the superior-anterior rim to be the least important, since the device will wrap around the wall of the aorta.

3D reconstruction significantly aided in patient selection.[14] The true shape and position of the defect were best seen from direct right atrial *en face* views (Fig. 40.3). Moreover, all rims surrounding the defect could be simultaneously displayed. In a preliminary comparison with 2D imaging studies, 3D echo provided improved information concerning the shape, position and surrounding rim tissue.[14]

Closure protocol

For optimum device deployment, closure was performed under general endotracheal anesthesia and transesophageal echocardiography guidance. Routine right and left heart catheterization was performed and assessment of the degree of left-to-right shunt was done by oxymetry measurements. Angiography was performed in the left atrium in straight anteroposterior (AP) projection to assess the size of the left atrium, and in the hepatoclavicular view to

profile the atrial septum and the size of the defect. For PFOs angiography was performed in the right atrium in the AP view to assess the size of the right atrium and to document the right-to-left shunt.

Balloon sizing of the defect was performed using a Meditech sizing balloon catheter (Boston Scientific Corporation, Watertown, MA, USA). For patients with an ASD, the balloon was inflated with a mixture of contrast and saline. The balloon was pulled against the atrial septum and gradually deflated with slight tension until it suddenly protruded across the defect. The size of the balloon just prior to advancing it through the defect was determined as the occlusive diameter of the defect. For patients with PFO, the balloon was advanced from the right to the left atrium. The device size chosen to be deployed was usually 1.4–1.6× the size of the occlusive diameter of the defect. A long 11–13F sheath (Cook, Bloomington, IN, USA) was positioned in the left atrium. The side-arm of the sheath was connected to a high-pressure saline bag, running continuously at a rate of 150–200 ml/hr to prevent air embolism. Similarly, the side-arm of the delivery catheter was connected to a high-pressure saline bag running at a similar rate. Closure was done while the proximal portion of the sheath was submerged under water to prevent air embolism. The delivery catheter and device were advanced inside the sheath until they reached the distal tip of the sheath. The sheath was withdrawn back into the right atrium leaving the delivery catheter tip in the left atrium.

Under fluoroscopic and TEE guidance, the left atrial disk was deployed by rotating the rotary thumbscrew clockwise, making sure the disk was free in the left atrium, far from the left atrial appendage and the mitral valve. The delivery catheter was pulled against the septum until it was parallel to the septum. With gentle traction, after ensuring all left atrial disk corners were in the left atrium, the right atrial disk was deployed by rotating the rotary thumbscrew clockwise until it could no longer advance; continuous traction was maintained to ensure that the disks were on their corresponding sides. Once satisfied with position, using TEE and fluoroscopy in different views, the release button was triggered. Assessment of device position and residual shunt was performed by TEE (Fig. 40.4). Hemostasis was assured and the patient awakened to recover overnight in the hospital. The following day, a chest radiograph, an electrocardiogram and a transthoracic color Doppler echocardiogram were performed prior to patient discharge. All patients were discharged on 81 mg of aspirin for a period of 3–6 months.

Results

Seventeen patients (6 males/11 females) with secundum ASDs (9 patients) and PFOs (8 patients) with a paradoxical

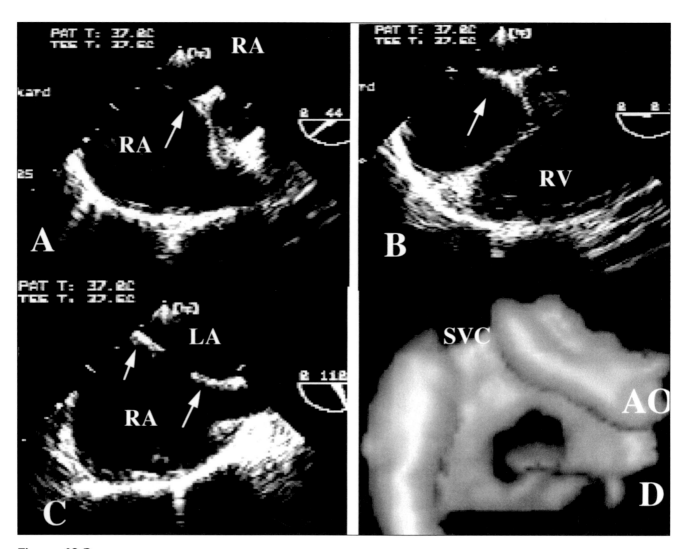

Figure 40.3

((a), (b) and (c)) Transesophageal 2D images for patient preselection. (a) Short-axis view revealing the superior-anterior rim (arrow).
(b) Four-chamber view at the level of tricuspid valve demonstrating the inferior-anterior rim (arrow). (c) Longitudinal view
demonstrating the superior-posterior (long arrow) and the inferior-anterior (short arrow) rims. (d) 3D transesophageal image showing
en face view of the atrial septum from the right atrium and the defect. (RA: right atrium; RV: right ventricle; LA: left atrium; SVC:
superior vena cava; AO: aortic valve.)

embolus and cryptogenic stroke underwent an attempt at
transcatheter closure of their defects (Table 40.1). The
median age was 29 yr (range: 7–50 yr) and median weight
60 kg (range: 23–91 kg). The median size of the defect by
2D TEE was 11 mm (range: 2.5–20 mm) and the median
occlusive diameter of the defect was 16 mm (range:
12–23 mm). Based on the occlusive diameter of the defect,
the median diameter of the device used was 23.5 mm
(range: 18–35 mm) and the median ratio of the device

implanted to the occlusive diameter of the defect was 1.56
(range: 1.19–2.2).

There was immediate complete closure of the defect
documented by color-flow echocardiography in 5 of 9
patients (56%) with ASD and by contrast echocardiography during Valsalva maneuver in 7 of 8 patients (87.5%)
with PFO. In one patient with ASD (no. 7), both device
disks were opened unintentionally in the left atrium. The
device was pulled into the right atrium and snared using

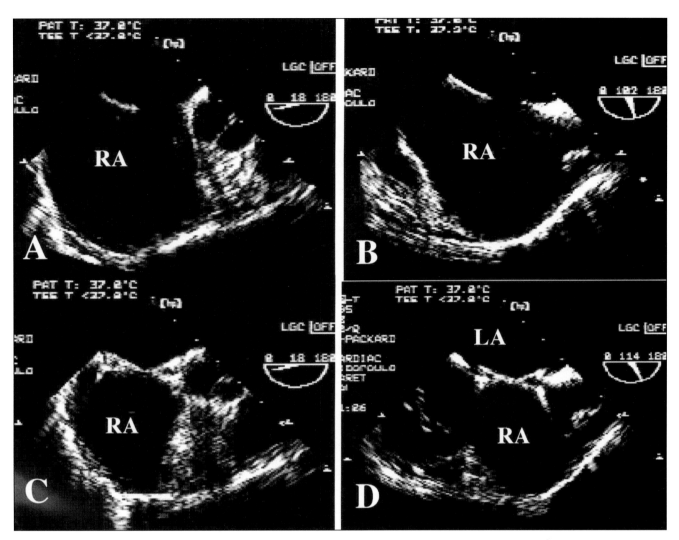

Figure 40.4
Transesophageal 2D images.   ((a) and (c)) Short-axis images pre- and postclosure with the Angel Wings.   ((b) and (d)) Longitudinal views pre- and postclosure with the Angel Wings device. (RA: right atrium; LA: left atrium.)

Amplatz gooseneck snare (Microvena, Vadnais, MN, USA). Another device was deployed successfully with complete closure. In two patients with ASD (nos. 4 and 8) one of the disks (left atrial in no. 4; right atrial in no. 8) did not open fully and was folded. Multiple attempts to unfold the disk were unsuccessful. The devices were released uneventfully in all except one patient (no. 14) with a mild degree of residual shunting. In patient no. 10, the inferior anterior corners of the left atrial disk prolapsed through the defect

leaving a significant residual shunt. In this patient, the device-to-occlusive-diameter ratio was 1.19. Subsequent to this patient, we chose a ratio of at least 1.4×. In another patient with ASD (no. 14), the device did not disconnect easily from the delivery catheter upon activation of the release button. A jerking movement used to deliver the device resulted in pulling of the superior posterior corner of the left atrial disk into the right atrium, resulting in a significant residual left-to-right shunt. No other complications

Table 40.1 Demographic characteristics of all patients and the results of closure.

Patient	Age (yr)	Wt (kg)	Dx	Esize	OD	D (mm)	D/OD	FT (min)	Result
1	16.1	56.8	PFO	5.0	12	22	1.83	19.0	CC
2	28.6	91.5	PFO	5.0	15	22	1.47	10.0	CC
3	29.3	58.0	ASD	12.0	15	25	1.67	28.4	CC
4	26.8	62.0	ASD	20.0	22	35	1.59	45.0	RS
5	21.9	80.0	PFO	5.0	15	22	1.47	25.6	CC
6	11.1	38.0	ASD	14.0	16	25	1.56	18.8	CC
7	13.8	40.0	ASD	11.0	16	25	1.56	50.0	CC
8	7.3	23.0	ASD	11.0	16	25	1.56	35.0	CC
9	10.9	64.0	ASD	11.0	12	18	1.50	22.8	CC
10	29.9	65.5	ASD	16.0	21	25	1.19	27.0	RS
11	50.2	63.6	PFO	11.0	23	30	1.30	39.7	RS
12	31.6	56.8	PFO	5.0	16	22	1.38	19.5	CC
13	41.8	69.0	PFO	3.0	15	22	1.47	17.3	CC
14	32.9	59.0	ASD	20.0	21	30	1.43	40.8	RS
15	37.5	52.2	PFO	2.5	14	22	1.57	20.0	CC
16	28.8	63.6	ASD	7.0	10	18	1.80	28.8	CC
17	48.2	91.0	PFO	3.0	10	22	2.20	20.0	CC

Notes:

DX: diagnosis; Esize: echocardiographic size of defect by TEE; OD: occlusive diameter of defect by balloon sizing; D: device size; FT: fluoroscopy time; ASD: atrial septal defect; PFO: patent foramen ovale; CC: complete closure; RS: residual shunt.

were encountered. The median fluoroscopy time was 26.3 min (range: 10–50 min). No patient required blood transfusion.

Follow-up: The following day, contrast echocardiography demonstrated no right-to-left shunt in all PFO patients resulting in 100% closure in the PFO group. In patients with ASD, color-flow Doppler demonstrated the same findings at the time of the procedure. At 6 months' follow-up, TEE with contrast echocardiography demonstrated complete closure of all PFOs. However, in patients with ASDs, there was complete closure in 6/9 (67%) patients. In patient no. 4, the degree of residual shunt decreased to mild. In patient no. 10 with significant residual shunt, an attempt at placing a second device was unsuccessful. The patient required surgical closure and excision of the old device. In patient no. 14, the device position has not changed, and the patient has a significant residual shunt.

Two patients (nos 1 and 17) developed an echogenic right atrial mass consistent with a thrombus or fibrous strands. In both patients, aspirin therapy was discontinued 2 months after the closure. Both patients were treated with anticoagulation for presumed thrombus. Patient no. 1 discontinued the treatment after 2 months. Repeat TEE after

6 months revealed no change in the size and location of the mass. Patient no. 7 is awaiting repeat TEE.

Chest radiography at 6 months revealed no fracture in the frame of the device. However, in one patient (no. 6) the device orientation changed slightly from the radiograph obtained the following day. This patient had complete closure of her ASD and the 6 months' TEE also revealed complete closure.

Discussion

The use of devices for transcatheter closure of ASDs/PFOs has intrigued cardiologists since the mid-1970s. Since that time, many devices have been developed for transcatheter closure with varying degrees of successful deployment and complete closure.

Results using a new device, the Angel Wings, from Microvena, have been reported in this chapter. For patients with PFO and a paradoxical embolus, the rate of complete closure was 100% at 24 hours after closure. Although the group studied is small, this is an improved rate of complete closure over the use of other devices.[15,16] For secundum ASDs, 67% had complete closure at the 6 months' follow-up. This rate is similar to rates achieved by other devices.[3,4] The device-to-occlusive-diameter ratio in the two patients with significant residual shunt was low, at 1.19 and 1.43. Now a larger ratio is employed. Moreover, in one patient, failure of the release mechanism caused the prolapse of one left atrial disk corner. Since then, the release mechanism has been improved to prevent such episodes. Our data indicate that the Das-Angel Wings is an effective device in closing PFOs. However, the use of this device to close moderate to large-sized ASDs in the initial phase requires more attention. Further clinical experience with this device is warranted before its commercial use. Careful selection of patients using TEE and the careful selection of device size (at least 1.4× the size of the occlusive diameter) should minimize the degree of residual shunt.

References

1   Carlgren LE. The incidence of congenital heart disease in children born in Gothenburg 1941–1950. *Br Heart J* 1959; **21**: 40–50.

2   King TD, Thompson SL, Steiner C, Mills NL. Secundum atrial septal defect. Nonoperative closure during cardiac catheterization. *J Am Med Assoc* 1976; **235**: 2506–9.

3   Justo RN, Nykanen DG, McCrindle BW, Boutin C, Benson LN. The clinical impact of catheter closure of secundum atrial septal defects with the double umbrella device: up to 56 months follow-up. *Circulation* 1995; **92 (Suppl I)**: I-308 (abstract).

4   Jenkins KJ, Newburger JW, Faherty C, et al. Midterm follow-up using the original Bard clamshell septal occluder. Complete experience at one center. *Circulation* 1995; **92 (Suppl I)**: I-308.

5   Rao PS, Sideris EB. Follow-up results of transcatheter occlusion of secundum atrial septal defects with the buttoned device, *Cathet Cardiovasc Diag* 1996; **38**: 112 (abstract).

6   Das GS, Voss G, Jarvis G, Wyche K, Gunther R, Wilson RF. Experimental atrial septal defect closure with a new, transcatheter, self-centering device. *Circulation* 1993; **88**: 1754–64.

7   Das GS, Hijazi ZM, O'Laughlin MP, Mendelsohn AM for the investigators. Initial results of the US PFO/ASD closure trial. *J Am Coll Cardiol* 1996; **27 (Suppl A)**: 119A (abstract).

8   Das GS, Shrivastava S, O'Laughlin MP, et al. Intermediate term follow-up of patients after percutaneous closure of atrial septal defects with the Das Angel Wings device. *Circulation* 1996; **95 (Suppl I)**: I-56 (abstract).

9   Sievert H, Babic UU, Ensslen R, et al. Transcatheter closure of large atrial septal defects with the Babic system. *Cathet Cardiovasc Diag* 1995; **36**: 232–40.

10 Hausdorf G, Schneider M, Franzbach B, Kampmann C, Kargus K, Goeldner B. Transcatheter closure of secundum atrial septal defects with the atrial septal defect occlusion system (ASDOS): initial experience in children. *Heart* 1996; **75**: 83–8.

11 Schneider M, Babic U, Franzbach B, Hausdorf G. Transcatheter closure of secundum atrial septal defects with the ASDOS device in children. *J Am Coll Cardiol* 1996; **27 (Suppl A)**: 119A (abstract).

12 Sharafuddin MJA, Gu X, Titus JL, Urness M, Cervera-Ceballos JJ, Amplatz K. Transvenous closure of secundum atrial septal defects. Preliminary results with a new self-expecting Nitinol prosthesis in a swine model. *Circulation* (in press).

13 Sharafuddin MJ, Gu X, Titus JL, Amplatz K. Secundum-ASD closure with a new self-expanding prosthesis in swine. *Circulation* 1996; **95 (Suppl I)**: I-56 (abstract).

14 Magni G, Hijazi ZM, Marx G, et al. Utility of 3-D echocardiography in patient selection and guidance for atrial septal defect (ASD) closure by the new Das-Angel Wings occluder device. *J Am Coll Cardiol* 1996; **27 (Suppl A)**: 190A (abstract).

15 Bridges ND, Hellenbrand W, Latson L, Filiano J, Newburger JW, Lock JE. Transcatheter closure of patent foramen ovale after presumed paradoxical embolism. *Circulation* 1992; **86**: 1902–8.

16 Ende DJ, Chopra PS, Rao PS. Transcatheter closure of atrial septal defect or patent foramen ovale with the buttoned device for prevention of recurrence of paradoxical embolism. *Am J Cardiol* 1996; **78**: 233–6.

Index